Atlas of Head/Neck and Spine Normal Imaging Variants

Alexander McKinney • Zuzan Cayci
Mehmet Gencturk • David Nascene
Matt Rischall • Jeffrey Rykken
Frederick Ott

Atlas of Head/Neck and Spine Normal Imaging Variants

Springer

Alexander McKinney, MD, CI/CIIP
Department of Radiology
University of Minnesota
Minneapolis, MN, USA

Mehmet Gencturk, MD
Department of Radiology
University of Minnesota
Minneapolis, MN, USA

Matt Rischall, MD
Department of Radiology
University of Minnesota
Minneapolis, MN, USA

Frederick Ott, MD
Department of Radiology
University of Minnesota
Minneapolis, MN, USA

Zuzan Cayci, MD
Department of Radiology
University of Minnesota
Minneapolis, MN, USA

David Nascene, MD
Department of Radiology
University of Minnesota
Minneapolis, MN, USA

Jeffrey Rykken, MD
Department of Radiology
University of Minnesota
Minneapolis, MN, USA

ISBN 978-3-030-07038-0 ISBN 978-3-319-95441-7 (eBook)
https://doi.org/10.1007/978-3-319-95441-7

This Springer imprint is published by the registered company Springer Nature Switzerland AG
The registered company address is: Gewerbestrasse 11, 6330 Cham, Switzerland

Alex McKinney: *This is dedicated to my nuclear and extended family, who have been very patient and attempt to keep me balanced, including Jennelle, Amina, Aliya, Zaki, and Nura. Also, to my parents Alex and Roni, and my brother Zeke who have helped me focus in more ways than I could imagine.*

Fred Ott: *This is dedicated to my girlfriend and soulmate Heather who has encouraged and supported me, more than I have ever been in the past. To my children Brent, Brittany, and Brooke, my grandson Winston, and son-in-law Nicholas who have brought me my share of joy. My father Wilbert and my mother Vivian who passed in 2017. They were always there for me whenever I needed them and taught me what really counts in life: family. My brother Robert, sisters Sheila and Connie, Heather's children James and Sophia. And of course, I praise and thank God for everything He's done for me. "I can do all things through Christ who strengthens me" Philippians 4:13.*

Zuzan Cayci: *This is dedicated to Cenk, my husband, who has always supported and encouraged me during any challenge I face, to my children Lara and Kaya who are the joys of my life, and to my mother, father, and brother who have always been there whenever I needed them.*

Jeff Rykken: *This is dedicated to my family, who continue to give me the most joy in my life. Especially to my lovely wife, Erin, who helps me stay grounded and achieve the balance that I need. To my kids Jaxson and James, who keep me young and challenge me in the ways that all good kids do. And certainly my parents, Janis and Bruce, who have supported and encouraged me always. Lastly, to the creator of the coffee bean, without which this project would not have been possible.*

Matt Rischall: *This work is dedicated to my wife Megan, the inspiration, sounding board, and backbone for so many things in my life. I thank my children Rosemary and Maeve for giving me more love and more to love than I ever thought possible. I am forever indebted to my parents Daniel and Karen for providing me with endless patience and compassion, for being my role models for life, and especially for availing themselves for all of the babysitting of late. To my brother Andrew, your humor and company continue to provide me with great joy.*

Mehmet Gencturk: *This is dedicated to my wife Nurhan, who has always supported me during my education in the USA, and to my daughter Su Ada, who came into our lives a year ago and brought joy, happiness, and energy.*

David Nascene: *My work in this book is dedicated to my family, including my wife Shannon, who has been through it all with me; my kids Laurel, Sophie, and Ben, who keep life interesting and make it all worthwhile; and my parents, Kevin and LeeAnn, who started me on my path. I would also like to thank all of my teachers along the way, each of whom has placed their mark on me, who collectively have made me into the educator that I am proud to be (especially my most important teacher, my mother).*

We mutually dedicate this to our past, current, and future residents, fellows, medical students, and research assistants who we have learned from as much as they have learned from us. Without an academic environment and individuals who are eager to learn, we would lose the initiative to improve. Finally we dedicate this to Bibi Husain, our administrator, who shows more patience than all of us combined and helps to keeps us as a hardworking and cohesive group!

Preface

In my previous atlas, *Atlas of Normal Imaging Variations of the Brain, Skull, and Craniocervical Vasculature*, released a year before this atlas, I opined "art can be work" and "work can be art." I developed this adage, but it is certainly predicated on how much someone is both committed to, while simultaneously deriving enjoyment from, their profession. I can say with certainty that both myself and the other six authors of this book feel this way about the field of neuroradiology. This is why we opted for a rather experimental and uncommon "multiauthor" approach to this book; we felt as a neuroradiology division that if we each shouldered a section of the book, we could complete the first edition in a much shorter time than my previous book, which took more than 10 years to compile. I therefore salute each of my coauthors, who are also my work colleagues. As their Division Director, I have been honored and fortunate to work with a group of my peers who both have mutual respect for each other and feel open to approach each other with suggestions and peer review for both clinical care and research. Below I summarize our approach to the six subsections/chapters of the book, which very much parallels the approach in my prior book and which our readership audience is focused on.

As with the abovementioned reason that this might be akin to composing "art" and as with my former work, this book is not a matter of just finding references for a particular normal variant. In many ways, it is more difficult than composing a peer-reviewed journal article or review, which I feel are more straightforward, since there is a limited range of possibilities and defined subject matter. The subject of *normal variations* can be difficult to address (as discussed in the prior book), because (1) a normal or "don't touch" variant may be either not visualized or not mentioned as it is of no consequence; (2) a variant is seen but constantly called abnormal but never proven to be so, as it is not a surgical entity; and (3) in the reverse of #1, the variant is thought as abnormal, but dedicated imaging is necessary to "put one's shoulder against the ocean liner" of physicians wanting to perform unnecessary therapy. Scenario #3 is more clinically important scenario for normal variants, as operating on a potentially normal variant that was initially suspected to be abnormal may lead to serious iatrogenic complications. Thus, depicting and confirming a normal variation can be an art form, as it may require using one's critical thinking skills and imagination to prove the variant as normal. To prevent situation #3 (and thus *expectation bias*), trainees and fellows are urged initially, prior to reviewing the clinical history, to first simply "say what they see" about an image (borrowing the words of our pioneer/predecessor and one of the original founders of the field of Neuroradiology in Minnesota, Dr. Harold O. Peterson). It seems that what a radiologist or clinician suspects to be a normal may be just that, but it needs proof. Therefore, the goal of this book is to compile the most common, identifiable, or interesting variants and to provide facile methods to identify them, as well as a range of imaging appearances to augment the provider's ability to identify such normal variations. Some variants are accompanied by "Comparison Cases," which cement the appearance of a normal variant in one's mind to compare/contrast the actual abnormality that the radiologist is worried about. Hence, such cases are intended to create a "spectrum of normal" within the radiologist's mind for comparison with the case they are interpreting.

The intended audience for this text includes radiologists, non-radiologists clinicians, and care providers, as well as their trainees. This may be a wider audience than in my previous text that covered predominately the brain, skull, and craniocervical vasculature, as this text covers a much wider anatomic range that includes the skull base, head/neck, orbits, sinuses, facial bones, and the entire spine. These other non-radiologist providers include, but are not limited to, neurologists, neurosurgeons, general surgeons, orthopedic surgeons, radiologic technologists, and others. We have chosen to reference and describe each particular subject in what we considered a brief fashion while simultaneously attempting to cover the most important aspects of each subject. For this purpose, the references are quoted at the end of each section, and we quote a range of numbers regarding the incidence of a variant rather than the exact percentage. Otherwise, our attempt to keep such descriptions under the length of 1–2 pages would have been rendered futile and would have disrupted the intent of the publisher and ourselves to have "more pictures than text." We opine that the purpose of the References, which are overall given in the order that the topic is described, is for more detailed analysis at the reader's discretion. Hence, we admit that this book is not intended for as much of an in-depth analysis of each variant but rather a review for a particular picture or imaging appearance. If mistakes are identified (which we are confident will occur) or if there are topic suggestions, we are open to an email to improve this work. Please provide a reference, and upon the release of a future version, we intend to acknowledge such a contribution.

Minneapolis, MN, USA Alexander M. McKinney IV, MD, CI-CIIP

Contents

1 Head/Neck and Spine Imaging Variants: Introduction

This book is separated into six different sections based on regional anatomy for the purpose of addressing the common modalities (such as CT or MRI), imaging sequences (particularly various MR sequences), and protocols (such as slice thickness or windowing) in order to identify each imaging variant in that region. These include: *Sinonasal Variants* (Chap. 2), *Orbital Variants* (Chap. 3), *Head and Neck Variants* (Chap. 4), *Temporal Bone Variants* (Chap. 5), *Cervical and Thoracic Spine Variants* (Chap. 6), and *Lumbar Spine Variants* (Chap. 7). Notably, the *Head and Neck Variants* chapter covers a wider range of anatomy and physiology (e.g., mucosal abnormalities, thyroid variants, salivary gland variants, Eagle syndrome, vascular variants and PET-CT variants) and thus is a bit more cursory because of the way neck CT imaging is routinely interpreted; perhaps this will be expounded on further in future editions, since some topics are quite vast in that region, and the anatomy is relatively compact. Furthermore, each of the above-mentioned six subjects tend to be subdivided further by sub-anatomic regions (e.g., "ossicular variants" within the *Temporal Bone Variants* chapter, "lacrimal gland" within the *Orbital Variants* chapter), and thus the variants of such regions are grouped together so that the differential diagnosis for true pathology and comparison to a known variant is practical; i.e. so a confident identification of the variant can be reached during routine image interpretation. Relevant references are provided for each subject. The goal of this text was to provide a quick, pictorial review with critical anatomy and imaging characteristics to facilitate prompt recognition of each variant, the reader is encouraged to review any of the numerous references included in each section for more in-depth learning.

Within the text of each chapter, each section attempts to first briefly address the frequency or incidence of each variant in the population or on certain routine imaging modalities (if known), the relevant anatomy and embryology (if necessary), and whether a particular gender or age group (children, adults, or the elderly) is more likely to have that variant. Many normal variants are congenital (e.g., *spina bifida occulta* in the spine), others are acquired (e.g., *retropharyngeal internal carotid arteries* in the neck, *epidural lipomatosis* in the spine), and some are developmental and thus often temporary (e.g., *normal vertebral marrow and sclerotome development* in neonates and infants). Additionally, there are a number of "don't touch lesions" that are not actually "normal variants," whether they are congenital abnormalities in development (e.g., *ectopic thyroid tissue* in the head/neck) or postsurgical/therapy changes that may mimic pathology (e.g., *denervation atrophy* in the neck or *ocular injections or implants* in the orbit). Such "don't touch lesions" should not undergo intervention to prevent iatrogenic injury, and the knowledge of implants, devices, or postsurgical changes prevents embarrassing "misdiagnoses" by the radiologists.

Finally, various artifacts on imaging modalities can simulate pathology in any of these six regions. These include artifacts commonly arising from *patient motion* or regionally on certain MRI sequences or imaging modalities (such as *Gibbs artifact* or *CSF flow artifact* simulating cord pathology on cervico-thoracic MRI, or *quantum mottle* simulating otospongiosis on HRCT of the temporal bone). While causes of these artifacts can be numerous, those most commonly causing confusion or likely to mimic pathology and subsequent unnecessary therapy or imaging are presented in each section.

When appropriate, a relevant differential diagnosis is provided for each variant, as the variants depicted herein can mimic true pathology, with pertinent "**Comparison Cases**" that the variant may imitate. Additionally, surgical considerations are noteworthy in many such variants (e.g., the presence of an aberrant internal carotid artery in middle ear surgery) in order to help prevent iatrogenic complications. It cannot be overstated how critical it is to recognize such variants, as typically benign procedures (although uncommonly) may lead to devastating iatrogenic complications when recognition of a normal variant or a benign or "don't touch

A. McKinney et al., *Atlas of Head/Neck and Spine Normal Imaging Variants*, https://doi.org/10.1007/978-3-319-95441-7_1

lesion" is not promptly recognized. As such, the intent of this text is to serve as a quick pictorial comparison for the radiologist, general surgeon, neurosurgeon, neurologist, radiation oncologist, orthopedic surgeon, or otolaryngologist prior to a procedure or other therapy when a variant is being considered clinically.

Some basic terminology and abbreviations regarding standard sequences are necessary, as MRI manufacturers unfortunately have not yet uniformly adopted a single standard for sequences outside of the routine sequences such as T1-weighted images (T1WI), T2-weighted images (T2WI), fluid-attenuated inversion recovery (FLAIR), and diffusion-weighted images (DWI). Thus, relatively standard terminology used throughout this section and the remainder of the book is described below. Notably, certain terms, such as "HRCT" and "HRMRI" for the *Temporal Bone Variants* chapter predominantly apply to one region of anatomy where that modality/sequence is most frequently implemented.

Terminology for this Book

- 1.5T and 3T = 1.5 Tesla and 3.0 Tesla MRI magnet field strengths
- 3D = Three dimensional
- 3D T2WI = Three dimensional T2-weighted imaging
- AP = Anterior-posterior view (plain films or 3D volume-rendered images)
- CECT = Contrast-enhanced CT
- CSF = Cerebrospinal fluid
- CT = Computed tomography
- DWI = Diffusion-weighted image
- FLAIR = Fluid-attenuated inversion recovery imaging
- FS = Fat-suppressed
- GE = Gradient echo
- GE T2*WI = Gradient echo T2*-weighted imaging
- HRCT = High-resolution CT (*regarding temporal bone CT*)
- HRMRI = High-resolution MRI (*for temporal bone/posterior fossa MRI*)
- IR = Inversion recovery imaging;
- MIP = Maximum intensity projection
- MPR = Multiplanar reformat
- MRA = MR angiography; TOF MRA = Time-of-flight MRA
- MRI = Magnetic resonance Imaging
- NECT = Non-enhanced CT
- SET1WI = Spin-echo T1-weighted imaging
- SET2WI = Spin-echo T2-weighted imaging
- STIR = Short tau inversion recovery imaging
- SWI = Susceptibility-weighted imaging
- T1WI = T1-weighted imaging
- T2WI = T2-weighted imaging
- T2*WI = GET2*-weighted imaging
- T2-SPACE and 3D T2-SPACE = 3D T2WI acquisition (*isotropic acquisition*)
- US = Ultrasound

2 Sinonasal Variants

2.1 Introduction, Technique, and Basic Anatomy

Sinonasal normal variations are well described, but their degree of clinical import often depends on not just the type of variant but also the location and the presence of concomitant sinonasal disease, such as sinusitis. The majority of these variations are first noted on computed tomography (CT), as it is the most common modality used to initially evaluate suspected sinonasal disease. On CT, some of these variations have a propensity to simulate an abnormality. Also, one should be aware of certain variants on magnetic resonance imaging (MRI) (e.g., aerated pterygoid process as an extension of a sinus), as their presence may simulate disease or confound evaluation (e.g., such as in arrested pneumatization). Additionally, identifying the presence of certain variations can be critical prior to surgery or other procedures to prevent complications such as a sphenoethmoidal Onodi cell surrounding the optic nerve.

Regarding technique, for paranasal sinus CT, multiplanar reformats (MPR) are preferred to enable reconstructions in any desired plane, but direct axial and coronal reconstructions should be considered the minimum requirement to adequately evaluate the sinus walls, osteomeatal units, and important recesses (e.g., frontoethmoidal, sphenoethmoidal). Thus, spiral CT acquisition is preferred, with a maximum recommended reconstruction thickness of 3 mm; thicker reconstructions may not be able to delineate some variants such as accessory sinus ostia or can cause variants to simulate disease. For MRI, a minimum of noncontrast T1WI and T2WI is necessary to evaluate for the presence of debris and to confirm certain variations. It is important to note that a single sequence such as T2WI should not be evaluated in solitude to assess for sinus disease, since T2-dark inspissated debris may mistakenly appear normal. Also, certain sequences, such as fat-suppressed T1WI (FS T1WI) or FLAIR, may enable rapid identification of some potentially problematic variants (e.g., arrested aeration/pneumatization). Plain films, the traditional mainstay of sinus imaging at the turn of the century, are now used much less frequently, and therefore such appearances of variants are not addressed here.

An in-depth description of normal anatomy is beyond the scope of this text as numerous references abound (please see the *Suggested Reading* section of this chapter), but an understanding of basic sinonasal anatomy and of the configuration of the osteomeatal units assists in recognizing such variants.

A. McKinney et al., *Atlas of Head/Neck and Spine Normal Imaging Variants*, https://doi.org/10.1007/978-3-319-95441-7_2

2.2 Pattern of Serial Paranasal Sinus Development and Sequential Pneumatization

The pneumatization pattern is unique to each group of sinuses, and the continuous change in the size and aeration of the sinus as a child grows has a significant impact on the treatment/surgery of sinus pathology in the pediatric age group. The ethmoid sinus is the only sinus seen on imaging at birth. It rapidly pneumatizes between 1 year and 4 years of age. However, ethmoid air cell growth slows between 4 and 8 years of age and reaches adult appearance by the age of 12. The next to develop are the maxillary sinuses, which are present as a shallow rounded sac at birth and are also not well-visualized on imaging at this time. They have rapid pneumatization between 1 and 4 years of age and attain an adult appearance between 12 and 14 years of age. The next sinus to pneumatize is the sphenoid. The sphenoid sinus is present as a tiny mucosal sac posterior to the nasal capsule at birth; it then rapidly pneumatizes between 1 and 3 years of age and grows progressively between 7 and 14 years. It may continue to pneumatize further into adulthood. Thereafter, the frontal sinuses are present as a small pit or furrow at birth and are not well seen on imaging, while there is slow pneumatization of the frontal sinuses between 1 and 4 years with rapid growth between 4 and 8 years. The frontal sinuses ultimately attain an adult appearance by approximately 12 years of age. Please note that variations in incomplete development (hypoplasia or aplasia) of each sinus are covered under the following topics for each respective sinus (Figs. 2.1, 2.2, 2.3, 2.4, and 2.5).

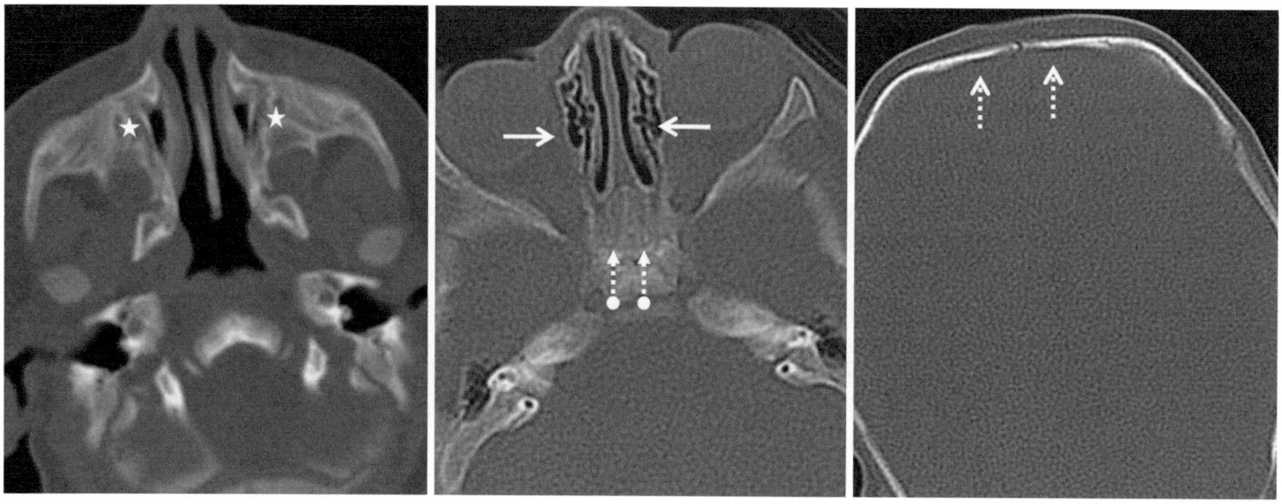

Fig. 2.1 A newborn baby with a history of birth trauma. Axial images at the level of the maxillary sinuses (*stars, left*), ethmoidal air cells (*arrows, middle*), sphenoid sinus (*dashed arrows, middle*), and frontal sinuses (*dotted arrows, right*) demonstrate pneumatization of only the ethmoidal air cells at this time

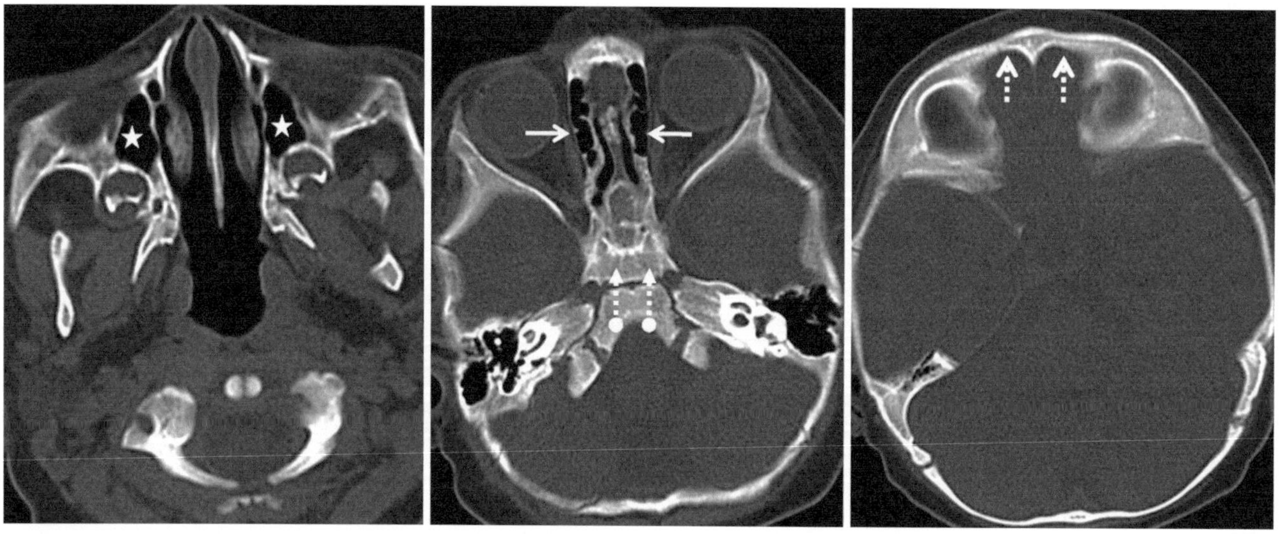

Fig. 2.2 Sequential axial head CT images of a 7-month-old infant obtained to "rule out" subdural hemorrhage demonstrate partial pneumatization of the maxillary sinuses (*stars, left*). While the ethmoid air cells (*arrows, middle*) are pneumatized, the sphenoid sinus (*dashed arrows, middle*) is not aerated, nor is the frontal sinus (*dotted arrows, right*)

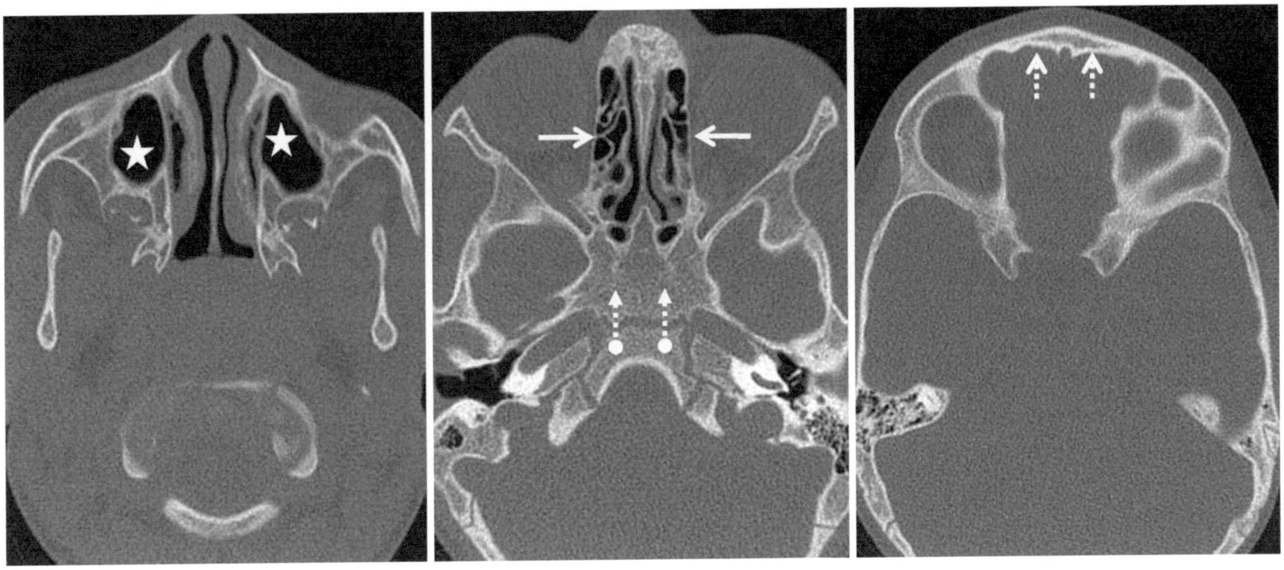

Fig. 2.3 Axial CT images of a 3-year-old male demonstrate near-complete pneumatization of the maxillary sinuses (*stars, left*), with partial pneumatization of the sphenoid sinus (*dashed arrows, middle*). Note that the ethmoids are already fully pneumatized/aerated (*arrows, middle*). The frontal sinuses are not yet pneumatized (*dotted arrow, right*)

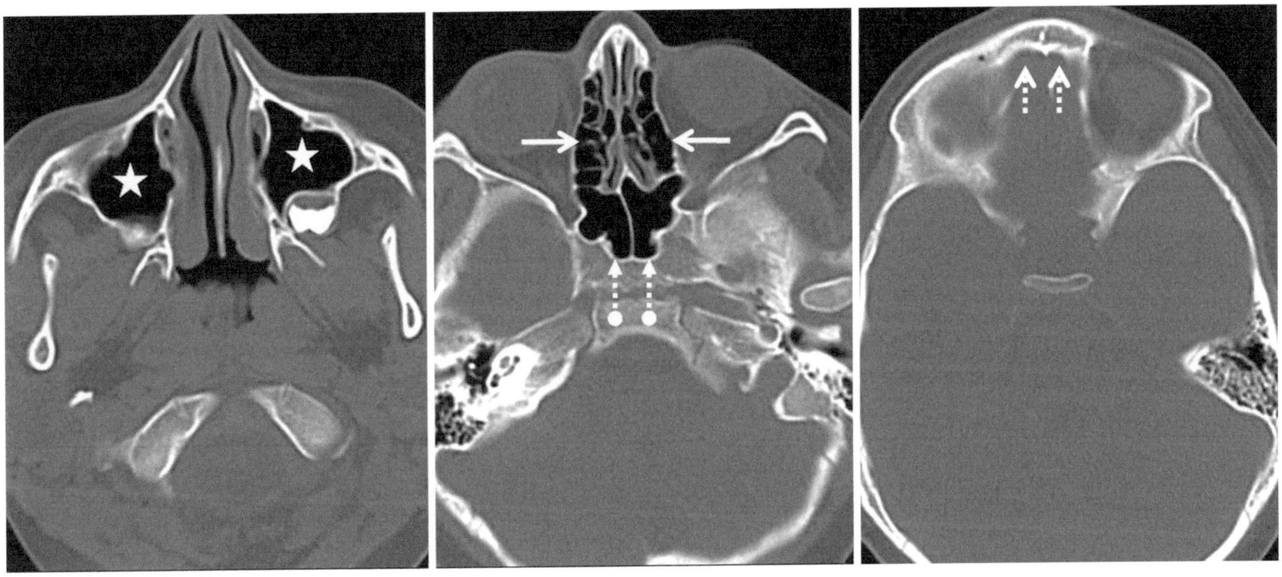

Fig. 2.4 A 7-year-old female with facial trauma. Axial head CT images demonstrate complete pneumatization of the maxillary sinuses (*stars, left*), ethmoidal air cells (*arrows, middle*), and the sphenoid sinus (*dashed arrows, middle*). Again, the frontal sinuses (*dotted arrows, right*) may not yet be pneumatized by this age

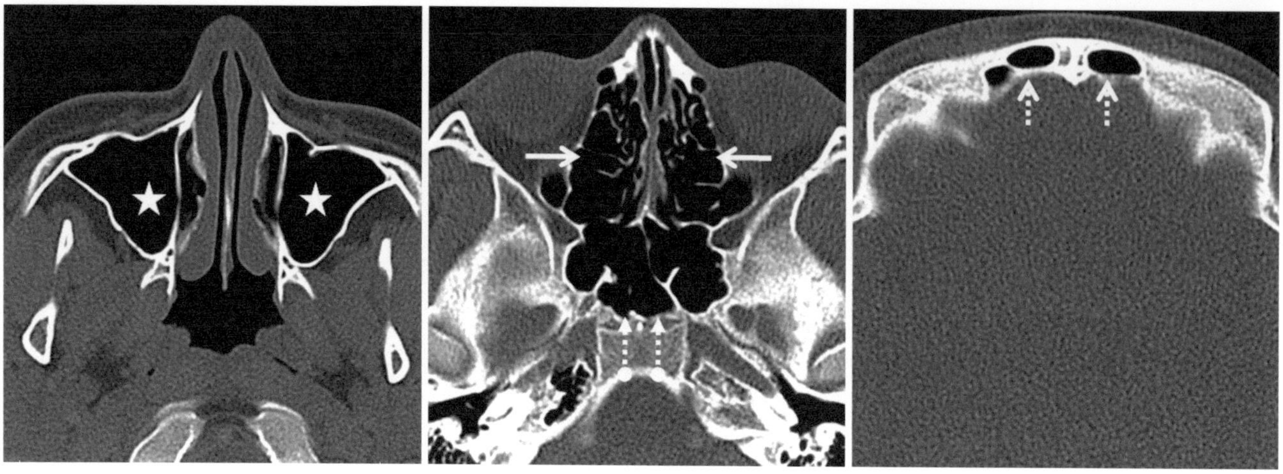

Fig. 2.5 Near completion of sinus pneumatization. Axial facial CT images of a 14-year-old male with facial trauma demonstrate complete development of the maxillary sinuses (*stars*, *left*), ethmoidal air cells (*arrows, middle*), and the sphenoid sinus (*dashed arrows*, *middle*). At this time, the frontal sinuses are also almost completely pneumatized (*dotted arrows*, *right*)

2.3 Maxillary Sinus

2.3.1 Maxillary Sinus Hypoplasia

The maxillary sinuses develop in the third month of intrauterine life. At the time of birth, the volume of each sinus is approximately 6–8 mm^3. The volume of the maxillary antrum increases in the vertical and lateral dimensions annually until puberty. Maxillary sinus hypoplasia may be seen in up to 10% of the population. The size of the maxillary sinus has relevance, particularly in the assessment for planned endoscopic surgery. If the size of the maxillary sinus is small, there is a higher chance of orbital penetration during surgery. Other conditions with a reduced size of the maxillary sinus are silent sinus syndrome, post-traumatic injury, and postoperative sequelae (Figs. 2.6, 2.7, and 2.8).

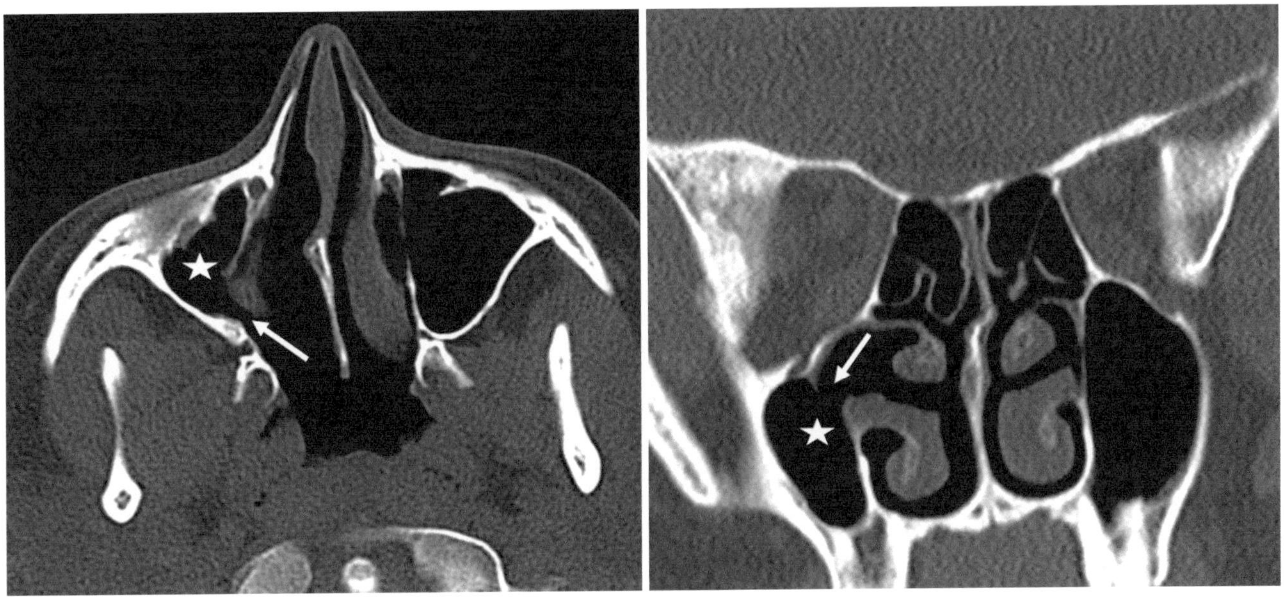

Fig. 2.6 A 19-year-old male with maxillary sinus hypoplasia and an accessory maxillary sinus ostium (AMSO). On axial (*left*) and coronal (*right*) 3-mm CT sections, there was incidental right maxillary sinus hypoplasia (*stars*) as well as a normal variant AMSO on the same side (*arrows*)

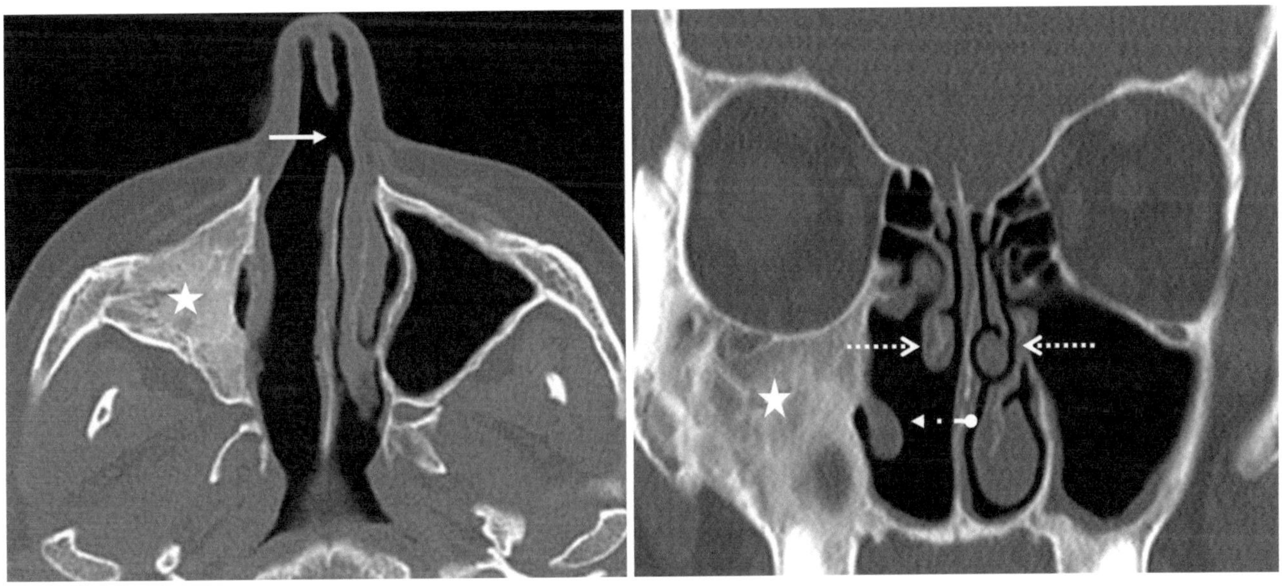

Fig. 2.7 Comparison case of a maxillary sinus ossification. Axial (*left*) and coronal (*right*) 3-mm CT sections in a 37-year-old male with a long history of maxillary sinusitis. The images demonstrate complete ossification of the right maxillary sinus (*stars*). In contrast to hypoplasia, the overall size of this sinus is normal, suggesting that this phenomenon is secondary to chronic inflammation or obstruction (less likely to have been caused by fibrous dysplasia). Also, note the incidental nasal septal perforation (*arrow, left*). Additionally, note normal variant paradoxical middle turbinates bilaterally (*dotted arrows, right*) and a hypoplastic (versus atrophied) right inferior turbinate (*interrupted arrow, right*)

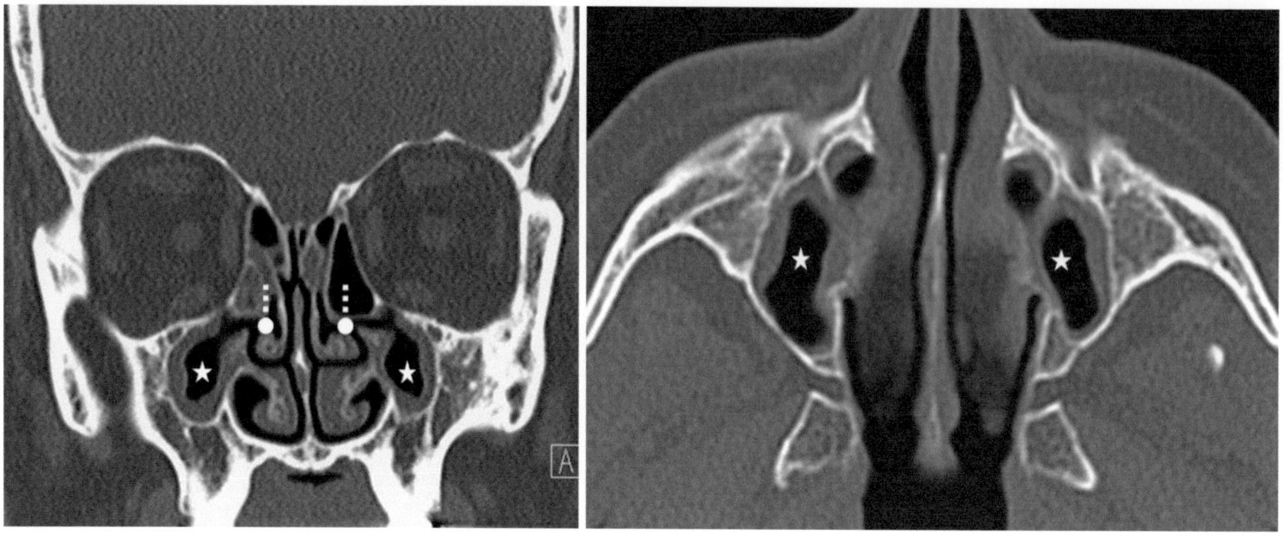

Fig. 2.8 Comparison case of sinusitis in maxillary sinus hypoplasia. A 45-year-old male suffering from "acute on chronic sinusitis" has bilateral moderately hypoplastic maxillary sinuses (*stars*) on coronal (*left*) and axial (*right*) 2-mm non-enhanced computed tomography (NECT) reconstructions, with a moderate amount of mucosal thickening/debris lining both maxillary and the right ethmoid sinus. Also note paradoxical middle turbinates (*circle tip dotted arrows, left*), another normal variant

2.3.2 Accessory Maxillary Sinus Ostia

As described in the Introduction section of this chapter, with regard to basic anatomy of the paranasal sinuses, the principal maxillary sinus ostium (PMSO) is present and patent in nearly all of the population. However, an accessory maxillary sinus ostium (AMSO) has been noted in about 12–37% of the population, being unilateral in approximately 6% of the population. This defect is typically situated posterior and inferior to the uncinate process of the maxilla and is usually less than 5 mm in caliber, although rarely it is larger. In much older literature it had been described as a "nasal fontanelle." The aforementioned wide variation in described prevalence probably relates to the identification of smaller defects with decreasing sub-millimeter slice thickness in more recent studies, whereas CT examinations before the year 2000 were typically of 3- to 5-mm thickness and often were nonspiral (i.e., sequential) in acquisition technique, preventing adequate isotropic reconstruction (Figs. 2.9, 2.10, 2.11, 2.12, 2.13, and 2.14).

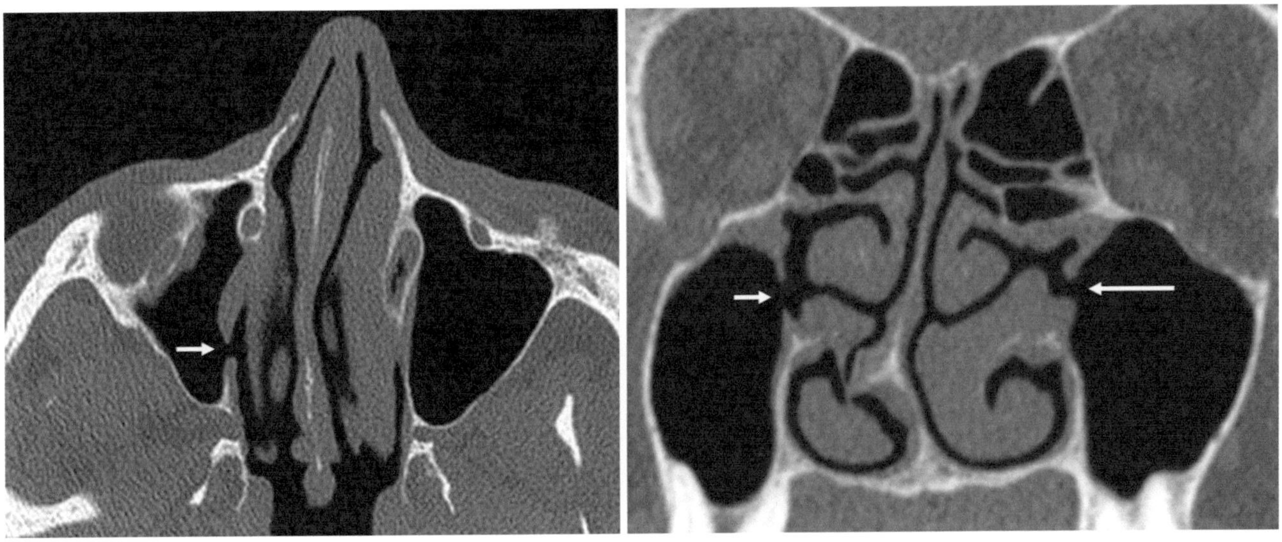

Fig. 2.9 A 59-year-old male with bilateral AMSOs. A 2.4-mm diameter on the right AMSO (*tiny arrows*) is noted on a temporal bone CT (0.6-mm thickness) performed for temporomandibular joint disease (*not shown*). Axial (*left*) and coronal (*right*) reconstructions demonstrate the right AMSO; note a smaller left-sided AMSO as well (*elongated arrow, right*)

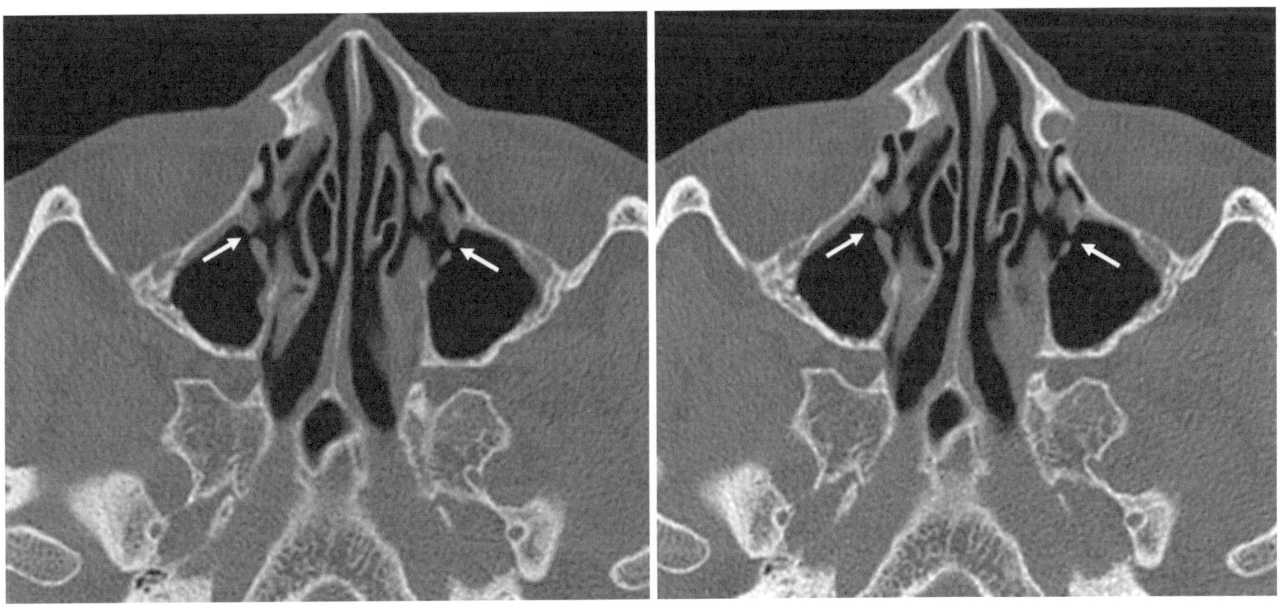

Fig. 2.10 A 67-year-old female with ~1-mm diameter incidental, bilateral tiny AMSOs (*arrows*) on axial reconstructions from a temporal bone CT (0.6-mm slice thickness) performed for hearing loss. Such tiny AMSOs may be invisible on routine thickness imaging, particularly if the images are 3–5 mm in thickness. These factors (small size and slice thickness) likely account for the widely varying prevalence of this variant in the literature

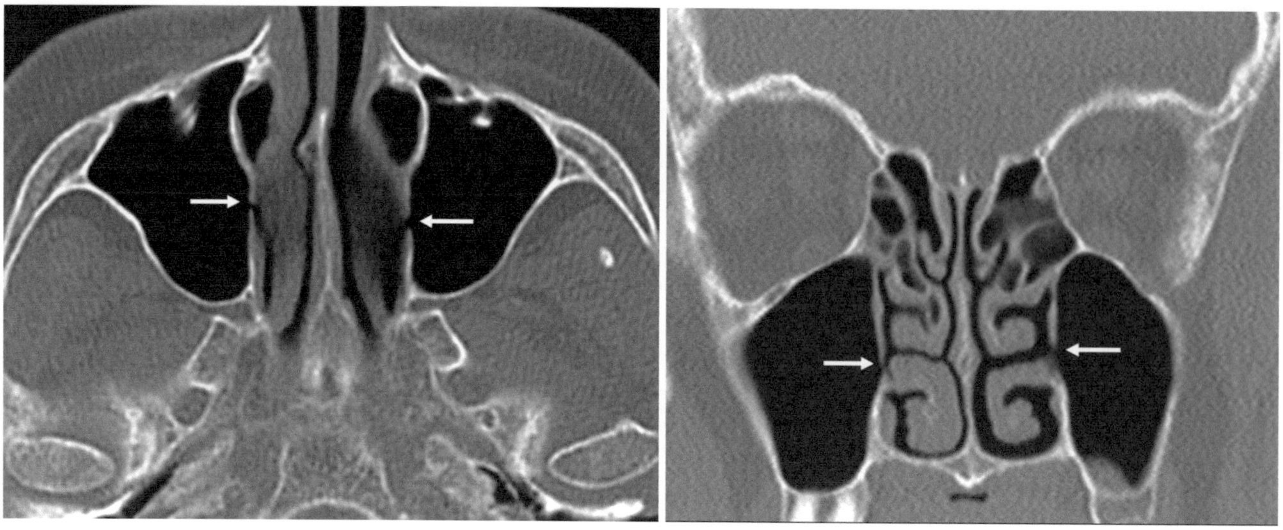

Fig. 2.11 A 78-year-old female with tiny, bilateral AMSOs (*arrows*), measuring 1 mm diameter on the right and 1.9 mm on the left on a sinus CT performed for a potential history of chronic sinusitis (only minimal mucosal thickening was noted). On a 2-mm thickness axial reconstruction (*left*), the bilateral AMSOs are tiny but evident. On coronal reformats (*right*), the AMSOs (*arrows*) are more difficult to visualize because of the increased 3-mm slice thickness as well as the volume averaging phenomenon

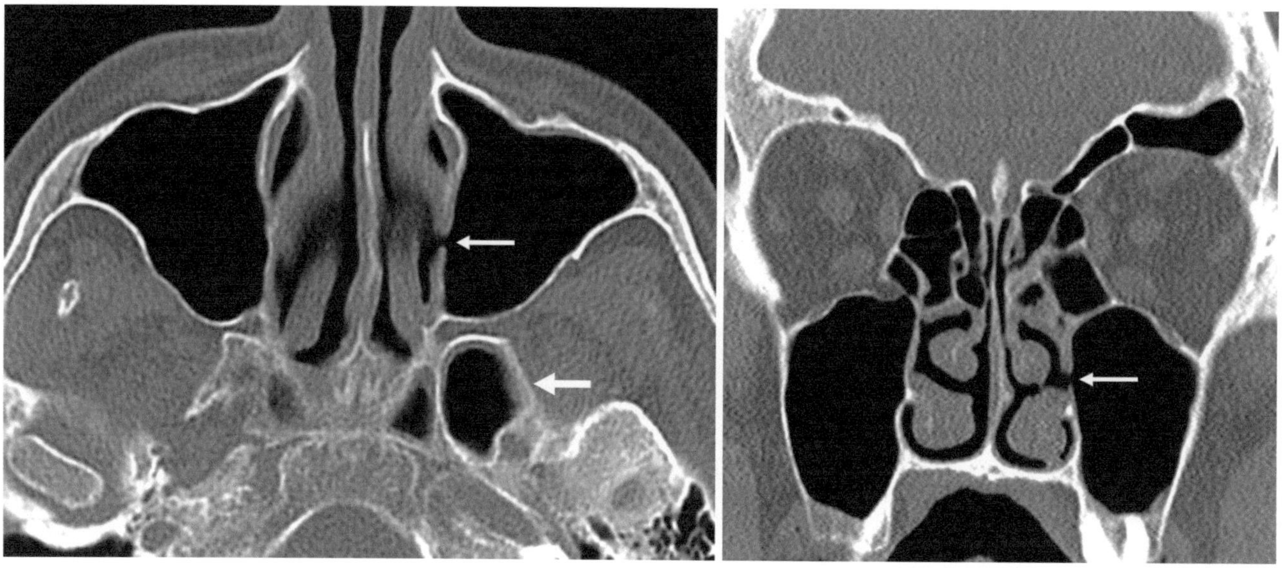

Fig. 2.12 A 74-year-old male had a unilateral left AMSO of 2.1 mm in diameter (*arrows*), as noted on 3-mm axial (*left*) and coronal (*right*) reformats of a CT performed for chronic sinusitis (negative examination). Note the lateral extension of sphenoidal pneumatization, also known as "pneumatized pterygoid" (*large arrow, left*), another normal variant in the absence of sinus inflammation

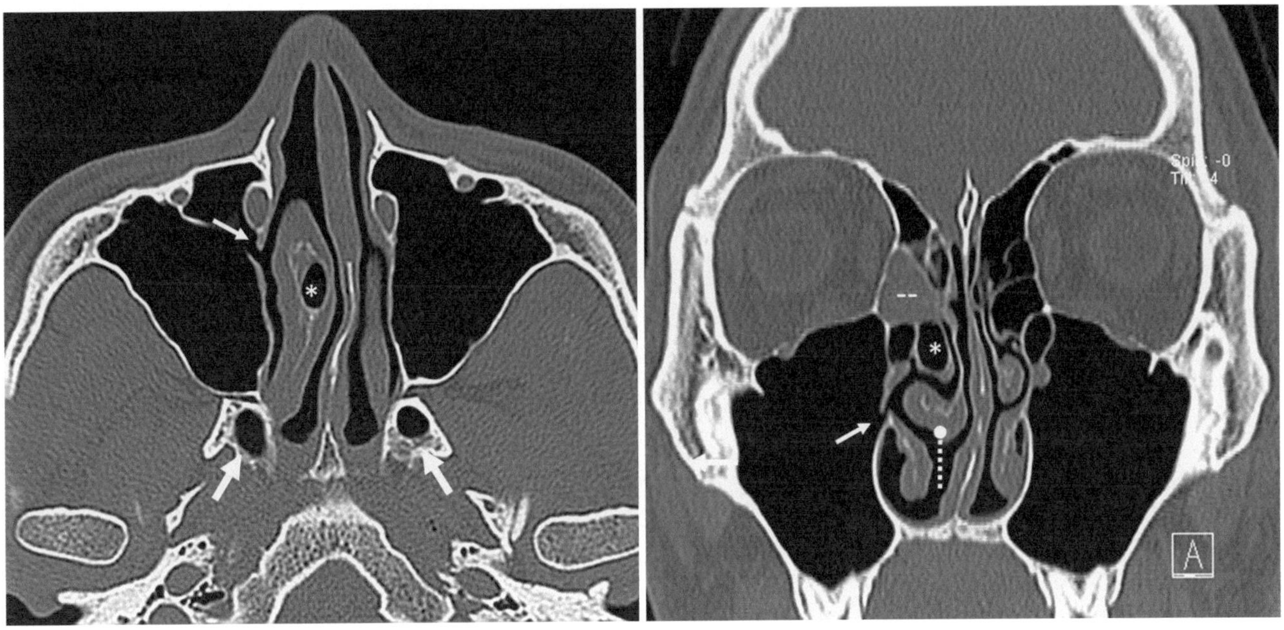

Fig. 2.13 A 33-year-old with rhinitis had a tiny (1.5-mm caliber) unilateral AMSO (*arrows*) on 0.6-mm thickness axial (*left*) and coronal (*right*) reconstructions for a sinus CT. Also note other normal variants, including the incidental aeration of the right middle turbinate (*, also known as conchae bullosa), a right paradoxical middle turbinate (*circle tip arrow*), and aerated-pneumatized pterygoids (*thicker arrows, left*). Finally, note a small amount of debris, or a focal mucous retention cyst, within the right ethmoid air cells (--)

Recent research has not only demonstrated a higher prevalence of AMSO than previously thought but also has evaluated its role in the circulation of mucus and air. This accessory ostium may be functional, since the presence of an AMSO may alter the normal "stream" of mucus and "ventilation" of the sinus as compared to when it is absent. Both air and mucus can be transmitted via this secondary accessory ostium from the maxillary sinus into the nasal cavity as well as through the PMSO and osteomeatal unit (OMU). This has led to theories for development of an AMSO that range from being purely embryologic (and thus congenital) in nature as opposed to being acquired; in the latter case an acquired AMSO would arise secondary to obstruction of the OMU or of the PMSO.

Anomalies that have been significantly associated with the presence of an AMSO include a mucous retention cyst (in 40–50% of AMSOs), mucosal thickening (40–45%), maxillary sinusitis (20–30%), and potentially nasal septal deviation, the last theoretically owing to altered ventilation and mucous flow (Fig. 2.15). AMSOs may be obscured in patients with maxillary sinusitis, polyposis, large mucous retention cysts, nasal intubation, or severe nasal septal deviation. Notably, there is likely no clinical significance related to the presence of an AMSO.

However, there can be confusion as to whether an AMSO is present when assessing whether a patent medial antrostomy defect is seen in a patient following functional endoscopic sinus surgery (FESS). Since certain FESS procedures focus on creating a medial antrostomy defect, postsurgical defects may simulate an AMSO; however, FESS defects are usually greater in caliber. Their diameter typically ranges from 1 to 2 cm, although they can be created much larger (a so-called "mega-antrostomy") to relieve chronic recurrent sinusitis, which is particularly helpful in patients with cystic fibrosis.

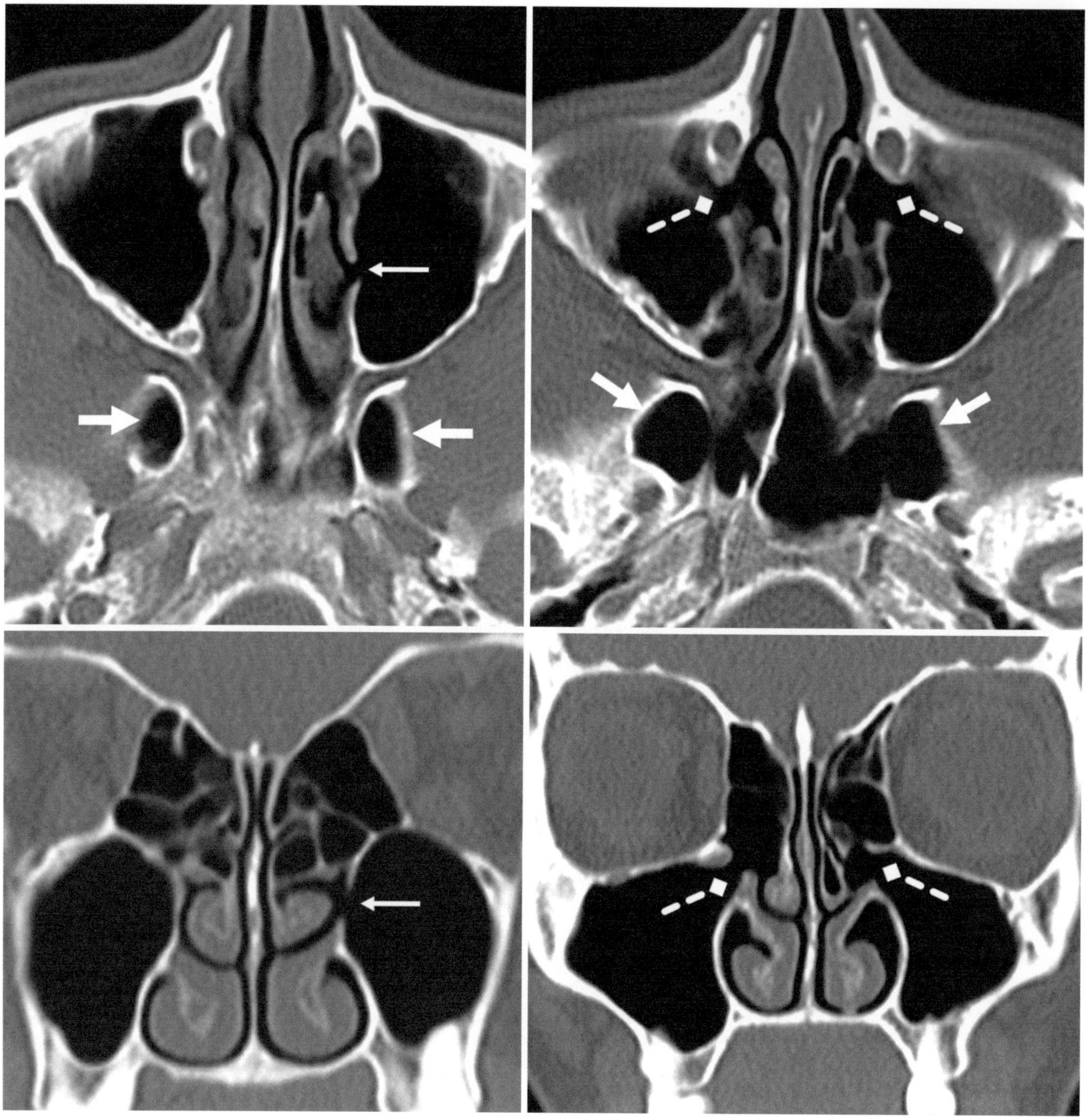

Fig. 2.14 A 35-year-old female with a history of chronic sinusitis with bilateral medial antrostomies and uncinectomies underwent a CT examination that demonstrated a unilateral left AMSO (*arrows*) measuring 2.8 mm in diameter on axial 3-mm thickness reconstruction (*top left*), and 3-mm thickness coronal CT (*bottom left*). On other axial (*top right*) and coronal (*bottom right*) slices, note that there are also medial antrostomy defects from endoscopy sinus surgery (*diamond tip dashed arrows*) that are larger, measuring 5.5 mm on the right and 8 mm on the left, with removal of the uncinate processes as well. There is also lateral pneumatization, also known as aerated pterygoid processes of the sphenoid, another normal variant (*thicker arrows, top row*). This case demonstrates how AMSOs may appear similar to but smaller than medial antrostomy defects on axial images, but they are in a different location and configuration from surgically-created deficits, which are often better defined on coronal images

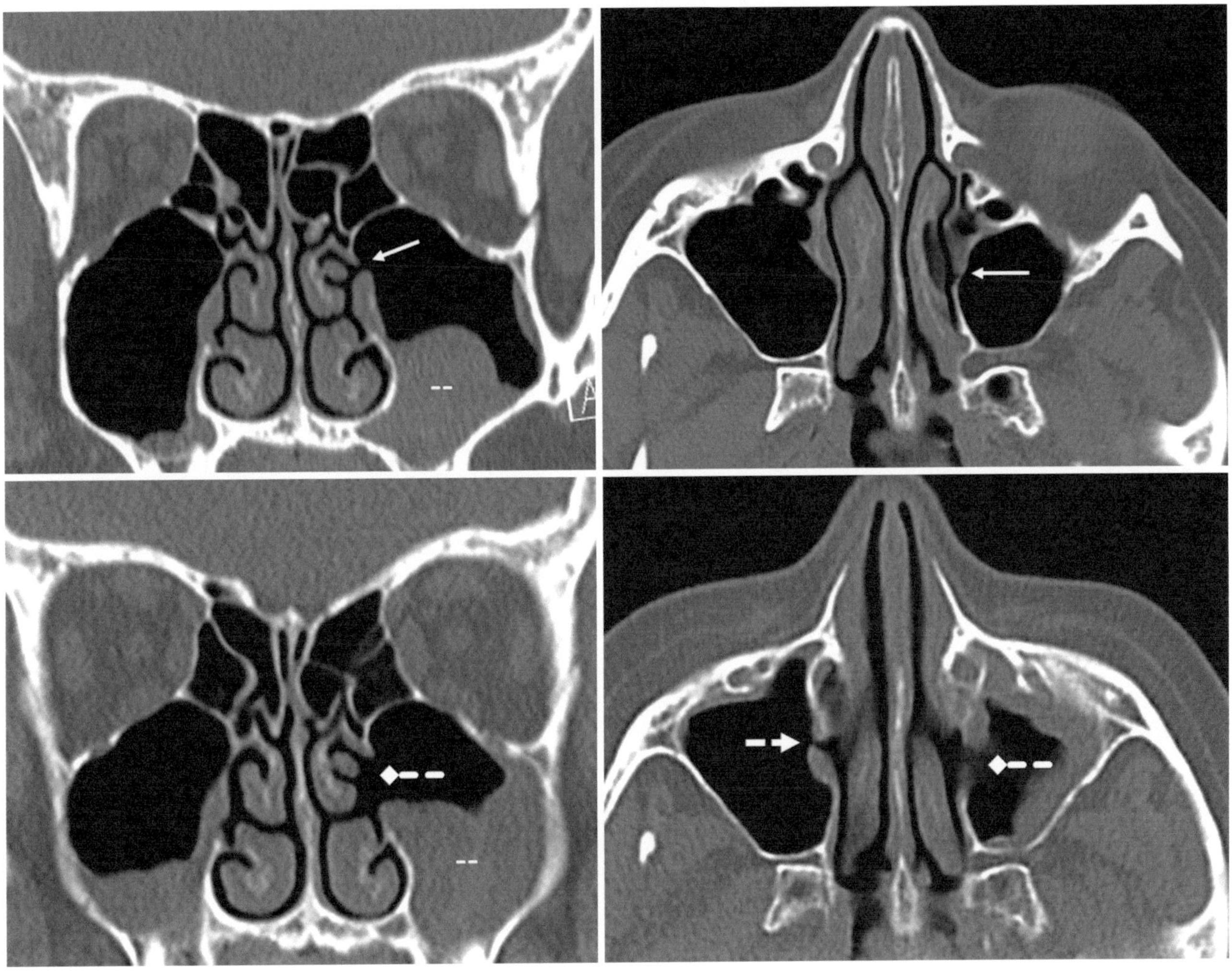

Fig. 2.15 Comparison case of medial antrostomy versus an AMSO. **Top row**: A 59-year-old female with a history of chronic maxillary sinusitis and debris (--) had an incidental 2-mm diameter left AMSO (*arrows*) on coronal (*left*) and axial (*right*) CT reconstructions. **Bottom row:** A repeat CT scan performed 11 years later several years after a left medial antrostomy (1.3 cm in diameter, *diamond tip dashed arrows*) via endoscopic surgery; mild residual mucosal thickening was present on coronal (*left*) and axial (*right*) reformats. The left AMSO is no longer visible, as it was at the site of the antrostomy. A new right medial antrostomy was also present (*dashed arrow, right*), which simulates an AMSO

2.3.3 Maxillary Sinus Septa

Septa (plural of septum) within the maxillary sinuses are common and may be fibrous or bony. They usually extend from the infraorbital nerve canal to the lateral wall (Figs. 2.16, 2.17, and 2.18). The prevalence of maxillary sinus septa ranges from 16% to 32% in the dental literature. These can affect the drainage of the maxillary sinuses and are also important in dental implant therapy. A procedure called maxillary sinus grafting has been used for occlusal rehabilitation,

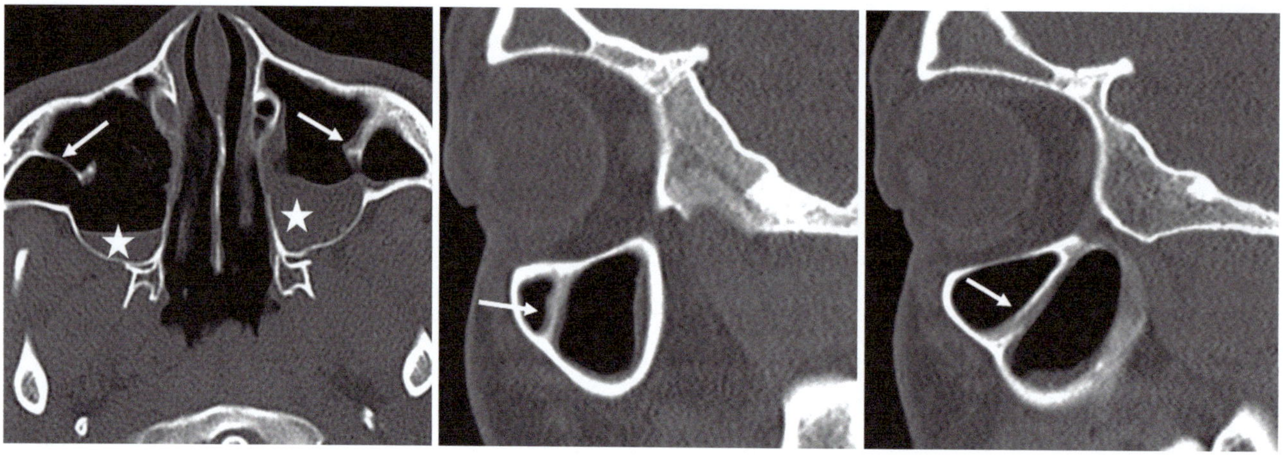

Fig. 2.16 A 32-year-old male with sinusitis. Incidental lateral septa are seen in both maxillary sinuses on axial section (*left*) as well as sagittal reformats of the right side (*middle*) and left side (*right*) on thin section CT. Also, note the layering fluid within the maxillary sinuses (*stars*), suggesting acute sinusitis

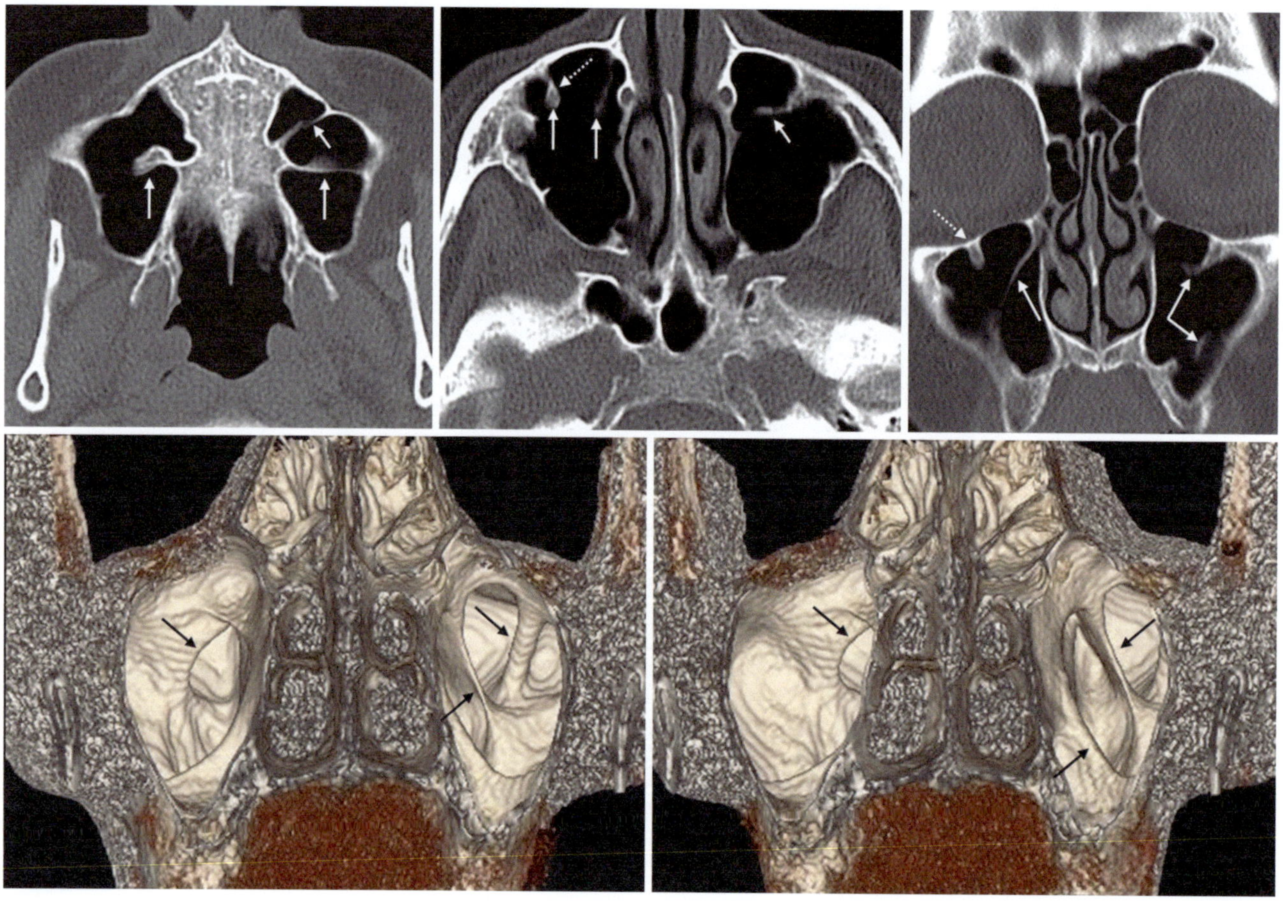

Fig. 2.17 A 65-year-old male with rhinitis underwent a preoperative sinus CT. **Top row:** Axial (*left, middle*) and coronal (*right*) 2-mm reconstructions demonstrated several maxillary sinus septa bilaterally (*thin arrows*). Note that one septum on the right contains the infraorbital nerve and foramen (*thin dotted arrows*). **Bottom row:** Two images of three-dimensional reconstructions with slightly different angles are viewed posteriorly (*left, right*), which depict how the septa (*thin black arrows*) create "pockets" of loculations within the maxillary sinuses

with prosthetic appliances placed over dental implants in the posterior maxilla. One of the complications during and after the sinus grafting procedure is perforation of the Schneiderian membrane (a membranous lining of the maxillary sinus), which is important in dental procedures because such perforations can predispose to recurrent inflammation; this complication is often associated with the presence of maxillary septa.

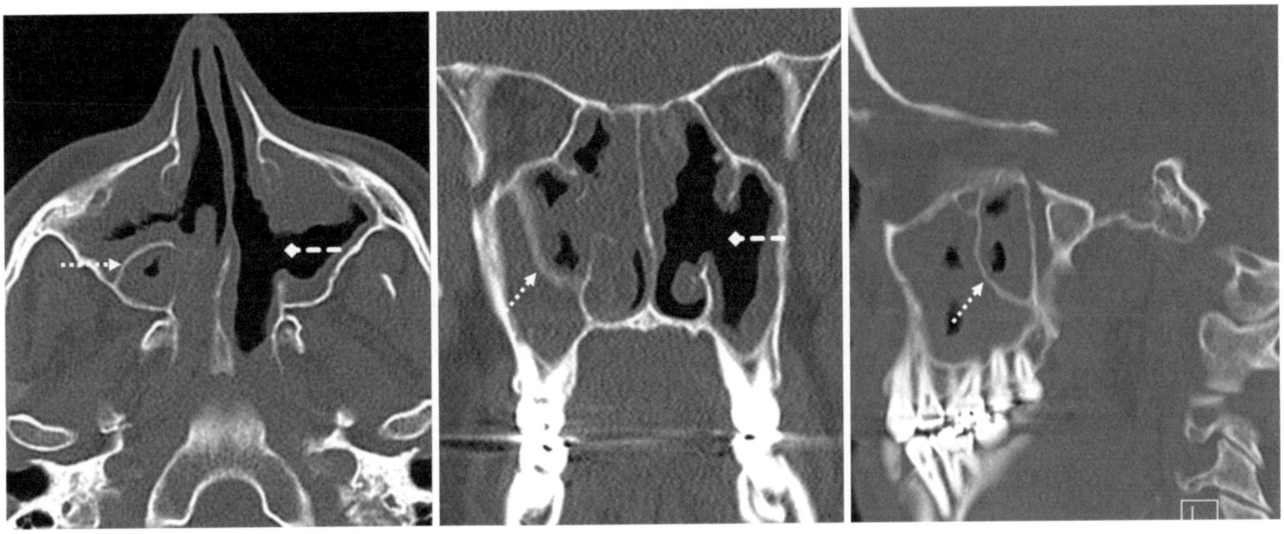

Fig. 2.18 Comparison case of obstructive sinusitis within a locule/septation. A 45-year-old male postendoscopic sinus surgery for a left medial antrostomy (*diamond tip arrows*) underwent a sinus CT with axial (*left*), coronal (*middle*), and sagittal (*right*) reconstructions that showed an obstructed right maxillary sinus locule owing to a bony septation (*dotted arrows*). This case demonstrates how a septum can contribute to obstruct portions of the maxillary sinuses

2.3.4 Dehiscence of the Infraorbital Nerve Canal

The infraorbital canal lies in the orbital part of the maxilla (floor of the orbit or below) and allows the passage of the infraorbital nerve. The infraorbital nerve, a branch of the maxillary division of the trigeminal nerve, is responsible for sensory innervation to the skin of the medial cheek, lateral nose and upper lip, the mucosa of the anteroinferior nasal septum and oral mucosa of upper lip. It traverses the antral roof but is usually completely encased in a bony canal. The antral wall of the infraorbital canal is particularly thin (even in normal patients), with an average thickness of 0.2 mm, while the thickness of the antral wall depends on age and the degree of pneumatization of the maxillary sinus. It has been reported that the incidence of a completely dehiscent infraorbital canal is between 12% and 16% in cadavers. In patients in whom the infraorbital nerve canal is completely dehiscent, the nerve may be easily irritated by mucosal inflammation or a mass and can cause facial pain in the distribution of the nerve (Fig. 2.19).

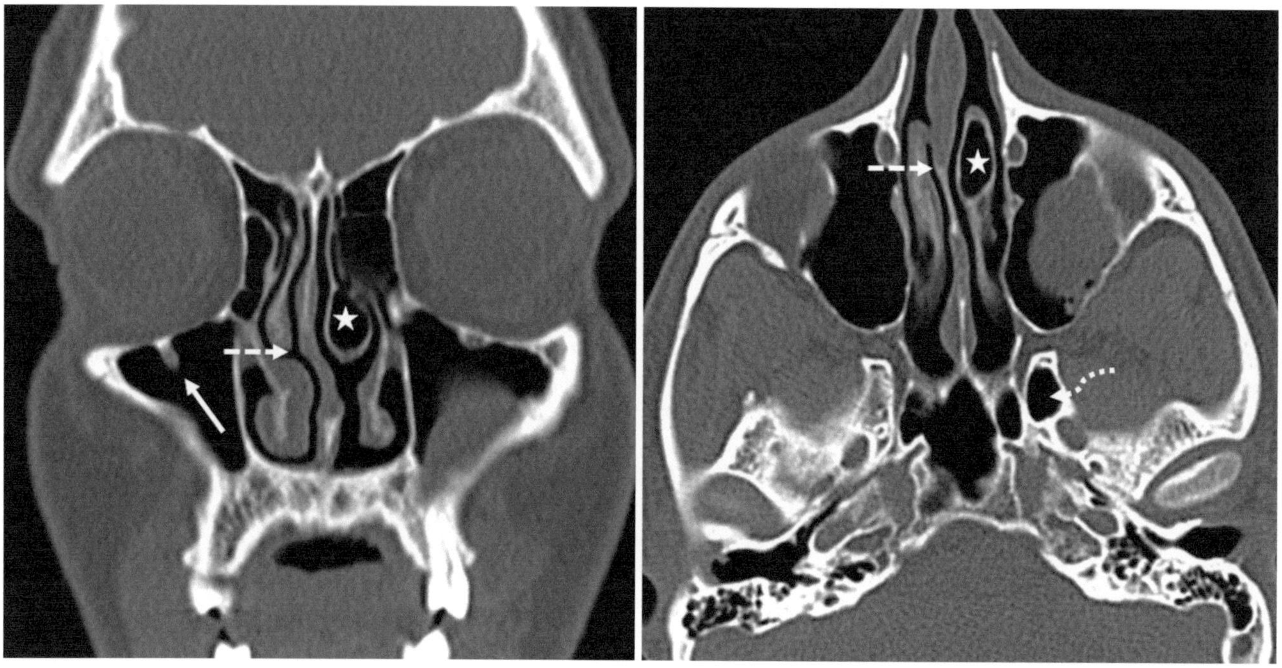

Fig. 2.19 Coronal (*left*) and axial (*right*) thin-section CT images of a 35-year-old male with headaches demonstrated right infraorbital nerve dehiscence with protrusion into the maxillary sinus (*arrow, left*). Also note the incidental mild deviation of the nasal septum (*dashed arrows*), a concha bullosa of the left middle turbinate (*stars*), and incidental normal variant aeration of the left sphenoidal pterygoid process (*curved dotted arrow, right*)

2.3.5 Maxillary Sinus Teeth ("Ectopic Teeth")

Any abnormal tissue interaction during odontogenesis may result in ectopic tooth development and eruption. One of the ectopic sites, although rare, is the maxillary sinus. The displacement of the tooth may be caused by the pressure caused by cystic enlargement of the sinus. Other etiologies that may predispose to ectopic maxillary teeth may include trauma in the setting of an underlying congenital/developmental anomaly (such as cleft palate) causing displacement of the teeth; maxillary infection; crowding of the teeth of the maxilla; genetic factors; and high bone density (according to the literature). The tooth can also entirely migrate superiorly into the sinus and even become dislodged from the bony maxilla to "float" within the inflammatory debris within the sinus. Symptoms may include recurrent or chronic sinusitis or purulent discharge from the nose, elevation of the floor of the orbit (uncommon), or even obstruction of the nasolacrimal duct (Figs. 2.20, 2.21, 2.22, and 2.23).

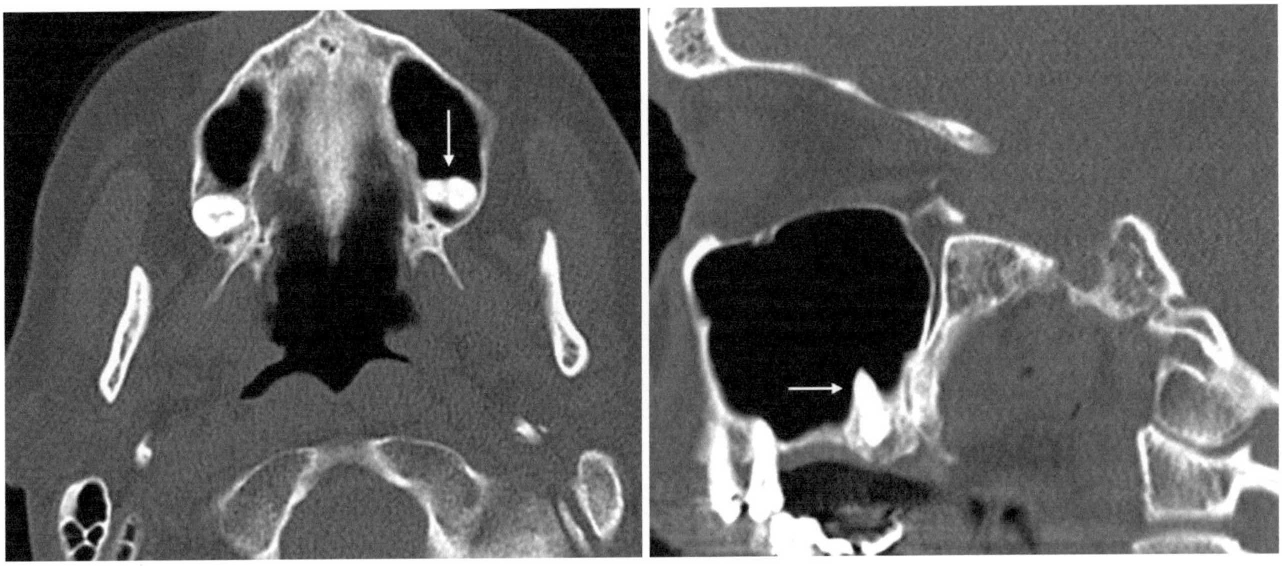

Fig. 2.20 A 45-year-old female with facial trauma. Axial (*left*) and sagittal (*right*) CT images demonstrate a normal variant ectopic molar tooth (*arrows*) within the left maxillary sinus

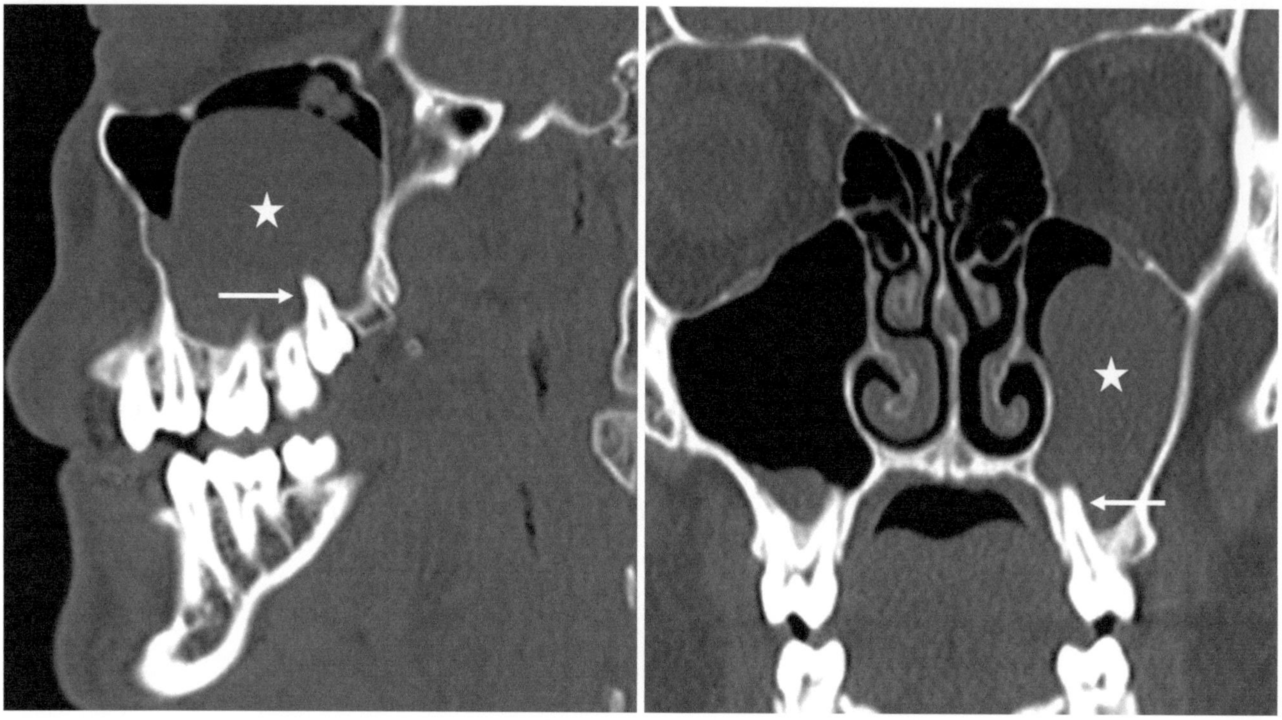

Fig. 2.21 A 35-year-old male with sinusitis. Sagittal (*left*) and coronal (*right*) CT images demonstrate a normal variant ectopic molar tooth (*arrows*) partially within the left maxillary sinus, abutting a large mucous retention cyst (*stars*)

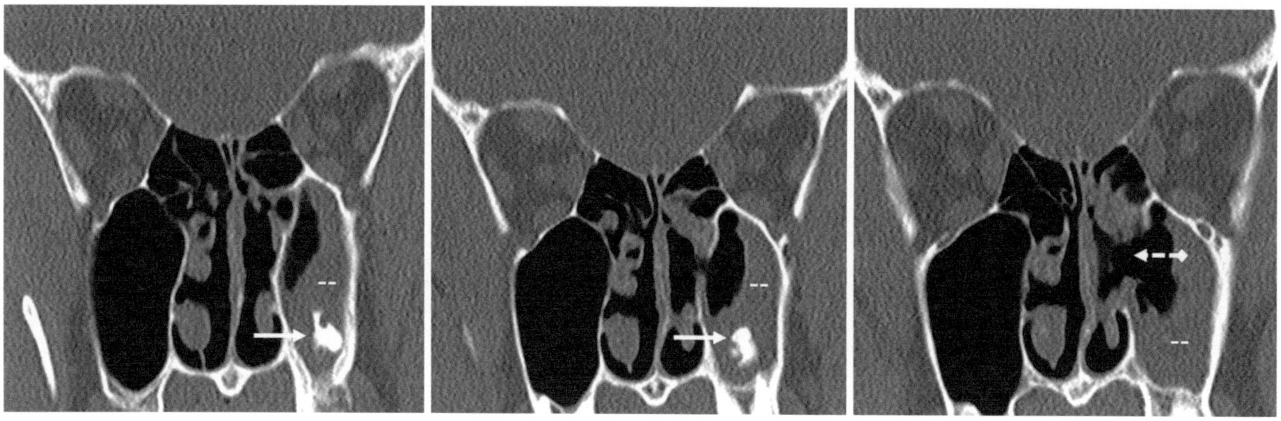

Fig. 2.22 Comparison case of recurrent sinusitis from a "floating" (ectopic) maxillary tooth. In a 44-year-old male with recurrent sinusitis, sequential 3-mm coronal CT reconstructions show a maxillary sinus tooth remnant (*arrows, left and middle*) "floating" within the debris of the inflamed left maxillary sinus. Notably, the patient had already undergone a left maxillary antrostomy for a 10- to 12-mm diameter antrostomy defect (*dashed arrow, right*). Hence, he suffered recurrent sinusitis (*dashes*) despite the medial antrostomy, since the source of the chronic sinusitis was most likely the dislodged ectopic tooth remnant

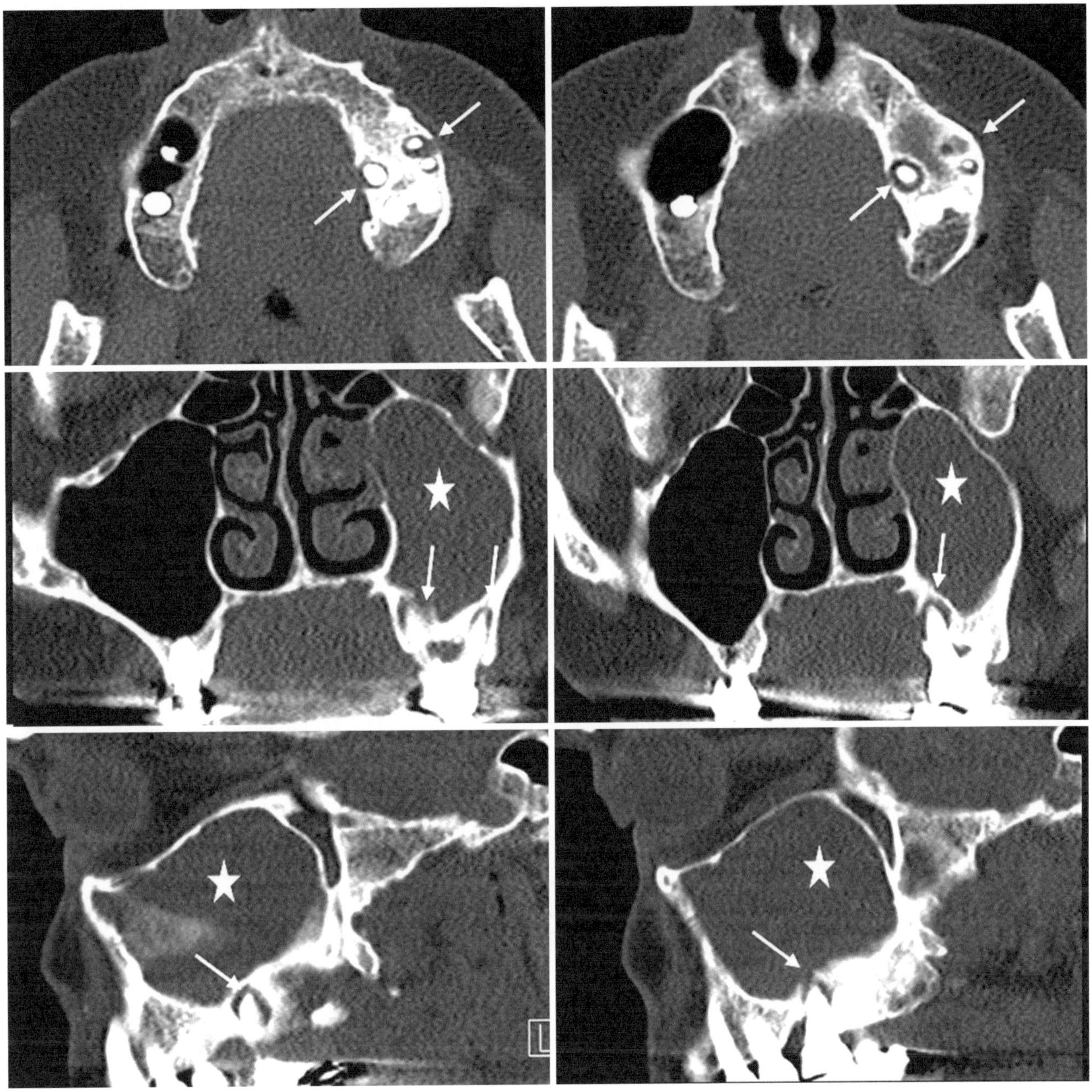

Fig. 2.23 Comparison case of odontogenic sinusitis. A 54-year-old female with a history of chronic, recurrent left maxillary sinusitis underwent paranasal sinus CT. Sequential axial (*top row*), coronal (*middle row*), and sagittal (*bottom row*) 3-mm CT images showed periapical lucencies surrounding both roots of a left maxillary premolar tooth (*arrows*). There is also complete obliteration of the left maxillary sinus from inspissated fluid/debris (*stars*), suggesting sinusitis secondary to periapical abscess, also known as "odontogenic sinusitis." On one sagittal image, the periapical abscess appears to cause dehiscence of the bony wall (*arrow, bottom right*), separating the tooth socket from the maxillary sinus, thus confirming that this abscess is a contributor to the chronic left maxillary sinusitis

2.4 Sphenoid Sinus

2.4.1 Sphenoid Sinus Pneumatization: Aerated-Pneumatized Clinoid (Onodi Cell), Pterygoid Processes, and Dehiscent Neural Structures

The normal pneumatization (i.e., "aeration") of the sphenoid sinus is quite variable and along a vast spectrum, while agenesis of the sphenoid sinus (nonpneumatization) is rather rare in adults. Agenesis or hypogenesis of the sinus is important to be aware of, since the sphenoid sinus forms and pneumatizes in a fashion that differs from the other paranasal sinuses, and such developmental variations lead to several other common variants. The sinus and its pneumatization begin in the embryo at about 4 months of gestational age as an evagination of the posterior nasal capsule into the sphenoid bone; it then develops in close proximity to the vomer at a site of paired ossification centers (the "bones of Bertin"). These two bones encompass and enclose a point in the body of the sphenoid bone (specifically in the rostral basisphenoid), where in the neonate it exists as a small "recess" bordered by the presphenoid and sphenoid conchas. Over the first few years of life, pneumatization increases with fusion of the presphenoid to the concha, and it continues later in adolescence as aeration extends further into the presphenoid and basisphenoid.

The progressive pneumatization of the sphenoid has led to the identification of three general types of sphenoidal pneumatization. Type I is the "conchal" type, which is essentially a solid block of bone without an air cavity; it is rare in adults (<1–2%). Type II is the "presellar" type, where the sphenoid sinus has air within but neither extends to nor indents the bony contour of the sella (~10–20%). Type III is the sellar type, which is the most common (~75–85%) and consists of the majority of the sphenoidal body being pneumatized, with the aeration both indenting and extending along the sellar contour. Notably, such pneumatization can appear rather extensive by seeming to involve nearly the entire sphenoid bone (including the greater and lesser wings) and even at times seeming contiguous with the remainder of the paranasal sinuses.

Lateral pneumatization is the general term for lateral extension of the aeration from the basisphenoid into varying degrees of the pterygoid plates and wings. This lateral pneumatization or lateral extension variant often involves or coexists with pneumatization of sphenoid or parasphenoidal bony structures other than the pterygoids, such as the anterior clinoid, posterior clinoid, or crista galli. Such extensions of pneumatization have also led to further proposed classifications of sphenoid sinus pneumatization, one of which involves six types based on the direction of pneumatization, including the sphenoid body, lateral (i.e., pterygoidal), clival, lesser wing (e.g., anterior and posterior clinoids), anterior, and combined.

As a subtype of lateral extension/pneumatization of the sphenoid sinus, aerated-pneumatized pterygoid processes are perhaps the most common variant of sphenoid pneumatization; they are present in about 25–40% of the population. There is wide variation in what this variant comprises, probably since the overall larger designation (particularly within neurosurgery and otolaryngologic literature) is termed "lateral pneumatization of the sphenoid"; thus, the incidence of this variant depends on how far the pneumatization extends later and to what extent it involves the pterygoid plate.

An aerated-pneumatized anterior clinoid process can extend from the posterosuperior ethmoidal air cell (i.e., the Onodi cell) or from the posterosuperior sphenoid sinus. This is an extension of either the ethmoid or sphenoid air cells into the lesser wing of the sphenoid's clinoid processes. It exists in 6–17% of the population, and about 30% to 40% are bilateral. Such pneumatization can also extend into the posterior clinoid process or optic strut, but these variants are less common (~3–7%). Thus, as this can extend from either the ethmoidal or sphenoid sinuses, which can be difficult to discern posteriorly and superiorly, they are grouped for the purpose of this text under the terms "aerated" (or "pneumatized") "clinoid process" (Figs. 2.24, 2.25, 2.26, 2.27, and 2.28). This aerated air cell typically partially or completely surrounds the optic nerve (so-called Onodi cell), which is usually an incidental finding but can occasionally become a clinically significant anatomic finding, particularly in presurgical evaluations. Thus, the grouping as "aerated clinoid" is also utilized for this text, since the potential clinical significance is that obstruction or filling of this air cell with fluid, inspissated debris, or tumor can lead to optic nerve dysfunction, whether caused by direct involvement by a pathologic process or by attempted surgical decompression that leads to iatrogenic injury. Furthermore, another less common but potentially fatal complication is that aeration of either the clinoid or posterior superior wall of the sphenoid is often associated with a thinner bony wall separating the air cells/sinus from the cranial vault. This may predispose to thinning or dehiscence, which ultimately can lead to craniospinal fluid leak or meningitis in the setting of acute or chronic sinusitis.

Kazkayasi et al. have noted that the presence of the aerated clinoid or pterygoid processes is significantly associated with the presence of *vidian nerve/canal* or *foramen rotundum protrusion* into the sphenoid sinus (Fig. 2.29). It is important to note the presence of a nerve or vasculature into the sphenoid sinus, especially in the presence of a sinus wall dehiscence. However, aerated clinoids or pterygoids are not necessarily associated with internal carotid artery protrusion into the sinus, although this is a critical variant to note before surgery and is present in a small minority of patients. Thus, in addition to noting the above-mentioned variations in pneumatization, it can be important to note the protrusion of critical neural or vascular structures into these sinuses as well, particularly in the presurgical setting of sinus surgery or in the setting of dehiscence related to inspissated/obstructive sinusitis (Figs. 2.30, 2.31, 2.32, 2.33, 2.34, and 2.35).

Finally, if such pneumatization is present adjacent to cerebral parenchyma or critical vascular structures, it can create pseudo-abnormalities on MRI, such as mimicking aneurysms or thrombi.

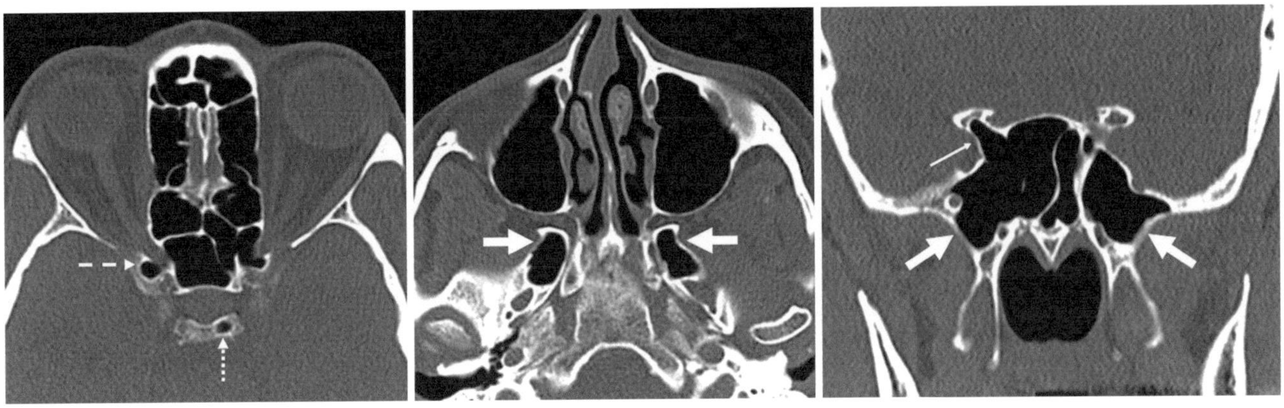

Fig. 2.24 A 51-year-old female with aerated pterygoids, optic strut, and anterior and posterior clinoid processes with unrelated infraorbital swelling (*not shown*). On axial (*left, middle*) and coronal (*right*) 2-mm CT sections, there was incidental lateral pneumatization of the sphenoid sinus bilaterally, with resultant aeration of the pterygoid processes (*large arrows, middle*) as well as pneumatization of the right optic strut (*thin arrow, right*), right anterior clinoid process (*dashed arrow, left*), and left posterior clinoid process (*dotted arrow, left*)

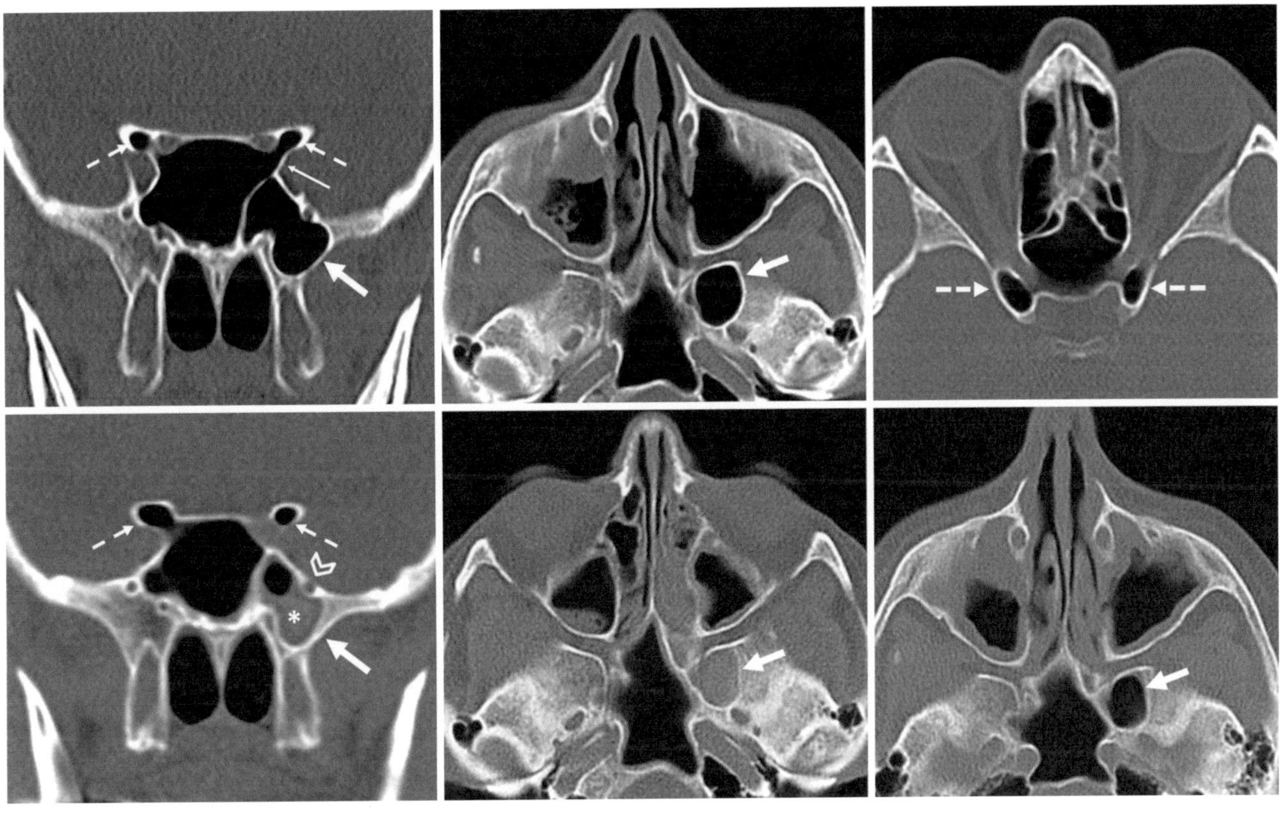

Fig. 2.25 A 60-year-old female with recurrent sinusitis, rhinorrhea, and left facial pain. **Top row:** On coronal (*left*) and axial (*middle, right*) 2-mm sections, aeration-pneumatization is noted of both anterior clinoid processes (*dashed arrows*), the left optic strut (*thin arrow, left*), and unilaterally of a left pterygoid process (*large arrows*). The maxillary sinuses have inflammatory mucosal thickening bilaterally, the right greater than the left. **Bottom row:** One year later, the patient's sinusitis and left facial pain worsened where the pneumatized left pterygoid (*large arrows*) had filled in with obstructive inflammatory debris (*, *left*) on coronal (*left*) and axial (*middle*) CT images, while the mucosal thickening of the maxillary sinuses had increased. On this examination, note new bony thickening from chronic inflammation surrounding the left foramen rotundum (V2, *chevron, at left*), which likely contributed to the patient's facial pain. Notably, following treatment, the debris within the aerated left pterygoid had cleared on an axial CT 2 years later (*right*), with improved facial pain as well. Thus, lateral pneumatization can be important to note as such patients can present with atypical orofacial pain, rhinorrhea, or other sensory symptoms

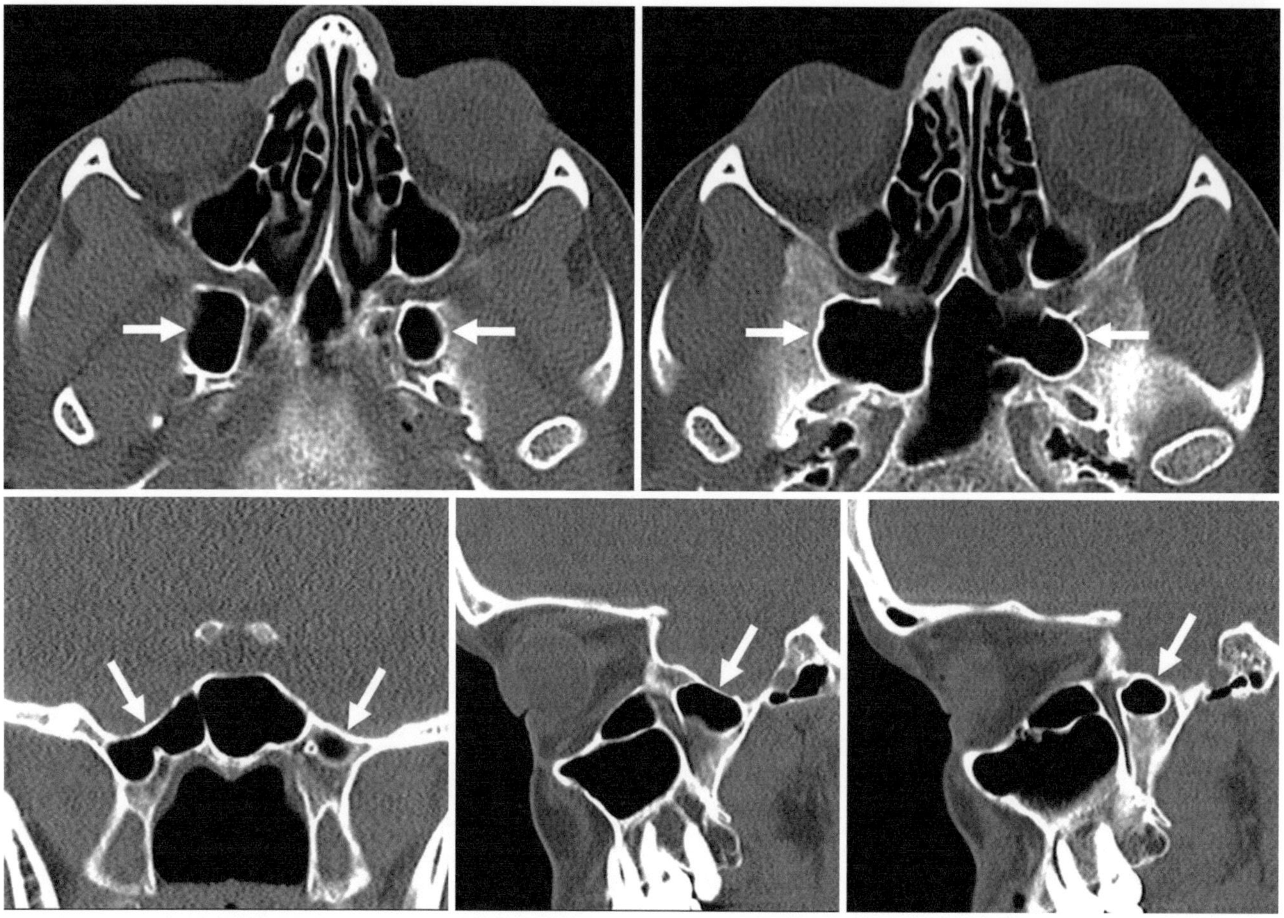

Fig. 2.26 A 34-year-old female with right facial pain. **Top row:** The patient had incidental bilateral although asymmetric lateral extension of sphenoid sinus pneumatization (*large arrows*) on 2-mm thickness axial CT images. **Bottom row:** The normal variant lateral pneumatization is also noted on coronal reconstructions (*left*), with aeration of the right pterygoid to a greater degree than the left, as demonstrated on right sagittal (*middle*) and left sagittal (*right*) reconstructions

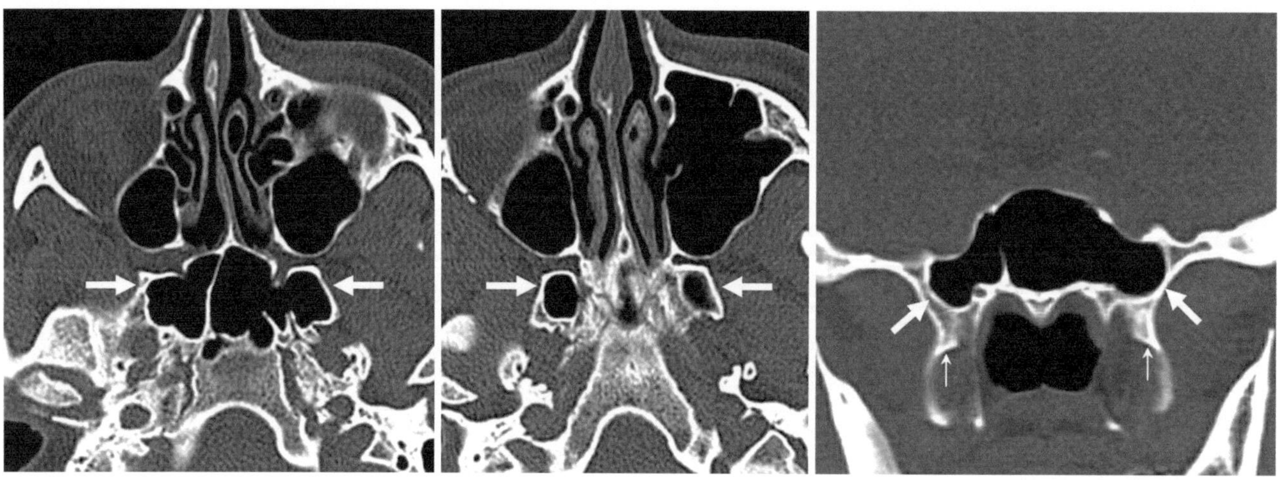

Fig. 2.27 A 37-year-old female with a history of intracranial hypotension underwent a head CT; 3-mm thickness axial (*left images*) and coronal (*right*) reconstructions demonstrated incidental lateral pneumatization of the sphenoid, resulting in aerated pterygoid processes bilaterally (*large arrows*). Note that this pneumatization does not extend completely to the base of the pterygoid wings/plates (*tiny arrows, right*)

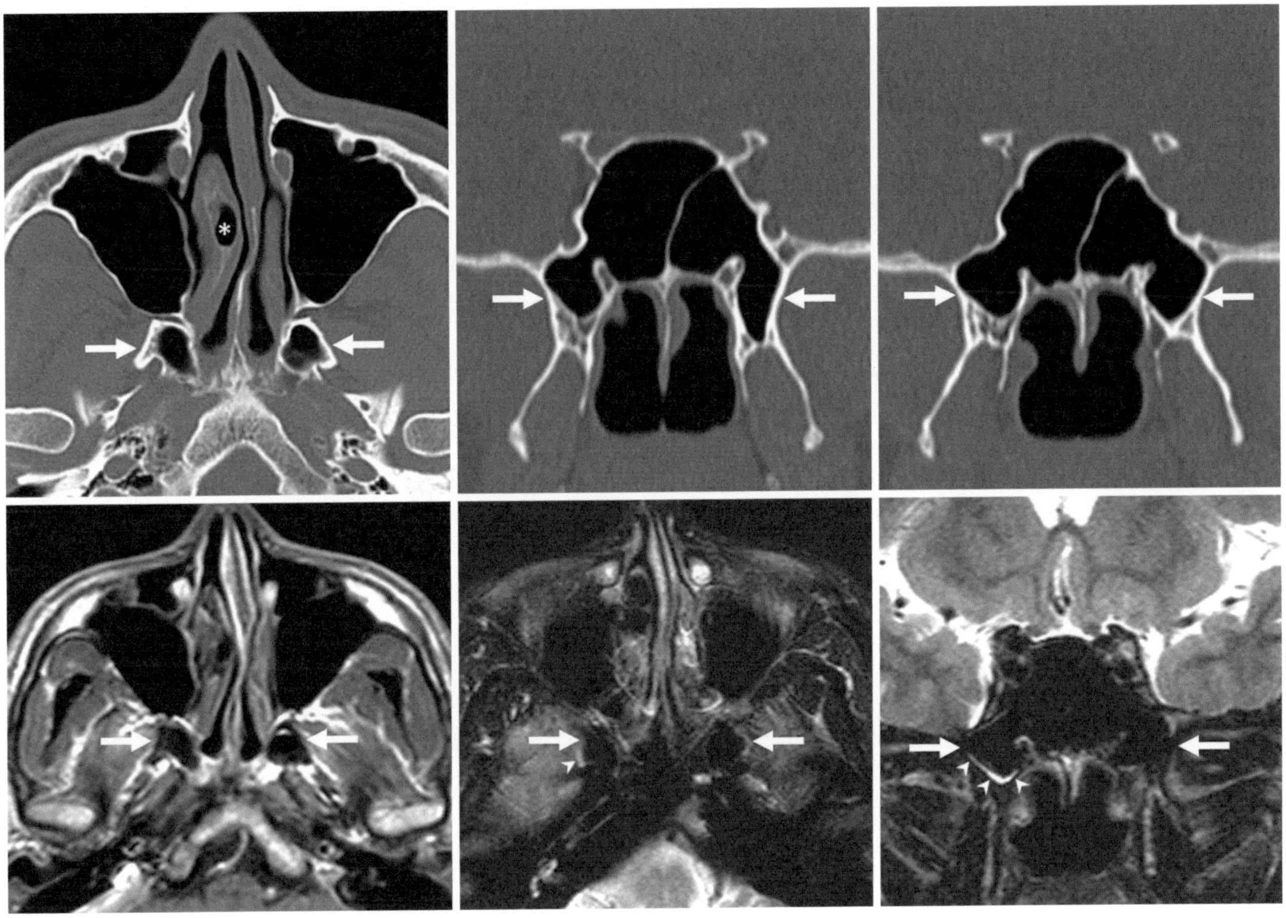

Fig. 2.28 A 36-year-old with rhinitis; bilateral aerated pterygoids cause artifacts on 1.5 T MRI. **Top row:** On axial (*left*) and coronal (*middle, right*) CT reformats, there is incidental lateral extension of pneumatization of the sphenoid sinus (*large arrows*), which extends inferiorly to the base of the pterygoid plates, particularly on the left side. There is also incidental normal variant aeration of the right middle turbinate (*, or conchae bullosa, *left*). **Bottom row:** Axial T1WI (*left*), T2WI (*middle*), and coronal T2WI (*right*) also depict the normal variant pneumatized pterygoids; note the air-related susceptibility artifact causing a hyperintense signal at the interface between bone, gas, and soft tissue (*tiny arrowheads, middle and right*). This can occasionally mimic disease, particularly if it is near vasculature or other vital structures, or it can obscure their adequate visualization on MRI

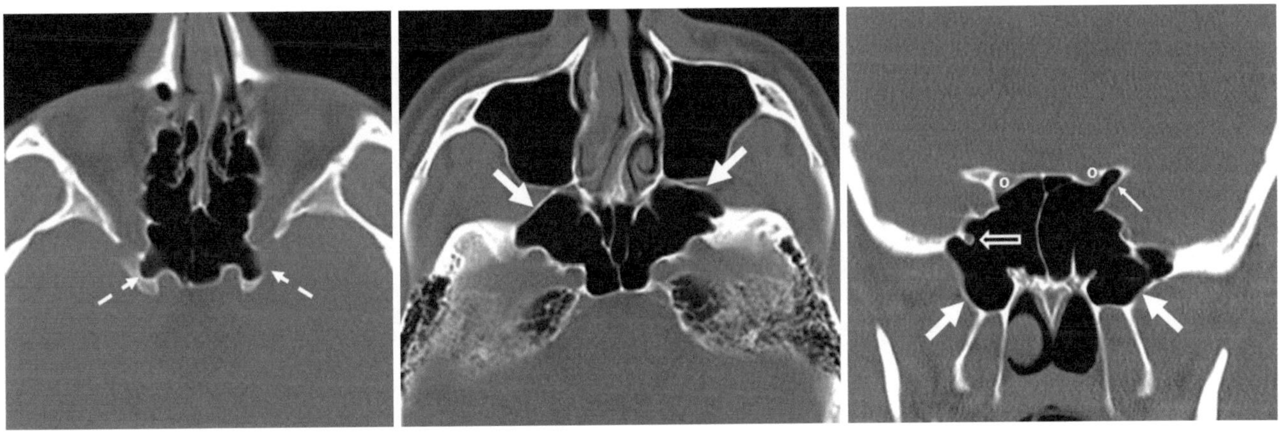

Fig. 2.29 A 17-year-old male with autism and a questionable prior history of sinusitis. Although the axial (*left, middle*) and coronal (*right*) 3-mm CT reformats were negative for sinusitis, there is incidental lateral extension of sphenoid sinus pneumatization, extending inferiorly all the way to the base of the pterygoid plates (*large arrows*). There is also aeration of the anterior clinoids (Onodi cells, *dashed arrows, left*) and especially of the left optic strut (*thin arrow, right*), while the right vidian nerve (*open arrow, right*) protrudes into the sphenoid sinus. Note the optic foramina bilaterally (*denoted as "o," right*), which transmit the optic nerves

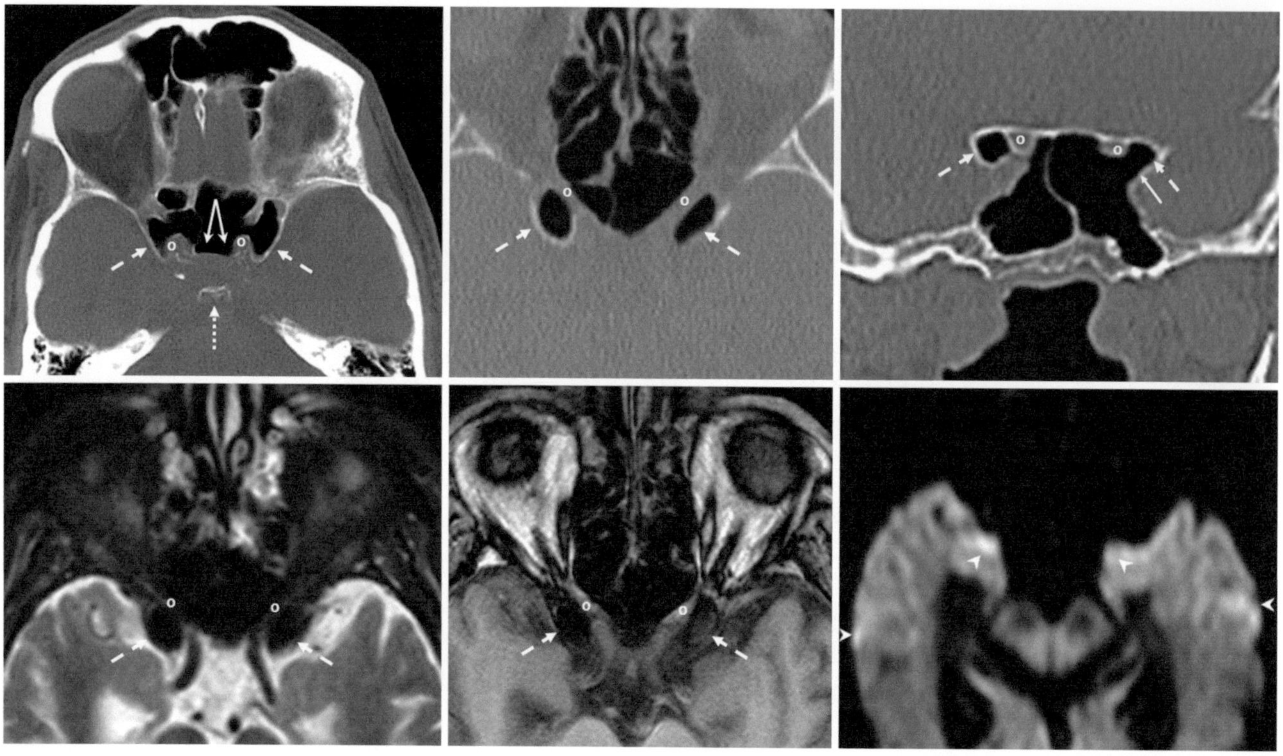

Fig. 2.30 A 75-year-old male who fell, with bilateral aerated anterior clinoid processes (Onodi cells) causing an artifact. **Top row:** The CT scan was negative for fracture on axial 2-mm (*left*) and other magnified axial reformats (*middle*), but aerated-pneumatized anterior clinoid processes (*dashed arrows*) adjacent to the optic nerves (*o*) and tuberculum sella (*double arrows, left*) were present, being normal variants. Also note a nonpneumatized posterior clinoid process (*dotted arrow, left*), with normal variant pneumatization of the left optic strut (*thin arrow*) on a coronal reconstruction (*right*). **Bottom row:** On a 1.5 T MRI, axial T2WI (*left*) and T1WI (*middle*) depict a dark signal within the anterior clinoids (*dashed arrows*) related to susceptibility effect from air. On DWI (*right*), the susceptibility artifact at air-bone-fluid interfaces causes hyperintensity (*arrowheads*) that can create mimics of cerebral parenchymal pathology such as infarcts, also noted along the inferior temporal lobes laterally, just above the mastoid air cells (also depicted by *arrowheads, right*). On the aforementioned images, note the position of the optic canals (*o*), which contain the optic nerves and are mostly surrounded by pneumatized bone on both sides

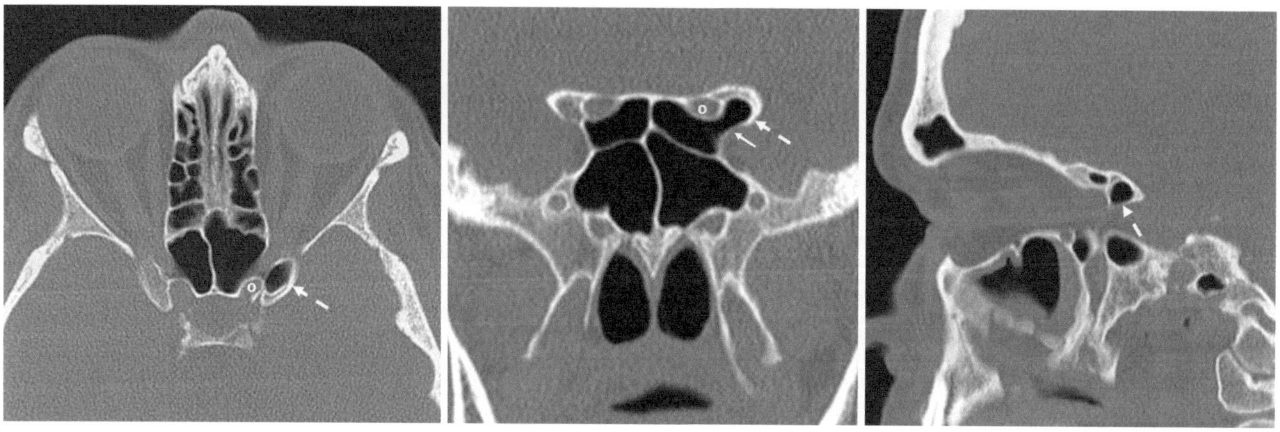

Fig. 2.31 In a 60-year-old male with a history of cancer of the soft palate (*not shown*), CT 2-mm thickness sections in axial (*left*), coronal (*middle*), and left-sided sagittal (*right*) planes demonstrate normal variant unilateral aeration-pneumatization of the left anterior clinoid process (*dashed arrows*) and left optic strut (*thin arrow, middle*). Note the left optic canal (*o, left and middle*), which contains the optic nerve

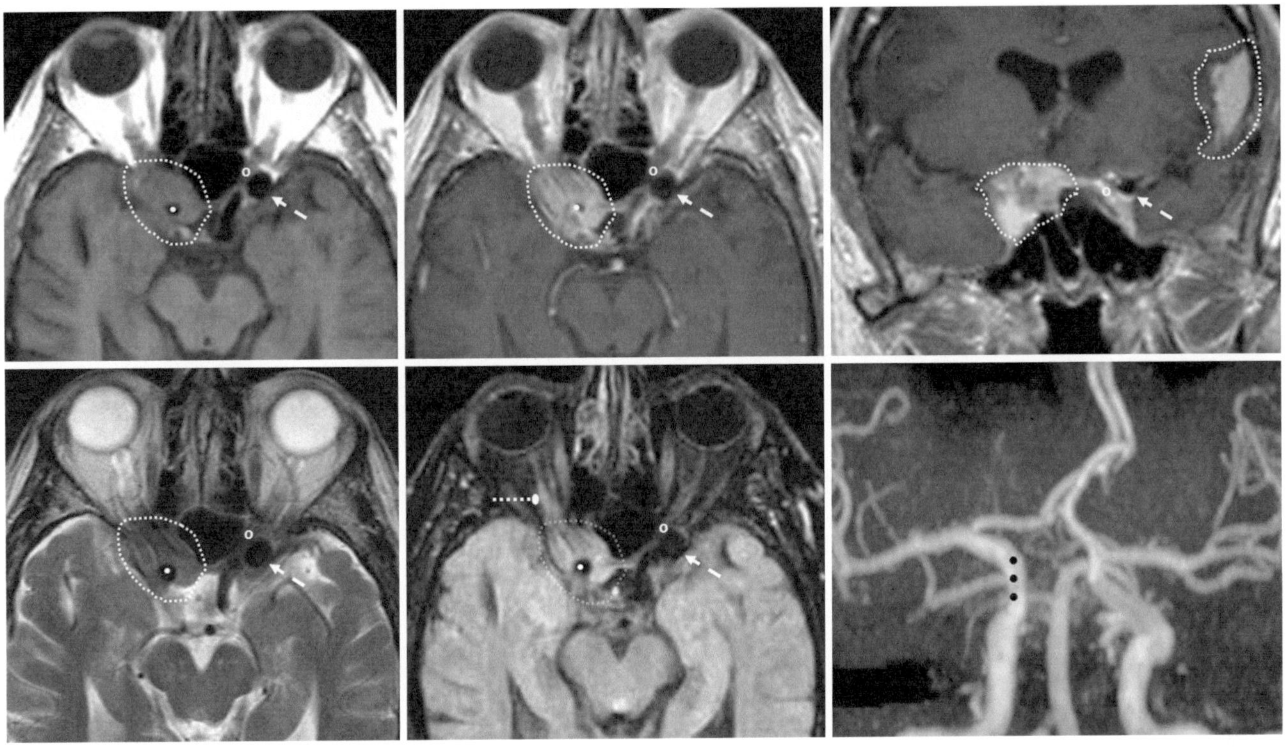

Fig. 2.32 Comparison case of paraclinoid meningioma, with a concomitant pneumatized anterior clinoid process simulating aneurysm. An 83-year-old male had both right paraclinoid and left convexity meningiomas (*dotted outlines*) for many years. On a 1.5 T MRI, a pneumatized left anterior clinoid process (*dashed arrows*) is present that simulates a flow void from an internal carotid artery (ICA); a resident physician initially suspected this to represent an ICA aneurysm. Note that a normal right ICA flow void (●) is present on the right side and is surrounded by tumor (tumor is delineated by *dotted outline*), as shown on axial noncontrast T1WI (*top left*), postcontrast T1WI (*top middle*), and coronal postcontrast T1WI (*top right*). Axial T2WI (*bottom left*) and fat-suppressed FLAIR (*bottom middle*) better depict a patient's right ICA flow void; on FLAIR, there may be extension of the meningioma anteriorly along the right optic nerve (*oval tip arrow, bottom middle*). On a three-dimensional noncontrast MRA anteroposterior view (*bottom right*), the right ICA (●) is minimally narrowed; although it is completely surrounded by tumor, there is no ICA aneurysm. This case demonstrates how an aerated anterior clinoid process can mimic vascular flow voids on MRI such as from an aneurysm if a CT is not performed

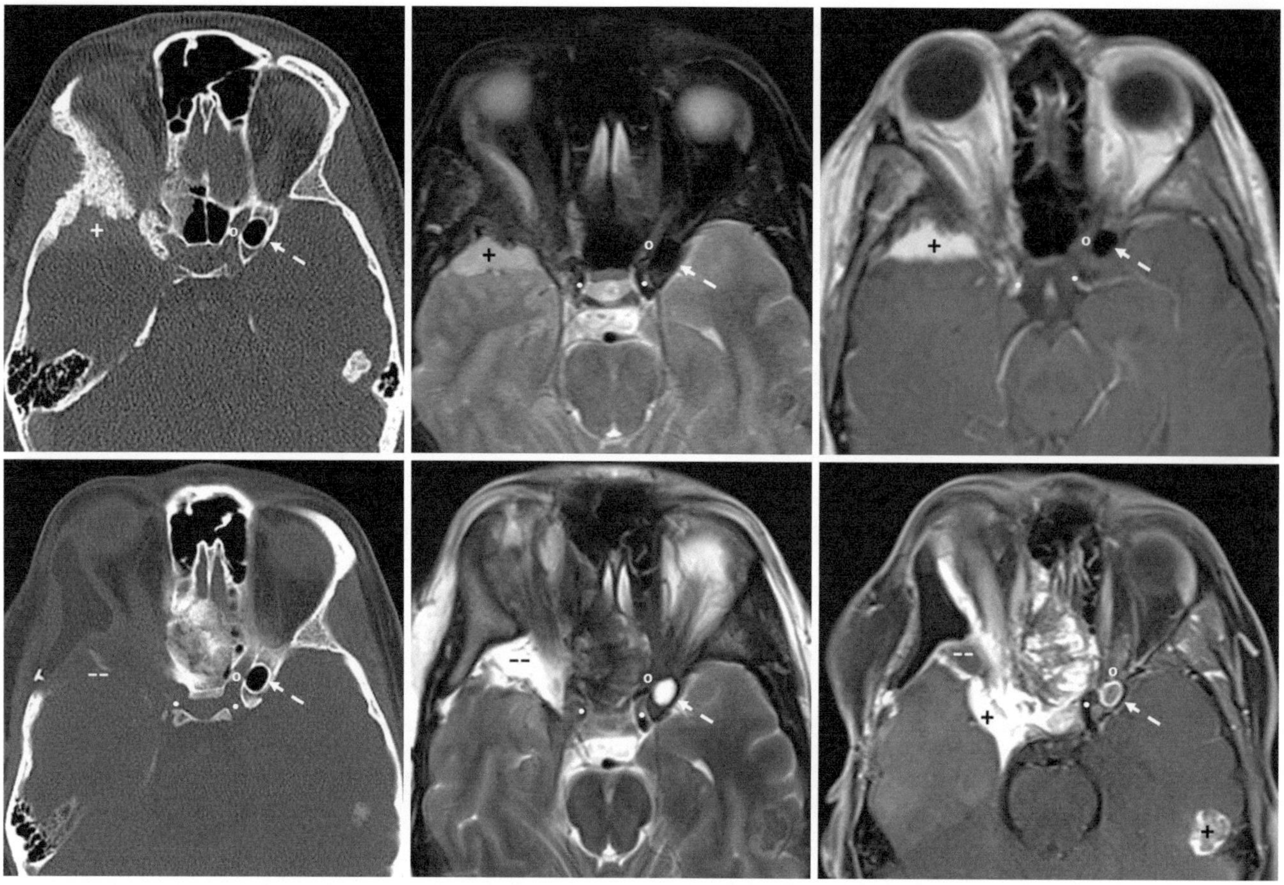

Fig. 2.33 Comparison case of sphenoid wing meningioma in a patient with meningiomatosis, with a concomitant pneumatized anterior clinoid process simulating recurrent tumor. **Top row:** A 35-year-old female had a rather extensive (but solitary at the time) meningioma (+) along the right sphenoid's greater wing, which caused a hyperostotic reaction of the bone on axial 1-mm thickness CT (*left*) and mildly displaced the anterior temporal lobe on 1.5 T MRI T2WI (*middle*) and postcontrast T1WI (*right*). A normal variant aerated and clear left anterior clinoid is present (*dashed arrows*) with a patent optic canal (*o*), while the right optic canal is narrowed and hardly visible due to the tumor. Notably, both ICA (●) flow voids are patent. **Bottom row:** One year later and postresection of the tumor, axial CT (*left*) demonstrates removal of the right sphenoidal greater wing (--), while the pneumatized left anterior clinoid is still patent and without debris (*dashed arrows*). Three years postsurgery, 1.5 T axial T2WI (*middle*) and postcontrast fat-suppressed T1WI (*right*) demonstrate a resection cavity at the site of tumor removal (--). However, the tumor recurred medial and posterior to the initial site (+, *right*), extending along the petroclinoid ligament and involving the right cavernous sinus. Note that the previously pneumatized left anterior clinoid process had filled in with T2-bright fluid (*dashed arrow, middle*) and the rim of the fluid enhanced with contrast (*dashed arrow, right*), indicating obstruction, although initially this obstructed, pneumatized clinoid process was thought to represent another focus of enhancing meningioma. However, a new, second tumor was noted along the floor of the left middle cranial fossa (+, *right*) as well as several other new extra-axial tumors (*not shown*), consistent with meningiomatosis. Note the close proximity of the aerated anterior clinoid to the left ICA (●). This case demonstrates how pneumatized and obstructed/inflamed anterior clinoid processes can simulate tumor

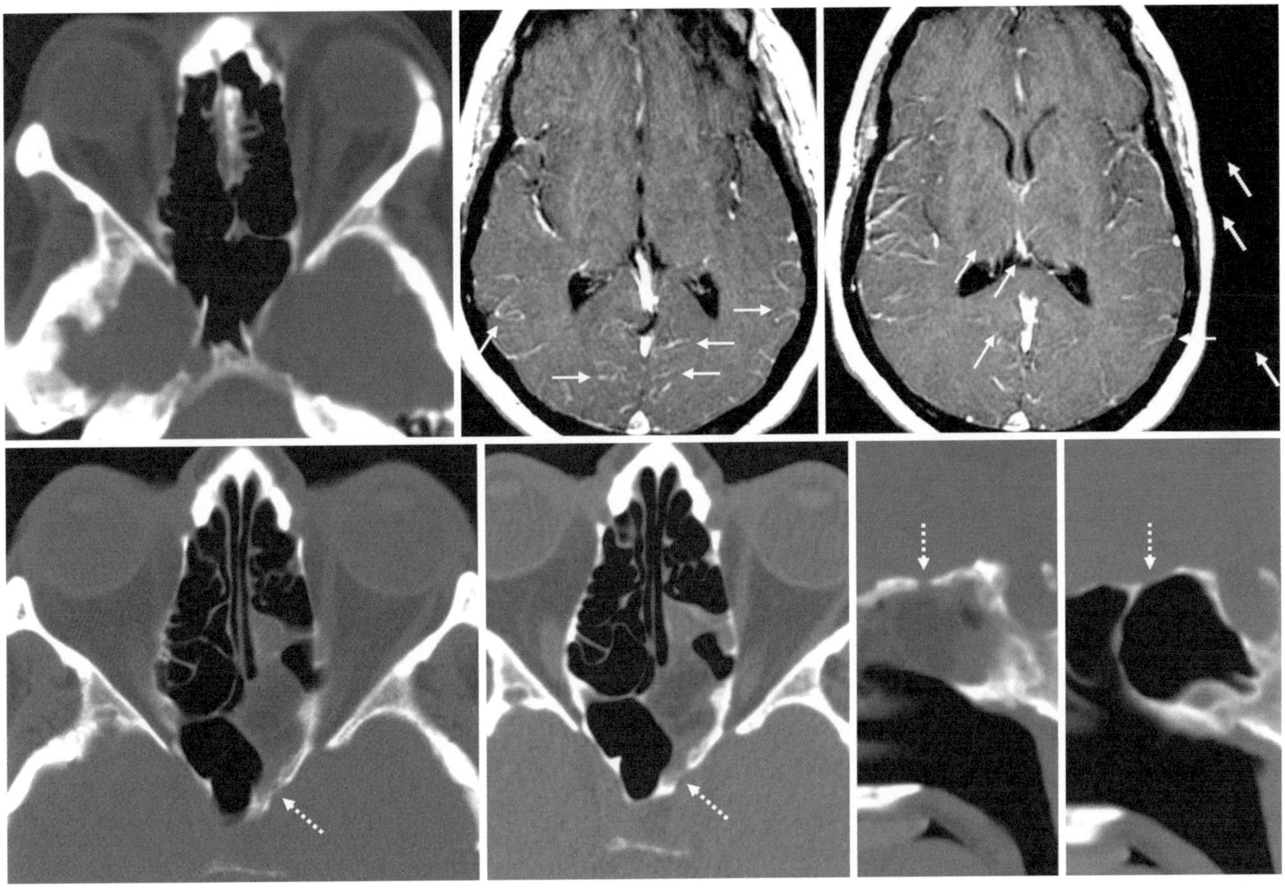

Fig. 2.34 Comparison case of sphenoid sinus wall dehiscence leading to CSF leak and meningitis. **Top row:** A 53-year-old female with recurrent nasal dripping (confirmed to be CSF leakage) underwent a 5-mm thickness head CT (*left*), which was negative, while a 1.5 T MRI soon after demonstrated abnormal mild diffuse leptomeningeal enhancement (*thin arrows*) on postcontrast T1WI (*middle, right*). Lumbar puncture confirmed that the patient had meningitis, and her symptoms improved after therapy. **Bottom row:** Several months later, the patient's symptoms, CSF leakage, and meningitis recurred, while a repeated axial CT at 4-mm thickness showed new left-sided sphenoid sinusitis, new focal bony thickening (suggesting chronicity) of the postero-superolateral wall, and a suggestion of focal thinning of the wall (*dotted arrow, left*). The source data was obtained, and axial images then reconstructed at 0.6 mm (*left middle*) confirmed focal dehiscence in that location as well as several other areas on sagittal images at left of midline (*dotted arrow, right middle*) and right of midline (*dotted arrow, right*). These three foci were surgically repaired and reinforced with no recurrence thereafter of the patient's CSF leakage or meningitis. This case demonstrates that although extensive aeration/pneumatization of the sphenoid sinus is a normal variation, even if occurring with varying degrees of bony wall thinning, this phenomenon can predispose to the development of CSF leakage and subsequent meningitis

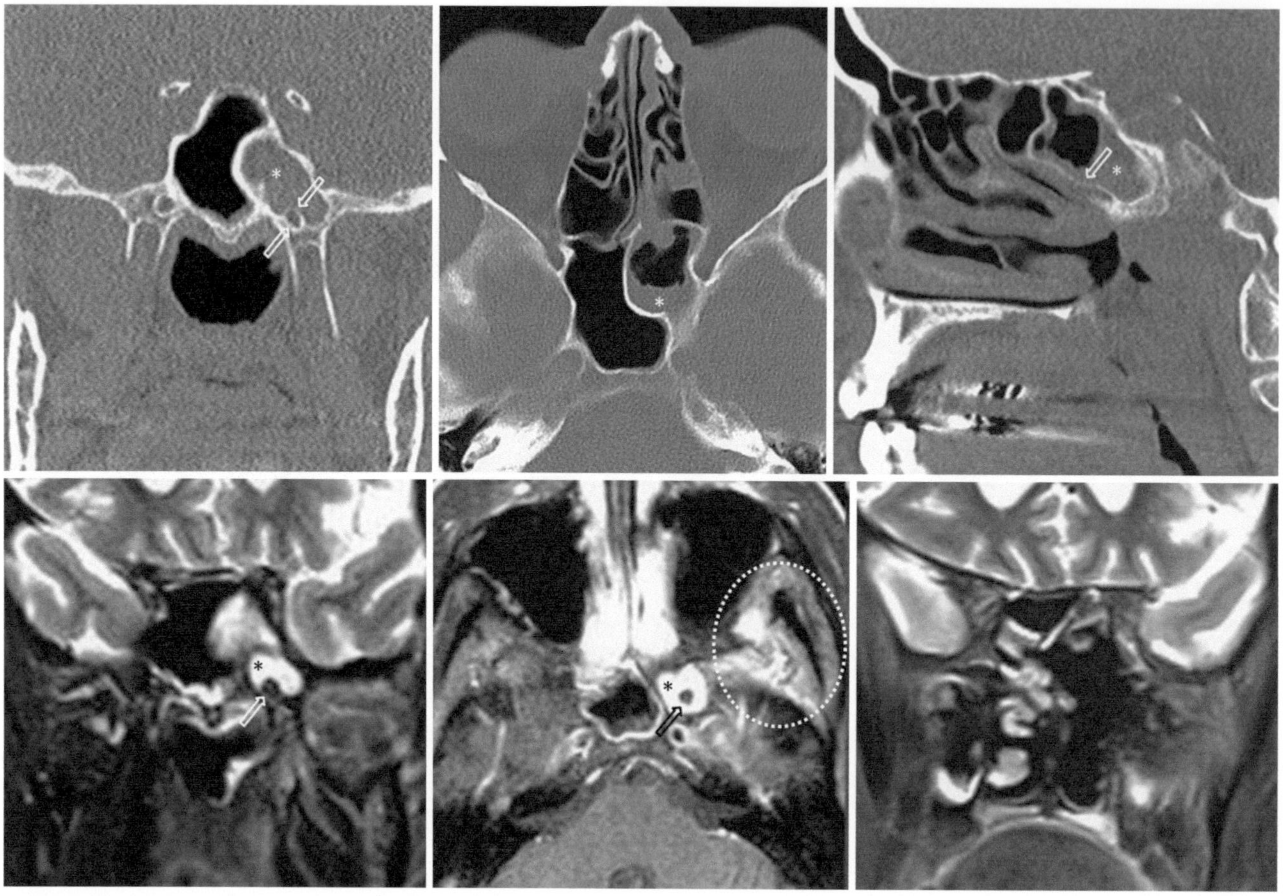

Fig. 2.35 Comparison case of vidian canal dehiscence from invasive fungal sinusitis. A 69-year-old female with type II diabetes had severe left orofacial pain-paresthesias with nasal discharge. **Top row:** 2-mm thickness coronal (*left*), axial (*middle*), and sagittal (*right*) CT reformats depict an obstructed left sphenoid locule with an air-fluid level (*asterisks*) and thinning of the left vidian canal's bony margin (*open arrows*), suggesting early bony dehiscence. **Bottom row:** A 1.5 T MRI coronal T2WI (*left*) also depicts the air-fluid level (*asterisks*) within the obstructed sinus surrounding the vidian canal (*open arrows*), while axial postcontrast T1WI (*middle*) shows that abnormal contrast enhancement extends into the left masticator space (*dotted circle*), representing extension of the infection. One week later, following surgical debridement, coronal T2WI (*right*) showed resolved sinusitis. A fungal culture was positive for Zygomycetes (i.e., mucormycosis). This case demonstrates that, while thinning of the bony wall of the vidian canal protruding into the sinus can be a normal variant, it can predispose to dehiscence with symptoms, and worsen with invasive sinusitis

2.4.2 Arrested Pneumatization of the Sphenoid Sinus

Arrested pneumatization is less recognized among radiologists and can sometimes cause significant confusion in differentiating pathologies that can occur in this region. It is known that the sphenoid bones undergo early fatty marrow conversion before normal pneumatization. However, in some individuals there can be a failure of normal pneumatization before the respiratory mucosa has fully extended into sites of early fatty marrow conversion; thus, the development in the sinus, whether focal or diffuse, persists as interspersed fatty marrow. The reason for this arrest is not understood. Such individuals are then left with persistent atypical fatty marrow adjacent to the aerated-pneumatized portion of the sinus, which persists into adulthood (Fig. 2.36). If unrecognized, arrested pneumatization may create diagnostic difficulties in the interpretation of skull base CT and MRI scans. It can be confused with several pathologies that affect this region, such as metastases, chordoma, chondrosarcoma, inspissated debris, or sinusitis.

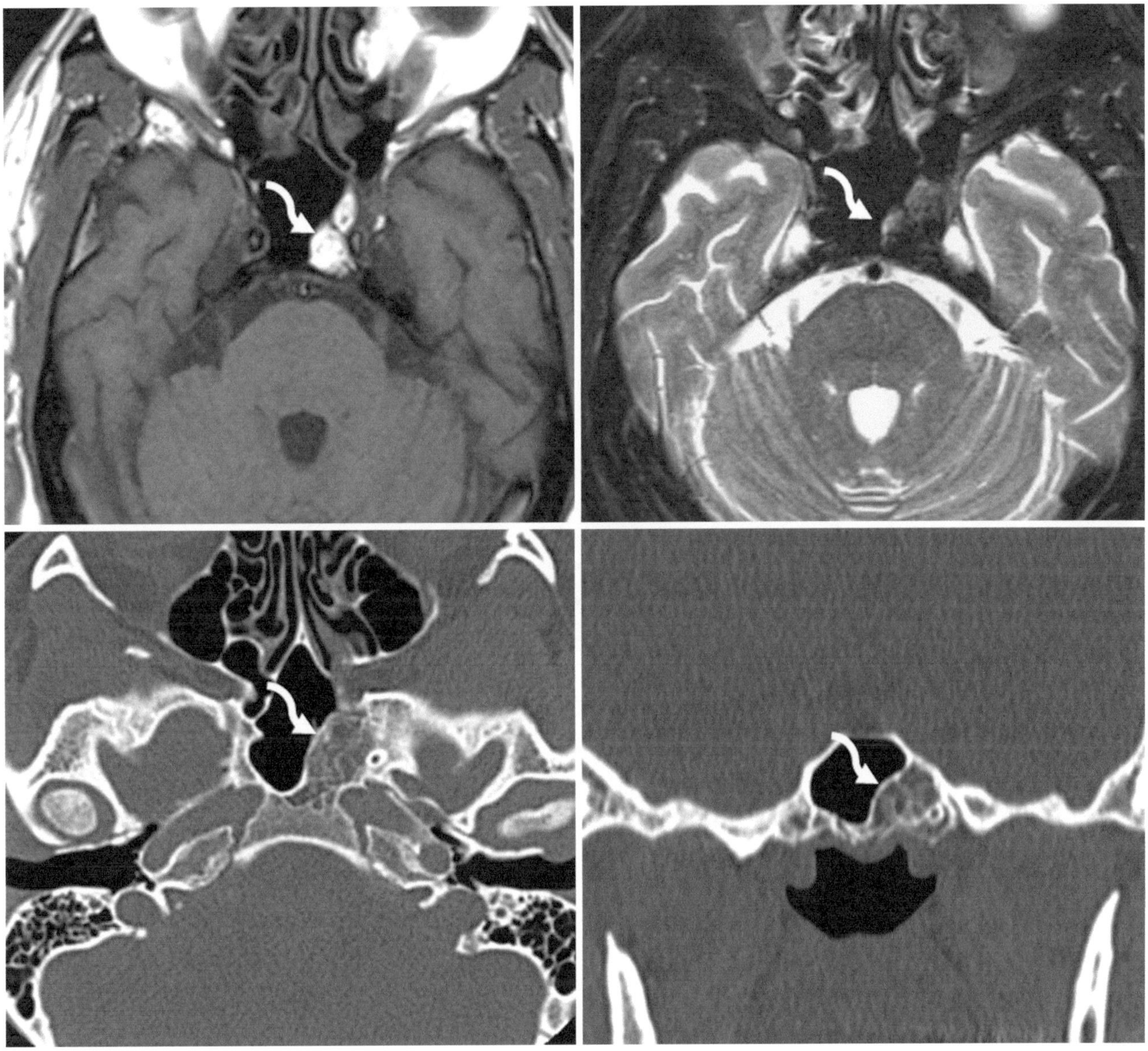

Fig. 2.36 Arrested sphenoid sinus pneumatization on CT and MRI in a 26-year-old male. **Top row:** On 1.5 T MRI, axial T1WI (*left*) demonstrates hyperintense fatty bone marrow (*curved arrows*) within the left aspect of the sphenoid sinus, which suppresses/darkens on fat-saturated T2WI (*right*). This was initially questioned by an outside radiologist to represent a sinus mass or hemorrhage within the sinus, but no fat-suppressed T1WI or postcontrast T1WI sequences had been obtained. **Bottow row**: Axial (*left*) and coronal (*right*) CT images demonstrate nonpneumatization of the left aspect of the sphenoid sinus with heterogeneously trabeculated bone and interspersed regions of fatty density (*curved arrows*). This finding and location are typical of arrested pneumatization of the sphenoid, a normal variation

2.5 Frontal Sinus

2.5.1 Frontal Sinus Aplasia and Hypoplasia

The frontal sinuses may develop from the anterior part of the nasal capsule, the frontal furrow, the anterior ethmoidal cells, or the frontal recess around the fourth fetal month. They may appear by the age of 1 year, and their growth continues after puberty, reaching their maximum volume at the age of 20 years. The volume of the frontal sinus is highly variable, ranging from a couple of cubic centimeters to 37 cm with an average of 10 cm^3. The phenomenon of frontal sinus aplasia occurs when no pneumatization happens in the frontal bone. This is typically unilateral but can be bilateral. The surgeon may need to be made aware of such variability in size of the frontal sinus or congenital dehiscence of the posterior wall on preoperative CT examinations if an external drainage procedure is planned (e.g., frontal sinus trephination) in order to prevent iatrogenic cerebral injury or the subsequent development of a cephalocele. The frequency of frontal sinus agenesis-aplasia varies (ranging from 1% to 5%) based on studies of different populations and cultures (Figs. 2.37, 2.38, 2.39, and 2.40).

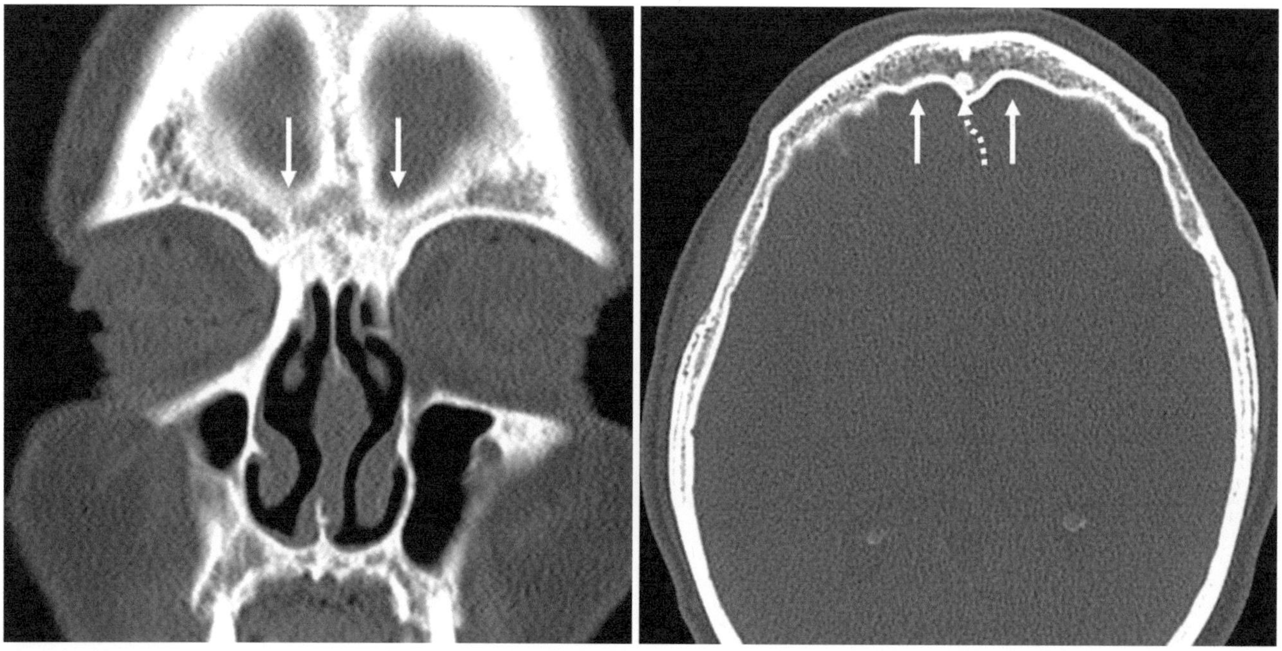

Fig. 2.37 Frontal sinus aplasia in a 46-year-old female with headaches and clinical suspicion of sinusitis. Coronal (*left*) and axial (*right*) 3-mm CT slices demonstrate congenital absence of frontal sinuses (*arrows*). Also, note an incidental bone island of the midline of the frontal bone on axial images (*curved dotted arrow, right*)

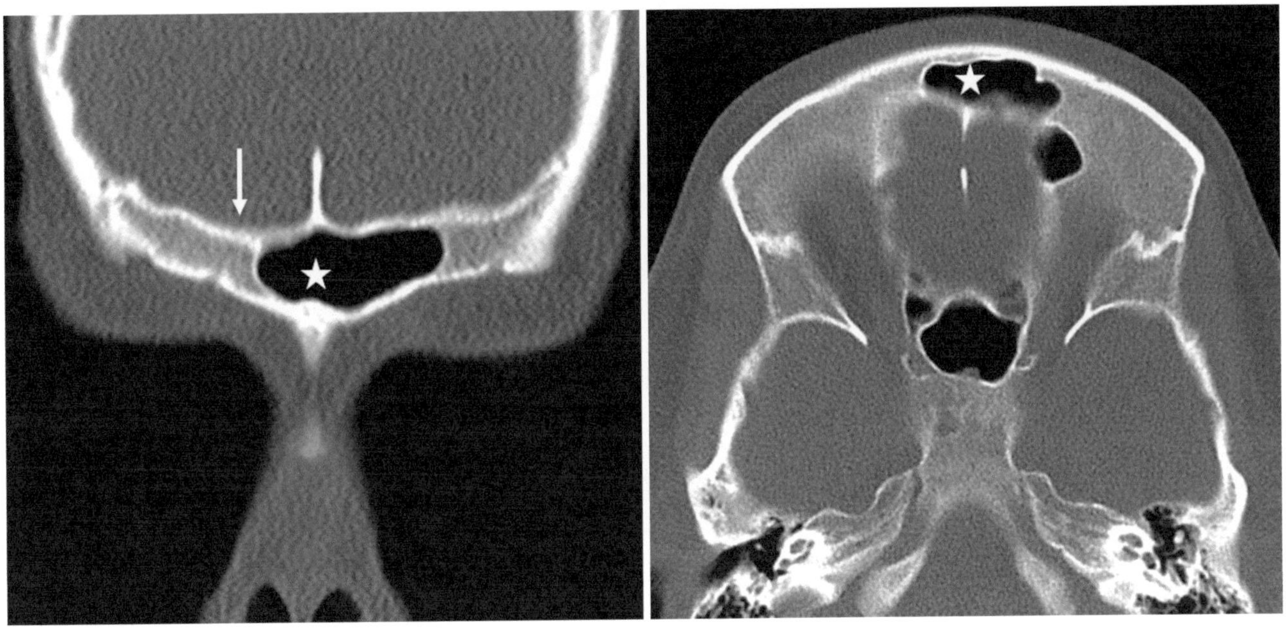

Fig. 2.38 Unilateral right frontal sinus aplasia in a 33-year-old male with headaches (negative CT). The right frontal sinus is hypoplastic (*arrow, left*) on coronal (*left*) and axial (*right*) 3-mm reconstructions. The more normal left frontal sinus (*stars*) partially extends across the midline to the right side, which is another normal variation

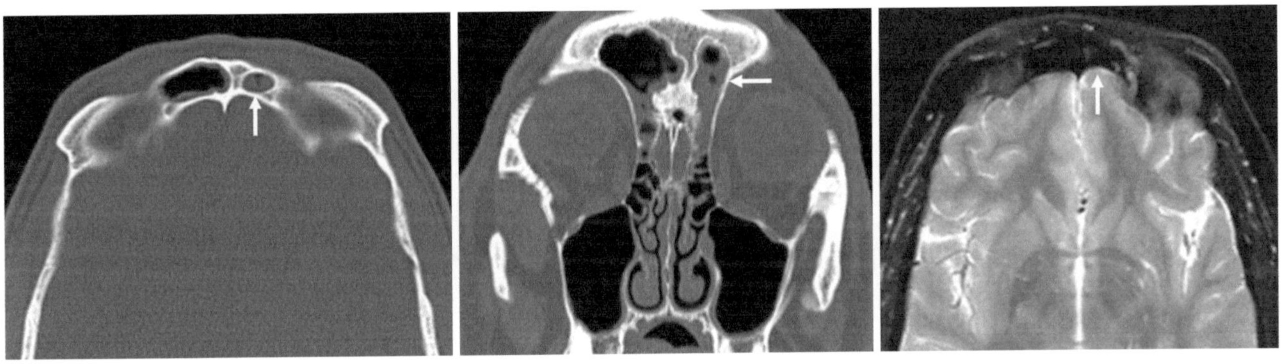

Fig. 2.39 Comparison case of hypoplastic frontal sinusitis. A 35-year-old male came to the Emergency Room with a severe left frontal headache ("worst headache of my life"). A sinus CT demonstrated mild to moderate left frontal sinus hypoplasia (*arrows*) on 2-mm thickness axial (*left*) and coronal (*middle*) reconstructions, with obstruction of the frontoethmoidal recess; notably, 5 years earlier a 1.5 T axial T2WI MRI was normal (*right*). The patient's symptoms markedly improved with urgent high intranasal-ethmoidal phenylephrine via a nasal endoscope. This case demonstrates how obstruction of a hypoplastic sinus can be quite symptomatic

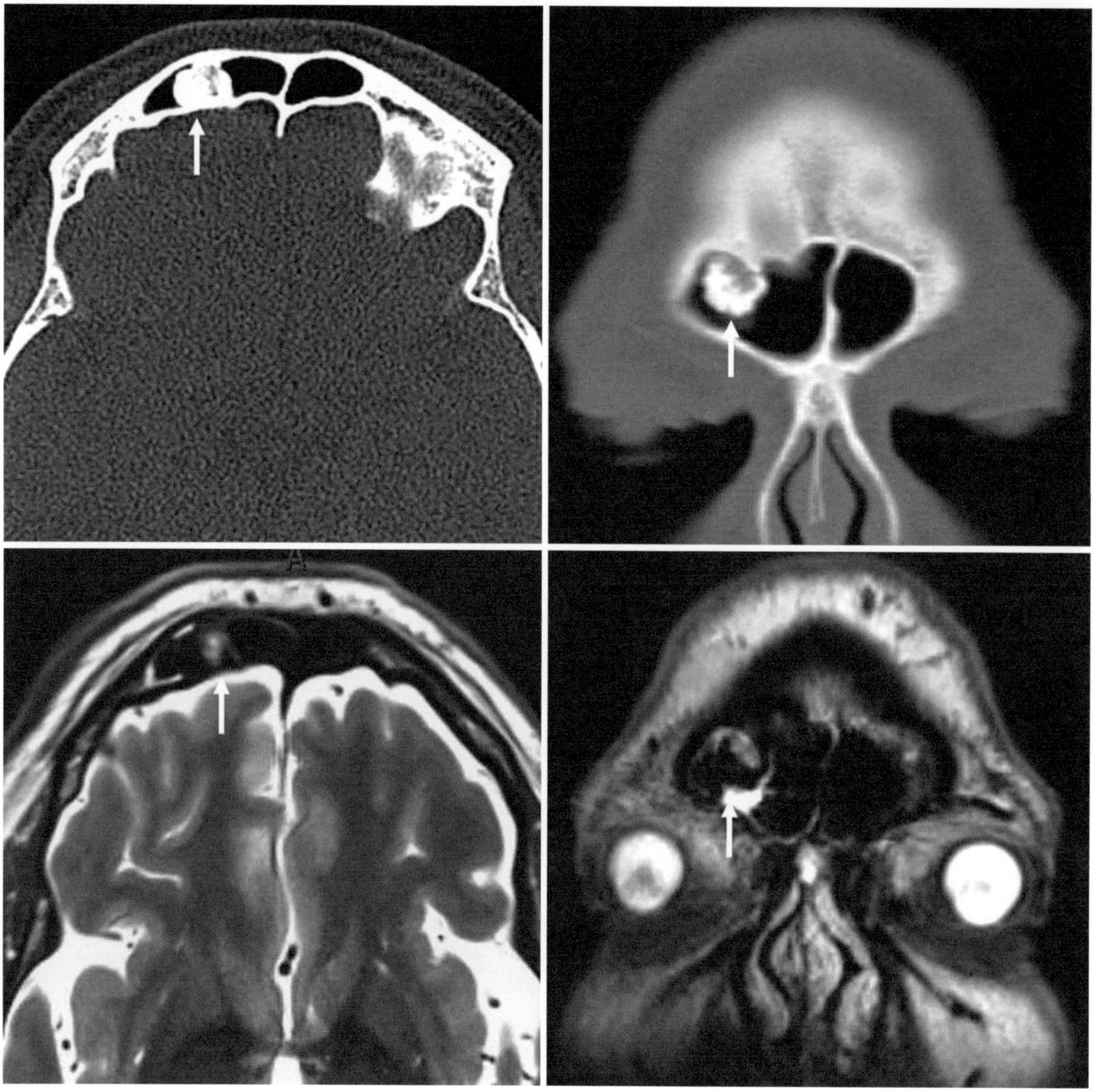

Fig. 2.40 Comparison case of a frontal osteoma filling most of a frontal sinus. In a 6-year-old male with Parkinson disease, a presurgical stereotactic CT with axial (*top left*) and coronal (*top right*) reconstructions as well as 1.5 T MRI axial (*bottom left*) and coronal (*bottom right*) T2WI demonstrate an incidental right frontal sinus osteoma (*arrows*)

2.5.2 Crista Galli Aeration-Pneumatization and Other Forms of Frontal Sinus Midline Extension

The crista galli is a midline, superior protrusion of the ethmoid bone, which is situated just above the cribriform plate. Intracranially, the anterior edge of the falx cerebri attaches to the posterosuperior tip of the crista. Occasionally, the crista can be aerated (pneumatized), as described in about 5–15% of the population. This variant (pneumatized crista galli) was initially (and traditionally) thought to represent extension from the ethmoid air cells based on the embryologic origin of the crista, but recent literature based on higher resolution and thin section (<1 mm) CT scans have demonstrated that such aerated cristae typically represent extensions from the frontal sinus or frontal-ethmoidal recesses. Additionally, sinus pneumatization has been shown to cross from one bone to another, which makes the concept of extension from the normally aerated frontal sinus seem plausible.

Thus, crista galli aeration-pneumatization (i.e. a form of frontal sinus extension) is a normal variation that is most commonly asymptomatic (Figs. 2.41, 2.42, and 2.43). However, the uncommon scenario arises when sinusitis and the resultant debris can involve the crista, and the debris can become inspissated owing to a difficult or tortuous drainage pathway. This is of import in recurrent sinusitis, in which the sinusitis-related debris within the crista persists despite therapy that has alleviated the frontal and ethmoidal sinusitis; occasionally, the sinusitis component within the crista necessitates direct surgical drainage. Also, a rare complication is

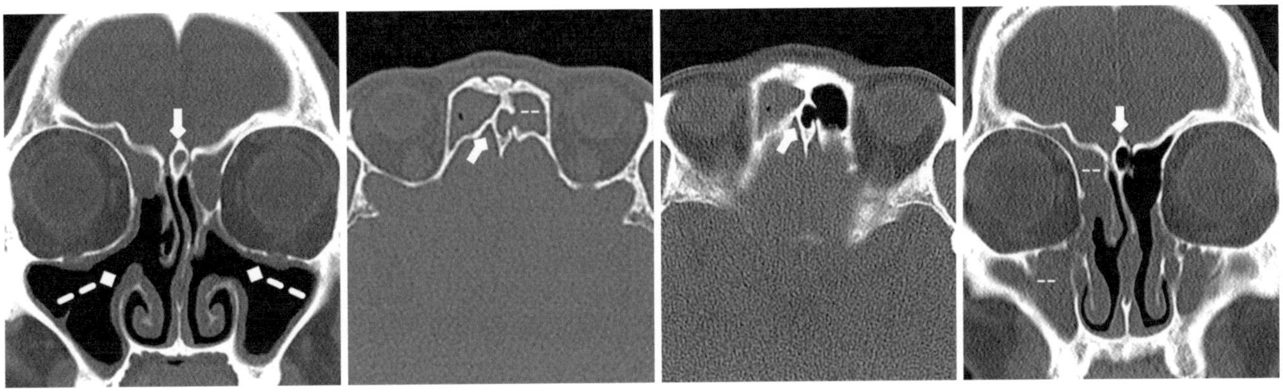

Fig. 2.41 In a 63-year-old male with a history of sinusitis, an aerated-pneumatized crista galli (*wide arrows*) is noted on coronal (*left*) and axial (*left middle*) 3-mm thickness CT images; the crista is filled with debris that is contiguous with left frontal sinusitis (--). The patient also has findings of a prior bilateral ethmoidectomy and medial antrostomies (*dashed diamond tip arrows*). One year later, on axial (*right middle*) and coronal (*right*) CT images, the pneumatized crista galli and left frontal sinus have cleared of debris, but the debris has worsened (--) within the right ethmoid and maxillary sinuses

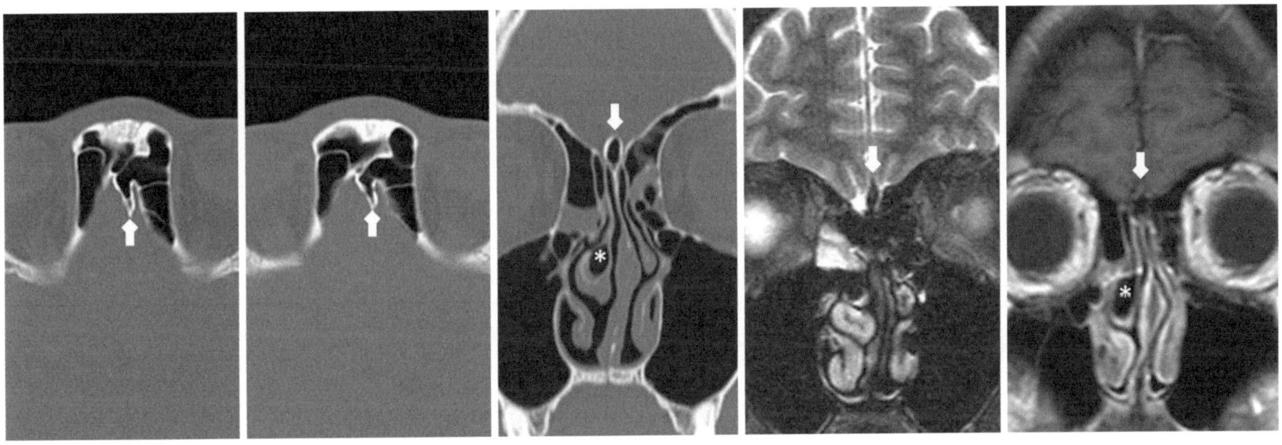

Fig. 2.42 A 35-year-old female with rhinitis had a pneumatized crista galli (*wide arrows*) on 2-mm thickness axial CT (*left, left middle*), coronal CT (*middle*), and on 1.5 T coronal T2WI (*right middle*) and post-contrast T1WI MRI (*right*). Note an incidental variant pneumatized right middle turbinate (concha bullosa) as well (*asterisks, middle and right*)

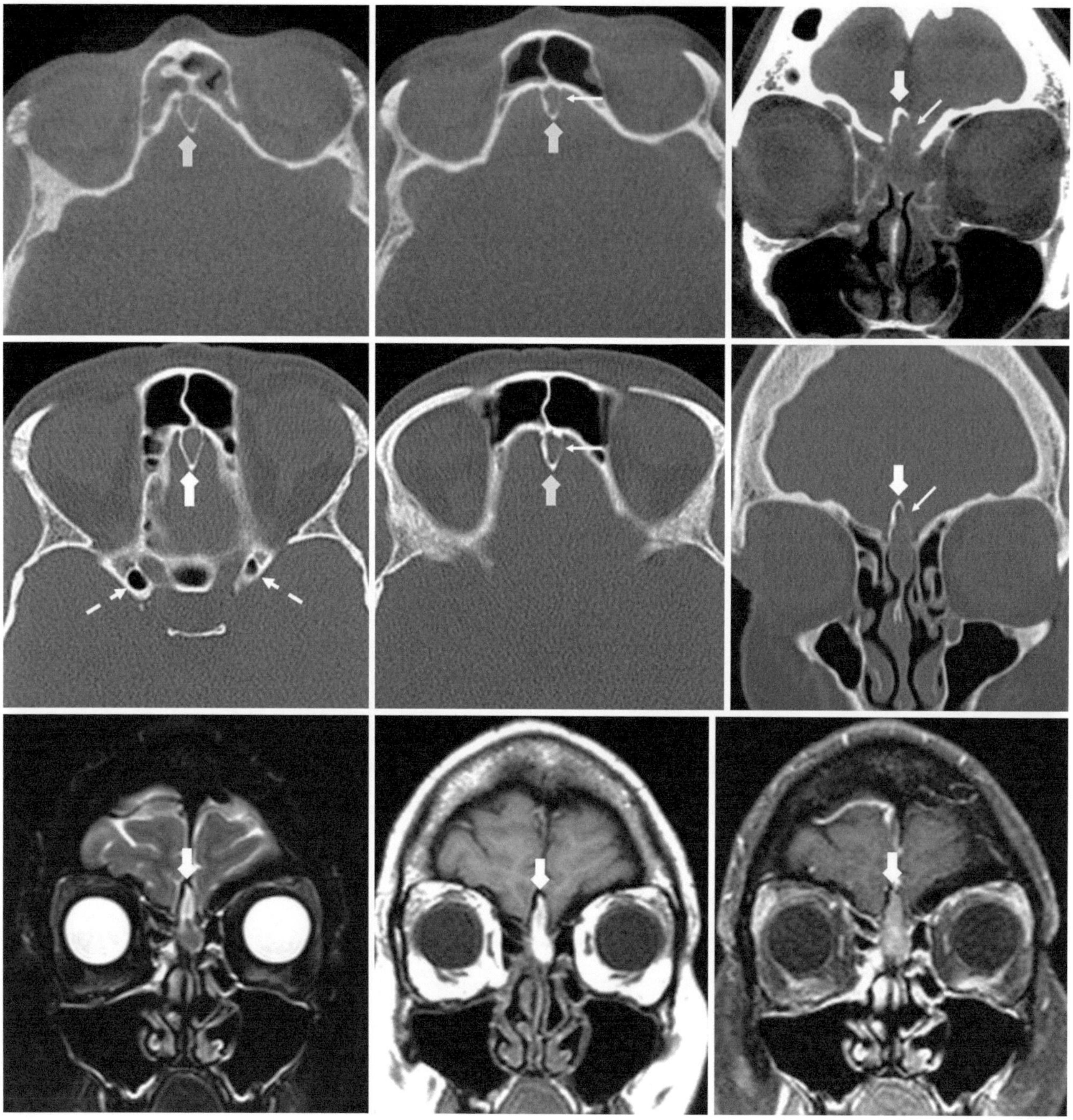

Fig. 2.43 A 54-year-old female with chronic ethmoidal sinusitis extending into a normal pneumatized crista galli. **Top row:** On a CT from an outside institution, an aerated crista galli (*wide arrows*) is filled with debris and is contiguous with the fronto-ethmoidal recesses of the ethmoid and frontal sinuses that also contain debris, as shown on axial (*left, middle*) and coronal (*right*) thicker section (5-mm) images. Note that the left side of the crista appears dehiscent (*thin arrows*). Incidentally, there were also prior maxillary sinus medial antrostomies bilaterally. **Middle row:** One month later, following medical therapy and partial ethmoidectomies bilaterally, the debris within the frontal and ethmoid sinuses improved, while the debris within the crista (*wide arrows*) remained. Thinner section (0.6 mm) axial (*left, middle*) and coronal (*right*) reformats depict that there is actually minimal remaining bone on the left side of the crista (*thin arrows, right*); thus, it is not entirely eroded. Also, note pneumatized anterior clinoid processes (*dashed arrows, left*), another normal variation. **Bottom row:** A 1.5 T MRI soon after demonstrates the T2- and T1- hyperintense inspissated debris within the crista galli (*wide arrows*) on coronal T2WI (*left*) and noncontrast T1WI (*middle*). On fat-suppressed postcontrast T1WI (*right*), the debris within the nearly dehiscent crista does not appear to enhance, and there is no evidence of intracranial dural invasion (i.e., no dural enhancement), confirming that the bony margin of the crista is likely still viable, although barely

either (1) dural extension from the crista causing intracranial infection (meningitis) due to dehiscence of the bony margin of the crista, whether from direct extension of the sinusitis or (2) caused by iatrogenic complication following surgical drainage of the crista (which can alternatively result in a CFS leak).

Another variation is that there are many forms of frontal sinus midline extension that do not involve pneumatization of the crista galli. These have been termed by Som et al. (2008) as "intersinus septal air cells" and as "extramural frontal sinus cells," which typically are extensions of pneumatization from the frontal recess that evaginate toward the midline (Figs. 2.44, 2.45, 2.46, 2.47, 2.48, and 2.49). This phenomenon has been described in about 30% of the population and has alternatively been colloquially termed a "frontal wishbone." The hypothesis is that rudimentary ethmoid air cells situated anteriorly can potentially form into or become incorporated into the frontal sinus. Again, the phenomenon of an intersinus septal cell representing an extension from or incorporation by the frontal sinus likely contradicts the traditional hypothesis that such midline extensions of pneumatization relate to ethmoid cell variation in aeration-pneumatization.

Crista galli deviation is yet another variant, which is likely of no clinical significance other than that it may simulate a traumatic fracture.

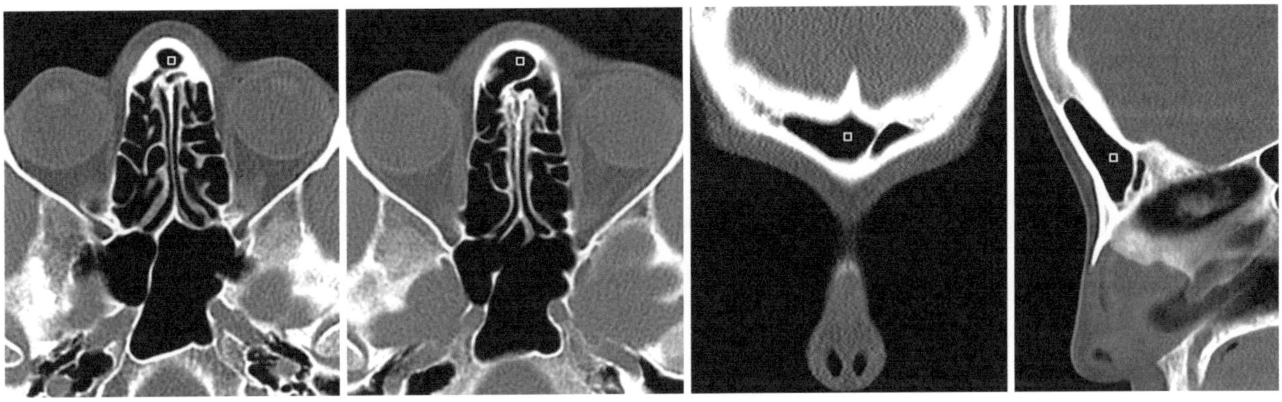

Fig. 2.44 A 34-year-old female with a history of facial pain had a negative CT, but a prominent intersinus septal air cell (□) is demonstrated on axial (*left images*), coronal (*right middle*), and sagittal (*right*) 2-mm CT reconstructions. This extramural air cell represents midline extension of the right frontal sinus

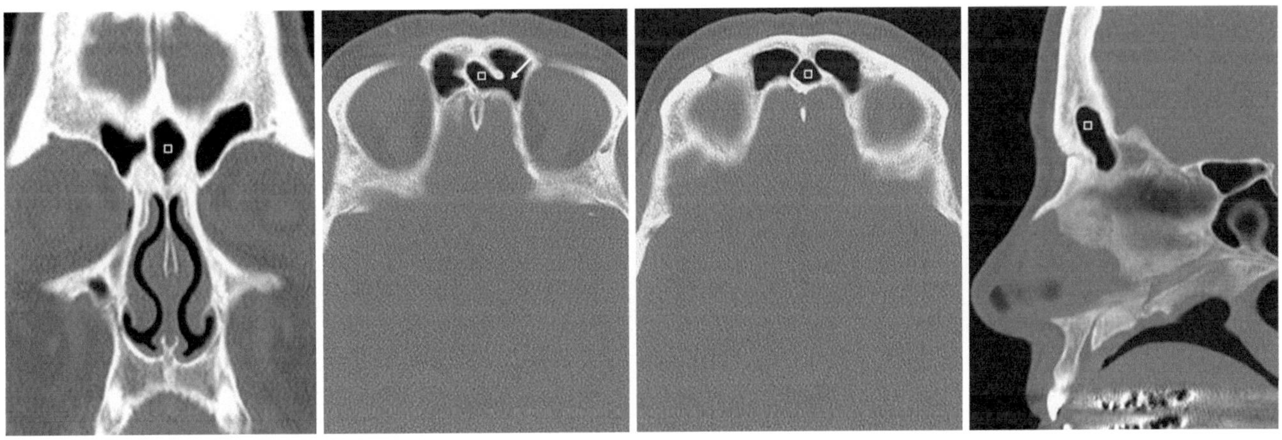

Fig. 2.45 A 60-year-old female with a history of palatal cancer (*not shown*) had an incidental midline interseptal sinus (□), as depicted on coronal (*left*), axial (*middle images*), and sagittal (*right*) 2-mm reconstructions from a facial bone CT. Note the small hole (*thin arrow, left middle*) that denotes the site of communication with the left frontal sinus

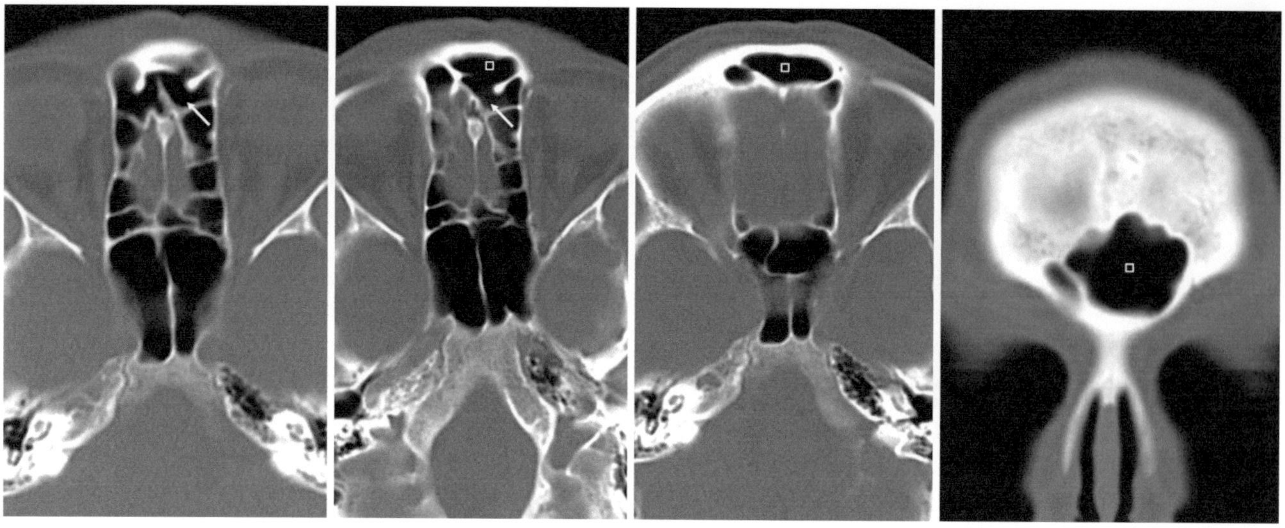

Fig. 2.46 A 62-year-old male with a headache and weakness had a negative head CT (5-mm thickness). Axial (*leftmost three images*) and coronal (*right*) reconstructions demonstrate midline frontal extension to an interseptal sinus (□), which had a small site of communication (*thin arrows, left and left middle*) with the left frontoethmoidal recess

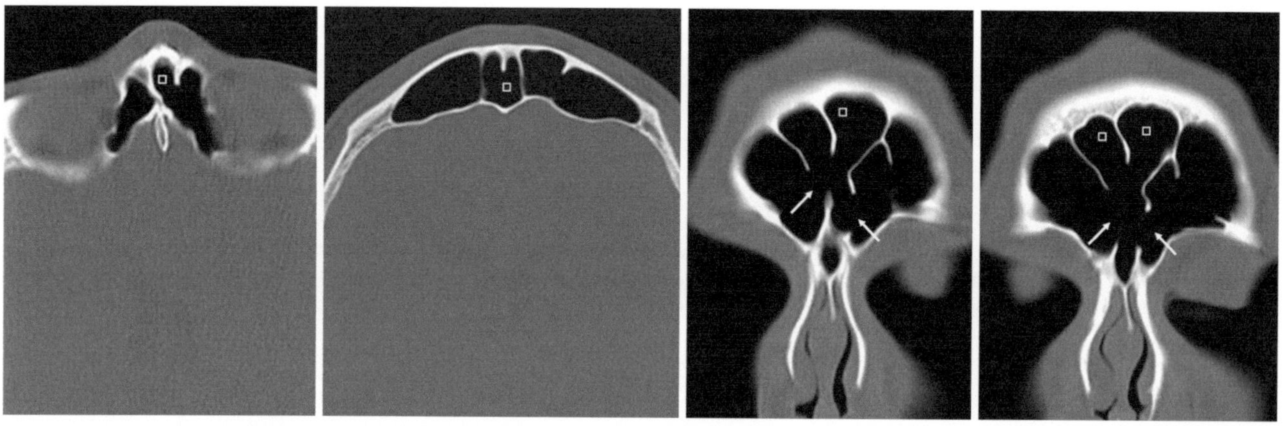

Fig. 2.47 An 18-year-old male with a remote history of sinusitis (although a negative CT) had hyperpneumatization of the sinuses diffusely. An incidental interseptal sinus (□) is shown on axial (*left images*) and on coronal (*right images*) 3-mm reconstructions of a sinus CT. This interseptal sinus appears to communicate (*thin arrows*) with the frontal sinuses bilaterally

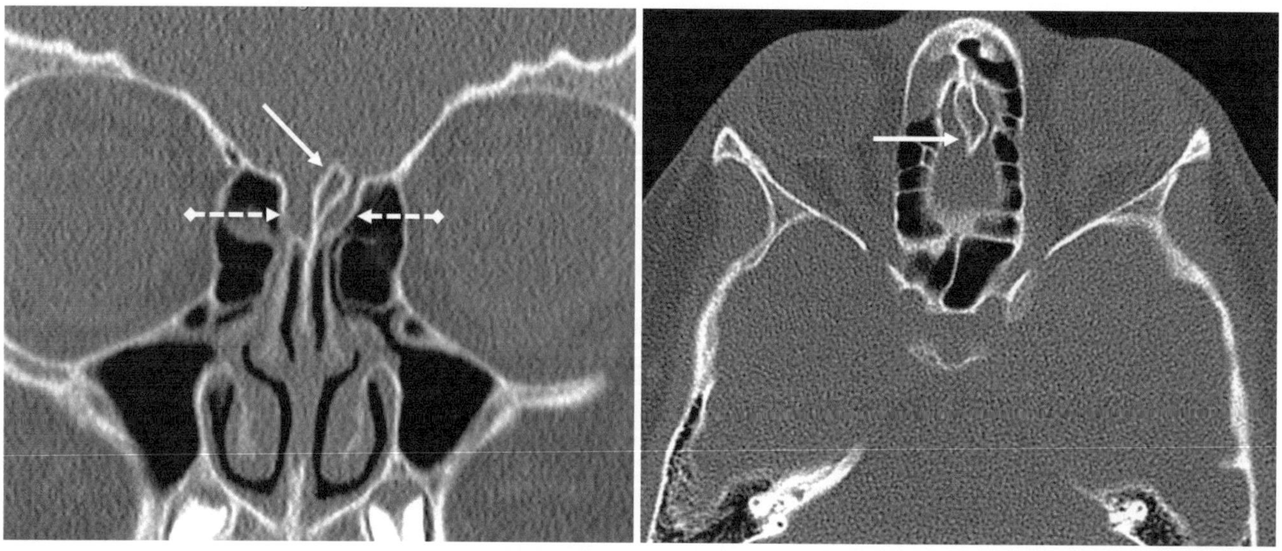

Fig. 2.48 An 8-year-old boy after a motor vehicle accident. Coronal and axial thin section (3-mm) images demonstrate incidental leftward deviation of the crista galli (*long arrows*). Also, note asymmetry of the olfactory sulci (*dashed arrows*), with the left side being narrower and slightly higher than the right; these are other normal variations that are of doubtful clinical significance

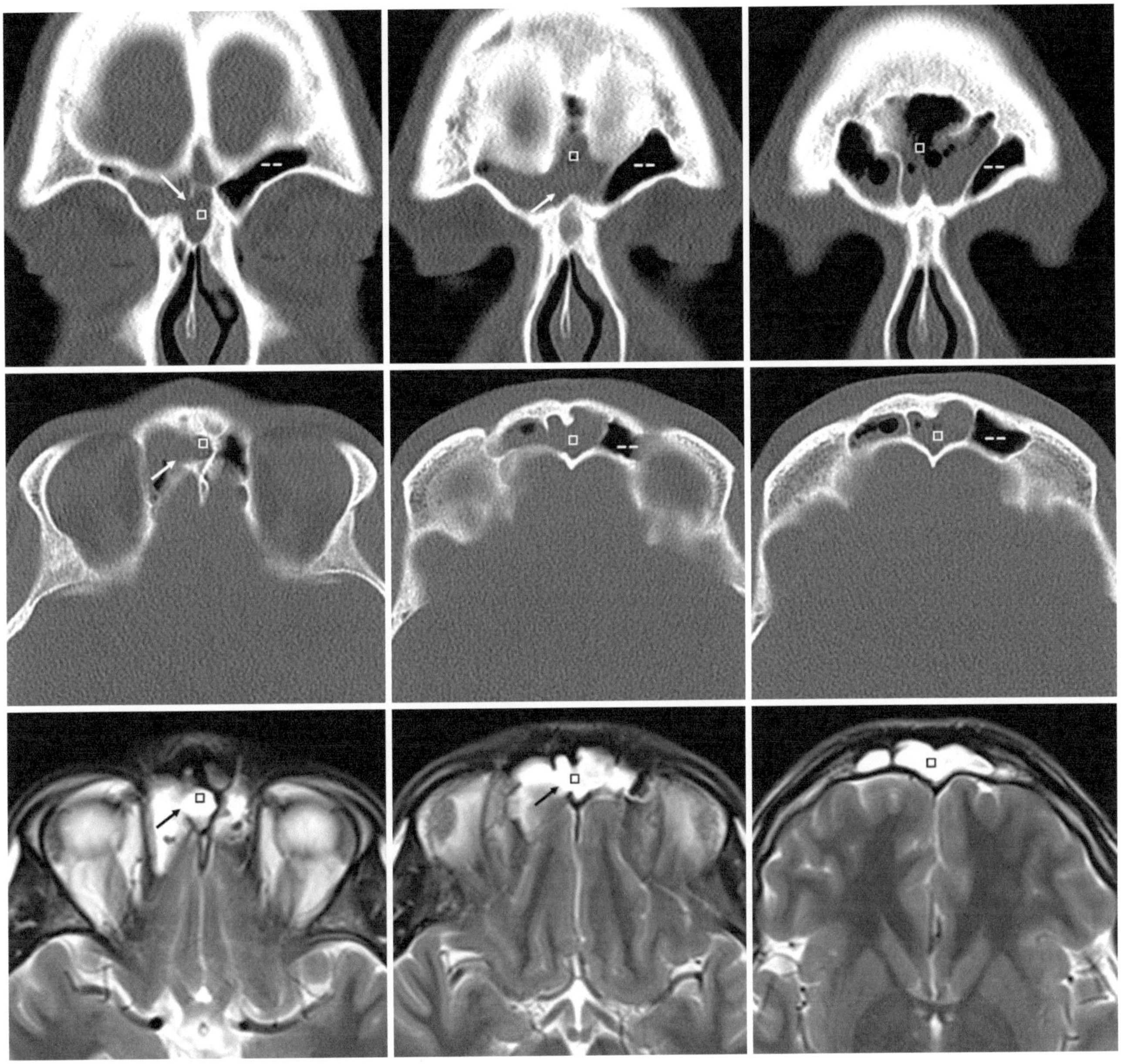

Fig. 2.49 Comparison case of recurrent sinusitis involving an interseptal sinus. A 20-year-old male with a history of recurrent sinusitis. **Top row:** 3-mm thickness serial coronal CT images demonstrate that the right frontal sinus extends toward the midline into an interseptal sinus (□) via a tract of communication (*thin arrows*), with sinusitis-related debris in both regions. The left frontal sinus (--) is relatively clear, probably confirming that it does not communicate with the interseptal sinus. **Middle row:** Axial 3-mm thickness CT images confirm such findings of the interseptal sinus. **Bottom row:** 1.5 T Axial T2WI MR images 3 months later similarly depict the interseptal sinus (□) and the tract of communication (*thin arrows*) from the right frontal sinus; however, the left frontal sinus is now also involved by debris from worsening bilateral frontal sinusitis

2.6 Ethmoidal Air Cells

2.6.1 Agger Nasi Cell, Haller Cell, Bulla Ethmoidalis, and Suprabulbar Recess

The ethmoid sinus can have a variable number of air cells. Additionally, the ethmoid sinuses are divided into groups of cells by bony basal lamellae. The most important one is the basal lamellae of the middle turbinate, which separates the ethmoid into anterior and posterior groups with different drainage patterns.

Agger nasi cells are the most anterior ethmoidal air cells, lying anterolateral and inferior to the frontoethmoidal recess and anterior and above the attachment of the middle turbinate. They are located within the lacrimal bone and therefore have as lateral relations with the orbit the following structures: the lacrimal sac and the nasolacrimal duct. They are seen in up to 93% of the population. Although some studies suggest that agger nasi cells may play a role in chronic frontal sinusitis, there is insufficient evidence to support this theory (Figs. 2.50 and 2.51).

Haller cells are the ethmoidal air cells extending along the floor of the orbits, lateral to the sagittal plane of the lamina papyracea. These are also called infraorbital ethmoidal air cells or maxilloethmoidal cells and have been reported in up to 45% of patients. These cells may narrow the maxillary sinus ostium, and thus the ostiomeatul unit (OMU) may become infected or inflamed, with the potential for extension into the orbit. Iatrogenic orbital injury may occur if this variant remains unrecognized prior to endoscopic sinus surgery (Figs. 2.52, 2.53, and 2.54).

The largest anterior ethmoidal cell is the bulla ethmoidalis, which is a key surgical landmark during endoscopic sinus surgery. It is of variable size and is underdeveloped in approximately 8% of the population. An underdeveloped bulla ethmoidalis may also predispose to inadvertent iatrogenic orbital injury. The suprabullar recess lies between the superior wall of the bulla ethmoidalis and the roof of the ethmoid sinus. This recess can extend laterally as supraorbital cells, which may be of consequence since large supraorbital cells can displace the bony canal or anterior ethmoidal artery posteriorly, thus potentially being mistaken for frontal sinus cells on imaging or during surgery.

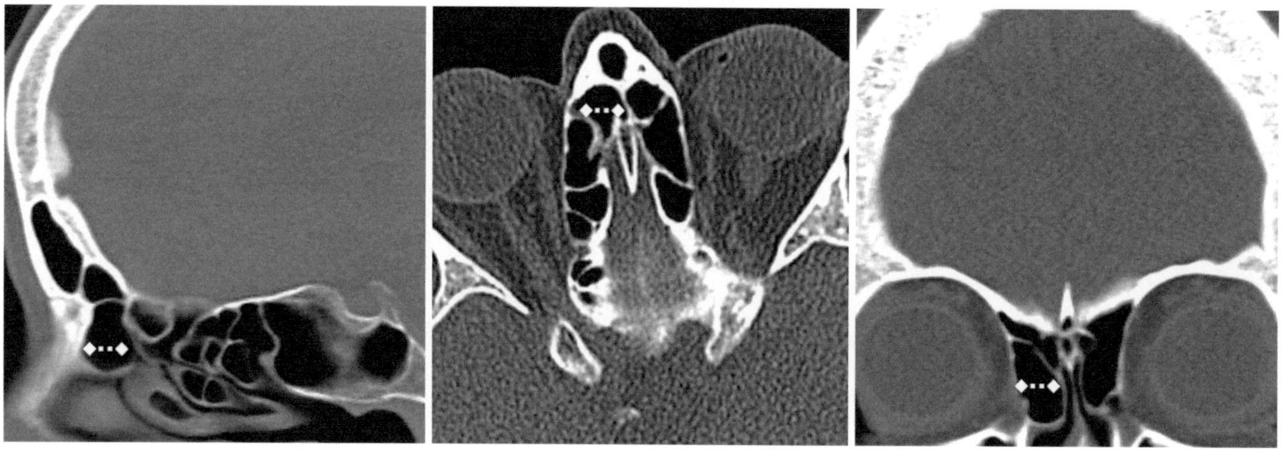

Fig. 2.50 Sagittal (*left*), axial (*middle*), and coronal (*right*) 1-mm reconstructed stereotactic CT images obtained prior to deep brain stimulator placement in a 65-year-old male with a history of Parkinson disease demonstrate incidental agger nasi cells on the right (*dotted arrows*)

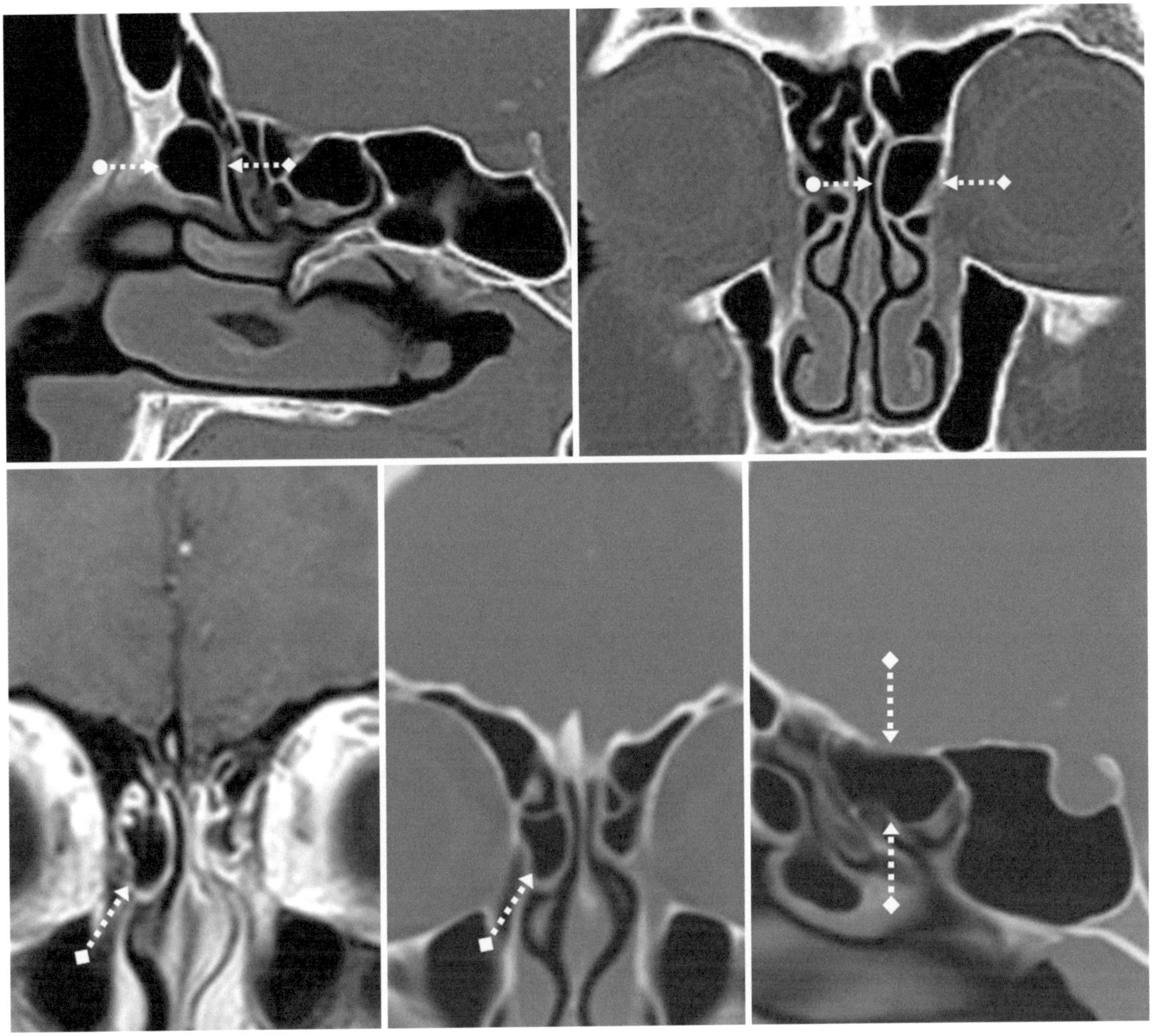

Fig. 2.51 Prominent agger nasi cells in two patients. **Top row:** a 24-year-old female with headache underwent paranasal sinus CT. Sagittal (*left*) and coronal (*right*) images show an incidental agger nasi cell on the left side (*dotted arrows*). **Bottom row:** a 23-year-old female suspected to have a stroke (negative MRI) had an incidental normally prominent agger nasi cell on the right side (*dotted arrows*) on postcontrast coronal SET1WI MRI at 1.5 T (*left*), and confirmed on coronal (*middle*) and sagittal (*right*) reformats from the CTA; note how normally enhancing sinus mucosa can cause a normal agger nasi cell to stand out on the postcontrast T1WI MRI, as in this patient

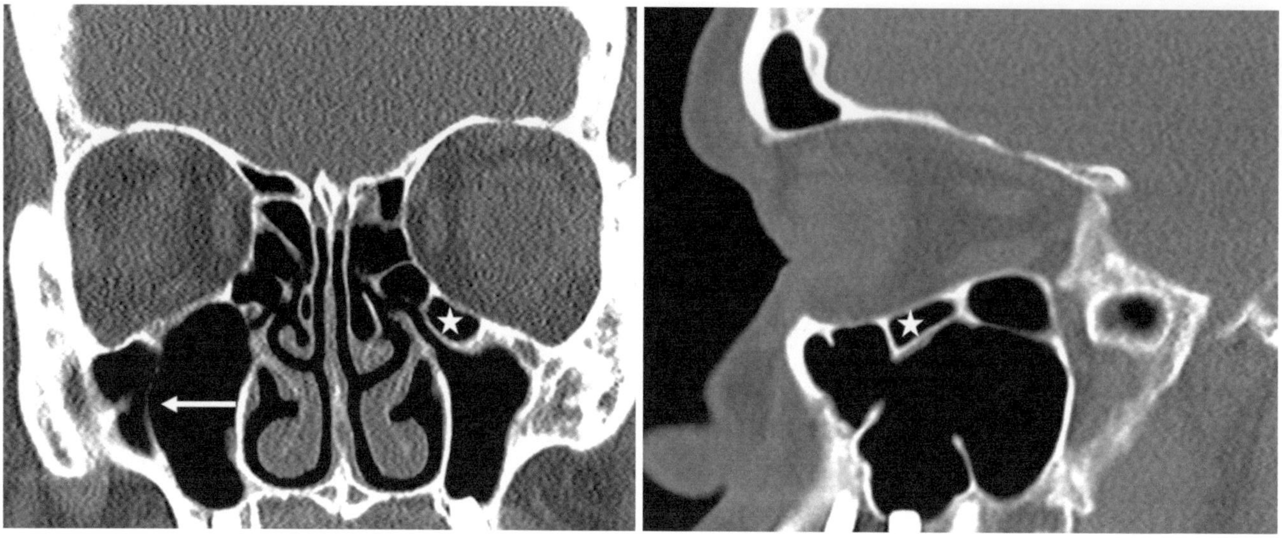

Fig. 2.52 A 23-year-old male patient with facial trauma was scanned to evaluate for facial fractures (negative examination). Thin-section (2-mm) coronal (*left*) and sagittal (*right*) CT images demonstrate an incidental Haller cell on the left (*star*), which is also known as an infraorbital ethmoidal air cell. Also noted is an incidental normal variant septum of the right maxillary sinus (*arrow, left*)

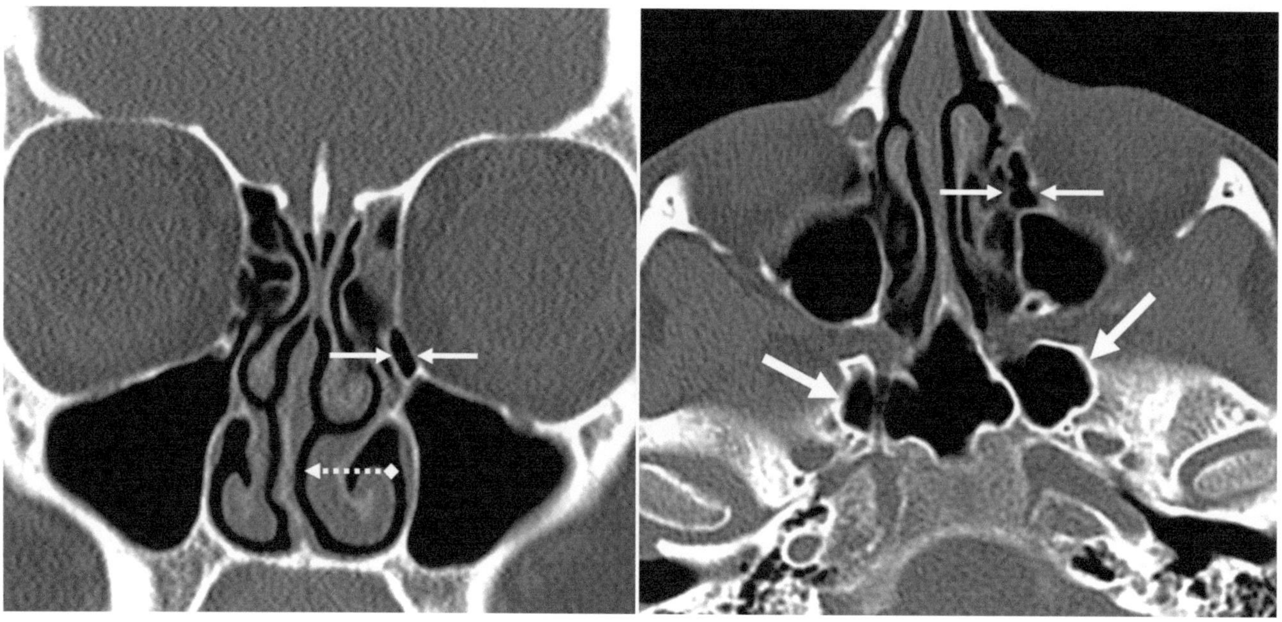

Fig. 2.53 Coronal (*left*), and axial (*right*) CT images of a 40-year-old female who underwent a maxillofacial CT for headaches (negative examination). There is a small Haller cell on the left (*thin arrows*). Also, note other normal variants, including mild rightward deviation of the nasal septum on the coronal image (*dotted arrow, left*) and pneumatization (*thick arrows*) of both pterygoid processes (lateral pneumatization) of the sphenoid bone on the axial image (*right*)

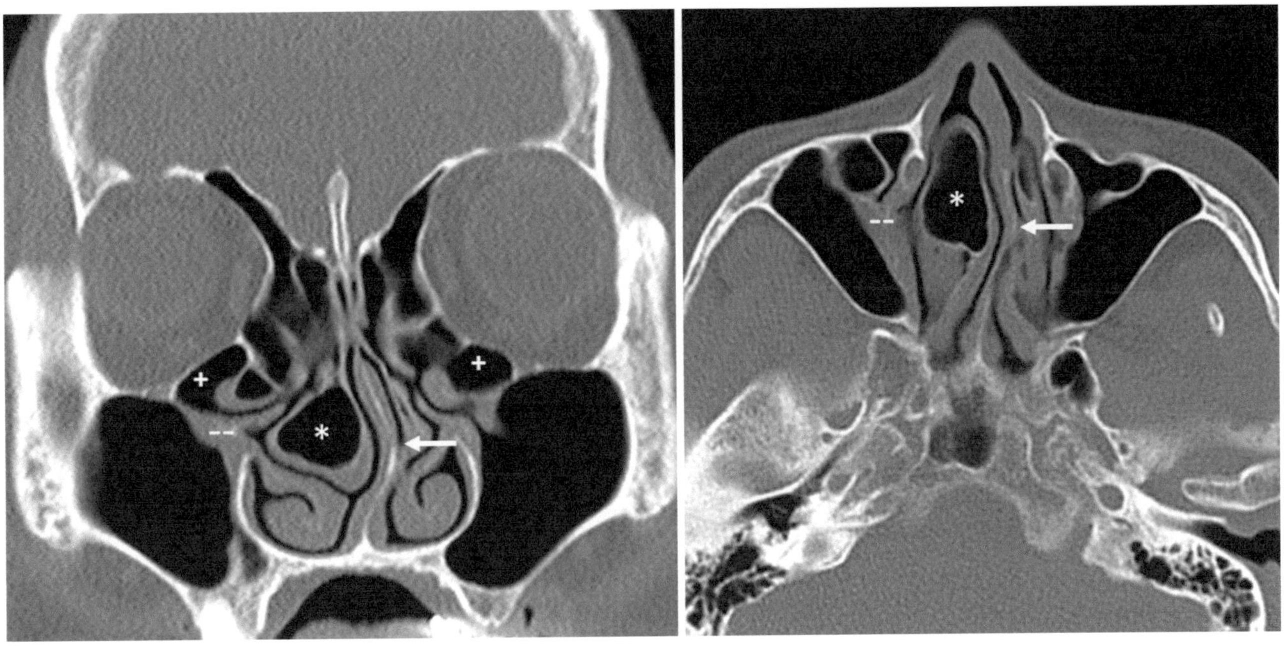

Fig. 2.54 Comparison case of enlarged Haller cells and concha bullosa (CB) enlargement, contributing to maxillary sinus ostium obstruction and nasal septal deviation. On coronal (*left*) and axial (*right*) 2-mm CT reformats, a 59-year-old female with right-sided sinus pain had obstruction of the right maxillary sinus outflow at the ostium caused by focal debris/mucosal thickening (--), likely from a combination of a prominent Haller cell (+) and an enlarged CB (*asterisks*). The large CB also caused leftward nasal septal deviation (*arrows*). Also note a small left-sided Haller cell (+)

2.7 Nasal Cavity

2.7.1 Concha Bullosa and Pneumatized Uncinate Process

Conchae bullosa (pneumatized middle nasal turbinate) is one of the most common sinonasal variants, being described in approximately 22–60% of the population (the upper range being related to the "partial pneumatization" subtypes), but it is typically incidental and usually of no clinical consequence. However, it can be associated with nasal septal deviation and can rarely be of clinical importance when the conchae bullosa and/or nasal septum together contribute to nasal airway and/or osteomeatal unit (OMU) obstruction (Figs. 2.55 and 2.56).

Pneumatization of the uncinate process of the maxilla is a less common variation. This has recently been described in up to 1–10% of the population. This is typically unilateral but is less commonly bilateral. This is of clinical import in the situation where occlusion of a pneumatized uncinate by debris can lead to obstruction of the OMU, whether caused by inflammation or infection from sinusitis, thereby causing swelling and potentially even an enlarging mucocele.

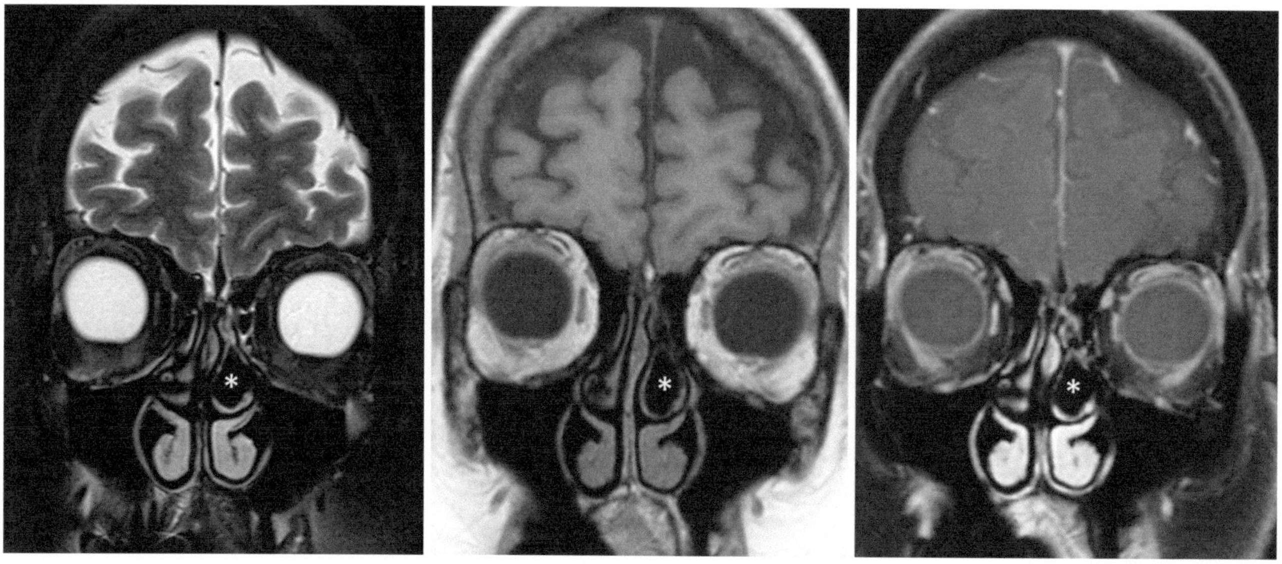

Fig. 2.55 A 47-year-old patient with visual loss. Coronal fat-saturated T2W (*left*), T1W (*middle*) and postcontrast fat-suppressed T1W images (*right*) demonstrate a unilateral concha bullosa (*asterisks*) on the left side

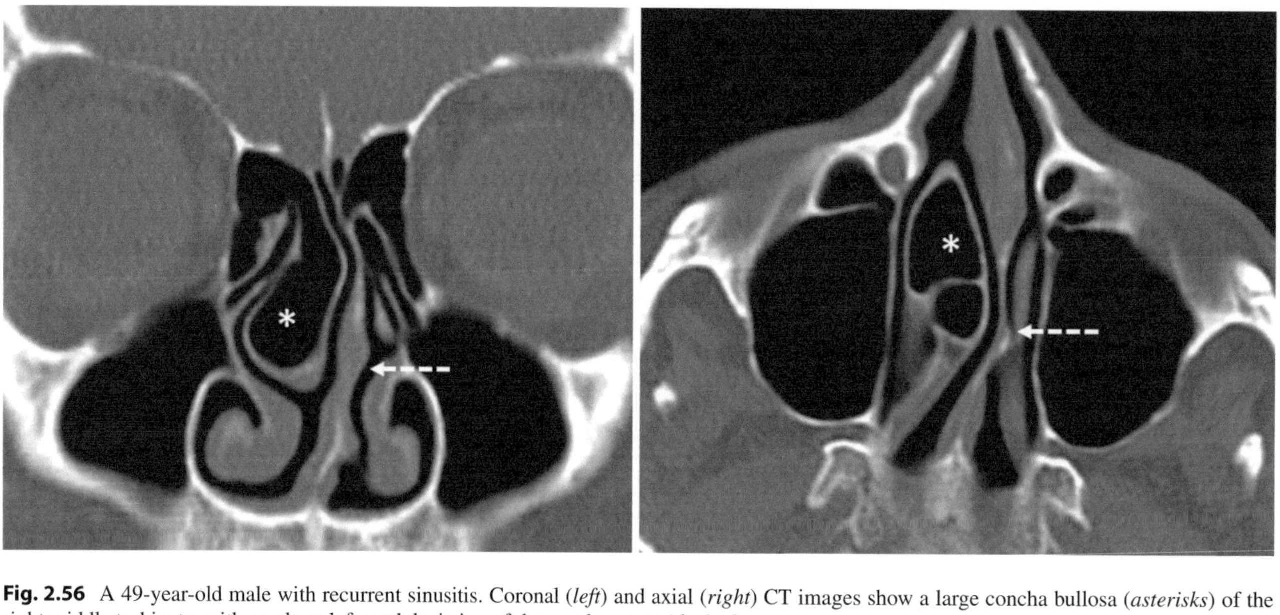

Fig. 2.56 A 49-year-old male with recurrent sinusitis. Coronal (*left*) and axial (*right*) CT images show a large concha bullosa (*asterisks*) of the right middle turbinate, with resultant leftward deviation of the nasal septum (*dashed arrow*)

2.7.2 Paradoxical Middle Turbinate and Turbinate Sinus

Paradoxical curvature of the middle turbinate is a common variation of doubtful clinical importance. This variant is estimated to occur in 10% to 16% of the population based on larger studies that implement dedicated multiplanar sinus CT techniques. It essentially consists of the middle turbinate curving in the opposite direction of the inferior turbinate. Normally, the convexity of the middle turbinate bone is directed medially toward the nasal septum. When paradoxically curved, the convexity is directed laterally, toward the lateral sinus wall. It has been theorized to be a possible cause for mucosal pathologies because of its convexity pointing toward the middle meatus, although there has not been much evidence of a significant association with any disease state to support such a relationship to sinonasal pathology (Figs. 2.57, 2.58, and 2.59).

A turbinate sinus is a reported deep invagination produced by acute curving of the inferior portion of the middle turbinate on itself. It is not commonly known and is likely of no clinical significance, so this variant is not depicted herein.

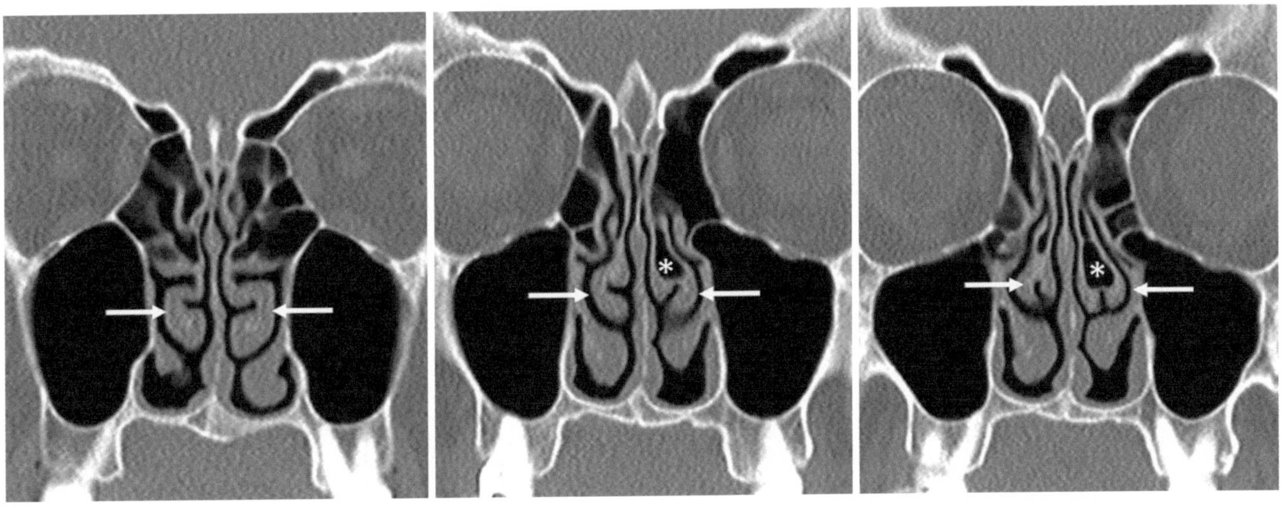

Fig. 2.57 Sequential coronal thin section CT images demonstrate bilateral paradoxical middle turbinates (*arrows*) as well as a normal variant concha bullosa (*asterisks*) of the left middle turbinate

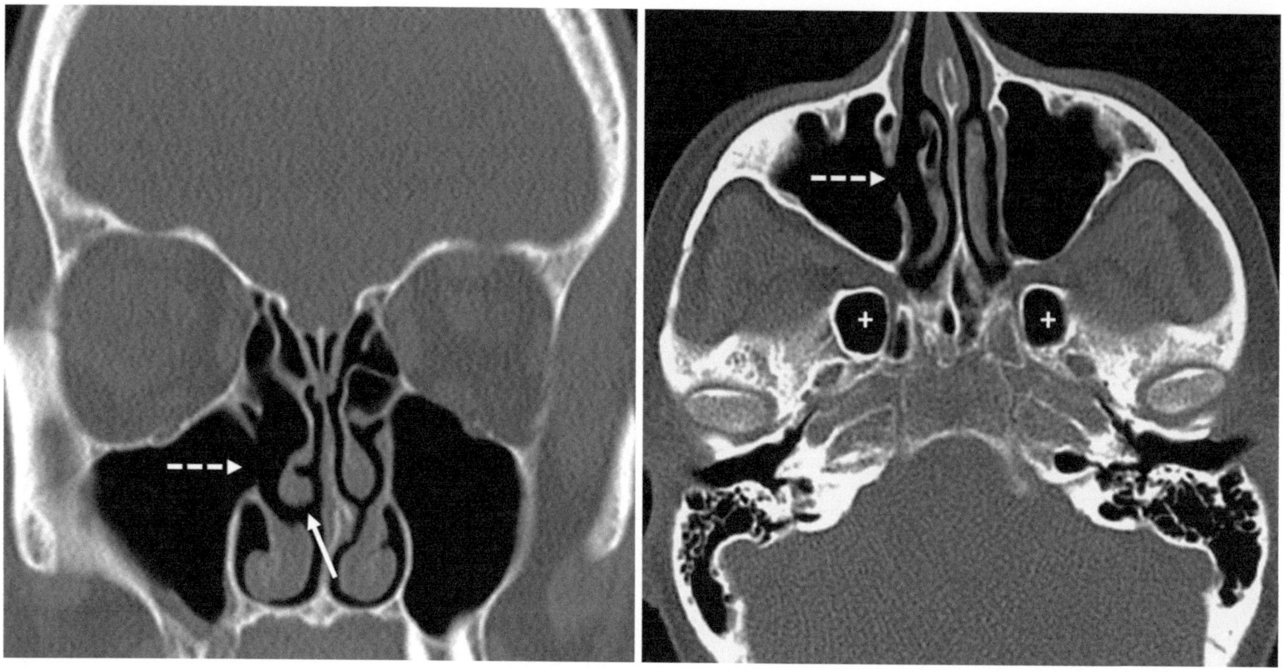

Fig. 2.58 A 35-year-old female with a history of functional endoscopic sinus surgery (FESS). Coronal (*left*) and axial (*right*) thin-section images demonstrate a paradoxical right middle turbinate (*arrow*) and a surgically created right maxillary antrostomy defect (*dotted arrows*). There is also normal bilateral pneumatization of the pterygoid processes of the sphenoid (+)

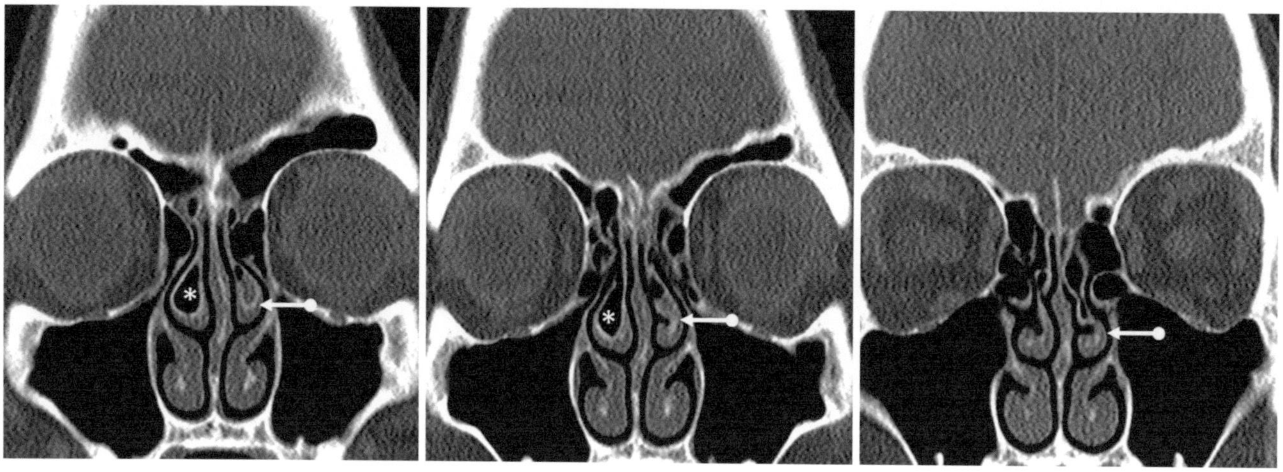

Fig. 2.59 Sequential coronal CT images of a 66-year-old male post–facial trauma show a paradoxical left middle turbinate (*arrows*), with a concha bullosa (*asterisks*) of the right middle turbinate

2.7.3 Nasal Septal Deviation, Septal Spur, and Septal Pneumatization

The nasal septum consists of an anterior cartilaginous and a posterior bony component. The bony septum is comprised of the vomer and the perpendicular plate of the ethmoid. Nasal septal deviation is a common variation that occurs to varying degrees and has been described variably and to differing degrees in up to 82% of the population. Based on multiplanar CT scans of a combination of sinus and head CT examinations, it has been demonstrated that the degree or presence of a septal deviation scan does not correlate with the patient's presence, absence, or severity of symptoms of nasal obstruction. Thus, it is usually an incidental "don't touch" finding.

The septum is commonly deviated in its inferior portion near the chondrovomeral junction and can also assume an S-shaped configuration with an undulating deviation to both sides of the midline. Nasal septal deviations may have various surgical implications: for example, gross septal deviations can displace the middle turbinate and interfere with surgical access to the middle meatus and may need to be addressed to improve surgical exposure. Septal spurs may be present and are typically associated with the presence of septal deviations; these spurs can occasionally form adhesions to the adjacent nasal turbinates.

Septal pneumatization is a variant that may occur anteriorly from the crista galli or posteriorly from the sphenoid sinus. Posterior septal pneumatization may occasionally narrow the sphenoethmoidal recess, which can impede drainage of inflammatory debris or can hinder surgical access to the sphenoid sinus ostium (Figs. 2.60, 2.61, 2.62, 2.63, and 2.64).

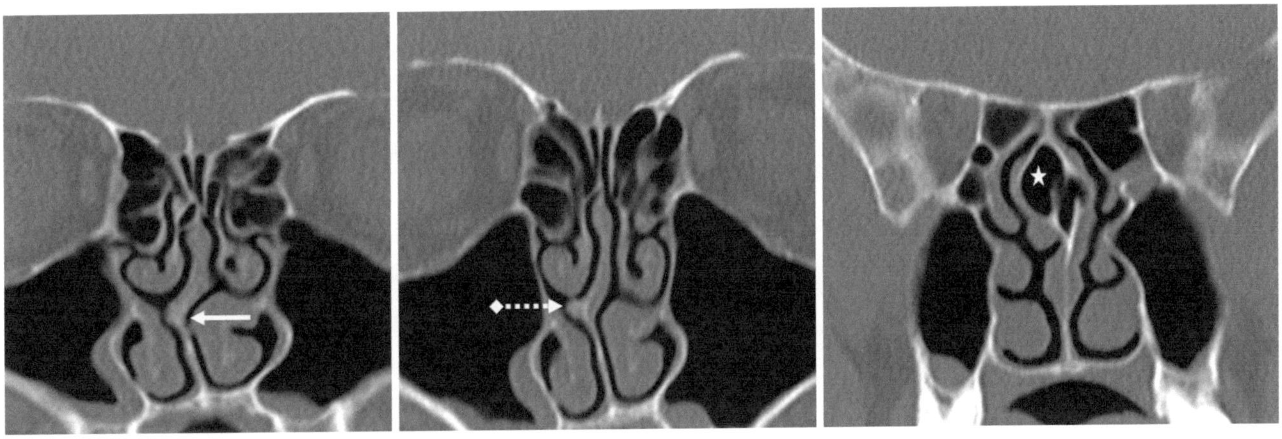

Fig. 2.60 Sequential coronal CT images of a 56-year-old female with orbital swelling. Incidentally noted nasal septal variations include nasal septal deviation to the right (*arrow, left*), septal spur (*dotted arrow, middle*), and septal pneumatization (*star, right*)

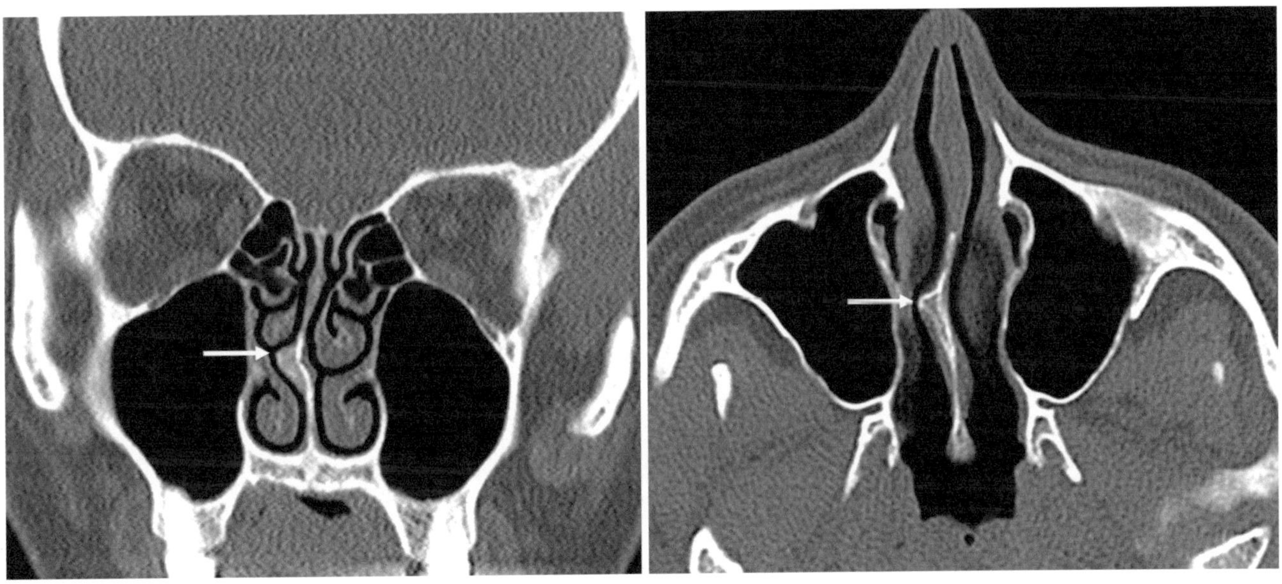

Fig. 2.61 A 55-year-old female with difficulty breathing. Coronal (*left*) and axial (*right*) 3-mm maxillofacial CT images demonstrate a variant nasal septal spur (*arrows*)

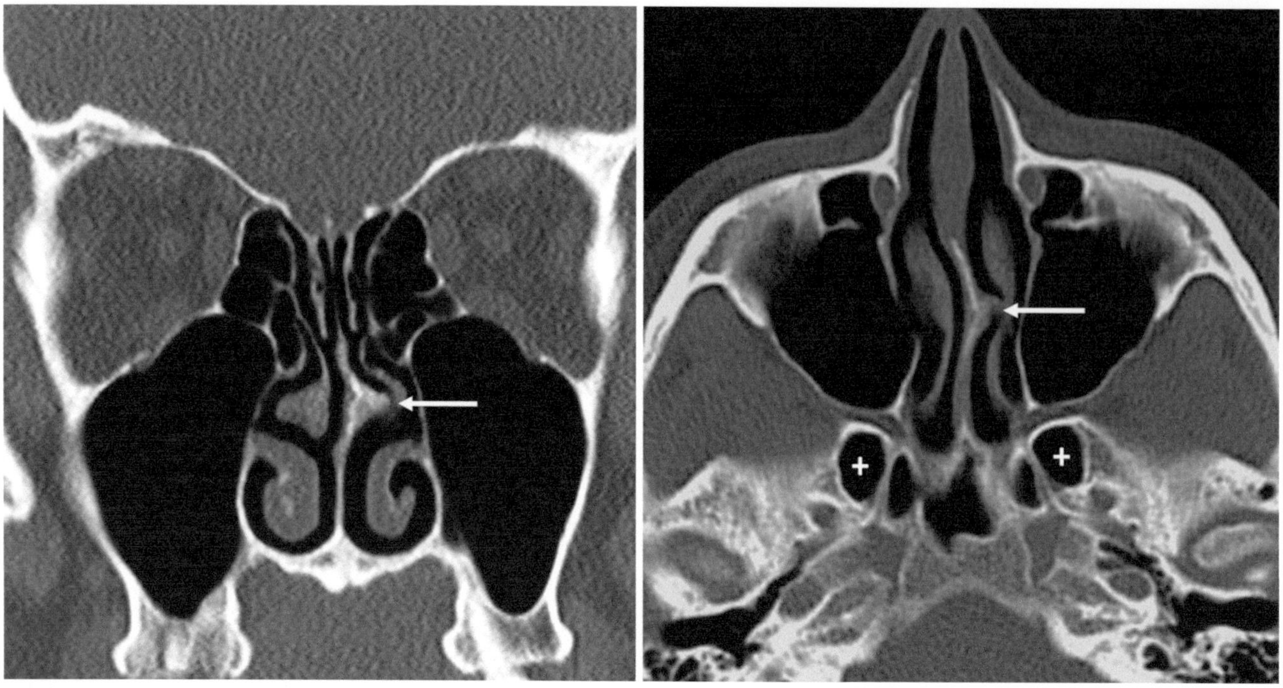

Fig. 2.62 Coronal (*right*) and axial (*left*) CT images of a 44-year-old male with a history of orbital trauma demonstrate a nasal septal spur (*arrows*). Also note normal pneumatization of the pterygoid wings of the sphenoid (+, *right*)

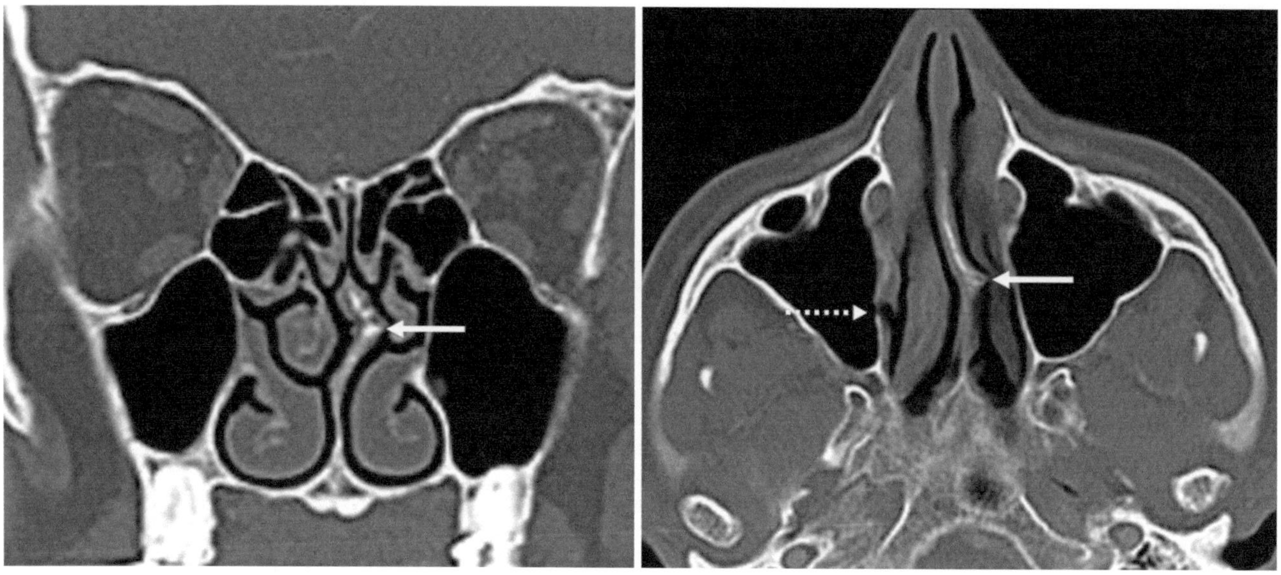

Fig. 2.63 A 28-year-old male with a history of tonsillar cancer underwent a neck CT. Coronal (*left*) and axial (*right*) reconstructions demonstrate incidental leftward deviation of the nasal septum, with a small septal spur (*arrows*). Also, note a tiny normal variant accessory maxillary sinus ostia on the right (*dotted arrow, right*)

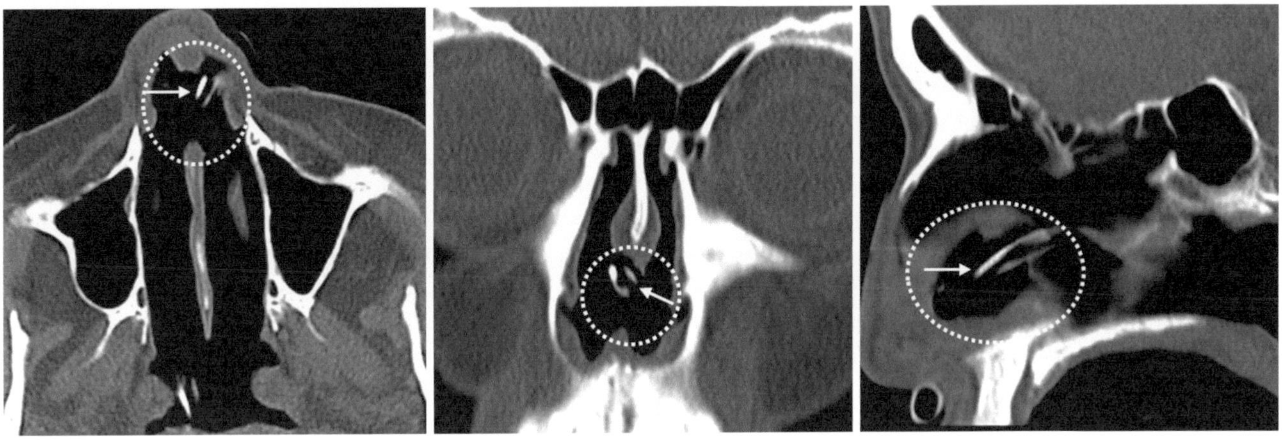

Fig. 2.64 Comparison case of a remote nasal septal perforation from an unknown cause. In a 75-year-old female post–motor vehicle accident, axial (*left*), coronal (*middle*), and sagittal (*right*) images show a large nasal septal defect (*outlined by dotted circle*). Note a nasogastric tube passing through the defect (*thin arrows*). Such remote defects have many possible causes

2.8 Anterior Skull Base

2.8.1 Lateral Lamellar Dehiscence and Asymmetry of the Olfactory Fossae

The olfactory fossa is formed by the crista galli medially, the medial lamella of the cribriform plate inferiorly, and the lateral lamella of the cribriform plate laterally. It contains the olfactory bulbs and olfactory tracts. The lateral lamella of the cribriform plate is structurally the thinnest bone in the anterior skull base and is dehiscent (or nearly dehiscent, based on CT) in up to 14% of patients. This is a relatively common variant, whose clinical significance is that there is a greater risk of intraoperative injury and iatrogenic CSF leak in this region or perhaps following trauma, especially in the case of congenital lateral lamellar dehiscence.

Another variation is that the depth of the olfactory fossa and the angle between the medial and lateral lamellae of the cribriform plate are not always symmetrical. Asymmetry of the olfactory fossa occurs in up to 10–30% of the population. This is usually of no clinical consequence but can be important in neurosurgical practice, as the complication of inadvertent/iatrogenic intracranial penetration is more common on the side where the olfactory fossa is lower and where the angle between the medial and lateral lamellae of the cribriform plate is greater (Figs. 2.65 and 2.66).

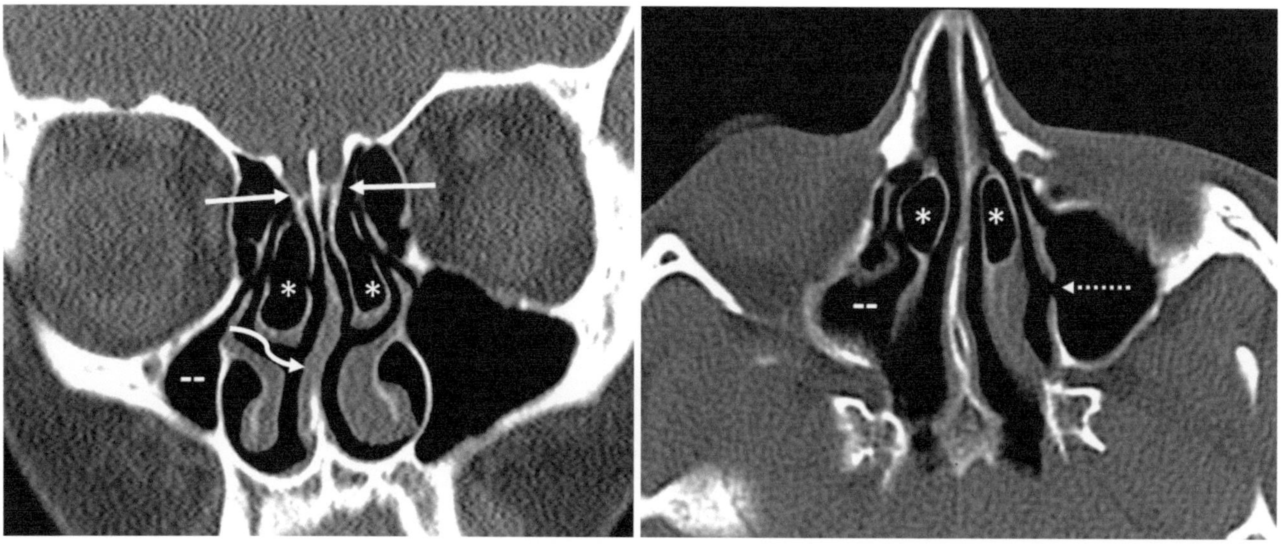

Fig. 2.65 Asymmetry of olfactory fossae with multiple other sinonasal variants. In a 44-year-old male with headaches, a 3-mm thickness paranasal sinus CT shows asymmetry of the olfactory sulci (*white arrows*), with the right being lower than the left on a coronal image (*left*). The angle between the lateral and medial lamellae of the cribriform plate is wider on the right side as well. There are also other normal variants, including: bilateral concha bullosae (*asterisks*), a hypoplastic right maxillary sinus (--), and mild rightward deviation of the nasal septum (*curved arrow, left*). On an axial CT image (*right*), note an accessory left maxillary ostium as well (*dotted arrow*)

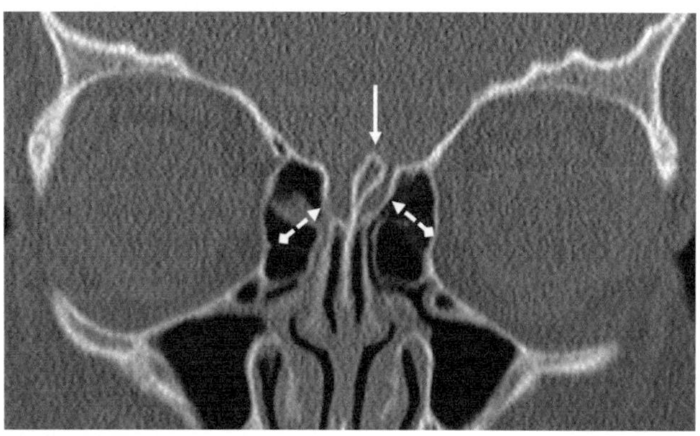

Fig. 2.66 An 8-year-old boy immediately following a motor vehicle accident (*from same patient as* Fig. 2.48). A 3-mm coronal reconstruction of a facial bone CT demonstrates normal leftward deviation of the crista galli (*arrow*) without evidence of fracture and no history of prior trauma. The olfactory fossae (*dashed arrows*) are asymmetric, with a narrower left side

2.8.2 The Nasal Cycle

The mucosal lining over the nasal septum and the nasal turbinates is influenced by the nasal cycle, which is responsible for alternating changes in the turbinate sizes caused by mucosal engorgement. This cyclic and physiologic enlargement of the turbinates is a normal variation that may alternate between both nasal cavities as frequently as every 45–60 min (while at least as often as once per 7–8 h) and thus should not be mistaken for a pathologic condition. In clinical practice, the radiologist may notice that the size or degree of swelling of the turbinates can change from side to side between follow-up and repeat examinations, even when performed on the same day (Fig. 2.67).

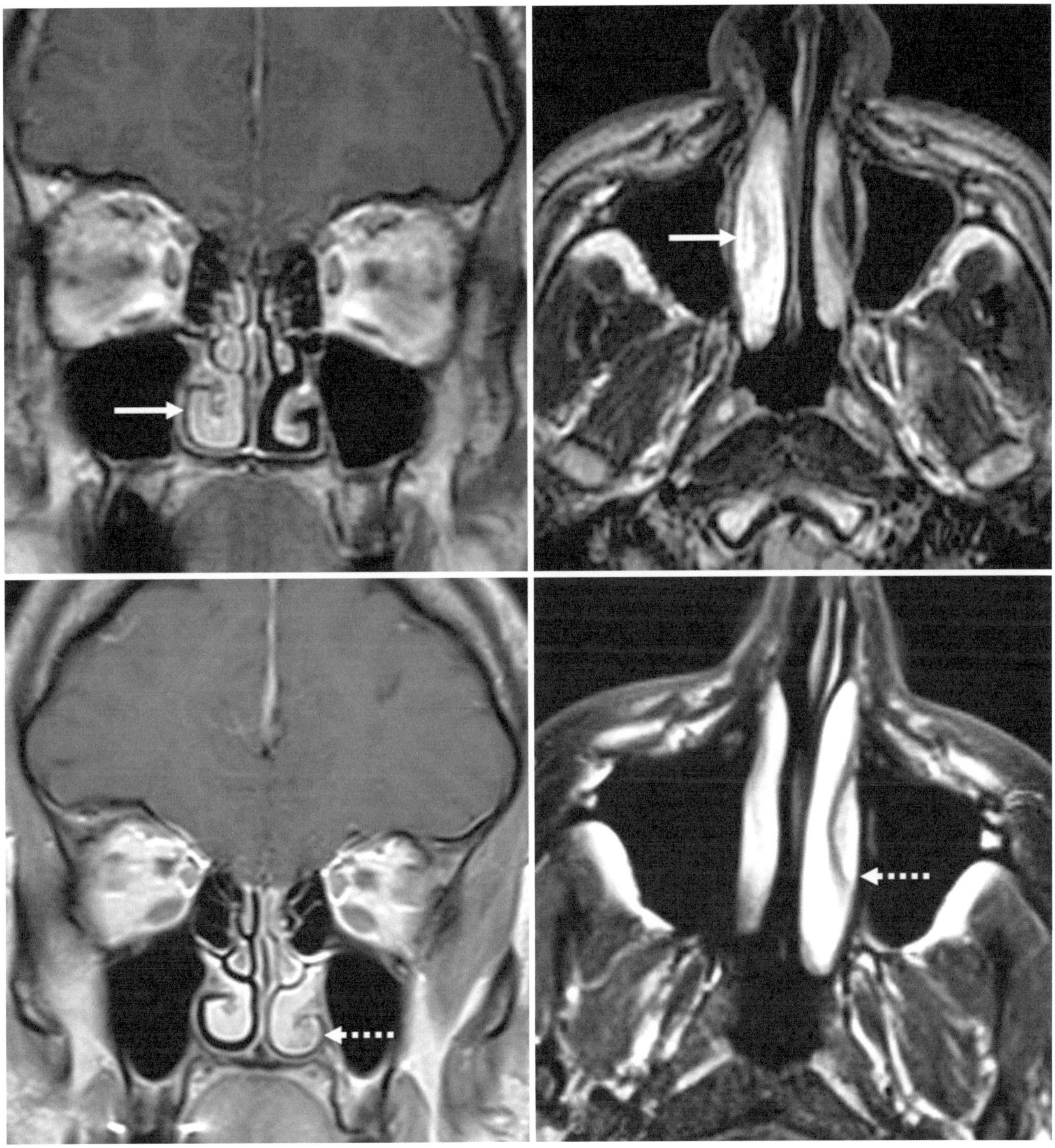

Fig. 2.67 Nasal cycling on MRI of a 36-year-old female with pituitary adenoma. **Top row:** Coronal contrast enhanced 1.5 T T1W (*left*) and axial FLAIR (*right*) images show prominence/congestion of the turbinates on the right (*arrows*). **Bottom row:** In the same patient, images 1 year later show greater prominence of the left-sided turbinates (*dotted arrows*), with relatively decongested (smaller) right-sided turbinates

Suggested Reading

Ahn JC, Lee WH, We J, Rhee C-S, Lee CH, Kim J-W. Nasal septal deviation with obstructive symptoms: association found with asthma but not with other general health problems. Am J Rhinol Allergy. 2016;30:17–20.

Aoki S, Dillon WP, Barkovich AJ, Norman D. Marrow conversion before pneumatization of the sphenoid sinus: assessment with MR imaging. Radiology. 1989;172:373–5.

Ardeshirpour F, McCarn KE, McKinney AM, Odland RM, Yueh B, Hilger PA. Computed tomography scan does not correlate with patient experience of nasal obstruction. Laryngoscope. 2016;126:820–5.

Aydinlioglu A, Kavakli A, Erdem S. Absence of frontal sinus in Turkish individuals. Yonsei Med J. 2003;44:215–8.

Bolger WE, Woodruff WW, Morehead J, Parsons DS. Maxillary sinus hypoplasia: classification and description of associated uncinate process hypoplasia. Otolaryngol Head Neck Surg. 1990;103:759–65.

Brunner E, Jacobs JB, Shpizner BA, Lebowitz RA, Holliday RA. Role of the agger nasi cell in chronic frontal sinusitis. Ann Otol Rhinol Laryngol. 1996;105:694–700.

Budu V, Mogoanta CA, Fanuta B, Bulescu I. The anatomical relations of the sphenoid sinus and their implications in sphenoidendoscopic surgery. Romanian J Morphol Embryol. 2013;54:13–6.

Çakur B, Sumbullu MA, Durna NB. Aplasia and agenesis of the frontal sinus in Turkish individuals: a retrospective study using dental volumetric tomography. Int J Med Sci. 2011;8:278–82.

Calhoun KH, Waggenspack GA, Simpson CB, Hokanson JA, Bailey BJ. CT evaluation of the paranasal sinuses in symptomatic and asymptomatic populations. Otolaryngol Head Neck Surg. 1991;104:480–3.

Capelli M, Gatti P. Radiological study of maxillary sinus using CBCT: relationship between mucosal thickening and common anatomic variants in chronic rhinosinusitis. J Clin Diagn Res. 2016;10:MC07–10.

Carver DD, Peterson S, Owens T. Intranasal teeth: a case report. Oral Surg Oral Med Oral Pathol. 1990;70:804–5.

Chao TK. Uncommon anatomic variations in patients with chronic paranasal sinusitis. Otolaryngol Head Neck Surg. 2005;132:221–5.

Cho DY, Hwang PH. Results of endoscopic maxillary mega-antrostomy in recalcitrant maxillary sinusitis. Am J Rhinol. 2008;22:658–62.

Chung SK, Cho DY, Dhong HJ. Computed tomogram findings of mucous recirculation between the natural and accessory ostia of the maxillary sinus. Am J Rhinol. 2002;16:265–8.

Earwaker J. Anatomic variants in sinonasal CT. Radiographics. 1993;13:381–415.

Genc S, Ozcan M, Titiz A, Unal A. Development of maxillary accessory ostium following sinusitis in rabbits. Rhinology. 2008;46:121–4.

Golden AL, Foote J, Lally E, Beideman R, Tatoian J. Dentigerous cyst of maxillary sinus causing elevation of the orbital floor: report of a case. Oral Surg Oral Med Oral Pathol. 1981;52:133–6.

Goldsztein H, Pletcher SD, Reh DD, Metson R. The frontal wishbone: anatomic and clinical implications. Am J Rhinol. 2007;21:725–8.

Hajiioannou J, Owens D, Whittet HB. Evaluation of anatomical variation of the crista galli using computed tomography. Clin Anat. 2010;23:370–3.

Hasegawa M, Kern EB. The human nasal cycle. Mayo Clin Proc. 1977;52:28–34.

Kainz J, Stammberger H. The roof of the anterior ethmoid: a locus minoris resistentiae in the skull base. Laryngol Rhinol Otol (Stuttg). 1988;67:142–9.

Kaplanoglu H, Kaplanoglu V, Dilli A, Toprak U, Hekımoğlu B. An analysis of the anatomic variations of the paranasal sinuses and ethmoid roof using computed tomography. Eurasian J Med. 2013;45:115–25.

Kasabah S, Krug J, Simunek A, Lecaro MC. Can we predict maxillary sinus mucosa perforation? ActaMedica. 2003;46:19–23.

Kazkayasi M, Karadeniz Y, Arikan OK. Anatomic variations of the sphenoid sinus on computed tomography. Rhinology. 2005;43:109–14.

Kayalioglu G, Oyar O, Govsa F. Nasal cavity and paranasal sinus bony variations: a computed tomographic study. Rhinology. 2000;38:108–13.

Kim JJ, Cho JH, Choi JW, Lim HW, Song YJ, Choi SJ, et al. Morphologic analysis of crista galli using computed tomography. J Rhinol. 2012;19:91–5.

Kreinnmair G, Ulm CW, Lugmayr H, Solar P. The incidence, location, and height of maxillary sinus septa in the edentulous and dentate maxilla. J Oral Maxillofac Surg. 1999;57:667–71.

Kumar H, Choudhry R, Kakar S. Accessory maxillary ostia: topography and clinical application. J Anat Soc India. 2001;50:3–5.

Leunig A, Betz CS, Sommer B, Sommer F. Anatomic variations of the sinuses; multiplanar CT-analysis in 641 patients. Laryngorhinootologie. 2008;87:482–9.

Lund VJ, Stammberger H, Fokkens WJ, Beale T, Bernal-Sprekelsen M, Eloy P, et al. European position paper on the anatomical terminology of the internal nose and paranasal sinuses. Rhinol Suppl. 2014;24:1–34.

Marquez S, Tessema B, Clement PA, Schaefer SD. Development of the ethmoid sinus and extramural migration: the anatomical basis of this paranasal sinus. Anat Rec (Hoboken). 2008;291:1535–53.

Nouraei SA, Elisay AR, Dimarco A, Abdi R, Majidi H, Madani SA, et al. Variations in paranasal sinus anatomy: implications for the pathophysiology of chronic rhinosinusitis and safety of endoscopic sinus surgery. J Otolaryngol Head Neck Surg. 2009;38:32–7.

Ohnishi T. Bony defects and dehiscences of the roof of the ethmoid bone. Rhinology. 1981;19:195–202.

Ozel HE, Ozdogan F, Esen E, Genc MG, Genc S, Selcuk A. The association between septal deviation and the presence of a maxillary accessory ostium. Int Forum Allergy Rhinol. 2015;5:1177–80.

Polavaram R, Devaiah AK, Sakai O, Shapshay SM. Anatomic variants and pearls--functional endoscopic sinus surgery. Otolaryngol Clin N Am. 2004;37:221–42.

Prasanna LC, Mamatha H. The location of the maxillary sinus ostium and its clinical application. Indian J Otolaryngol Head Neck Surg. 2010;62:335–7.

Ray B, Bandopadhyay SN, Das D, Adhikary B. A rare cause of nasolacrimal duct obstruction: Dentigerous cyst in maxillary sinus. Indian J Ophthalmol. 2009;57:465–7.

Scuderi AJ, Harnsberger HR, Boyer RS. Pneumatization of the paranasal sinuses: normal features of importance to the accurate interpretation of CT scans and MR images. Am J Roentgenol. 1993;160:1101–4.

Sevinc O, Is M, Barut C, Erdogan A. Anatomic variations of sphenoid sinus pneumatization in a sample of Turkish population: MRI study. Int J Morphol. 2014;32:1140–3.

Shpilberg KA, Daniel SC, Doshi AH, Lawson W, Som PM. CT of anatomic variants of the paranasal sinuses and nasal cavity: poor correlation with radiologically significant rhinosinusitis but importance in surgical planning. Am J Roentgenol. 2015;204:1255–60.

Singhal MD, Singhal DMK. Anatomy of accessory maxillary sinus ostium with clinical application. Int J Med Sci Public Health. 2014;3:327–32.

Smith RA, Gordon NC, De Luchi SF. Intranasal teeth. Report of two cases and review of the literature. Oral Surg Oral Med Oral Pathol. 1979;47:120–2.

Som PM, Lawson W. The frontal intersinus septal air cell—a new hypothesis of its origin. Am J Neuroradiol. 2008;29:1215–7.

Som PM, Park EE, Naidich TP, Lawson W. Crista galli pneumatization is an extension of the adjacent frontal sinuses. Am J Neuroradiol. 2009;30:31–3.

Spencer MG, Couldery AD. Nasal tooth. J Laryngol Otol. 1985;99:1147–50.

Stallman JS, Lobo JN, Som PM. The incidence of concha bullosa and its relationship to nasal septal deviation and paranasal sinus disease. Am J Neuroradiol. 2004;25:1613–8.

Stool S, Post J. Cranial growth, development and malformations: phylogenetic aspects and embryology. In: Bluestone CD, Stool SE, Kenna MA, editors. Pediatric otolaryngology. 3rd ed. Philadelphia, PA: W.B. Saunders Co.; 1996. p. 1–18.

Thulasidas P, Vaidyanathan V. Role of modified endoscopic medial maxillectomy in persistent chronic maxillary sinusitis. Int Arch Otorhinolaryngol. 2014;18:159–64.

Ulm CW, Solar P, Krennmair G, Matejka M, Watzek G. Incidence and suggested surgical management of septa in sinus-lift procedures. Int J Oral Maxillofac Surg. 1995;10:462–5.

Wang EW, Gullung JL, Schlosser RJ. Modified endoscopic medial maxillectomy for recalcitrant chronic maxillary sinusitis. Int Forum Allergy Rhinol. 2011;1:493–7.

Wang J, Bidari S, Inoue K, Yang H, Rhoton A Jr. Extensions of the sphenoid sinus: a new classification. Neurosurgery. 2010;66:797–816.

Wani AA, Kanotra S, Lateef M, Rafiq A, Sajad M, Qazi SA. CT scan evaluation of the anatomical variations of the ostiomeatal complex. Indian J Otolaryngol Head Neck Surg. 2009;61:163–8.

Yenigun A, Fazliogullari Z, Gun C, Uysal II, Nayman A, Karabulut AK. The effect of the presence of the accessory maxillary ostium on the maxillary sinus. Eur Arch Otorhinolaryngol. 2016;273:4315–9.

Zhu JH, Lee HP, Lim KM, Gordon BR, Wang de Y. Effect of accessory ostia on maxillary sinus ventilation: a computational fluid dynamics (CFD) study. Respir Physiol Neurobiol. 2012;183:91–9.

3 Orbital Variants

3.1 Introduction, Technique, and Basic Anatomy

Because of the anatomic scale of the globe, clinical examination remains the primary tool for diagnosis of ocular pathology, while cross-sectional imaging is often reserved for evaluation of the deep retrobulbar orbital structures. Knowledge of normal and variant appearances of the orbits is advantageous because they are commonly included on routine cross-sectional imaging of the head and neck and may be a source of incidental findings. Dedicated imaging is often necessary for accurate assessment of orbital pathology.

Plain films of the orbit have been largely relegated to the role of screening for retained metallic or foreign material for the purposes of MRI safety. Regarding the technique for orbital CT, whether nonenhanced CT (NECT) or contrast-enhanced CT (CECT), a multi-detector helical acquisition with multiplanar reformats has become standard. A slice collimation of 0.625 mm with a maximum reconstruction thickness of 3 mm is recommended, since thinner slices are often required for the detection of subtle fractures and can help reduce streak artifact. Radiation dose to the orbit is an important consideration in CT because of the sensitivity of the lens. Historically, gantry tilt techniques have been employed for head CT to minimize the dose to the orbit. However, with the increasing utilization of multi-detector CT units, alternative means of dose reduction, such as automated tube current modulation, are being more widely utilized.

Orbital MRI is an invaluable tool in the assessment of the globe and orbital soft tissues. MRI of the orbit should include thin slice small field-of-view T1-weighted imaging (T1WI), fat-suppression (FS)-T2WI, diffusion-weight imaging (DWI), and post-gadolinium fat-suppressed spin echo T1WI (FS-SET1WI), with a combination of axial and coronal planes. Orbital fat provides helpful background contrast on T1WI, although effective fat suppression is essential for spin-echo T2WI (SET2WI) and postcontrast imaging. There are multiple techniques for fat suppression (FS) that can be employed within the orbit, each with its own advantages and disadvantages. Chemical shift selective suppression (CHESS) utilizes a chemically-selective radiofrequency (RF) pulse signal centered on the resonant frequency of fat to suppress its signal. CHESS provides high signal-to-noise ratio (SNR) images with relatively quick acquisition time, especially when performed at higher field strengths; however, it is quite susceptible to magnetic field inhomogeneity. Fat-water separation technique (Dixon technique) utilizes the differing precession frequencies of fat and water to obtain "in-phase" and "out-of-phase" images, which can be summed to generate a fat-suppressed pure water image in the traditional "two-point" technique. This technique is relatively insensitive to B1 field inhomogeneity and has a high SNR, although is sensitive to B0 field heterogeneity. Three-point and four-point variations have been developed that reduce sensitivity to B0 field heterogeneity, but at the cost of longer acquisition times. Inversion recovery techniques such as short-tau inversion recovery (*STIR*) and hybrid inversion recovery techniques that also utilize spectral presaturation with or without an adiabatic pulse (e.g., *SPIR* and *spectral attenuated inversion recovery [SPAIR]*, respectively) may also be considered for use in the orbit. Notably, a SPIR-SPAIR combination may have more homogeneous fat suppression (due to a relative insensitivity to B1 field inhomogeneity) as compared to CHESS, with a potentially higher SNR than STIR since the SPIR-SPAIR combination is more selective of fat.

A. McKinney et al., *Atlas of Head/Neck and Spine Normal Imaging Variants*, https://doi.org/10.1007/978-3-319-95441-7_3

3.2 Bony Orbit: Normal Orbital Sutures, Orbital Roof Thinning, and Orbital Decompression

3.2.1 Normal Orbital Sutures

The bony orbit is a complex structure composed of seven bones that are separated by 12 sutures. The *orbital sutures* become increasingly fused with age, although the timing of fusion has not been well described. The orbit is frequently evaluated in the setting of trauma, making knowledge of orbital bony anatomy essential for the accurate interpretation of fracture. On thin-slice multidetector CT, the frontonasal, frontozygomatic, and sphenozygomatic sutures are present in a majority of adults. The zygomaticotemporal and zygomaticomaxillary sutures are relatively less common but are frequently visualized. The sphenofrontal and frontolacrimal sutures are only well visualized in 6% and 2% of adults, and thus their presence may be more likely to simulate a fracture relative to the other orbital/periorbital sutures, especially if they are asymmetrically fused. Sutures of the thin medial orbital wall (i.e., the lamina papyracea) are usually undetectable.

3.2.2 Orbital Roof Thinning

The orbital roof or superior wall is composed primarily of the orbital plate of the frontal bone with a smaller contribution from the lesser sphenoid wing. The orbital roof becomes increasingly thin with *normal aging*. In some instances the bone may become dehiscent, although this does not often have clinical implications in the nontraumatic setting because of the presence of the dense connective tissue of the periorbita and dura.

3.2.3 Postoperative Orbital Decompression

Thyroid eye disease has a prevalence of 0.25%; it has no significant ethnic predisposition. While surgical decompression of the orbit has historically been reserved for thyroid eye disease that is complicated by optic neuropathy or extreme corneal exposure, the indications for surgery have broadened over recent decades. Decompression may involve osteotomy of any of the four walls of the orbit (medial, lateral, roof, and floor) and aims to relieve proptosis and lid retraction. The orbital floor is typically decompressed in combination with the medial wall or both medial and lateral walls (i.e., three-wall decompression). Because of the symmetric appearance of the osteotomy defects, these can usually be differentiated from pathologic post-traumatic orbital injury (Figs. 3.1, 3.2, 3.3, and 3.4).

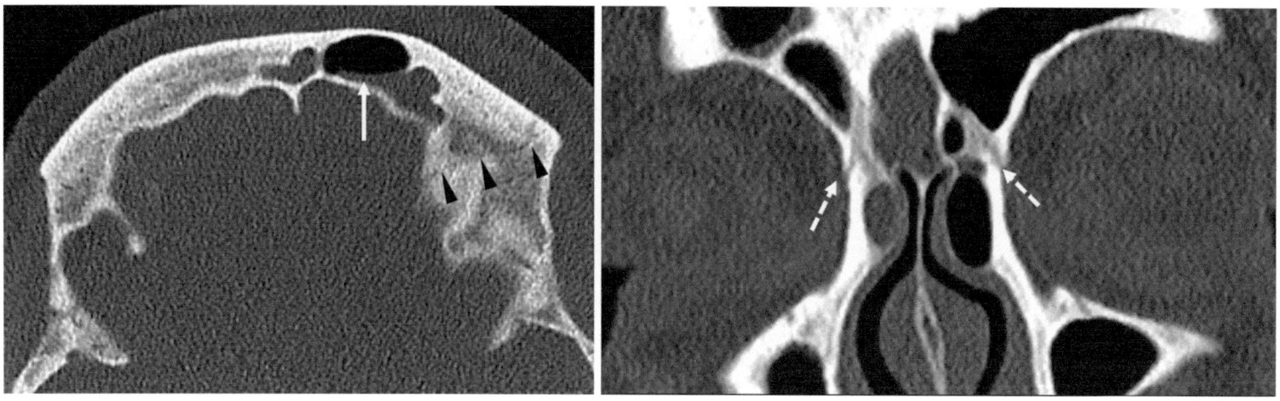

Fig. 3.1 Two different adult patients with persistent orbital sutures simulating fractures. **Left**: Axial NECT through the anterior cranial fossa of a 67-year-old male following a motor vehicle accident demonstrates a normal, asymmetric unfused left sphenofrontal suture (*arrowheads*), with an air-fluid level present within the left frontal sinus (*arrow*) caused by intrasinus hemorrhage from a left frontal sinus fracture (*not shown*). **Right**: coronal NECT of a 60-year-old female demonstrates patent bilateral frontolacrimal sutures (*dashed arrows*)

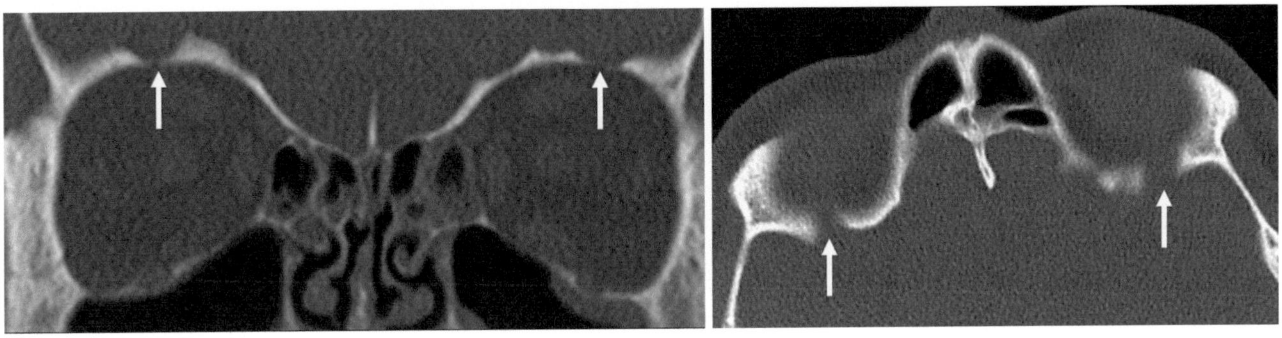

Fig. 3.2 Coronal (*left*) and axial (*right*) NECT images through the orbits of a 77-year-old male demonstrate normal variant focal bony thinning and dehiscence of the lateral to the middle third of the orbital roof bilaterally (*arrows*)

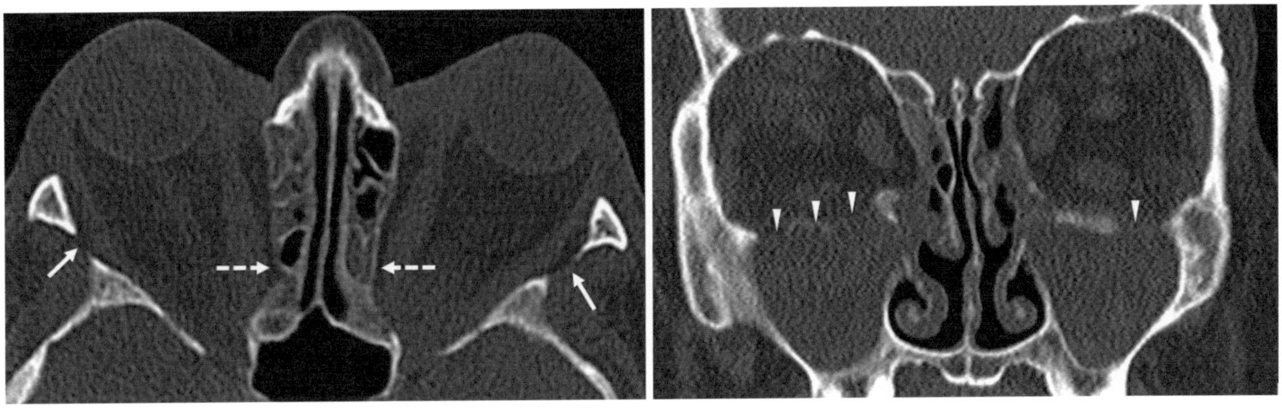

Fig. 3.3 A 66-year-old female with a history of thyroid eye disease had been treated with bilateral three-wall orbital decompressions. Axial (*left*) and coronal (*right*) NECT images demonstrate orbitotomy defects involving the bilateral lateral orbital walls (*arrows*), the medial orbital walls (*dashed arrows*), and the orbital floors (*arrowheads*). There is continued bilateral proptosis predominantly caused by an increased volume of the intraorbital fat

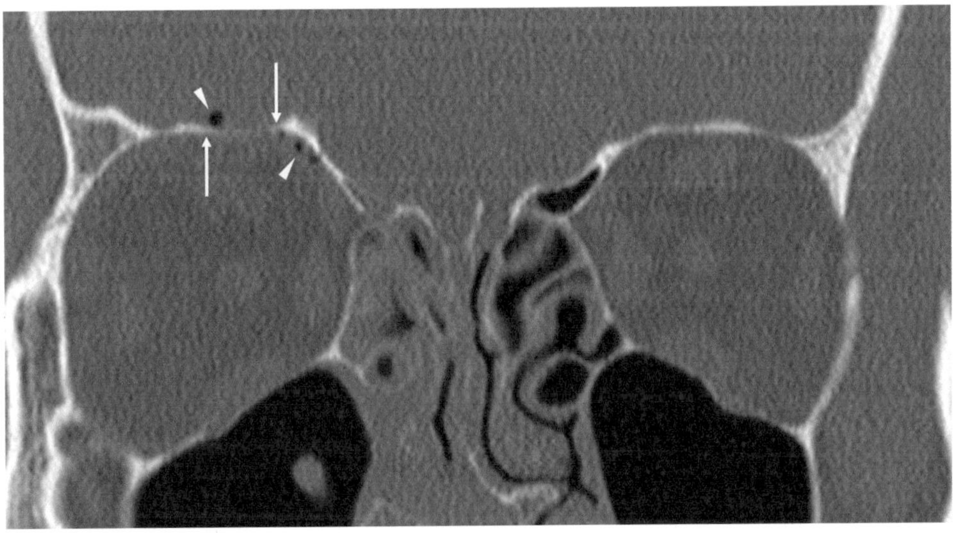

Fig. 3.4 Comparison case of orbital roof fracture. A coronal NECT image through the orbits of a 59-year-old male following a motor vehicle collision demonstrates a fracture through the right orbital roof. There is a subtle step-off in a thinned region between the medial and lateral aspects of the orbital roof (*arrows*). There is small amount of accompanied pneumocephalus and orbital emphysema (*arrowheads*) from ventral extension of the fracture through the right frontal sinus (*not shown*), typical of an orbital roof fracture

3.3 Globe

The most common cause of variation in appearance in the globe on cross-sectional imaging is the postoperative state, which should not be mistaken for orbital foreign body or injury. There is a wide array of ophthalmologic surgical techniques that are beyond the scope of this chapter; therefore we will focus on solely those procedures that have clear manifestations on cross-sectional imaging and are most frequently encountered in clinical practice.

3.3.1 Intraocular Lens Implant

Surgical removal of cataracts provides long-term improvement in patient vision and quality of life and as a result has become the most commonly performed surgical procedure in many developed nations. The cataractous native lens is first broken up by ultrasonic phacoemulsification with subsequent suction removal and placement of an artificial intraocular lens implant (pseudophakia), typically in the preserved native lens capsule. This artificial lens implant consists of two components: an optic component that replaces the native lens, and haptics that serve to anchor the optic component in position. Only the optic component is visible on cross-sectional imaging. An intraocular lens implant is a thin linear structure positioned posterior to the iris in the expected location of the native ovoid biconvex lens; it appears hyperdense on CT and hypointense on both T1WI and T2WI.

3.3.2 Glaucoma Shunt Implant

Glaucoma shunt implants are classically reserved for glaucoma that is refractory to medical therapy and trabeculectomy. The goal of shunting is to reduce intraocular pressure by creating a low resistance pathway for efflux of aqueous humor from the anterior chamber. Shunt implants are composed of a small tube that extends from the anterior chamber to a plate that is fixed to the sclera, which maintains a subconjunctival potential space. Aqueous humor is diverted into the subconjunctival space, often resulting in the formation of a periocular fluid bleb surrounding the plate of the shunt; it then diffuses into the surrounding soft tissues. The plate is usually placed in the superotemporal aspect of the globe because of the improved safety profile of the surgical exposure. The most common complication is globe hypotony, which is often diagnosed clinically. The plate component of the shunt is visualized on imaging as a curvilinear structure that is contiguous with a quadrant of the wall of the globe. Typically composed of nonmetallic material, the plate component usually appears as hyperdense on CT. On MRI, the plate demonstrates hypointense signal. However, the surrounding fluid bleb is more conspicuous on T2WI and should not be misconstrued as a pathologic orbital cystic lesion.

3.3.3 Scleral Buckle

Scleral buckles are utilized for the treatment of retinal detachment. They function by indenting the wall of the globe and thereby reducing the vector forces pulling on the retina. Scleral buckles are band-like structures that may completely or nearly completely encircle the entire globe, and they are usually oriented perpendicular to the extraocular muscles. They may be composed of (1) silicone rubber that demonstrates a hyperdense appearance on CT, or (2) porous silicone sponge that demonstrates air attenuation. On MRI, both types of scleral buckle material will appear as a uniformly hypointense band with associated mild circumferential indentation of the globe.

3.3.4 Ocular Injection of Gas or Silicone Oil

Vitrectomy is often necessary for repair of retinal detachment because it decreases traction on the separated retinal layers and the flow of vitreous into the intraretinal potential space. Subsequently, the posterior segment of the globe is often filled with either silicone oil or long-acting gas such as sulfur hexafluoride in order to tamponade the retinal defect while the retinal pigment cells resorb the intraretinal fluid, thus allowing the retinal layers to reappose. Intraocular gas will demonstrate air attenuation on CT and signal void on MRI. Ocular silicone is uniformly hyperdense on CT with attenuation ~ HU > 100, greater than would be expected for hemorrhage. On MRI, the signal characteristics of silicone may vary, depending on its concentration, although it typically demonstrates a hyperintense T1 signal and hypointense T2 signal.

3.3.5 Orbital Implant and Ocular Prosthesis

Following enucleation, spherical orbital implants are placed in order to add bulk to the anophthalmic socket and prevent a sunken appearance. Orbital implants may be made from a variety of materials, including silicone oil, polymethylmethacrylate (PMMA), and porous materials such as polyethylene. Orbital implants may be sutured to the extraocular musculature to allow for movement. An *ocular implant* may be placed anterior to the orbital implant between the eyelids, allowing for improved cosmesis. Silicone and PMMA are hyperdense on CT and hypointense on MRI and thus could mimic hemorrhage. Porous polyethylene demonstrates a varied appearance from the time of implantation owing to progressive fibrovascular ingrowth into the implant.

3.3.6 Eyelid Weights

Subcutaneous upper eyelid weight implants are placed in the setting of facial nerve injury with symptomatic lagophthalamos in order to prevent corneal damage and preserve vision. Metallic weights are frequently made from gold and have associated streak artifact. Their location, curvilinear appearance, and holes for suturing are characteristic, so these should not mimic pathology. However, associated dense streak artifact may obscure adjacent structures or pathology on CT.

3.3.7 Congenital Proptosis

Positioning of the globe within the orbit can be reliably measured on cross-sectional imaging using the interzygomatic line, a line drawn between the anterior aspects of the zygomatic arches on axial images as a reference point. Measurements should be made on axial images with the scan plane parallel to the optic nerve and lens with the eyes looking forward. The normal distance from the interzygomatic line to the posterior margin of the globe in asymptomatic patients has been reported as mean 9.4 mm and range 5.9–12.8 (±2 SDs), while the distance from this line to the anterior globe's surface should be less than 23 mm. However, multiple studies have demonstrated wide variation in normative exophthalmometry measurements across age in the pediatric population and race, notably with African American patients having typically higher values than reported for Caucasians. Hence, a nonacquired form of mild *congenital proptosis* is likely a normal variant and can be seen on routine head CTs in patients lacking orbital pathology or symptoms.

3.3.8 Pseudo-proptosis and Measurement Error Caused by Nonuniform Axial Plane

While measurement of globe position within the orbit on cross-sectional imaging is accurate and reproducible, it is dependent on having a uniform axial scan plane. Scans that are not tailored to the evaluation of the orbital structures may often be acquired or reconstructed in axial planes that are not parallel to the optic nerves and lenses and thus may result in an artefactual appearance of globe malposition (i.e., "pseudo-proptosis"). For example, head flexion will exaggerate an enopthalmic appearance, while head extension will exaggerate an exophthalmic appearance.

3.3.9 Sedation-Related Strabismus

Conscious sedation or general anesthesia may be employed during cross-sectional imaging as a means of reducing patient discomfort and motion. Sedation is routinely performed in the setting of patient agitation, claustrophobia, movement disorder, or early childhood, and it is most commonly utilized during MRI because of its relatively long acquisition time. However, many of the commonly administered anesthetics do not limit eye motion but rather result in large amplitude oscillatory sweeps and impairment of the normal involuntary gaze stabilizing and gaze shifting mechanisms. Thus, sedation may produce the appearance of or accentuate ocular misalignment. Such normal *sedation-related strabismus* may raise concern for orbital pathology. Interestingly, stroke has been cited as the most common cause of strabismus in adults; stroke-related strabismus is present in about one fifth of stroke patients (Figs. 3.5, 3.6, 3.7, 3.8, 3.9, 3.10, 3.11, 3.12, 3.13, and 3.14).

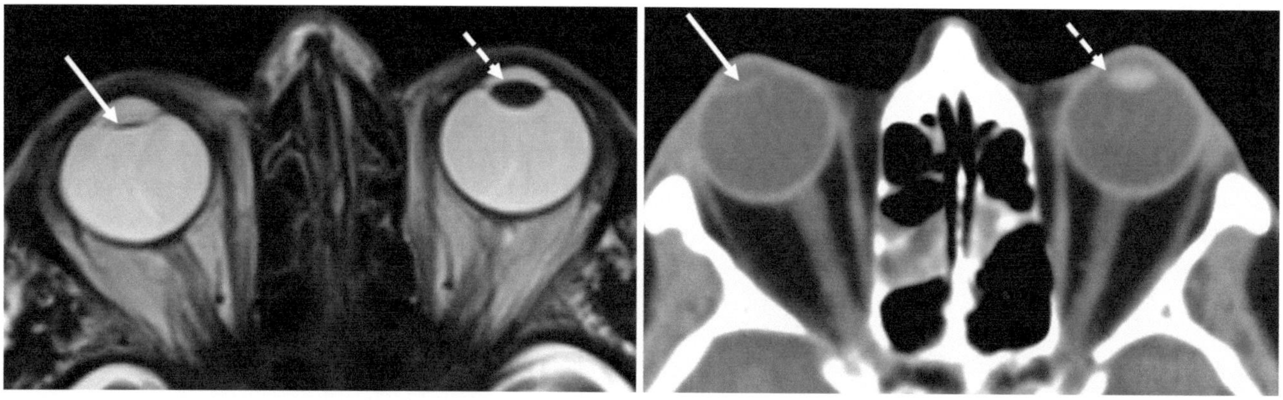

Fig. 3.5 Axial SET2WI MRI (*left*) and NECT (*right*) of a 72-year-old male with postsurgical changes of right cataract removal and intraocular lens implantation (pseudophakia). The visible optic component of the implant appears as a thin curvilinear band posterior to the iris that is hypointense on SET2WI and hyperdense on NECT (*arrows*), while the native left lens demonstrates normal expected biconvex morphology (*dashed arrows*)

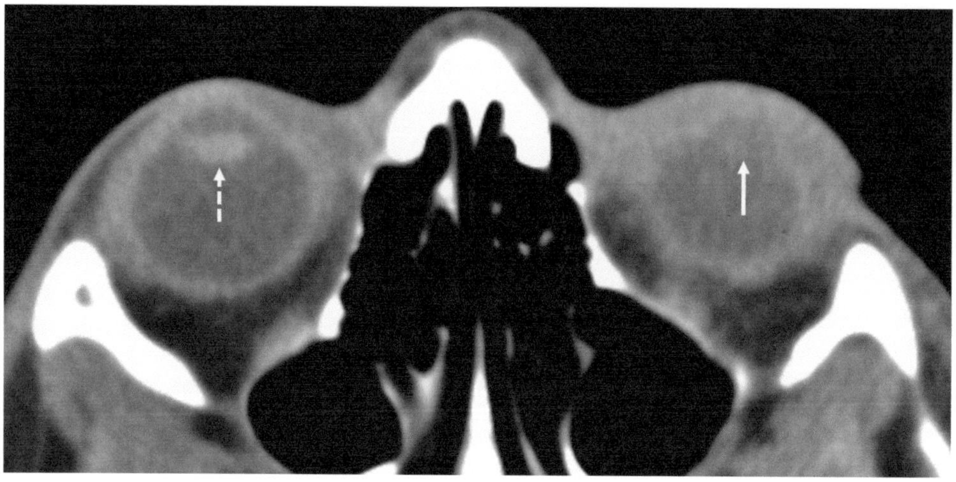

Fig. 3.6 Comparison case of traumatic cataract. Axial NECT of a 12-year-old female with a clinically evident globe rupture following blunt trauma to the left orbit demonstrates blurring and indistinctness of the left lens (*arrow*) relative to the normal biconvex right lens (*dashed arrow*) consistent with a traumatic left-sided cataract. In contrast to a pseudophakic globe, there is no discrete thin curvilinear optic component visualized

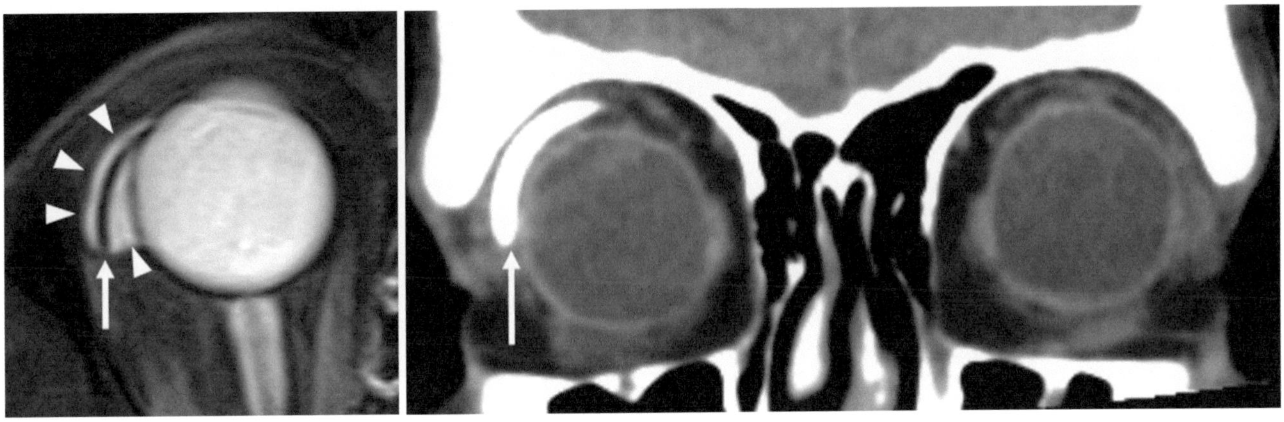

Fig. 3.7 Axial FS-SET2WI MRI (*left*) and coronal NECT (*right*) images through the right globe in a 76-year-old male demonstrate postsurgical changes of a right glaucoma drainage device (i.e., shunt) placement. The visible plate component appears as a thin curvilinear structure that is adherent to the superotemporal margin of the right globe and is hypointense on FS-SET2WI and hyperdense on NECT (*arrows*). FS-SET2WI best demonstrates the expected surrounding periocular T2-hyperintense fluid bleb (*arrowheads, left*) created by the shunted aqueous humor

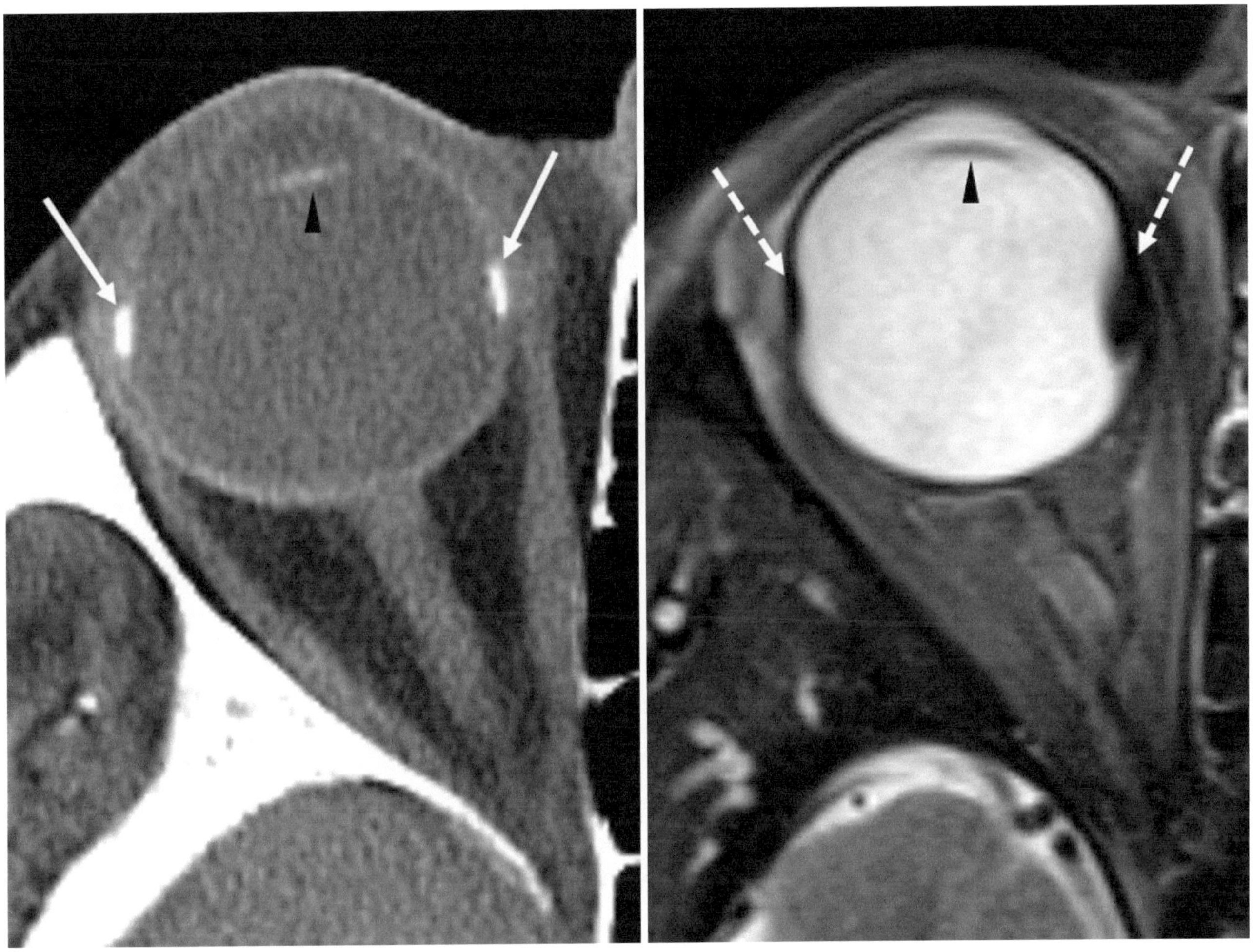

Fig. 3.8 Axial NECT (*left*) and FS-SET2WI (*right*) through the right orbit of a 66-year-old male demonstrate postsurgical changes of a scleral buckle. The silicone material appears as a circumferential band oriented perpendicular to the extraocular muscles that is hyperdense on NECT (*arrows, left*) and hypointense on SET2WI (*dashed arrows, right*). There is slight indentation of the sclera that is typically best appreciated on T2WI. Intraocular lens implants are also present (*black arrowheads*)

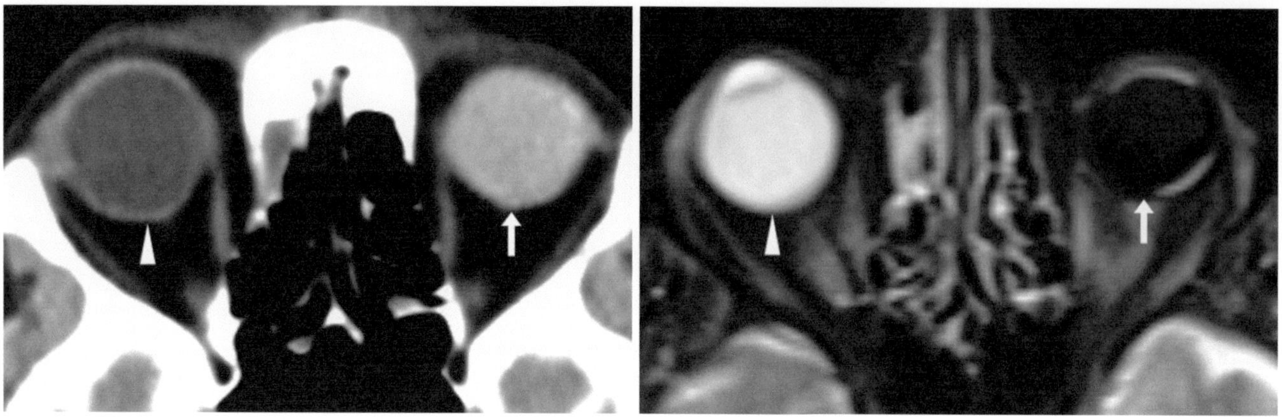

Fig. 3.9 Axial NECT (*left*) and FS-SET2WI (*right*) of a 92-year-old male with findings of prior left intraocular silicone injection. There is uniform hyperdensity and T2-hypointense signal throughout the posterior segment of the left globe (*arrows*) compared to the normal fluid attenuation and T2-hyperintense signal of the posterior right globe (*arrowheads*)

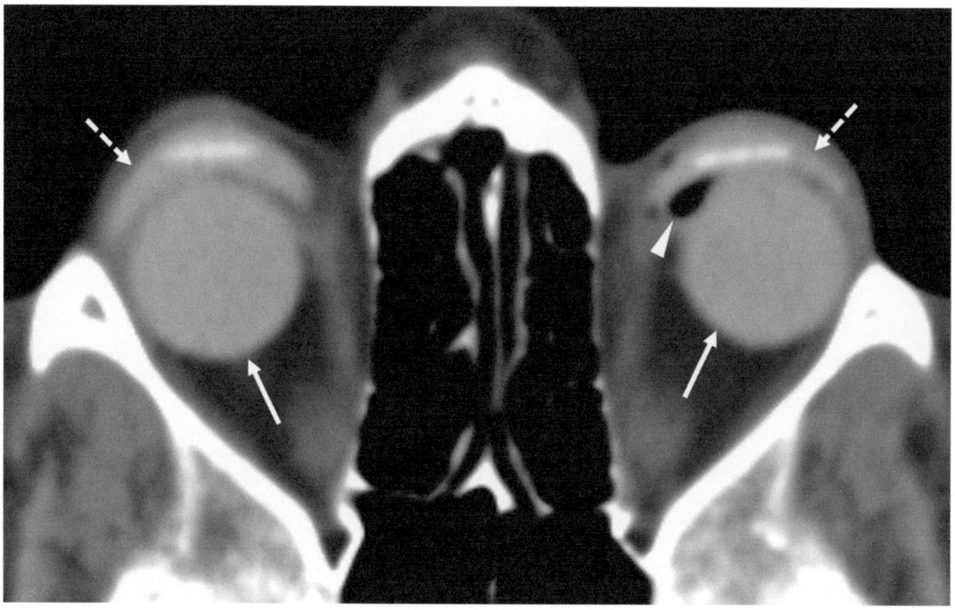

Fig. 3.10 Axial NECT image of a 36-year-old female demonstrating postsurgical changes of bilateral enucleation, orbital/globe implants (*arrows*), and overlying ocular prostheses (*dashed arrows*). Because of the superficial location of the ocular prosthesis below the eyelids and the' removable nature of the prosthesis, air may normally be visible surrounding the ocular prostheses (*arrowhead*)

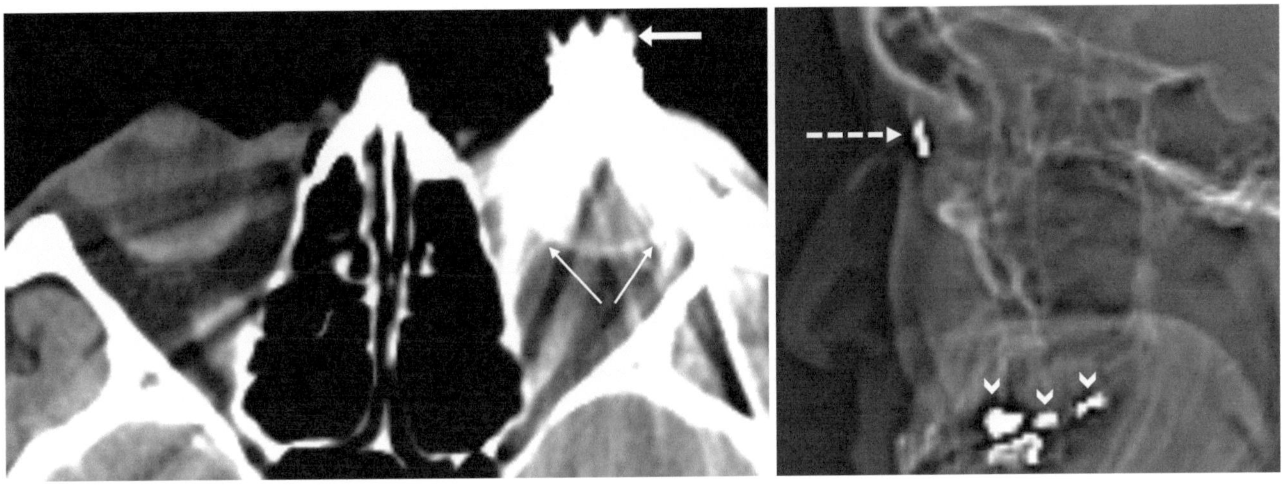

Fig. 3.11 Axial NECT (*left*) and accompanying lateral scout topogram for the CT (*right*) of a 62-year-old male with a left facial nerve palsy following a radical parotidectomy. The metallic density overlying the left globe (*arrow, left*) has the characteristic location and appearance of an eyelid weight in the region of the subcutaneous soft tissues of the upper left lid, with associated extensive streak artifact (*thin arrows, left*) and a curvilinear morphology (*dashed arrow, right*). Note that the density of the eyelid weight is similar to that of metallic dental amalgam inferiorly (*chevrons, right*)

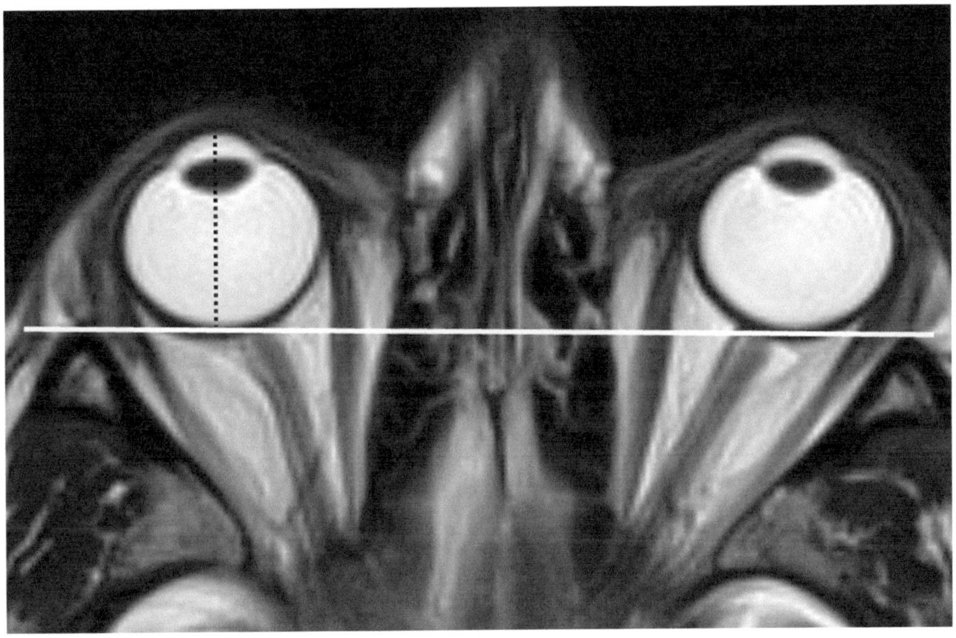

Fig. 3.12 Axial SET2WI of a 67-year-old African American female with no history of visual symptoms demonstrates relatively anterior positioning of the globes within the orbits. The interzygomatic line (*solid white line*) contacts the posterior margins of the globes (0 mm), and the distance to the elevated anterior margin of the globe (*dashed black line*) is 24 mm. Since the patient is asymptomatic and does not have an acquired orbital abnormality, this likely represents variant mild congenital proptosis, although the imaging appearance may mimic that of pathologic exophthalmos

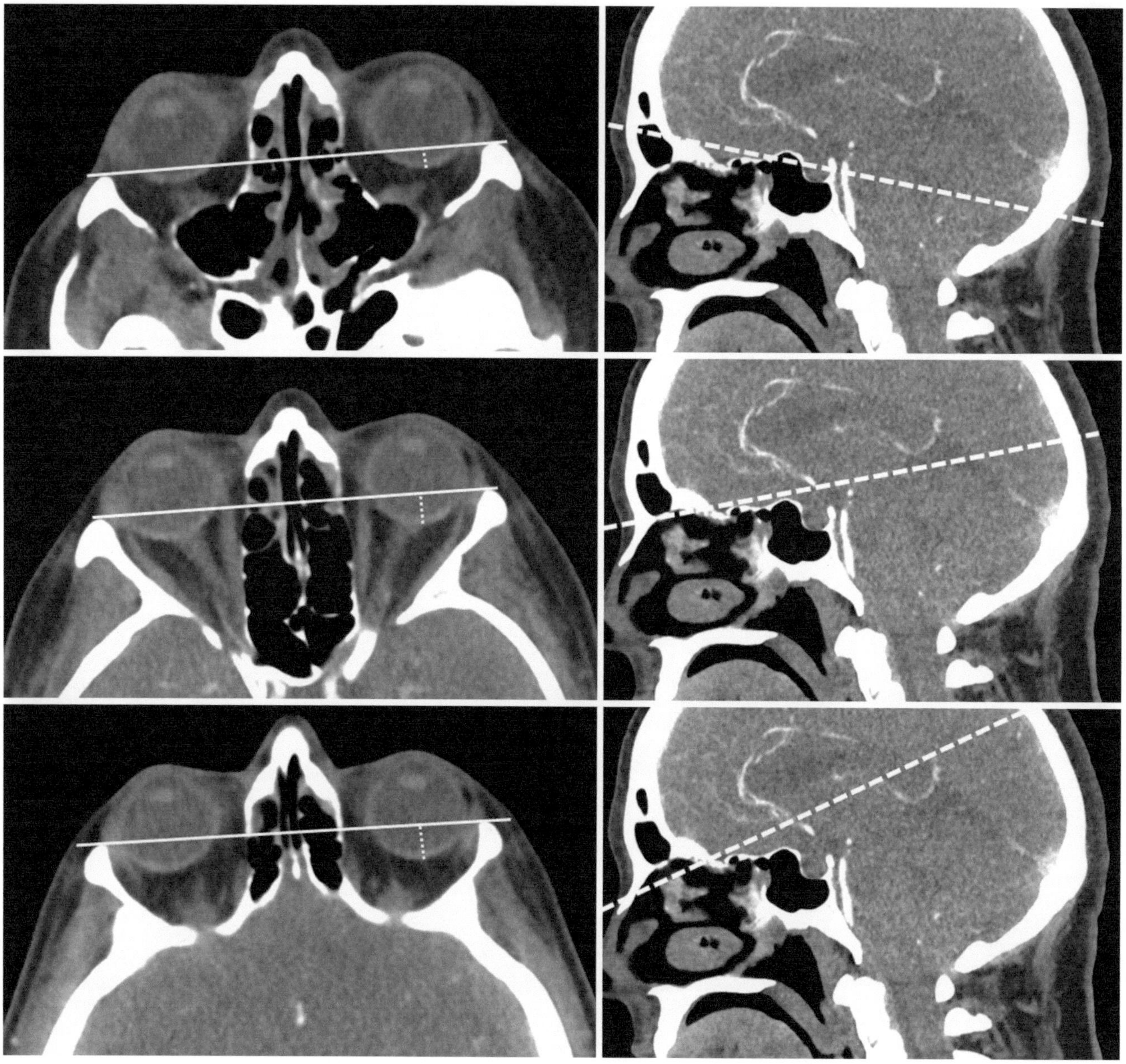

Fig. 3.13 Paired axial (*left column*) and sagittal (*right column*) reconstructed CT angiography (CTA) images demonstrate increasing distance from the interzygomatic line (*solid lines, left column*) to the posterior margin of the globe (*dotted line, left column*) with an increasing posterior to anterior downward slope of the axial scan plane as represented by the *dashed lines* (*right column*). Thus, such pseudo-proptosis (*top left image*) can result from suboptimal positioning or suboptimal reconstruction of the axial plane from CTA or NECT

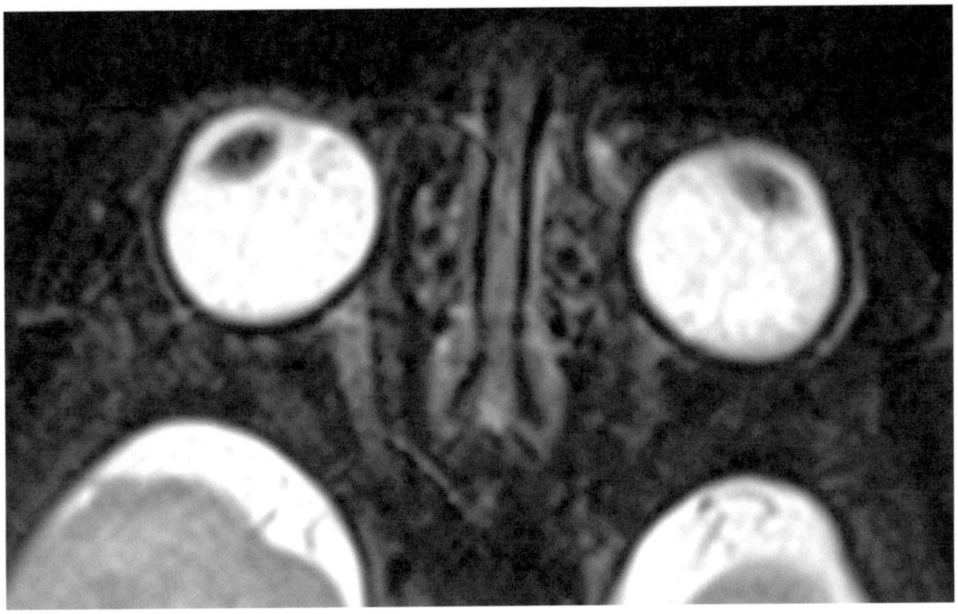

Fig. 3.14 Axial FS-SET2WI from an MRI performed under general anesthesia on a 1-year-old child demonstrates temporal deviation of both globes that was not noted on baseline clinical ophthalmologic examination or following the completion of the study and that is consistent with incidental exotropia (a form of strabismus) secondary to sedation

3.4 Extraocular Muscles

3.4.1 Normal Contrast Enhancement

There is normal marked enhancement of the extraocular musculature relative to background facial skeletal muscle. On MRI, *extraocular muscle enhancement* is best appreciated on fat-suppressed T1WI due to the surrounding T1 bright retrobulbar fat. The degree of enhancement may approximate that of the adjacent nasal mucosa. The physiologic explanation for this marked enhancement is thought to be related to the dense innervation and associated rich capillary supply of the extraocular muscles in combination with abundant extracellular space, which allows for the accumulation of contrast material. While the extraocular muscles typically demonstrate uniform enhancement on most imaging protocols, there may be differential enhancement of the central global layer and thin marginal outer orbital layer of muscle fibers on early phase imaging, creating a C-shaped pattern of enhancement oriented toward the globe. Pathologic entities that affect the extraocular muscles may enhance similarly or perhaps slightly more than background physiologic enhancement, although such pathologic entities (such as neoplasm or pseudotumor) may be discerned by the associated enlargement of the muscle and the deformity of its contour.

3.4.2 Physiologic FDG Uptake

The extraocular muscles demonstrate normal physiologic symmetric avid uptake of radiotracer on fluorodeoxyglucose–positron emission tomography (FDG-PET) relative to background skeletal muscle. Such *physiologic extraocular muscular uptake of FDG* is likely caused by the specialized function of the extraocular muscles and both voluntary and involuntary recruitment during the uptake phase prior to imaging. Normal standardized uptake values in the extraocular muscles can approximate those found in the brain, an obligate glucose metabolizer. This high level of background uptake may obscure extraocular muscle involvement by inflammatory or neoplastic processes on PET (Figs. 3.15, 3.16, and 3.17).

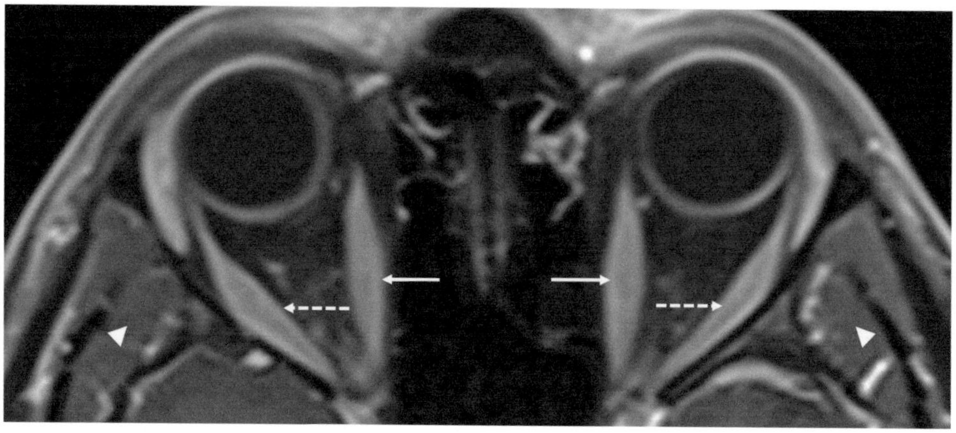

Fig. 3.15 Axial postcontrast FS-SET1WI image of a 40-year-old male demonstrates normal symmetric enhancement of the extraocular muscles. The medial recti (*arrows*) and lateral recti (*dashed arrows*) are shown in comparison to the temporalis musculature (*arrowheads*)

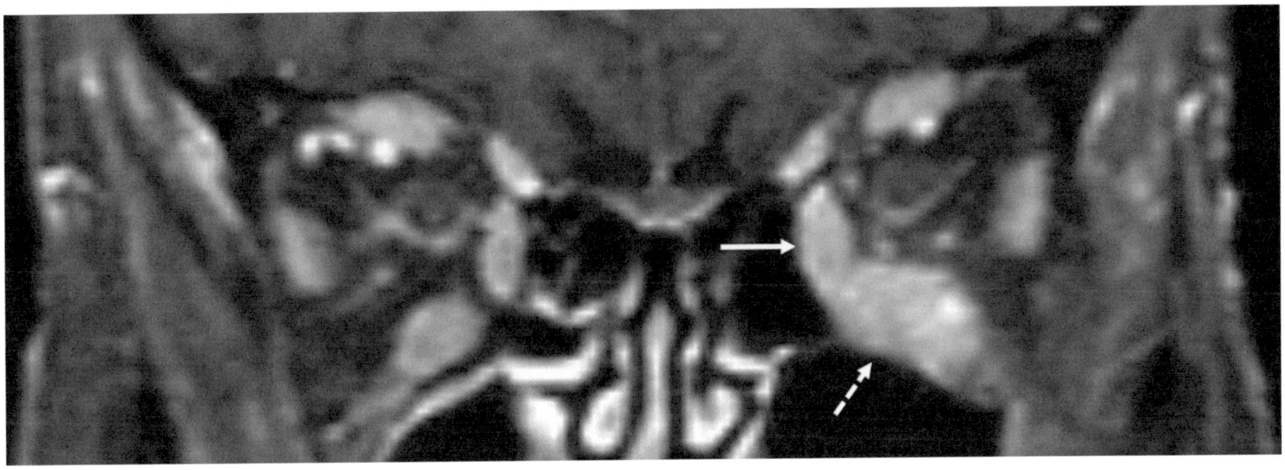

Fig. 3.16 Comparison case of orbital lymphoma. Coronal FS-SET1WI MRI of an 82-year-old male with orbital lymphoma demonstrates asymmetric enhancement and enlargement of the left lateral rectus (*arrow*) and inferior rectus muscles (*dashed arrow*) relative to the normal right orbital extraocular musculature

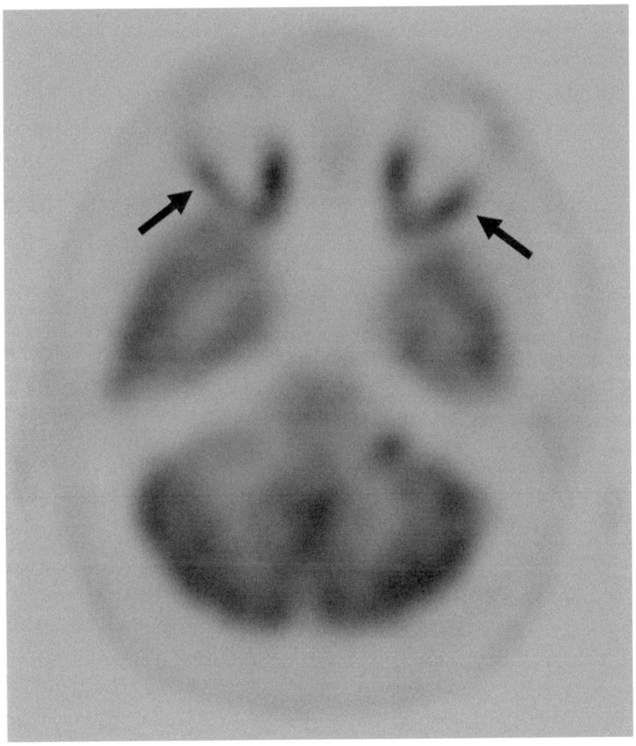

Fig. 3.17 Axial source PET data of a 65-year-old female with a complete therapeutic response of abdominopelvic marginal zone lymphoma demonstrates normal, symmetric FDG uptake within the extraocular muscles (*arrows*), similar to the degree of uptake of the brain

3.5 Optic Nerve Tortuosity, Diameter, Sheath Distention, and Normal Perineural Enhancement

3.5.1 Optic Nerve Tortuosity

While tortuosity of the orbital segment of the optic nerve has been associated with pathology such as neurofibromatosis type-1 (NF-1) and idiopathic intracranial hypertension (IIH), this finding is nonspecific and can be an incidental finding in patients without visual symptoms, especially if seen in isolation. While *optic nerve tortuosity* may be quantitatively assessed using a tortuosity index, it is typically assessed qualitatively in clinical practice. Lack of congruity of the optic nerves in more than one coronal section and subarachnoid space dilatation surrounding the optic nerves have been proposed as a practical radiologic definition of optic nerve tortuosity. Isolated tortuosity of the optic nerve should be considered a normal variant in the setting of a lack of clinically evident visual symptoms, ancillary findings of elevated intracranial pressure, or associated optic nerve enlargement or signal abnormality on MRI.

3.5.2 Optic Nerve Sheath Distention

The optic nerve sheath is a continuation of the intracranial meninges that envelops the optic nerve throughout its orbital segment. The subarachnoid space of the optic nerve sheath communicates with that of the intracranial space and is therefore subject to changes in intracranial pressure. While optic nerve sheath diameter has been positively correlated with intracranial pressure, there is variability in normal controls that can overlap with abnormal patients. Normal adult optic nerve sheath diameters have been reported as 5.52 ± 1.11 mm just posterior to the globe and 5.2 ± 0.9 mm at 4 mm posterior to the globe. The bulbar segment of the optic nerve sheath, located just posterior to the globe, is the most distensible segment and often demonstrates a bulbous appearance. Hence, optic nerve sheath fluid distention can be considered a normal variant in asymptomatic patients, but it can mimic the *optic nerve sheath distention* that can be seen in IIH (also called pseudotumor cerebri), NF-1, or rare inflammatory disorders such as sarcoidosis. Lack of dural venous sinus stenosis on postcontrast MR venography (MRV) and normal cerebrospinal fluid opening pressure on lumbar puncture can exclude IIH when nonspecific optic sheath distention is present in the setting of suggestive clinical symptoms.

3.5.3 Optic Perineural Enhancement: A Normal Variant

While orbital inflammatory, infiltrative, and neoplastic processes may result in abnormal thickening and enhancement on postcontrast T1WI (typically FS-SET1WI) of the optic nerve sheath, thin (≤1 mm) circumferential vascular enhancement of the sheath is often seen in normal asymptomatic patients. Perineural enhancement that is thick, nodular, eccentric, or demonstrates associated involvement of the retrobulbar fat or optic nerve T2 hyperintense signal abnormality (i.e., edema) and displacement is likely pathologic. Hence, mild *optic perineural enhancement* is often a normal variation in patients lacking visual symptoms, and the absence of central optic nerve swelling or enhancement excludes optic neuritis or optic neuropathy. In questionable cases of optic neuritis, dedicated less than 3 mm thickness coronal postcontrast fat-suppressed fluid-attenuated inversion recovery (FS-FLAIR) imaging (a relatively specific technique to evaluate for optic nerve edema) in comparison with postcontrast FS-SET1WI can confirm mild optic perineural enhancement, a normal variant that can mimic optic neuritis.

3.5.4 Optic Nerve Diameter and Normal Variation

Variation in *optic nerve diameter* may be seen with increasing age in the pediatric population, with the greatest growth seen in the first 2 years of life. Normal retrobulbar segment (immediately posterior to the globe) optic nerve diameter on coronal T2-weighted images measures 1.35 ± 0.82 mm in patients younger than 6 months, 2.03 ± 0.30 mm in patients 6 months to 2 years, and gradually increases up to 2.35 ± 0.40 mm for patients between 12 and 18 years. In adults, there are well-established normative values of the optic nerve sheath diameter, which is affected by cerebrospinal fluid (CSF) volume of the subarachnoid space, and a paucity of data regarding the diameter of the optic nerve proper on cross-sectional imaging. Studies have demonstrated adult optic nerve diameters in the range of 3.5–4.0 mm and slightly smaller (~0.5 mm less) at greater than 10 mm posterior to the globe. However, this data in adults varies, likely related to technique, plane (coronal section is best for measurement), and sequence (heavily T2-weighted sequences best separate the true optic nerve from the larger T2-bright CSF-containing optic sheath). The optic nerve diameter can be abnormally enlarged in cases of optic glioma, optic neuritis, or other inflammatory causes, while the nerve diameter can be decreased in cases of acquired optic neuropathy or congenital hypoplasia such as in septo-optic dysplasia (SOD) (Figs. 3.18, 3.19, 3.20, 3.21, 3.22, 3.23, 3.24, 3.25, and 3.26).

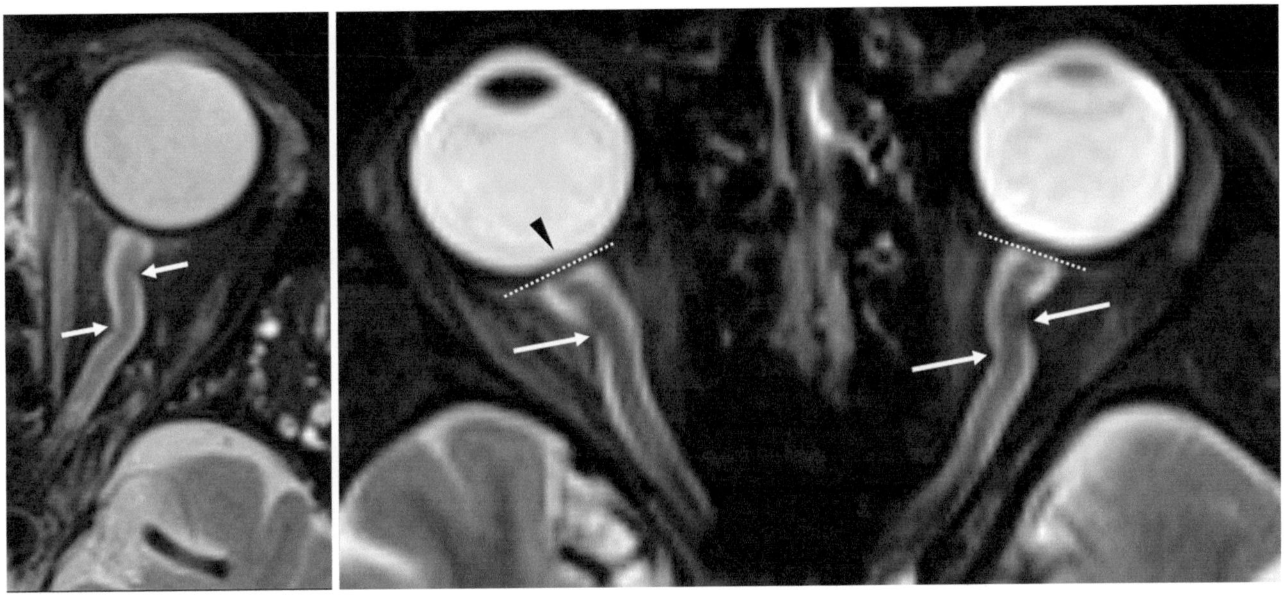

Fig. 3.18 Axial FS-SET2WI of two different patients with tortuosity of the optic nerve sheath complexes in the axial/horizontal plane. **Left**: In a 78-year-old male with right optic atrophy clinically (not evident radiologically) and normal CSF opening pressure, axial FS-SET2WI MRI demonstrates kinking of the left optic nerve sheath (*arrows*), a nonspecific finding in isolation. **Right**: Comparison case of idiopathic intracranial hypertension (IIH). On axial FS-SET2WI MRI, a 20-year-old female with IIH (aka pseudotumor cerebri) has kinking of the optic nerve sheaths bilaterally (*solid arrows*) and posterior scleral flattening (*dotted lines*) with slight bulging of the right optic disc (*black arrowhead*) typical of IIH. There were corroborative findings of elevated intracranial pressure on lumbar puncture. Hence, tortuosity of the optic nerve sheath in and of itself is nonspecific and is not necessarily abnormal if there are no findings of globe or optic nerve abnormalities

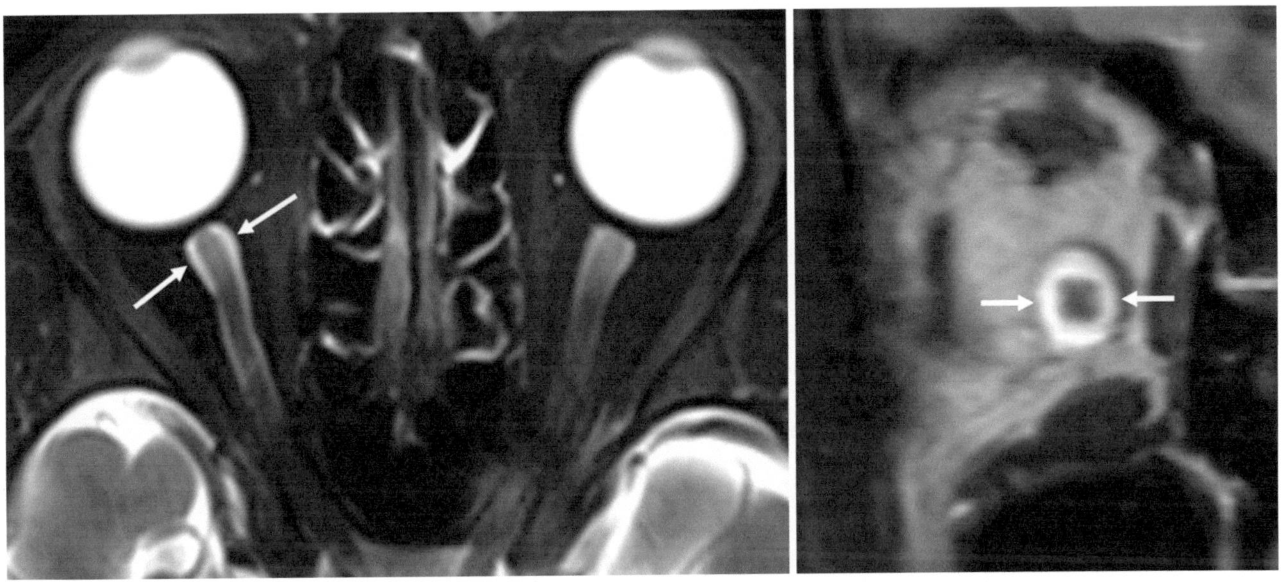

Fig. 3.19 An MRI with axial FS-SET2WI (*left*) and a coronal T2WI non-FS section through the level of the bulbar segment of the right optic nerve (*right*) of a 17-year-old male with no clinical suspicion of elevated intracranial pressure (history of developmental delay and no visual symptoms) demonstrates fluid distention of the optic nerve sheath and enlarged optic nerve sheath diameter (*sheath outlined by arrows*) measuring up to 8.5 mm, which is well above reported normal ranges. Thus, solitary mild distention of the optic nerve sheath without corresponding globe abnormalities or other radiologic findings or clinical symptoms can be considered a "don't touch lesion"

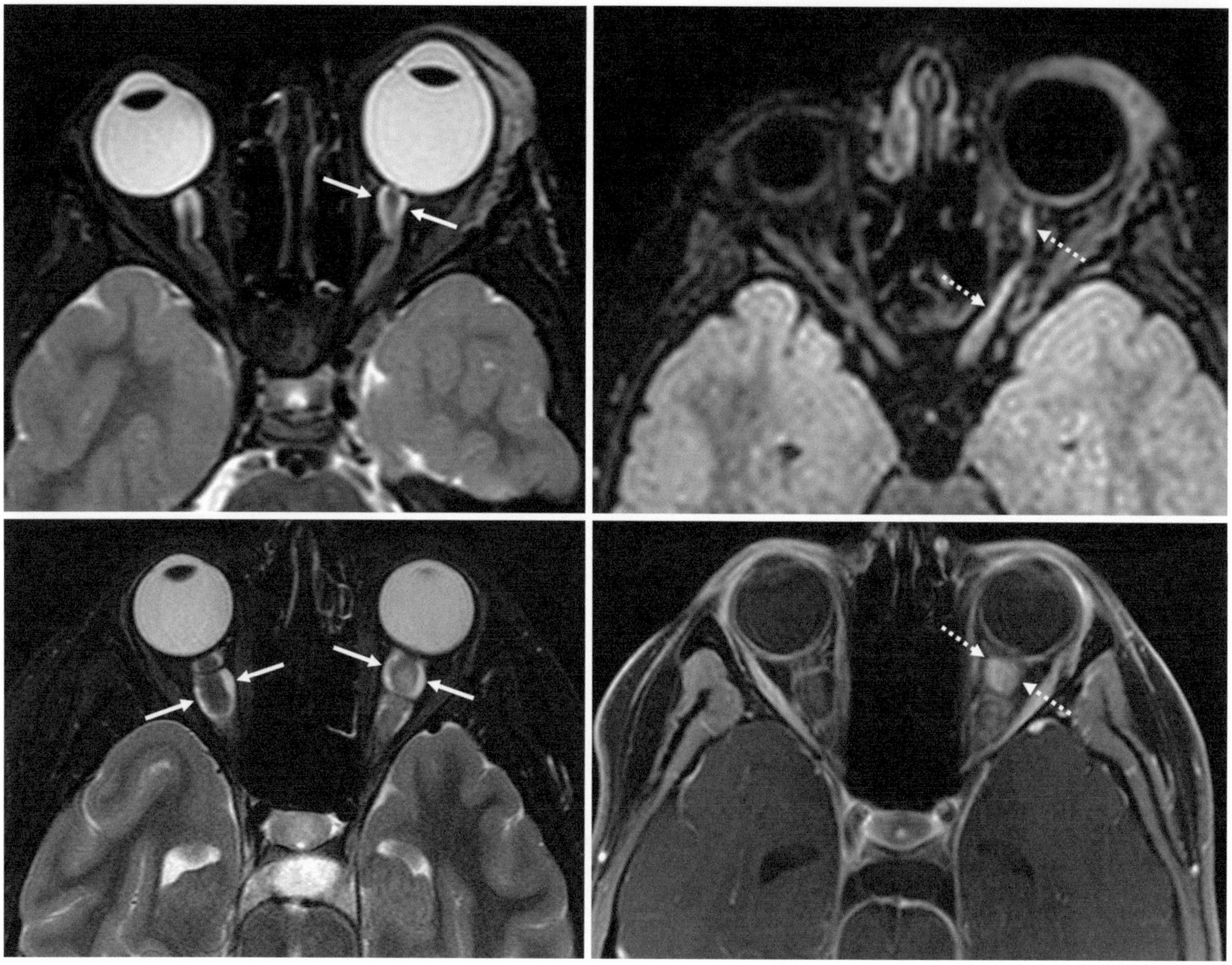

Fig. 3.20 Comparison cases of neurofibromatosis type 1 (NF-1) with optic sheath distention and tortuosity in two different patients. **Top row**: In a 5-year-old male on 3T MRI with axial FS-SET2WI (*left*) and FS-FLAIR (*right*), there is dilatation of the left optic nerve sheath (*outlined by arrows, left*), hyperintensity with mild enlargement of the left optic nerve from a subtle optic glioma (*dotted arrows, right*), and bupthalmos (enlarged globe), consistent with NF-1. **Bottom row**: In a 13-year-old female with NF-1 on 3T MRI with axial FS-SET2WI (*left*) and postcontrast FS-SET1WI (*right*) there is dilatation/distention of the optic sheaths bilaterally (*outlined by arrows, left*) and enlargement of both optic nerves but abnormal enhancement of only the left optic nerve (*dotted arrows, right*). This case demonstrates that optic gliomas, present bilaterally in this patient, may or may not enhance with contrast

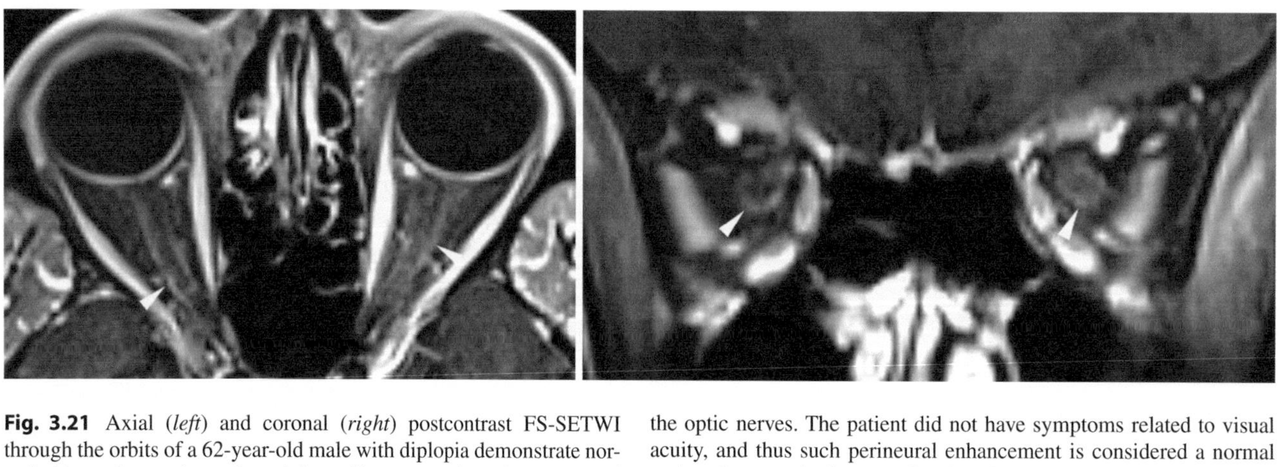

Fig. 3.21 Axial (*left*) and coronal (*right*) postcontrast FS-SETWI through the orbits of a 62-year-old male with diplopia demonstrate normal, thin, and near-circumferential curvilinear vascular enhancement of both optic nerve sheaths (*arrowheads*), with absence of enhancement in the optic nerves. The patient did not have symptoms related to visual acuity, and thus such perineural enhancement is considered a normal variant because it does not involve the optic nerves more centrally within the sheaths

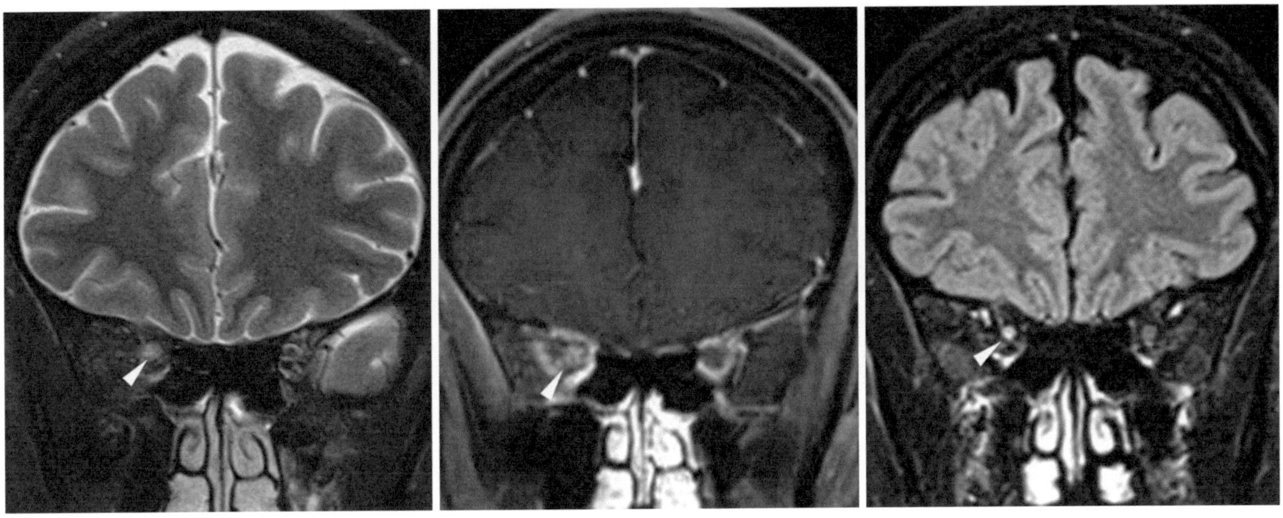

Fig. 3.22 Comparison case of isolated optic neuritis and ensuing optic neuropathy. In a 43-year-old female with sudden vision loss (later confirmed not to have multiple sclerosis or white matter lesions on MRI), an MRI demonstrated right optic nerve edema/swelling (*arrowheads*) on coronal FS-SET2WI (*left*) and enhancement on postcontrast FS-SET1WI (*middle*) consistent with optic nerve inflammation (i.e., acute optic neuritis). On a clinical follow-up 6 months later, the patient had improved but residual visual symptoms, while an MRI at that time demonstrated residual hyperintense signal and faint enhancement within the right optic nerve on coronal postcontrast FS-FLAIR (*right*); this was consistent with subsequent optic neuropathy as a sequela of the prior acute episode of optic neuritis

Fig. 3.23 Comparison case of orbital fibromatosis. Coronal postcontrast FS-SETWI of a 44-year-old male with orbital fibromatosis (biopsy proven) demonstrates pathologic thick, eccentric, mass-like left optic perineural enhancement (*arrowheads*), with involvement of the retrobulbar fat and associated inferior displacement of the left optic nerve (*arrows*) relative to the normal right optic nerve (*dashed arrows*)

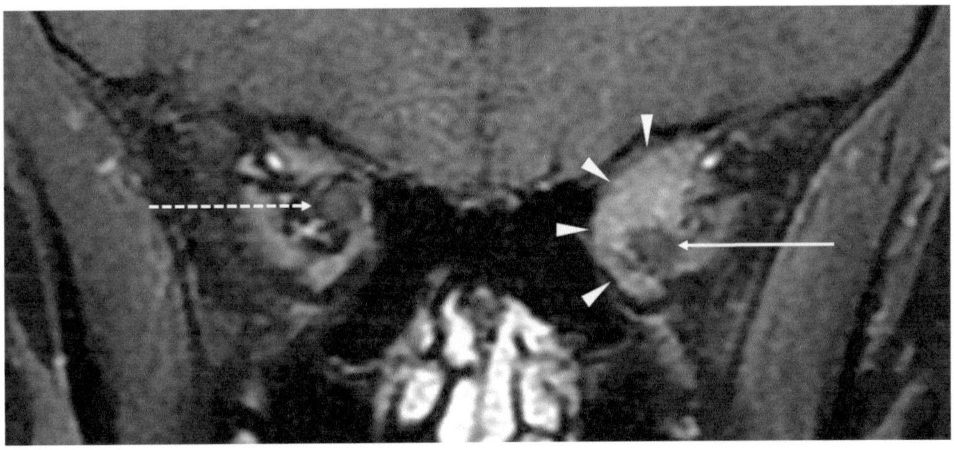

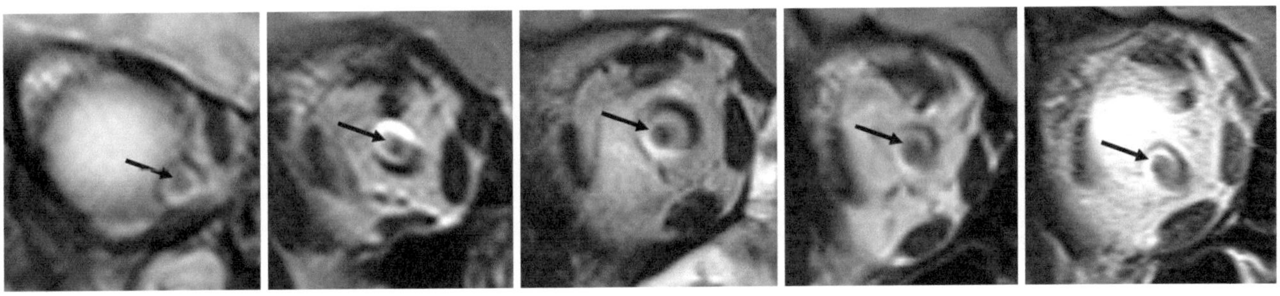

Fig. 3.24 Coronal T2WIs through the right orbit demonstrating normal retrobulbar segment optic nerve diameters (*arrows*) that normally slowly increase in size with patients of ascending age (*from left to right*): 5-day-old male (1.6 mm), 18-month-old female (2.3 mm), 3-year-old female (2.5 mm), 9-year-old male (2.5 mm), and 19 year old male (3.1 mm)

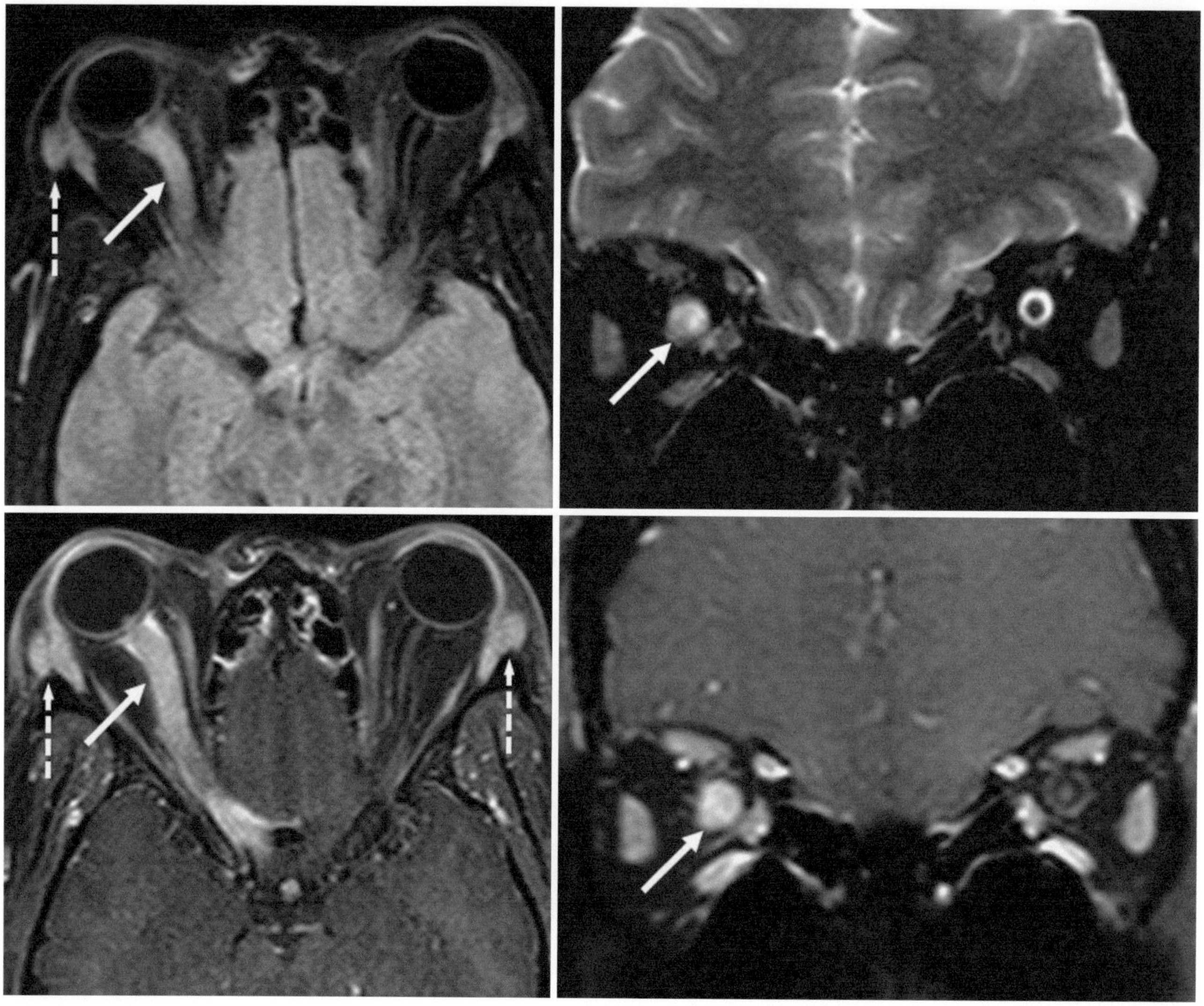

Fig. 3.25 Comparison case of optic and lacrimal sarcoidosis. A 38-year-old female with progressive visual loss on the right side underwent MRI. **Top row**: Noncontrast axial FLAIR (*left*) and FS-SET2WI (*right*) demonstrated moderate to severe enlargement and edema of the right optic nerve (*arrows*) measuring 7 mm in diameter; the right lacrimal gland also appears enlarged (*dashed arrows, left*). **Bottom row**: Postcontrast axial (*left*) and coronal (*right*) FS-SET1WI confirmed enhancement of the enlarged right optic nerve (*arrows*) as well as both lacrimal glands (*dashed arrows, left*). In order to evaluate for tumor, biopsy was performed of the optic nerve, and the pathology was confirmed to be sarcoidosis; notably, no lymphadenopathy was present in the cervical, thoracic, or abdominopelvic regions in this patient

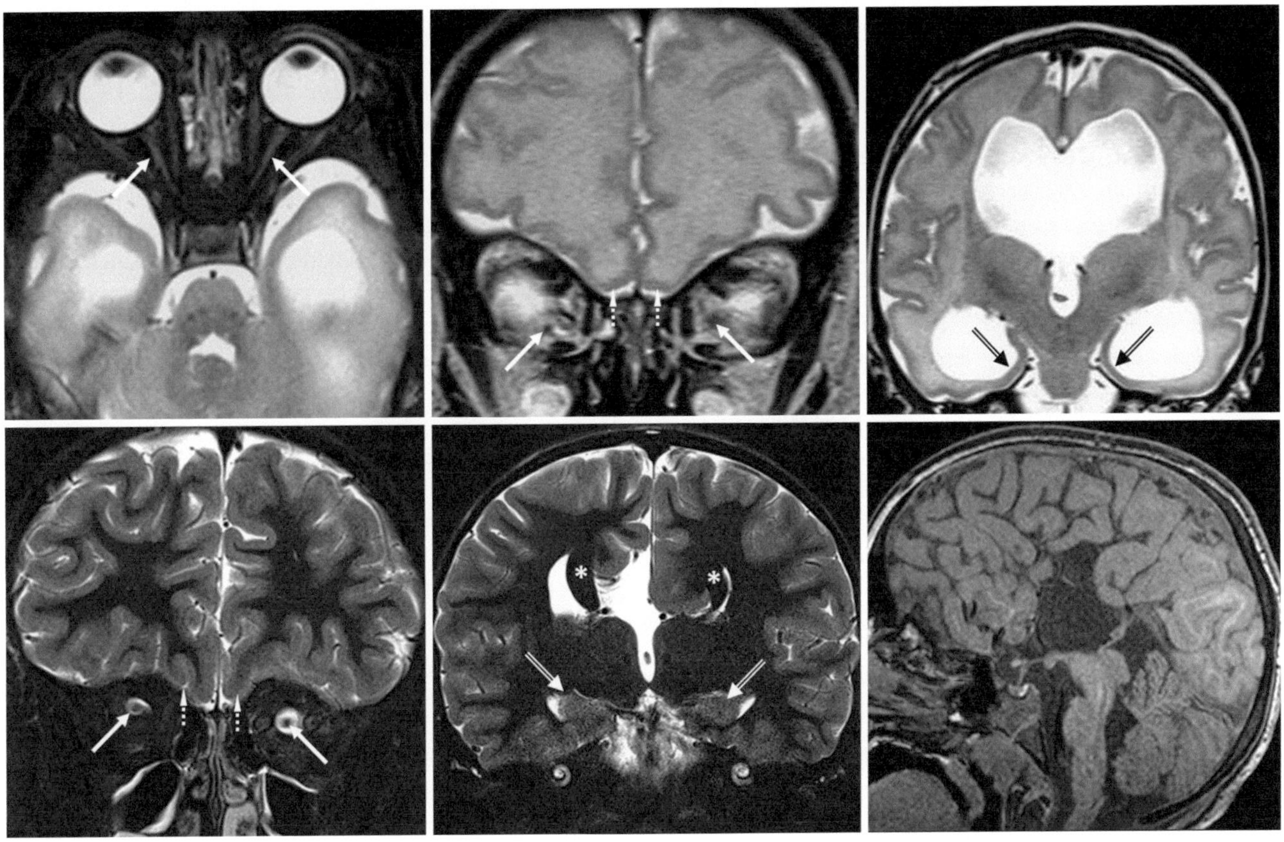

Fig. 3.26 Comparison cases of optic hypoplasia in two different patients with septo-optic dysplasia (SOD). **Top row**: In a 1-day-old neonate with SOD, axial (*left*) and coronal (*middle, right*) SET2WIs show that both optic nerves are tiny (*arrows*), being smaller on the right side, with lack of the olfactory bulbs or sulci (*small dotted arrows, middle*) and lack of the septum pellucidum; there are also bilateral severe hippocampal malformations/malrotations (*beveled arrows, right*). **Bottom row**: In an 8-year-old male with SOD, coronal FS-SET2WI MRI (*left, middle*) demonstrates that both optic nerves (*arrows, left*) are hypoplastic (the left being smaller than the right); the left olfactory sulcus is also hypoplastic as compared to the normal right side (*small dotted arrows, left*) and there are Probst bundles (*asterisks, middle*) typical of callosal agenesis. Note the normal hippocampi (*beveled arrows, middle*) as well as characteristic findings of callosal agenesis on sagittal gradient-echo T1-weighted imaging (GET1WI) (*right*)

3.6 Orbital Calcifications

Asymptomatic or benign *orbital calcifications* are common incidental findings. Familiarity with their characteristic appearance and locations is important because it allows distinction from radiopaque intraorbital foreign bodies. Confident exclusion of a retained metallic intraorbital foreign body is especially critical in the setting of screening prior to an MRI examination (which may require a minimum of an anteroposterior plain film for confirmation), since these can potentially lead to optic nerve or globe injury. Retinoblastoma, orbital vascular malformations, lacrimal apparatus tumors, optic nerve sheath meningiomas, and metastatic disease may also have associated calcifications, although each of these pathologies demonstrate some degree of soft tissue or vascular component and should be readily discernable from isolated orbital calcification.

3.6.1 Trochlear Calcifications

The trochlear apparatus is a hook-shaped cartilaginous sleeve that contains the superior oblique muscle tendon and its synovium-lined sheath. Incidental *trochlear calcifications* have been identified in 12–16% of asymptomatic patients and may be either unilateral or bilateral. Trochlear calcifications demonstrate a punctate or rounded appearance and measure in the range of 1–4 mm. The exact site of calcification within the apparatus has not been well characterized. While an early study suggested the possibility of an association of the presence of trochlear calcifications with advanced age, diabetes mellitus, and hypertension, subsequent larger population-based studies have contradicted this hypothesis. Trochlear calcifications demonstrate a bimodal peak distribution occurring in the second and fourth decades, while are not typically being present in pediatric patients less than 15 years old, and are thus likely acquired.

3.6.2 Drusen

Optic nerve head *drusen* occur along the surface of the optic disc within the posterior globe. These represent calcified hyaline bodies, thought to be byproducts of axonal degeneration. Optic nerve head drusen may be superficial and evident on funduscopic examination and may mimic optic nerve head edema, so-called "pseudo-papilledema." Calcified drusen are present in 3% of asymptomatic patients, although they increase in prevalence with age and are associated with age-related macular degeneration.

3.6.3 Senile Scleral Plaques

Calcified *senile scleral plaques* demonstrate a similar appearance, although they occur within the wall of the anterior globe at sites of focal senile thinning near the insertion of medial and lateral rectus muscles. Scleral plaques in this location are essentially nearly always asymptomatic and have been demonstrated to be present in 6% of patients, although they are associated with increased age. Calcified scleral plaques within the posterior globe or remote from sites of muscle insertion anteriorly may be the result of a prior scleral inflammatory process or hypercalcemic state. Calcified scleral plaques may be easily confirmed by slit-lamp examination, during which they demonstrate an associated characteristic grey scleral discoloration.

3.6.4 Arterial Atherosclerosis

Arterial atherosclerotic calcifications of the ophthalmic arteries are less commonly seen and are associated with typical vascular risk factors such as hypertension, diabetes, and end-stage renal disease. As with elsewhere in the body, atherosclerotic calcifications have a characteristic curvilinear appearance along the expected course of an artery. While these are not normal, they are considered "don't touch" lesions (Figs. 3.27, 3.28, 3.29, 3.30, and 3.31).

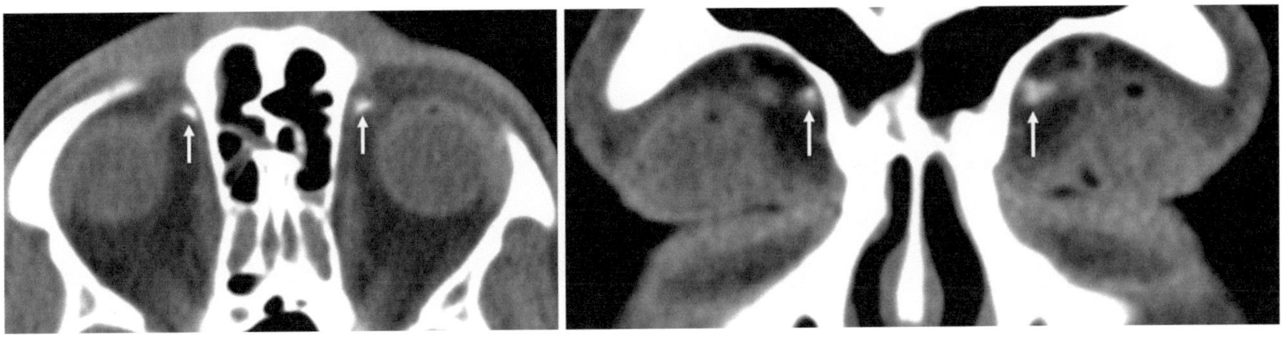

Fig. 3.27 Axial (*left*) and coronal (*right*) NECT images of a 43-year-old male (imaged because of concern for sinusitis) demonstrate incidental bilateral trochlear calcifications (*arrows*)

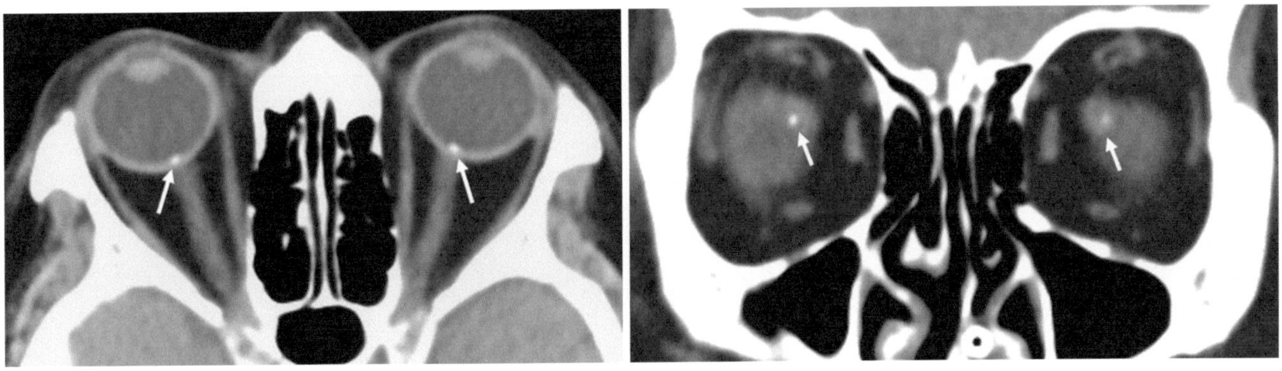

Fig. 3.28 Axial (*left*) and coronal (*right*) NECT of a 63-year-old female with altered mental status demonstrates incidental punctate calcified drusen at the optic nerve heads bilaterally (*arrows*)

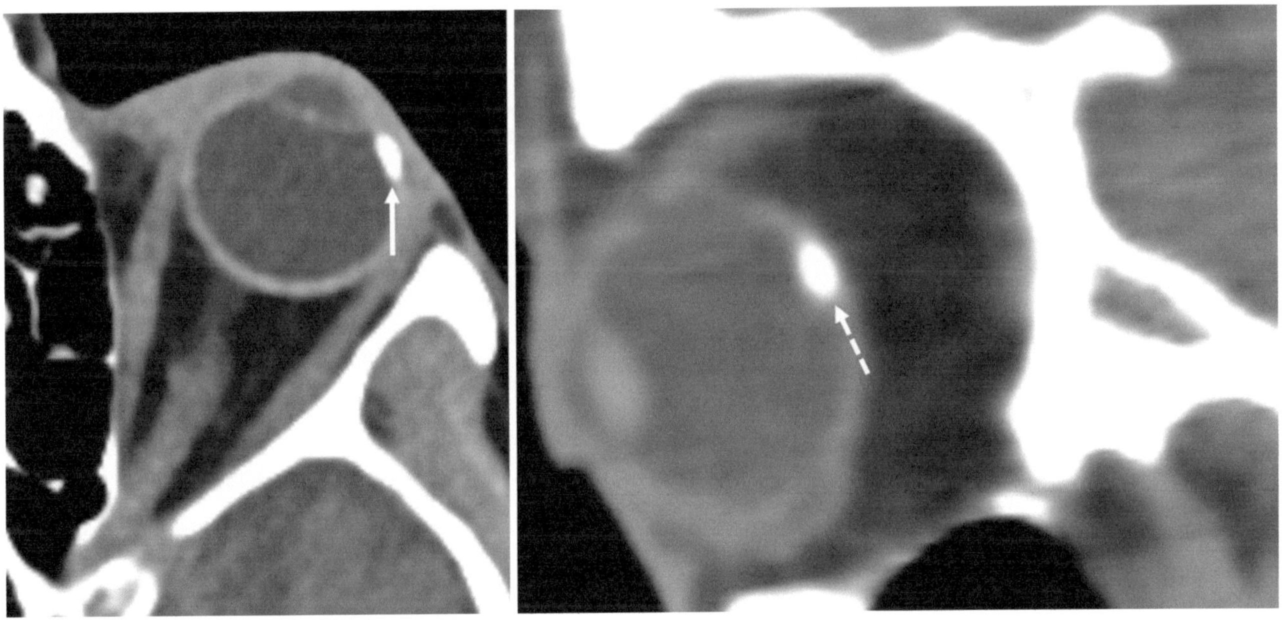

Fig. 3.29 Scleral plaques in two separate patients. **Left**: An axial (*left*) NECT of an 85-year-old female with acute cerebral infarct demonstrates incidental calcified scleral plaque in the typical location anterior to the insertion of the left lateral rectus muscle (*solid arrow*). **Right**: In a different patient, on a sagittal reformatted NECT (*right*), a 69-year-old male has scleral plaque in a less common location at the posterior temporal aspect of the right globe (*dashed arrow*)

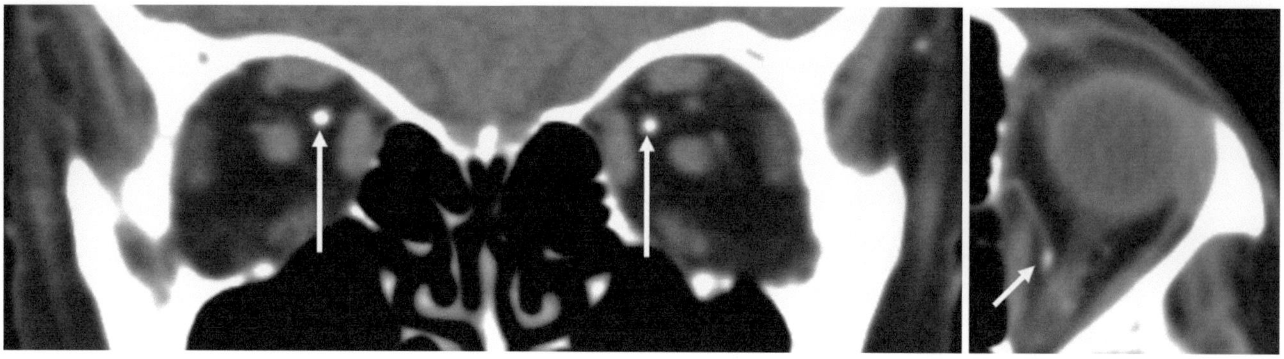

Fig. 3.30 Coronal (*left*) and axial (*right*) reconstructions of a NECT in an 80-year-old female with altered mental status demonstrates atherosclerotic calcifications of the ophthalmic arteries bilaterally (*arrows*). This patient had a history of type 1 diabetes mellitus complicated by advanced atherosclerotic disease, which required multiple arterial bypass surgeries

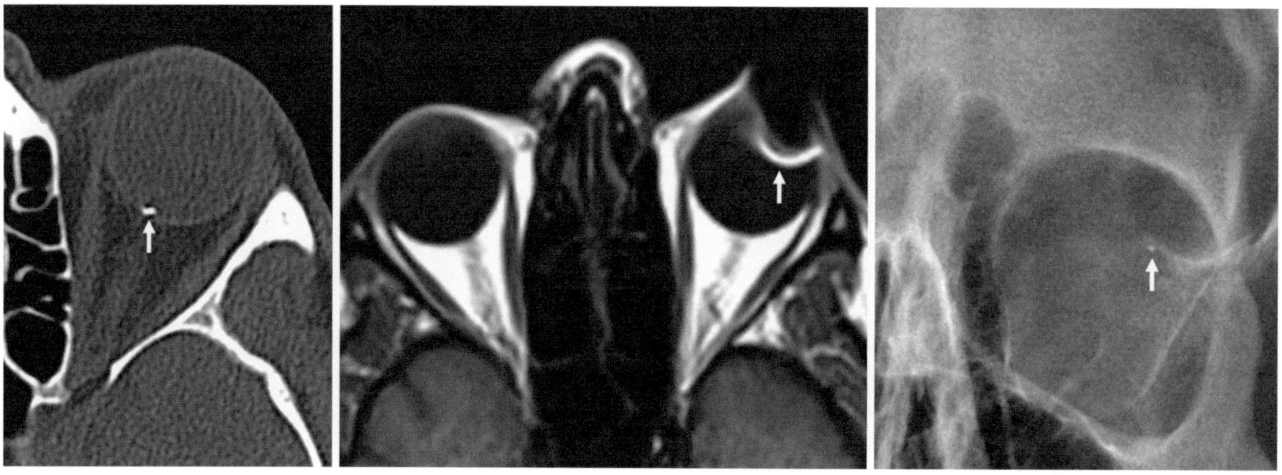

Fig. 3.31 Comparison cases in two patients of retained orbital metallic foreign bodies. **Left**: In a 50-year-old male who experienced sudden onset of left ocular pain while hammering a nail, axial NECT demonstrates an intraocular retained metallic density foreign body in the left vitreous near the optic nerve head. Note the linear morphology and increased density (*arrow*) with associated subtle streak artifact (tiny areas of darker density both anterior and posterior to the dense foreign body), which help to distinguish this foreign body from an optic nerve head drusen. **Middle and right**: In a different 57-year-old male imaged for facial pain, an MR screening form was negative for implants or metal exposure (such as welding), but susceptibility artifact (*arrows*) was noted overlying the anterior left globe on routine 1.5T MRI SET1WI (*middle*), and the patient complained of some feeling of heat in the orbit after that sequence. The patient was removed from the MRI scanner and a subsequent anteroposterior plain film (*right*) revealed a punctate, less than 1 mm sized metallic foreign body (*arrows*) of the left orbit

3.7 Orbital Venous System

3.7.1 Superior Ophthalmic Vein Asymmetry and Enlargement

The majority of the venous drainage from the orbit occurs via the superior ophthalmic vein, which is readily identifiable on routine cross-sectional CT or MR imaging. The superior ophthalmic vein courses medial to lateral within the orbit along the undersurface of the superior rectus muscle, receiving inflow from facial cutaneous veins via the supraorbital foramen and draining centrally into the cavernous sinuses via the superior orbital fissure. The mean diameter of the superior ophthalmic vein has been reported as 1.7 mm, although diameters may vary widely, ranging from 0.3 to 4.6 mm, with asymmetry present in up to 75% of the normal population. Pathologic unilateral enlargement of the superior ophthalmic vein can be seen in the setting of vascular shunts/malformations, venous thrombosis (e.g., cavernous sinus thrombosis), and inflammatory and neoplastic processes of the retrobulbar and paracavernous regions. The superior ophthalmic vein diameter has been shown to be positively correlated with CSF pressures, although vein diameters of patients with elevated intracranial pressure overlap with normative measurements. Thus, superior ophthalmic vein asymmetry and dilatation can be a normal variation but should merit attention for potential ancillary findings of pathologic increased venous pressure to exclude vascular pathology. When in question, MR or CT angiography or venography and dedicated pre- and postcontrast MR imaging of the orbits and cavernous sinuses can help elucidate or exclude such pathology.

3.7.2 Inferior Ophthalmic Venous Plexus

Compared to the superior orbital venous system, the inferior orbital venous system is highly variable and diminutive. On gross dissection of the orbit, approximately 30% of inferior ophthalmic veins, the dominant vein of the inferior orbital venous system, have been described as atretic, and hence likely a normal variation. Accordingly, the inferior ophthalmic venous plexus is much less commonly identified by cross-sectional imaging, and thus its presence as a normal variation may be misconstrued as a pathologic process. The inferior ophthalmic venous plexus starts as a network at the front floor of the orbit medially, and it drains posteriorly to combine with veins from the inferior rectus and oblique muscles and the lacrimal sac to become the inferior ophthalmic vein posteriorly. When present, the inferior ophthalmic vein courses along the superior and lateral margins of the inferior rectus muscle and may curve upward in the posterior orbit near the annulus of Zinn to communicate with the superior ophthalmic vein or, alternatively, drain directly into the cavernous sinus.

3.7.3 Orbital Venous Varix

An orbital venous varix is an enlarged and possibly tortuous venous channel that communicates with the normal orbital venous system and is a vascular malformation that is thought to be congenital in origin and thus asymptomatic in most (primary type); alternatively, it may be related to another vascular malformation (secondary type). While orbital varices may occasionally result in symptomatic orbital hemorrhage, thrombosis, or proptosis, particularly if they are of the secondary type, primary varices may be detected incidentally in asymptomatic patients. Dedicated cross-sectional orbital imaging typically demonstrates the characteristic features, thereby eliminating suspicion of an aggressive process and obviating an invasive work-up. On cross-sectional MR or CT imaging, orbital varices appear as distensible tubular structures that demonstrate dynamic increases in size with prone positioning, Valsalva maneuver and progressive contrast filling after intravenous contrast administration. MR signal characteristics and contrast filling depend on the presence or degree of thrombosis. Thus, in most patients primary orbital varices are "don't touch" lesions, although dedicated postcontrast CT or MR imaging can exclude secondary varices related to intracranial vascular pathology such as carotid-cavernous fistula, dural arteriovenous fistula, or arteriovenous malformation (Figs. 3.32, 3.33, 3.34, and 3.35).

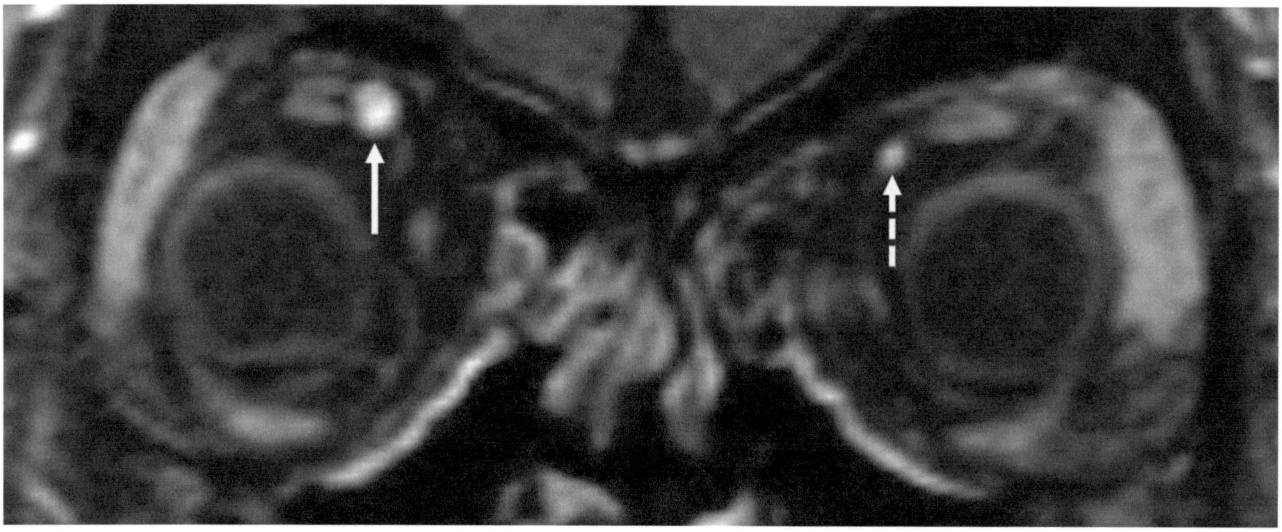

Fig. 3.32 Coronal postcontrast FS-SET1WI of a 54-year-old female with suspected ischemic neuropathy demonstrates normal variant asymmetry of the superior ophthalmic veins. The right superior ophthalmic vein (*arrow*) is approximately two to three times the diameter of the left superior ophthalmic vein (*dashed arrow*)

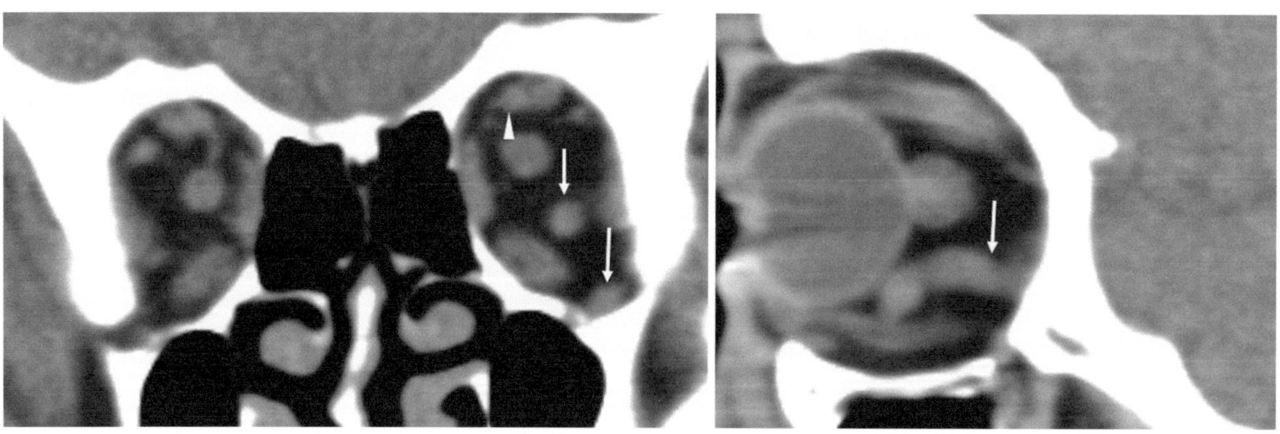

Fig. 3.33 Coronal (*left*) and sagittal (*right*) NECT reformats through the orbits of a 59-year-old male depict normal asymmetric distention of the left inferior ophthalmic venous plexus (*arrows*), which is enlarged relative to the typically dominant superior ophthalmic vein (*arrowhead, left*)

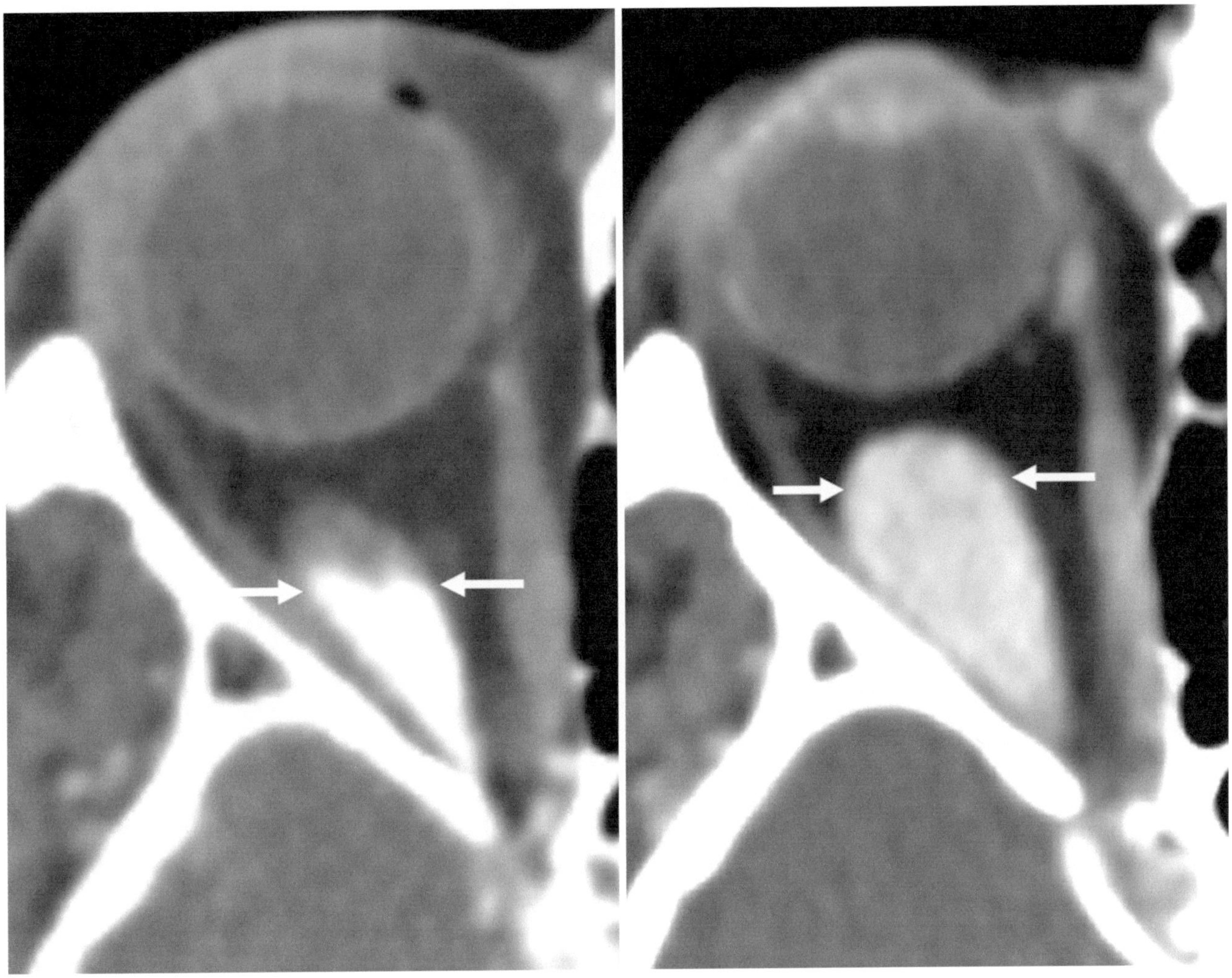

Fig. 3.34 Axial CTA (*left*) and 60-second delay CTV (*right*) images through the orbits in a 67-year-old female performed for characterization of an incidentally noted retrobulbar lesion on other imaging demonstrate a progressively enhancing and enlarging tubular structure within the right intraconal space (*arrows*) consistent with an orbital venous varix. This would be considered a primary (idiopathic or congenital) varix and is a "don't touch" lesion since the patient was asymptomatic

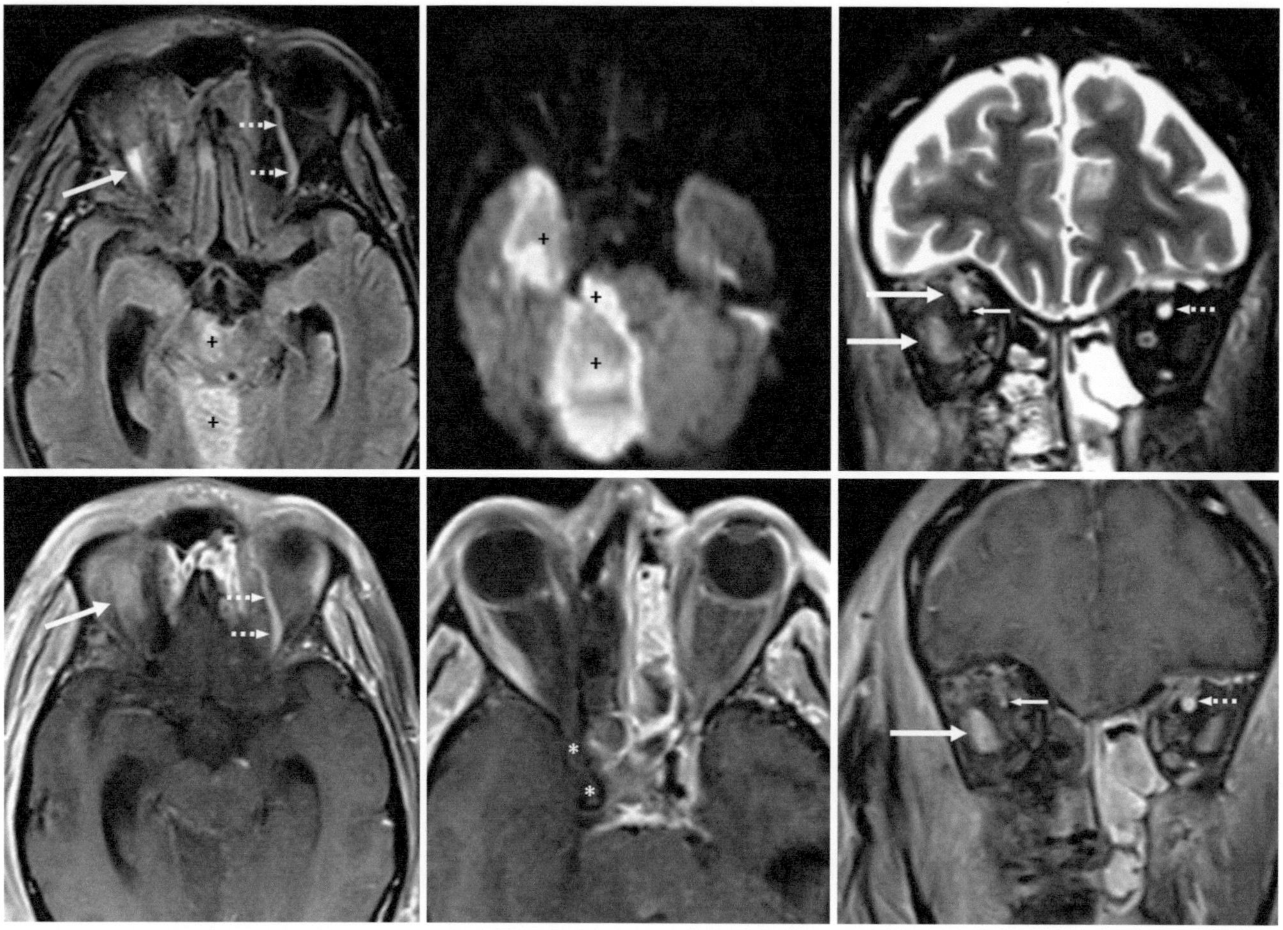

Fig. 3.35 Comparison case of cavernous sinus thrombosis from sinonasal mucormycosis. **Top row**: In a 36-year-old immunocompromised male on noncontrast 1.5T MRI there were findings of enlarged right superior and lateral rectus muscles (*arrows*), enlarged left superior ophthalmic vein (SOV, *dashed arrows*), and cerebral-brainstem infarcts (+), on axial FLAIR (*left*), DWI (*middle*), and coronal FS-SET2WI (*right*). The right SOV was very tiny (*tiny arrow, right*) and questioned as being either thrombosed or occluded. **Bottom row**: Given the above-mentioned findings, intravenous contrast was administered. This confirmed the SOV enlargement on the left side (*dashed arrows*) as compared to the SOV's being nearly occluded on the right (*tiny arrow, right*) as shown on postcontrast FS-SET1WI axial (*left, middle*) and coronal (*right*) images. Note the absence of expected contrast enhancement of the right cavernous sinus (*asterisks, middle*), with diffuse enlargement of the right temporal fossa musculature caused by impaired venous drainage. The cerebral infarcts were presumably related to direct extension from the diffuse sinusitis through the dura, and mucormycosis was confirmed on CSF analysis and surgical sinonasal decompression

3.8 Lacrimal Gland

3.8.1 Lacrimal Gland Size, Symmetry

The normal size of the *lacrimal glands* has been briefly described in the literature and varies widely, perhaps owing to a difference in cross-sectional imaging modality (e.g., CT versus MRI), technique/sequence (e.g., SET2WI versus SET1WI on MRI), and plane of imaging (e.g., axial versus coronal plane of measurement). Ranges of normal-sized lacrimal glands have been described as varying from approximately 10–20 mm in 90% of the population (they measure slightly larger on coronal imaging due to the gland's dimensions usually being greatest in the craniocaudal plane), which may differ slightly between men and women. There is expected gradual decrease in lacrimal gland size with normal aging. A senescent change in the MRI signal of the lacrimal gland may occur, in which increasing T1 signal and decreasing T2 signal have been described with advancing age. However, to represent a decreasing fluid content leading to a relative "desiccation" of the gland in the elderly may be the reason for keratoconjunctivitis sicca in the elderly population. Typically, there is symmetry in the size of the glands between sides, although minimal asymmetry in size may occur, which can be a normal variant. The glands should enhance on postcontrast T1WI, but the degree of enhancement varies. Hence, the size of the lacrimal glands and even the signal may vary, depending on age, gender, and cross-sectional imaging technique. Some general rules are proposed here to discern normal from abnormal glands: (1) the glands should be relatively similar in size, (2) they should not measure much larger than 2 cm in maximum size, and (3) the glands should have relatively well-defined margins. Therefore an enlarged, asymmetric gland may be of concern for the presence of a tumor (such as a pleiomorphic adenoma, lymphoma, carcinoma/adenocarcinoma, or metastasis), inflammatory disease (such as sarcoidosis), or an infectious process (such as dacryoadenitis or abscess). Careful evaluation of the surrounding structures and the remainder of the face/neck can aid in confirmation.

3.8.2 Lacrimal Gland Cyst

Lacrimal gland cyst, also known as dacryops, is an epithelial-lined fluid-filled cyst within normal lacrimal glandular tissue. It is an uncommon and benign entity that may be incidentally noted on cross-sectional imaging, or alternatively present as a painless superior lid mass. Hence, these are usually "don't touch" lesions. Lacrimal gland cysts have been reported in the post-inflammatory setting, although they may be idiopathic. On cross-sectional imaging, the cyst appears as a nonenhancing, well-circumscribed, thin-walled focus of simple fluid. Occasionally, these cysts may occur within sites of ectopic lacrimal tissue in the orbit. Lacrimal gland cysts may be clinically observed, although surgical excision is typically curative when necessary. These should be distinguished from lacrimal gland neoplasm, phlegmon, or abscess, which typically occur in an asymmetrically enlarged gland (Figs. 3.36, 3.37, and 3.38).

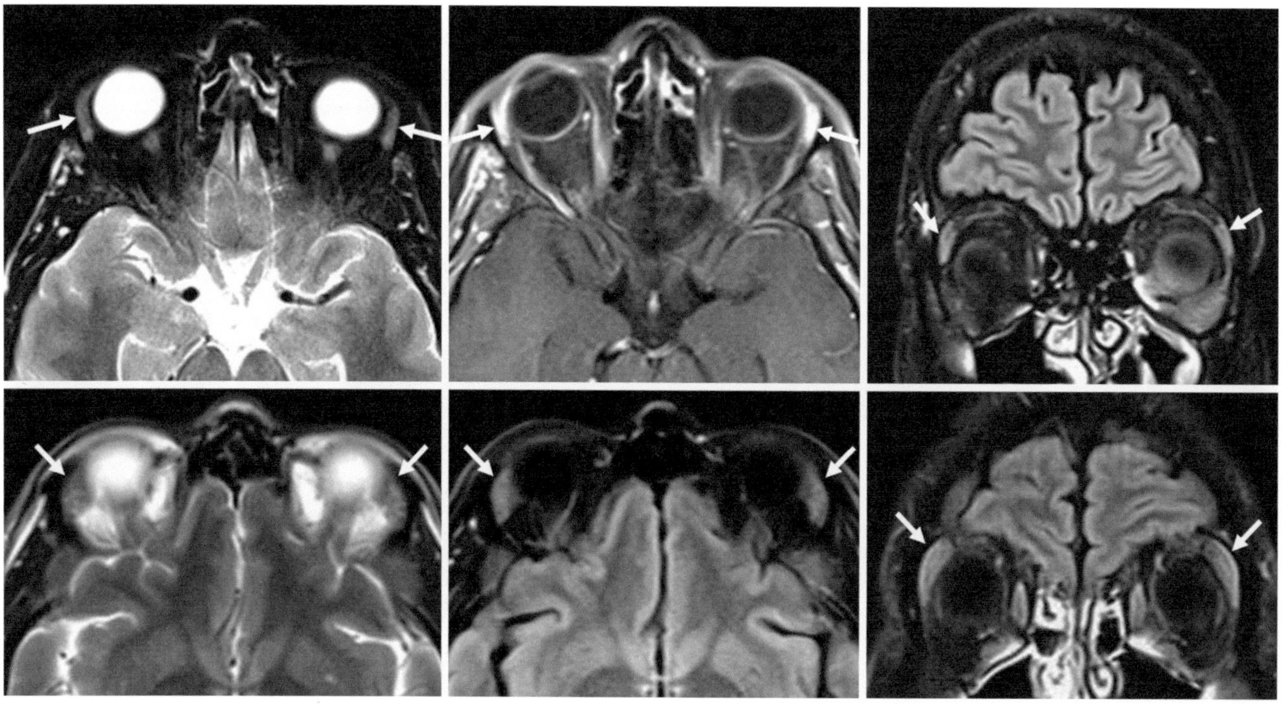

Fig. 3.36 Two different patients illustrating a typical lacrimal gland size and symmetric but prominent glands. **Top row**: In a 23-year-old male with an MRI for headaches, the lacrimal glands (*arrows*) are symmetric and typical in size, measuring 11 mm (craniocaudal) × 5 mm (transverse thickness) × 11 mm (anteroposteriorly), as visualized on axial FS-SET2WI (*left*), axial postcontrast FS-SET1WI (*middle*), and postcontrast FS-FLAIR (*right*). **Bottom row**: In a 43-year- old male with headaches, the lacrimal glands are bilaterally the upper limit of normal in size on MRI, being 21 mm (craniocaudal) × 9 mm (transversely) × 19 mm (anteroposteriorly). This was visualized on axial non-FS-SET2WI (*left*), axial noncontrast FLAIR (*middle*), and postcontrast FS-FLAIR (*right*). These two patients demonstrate a range of normal, symmetric gland size

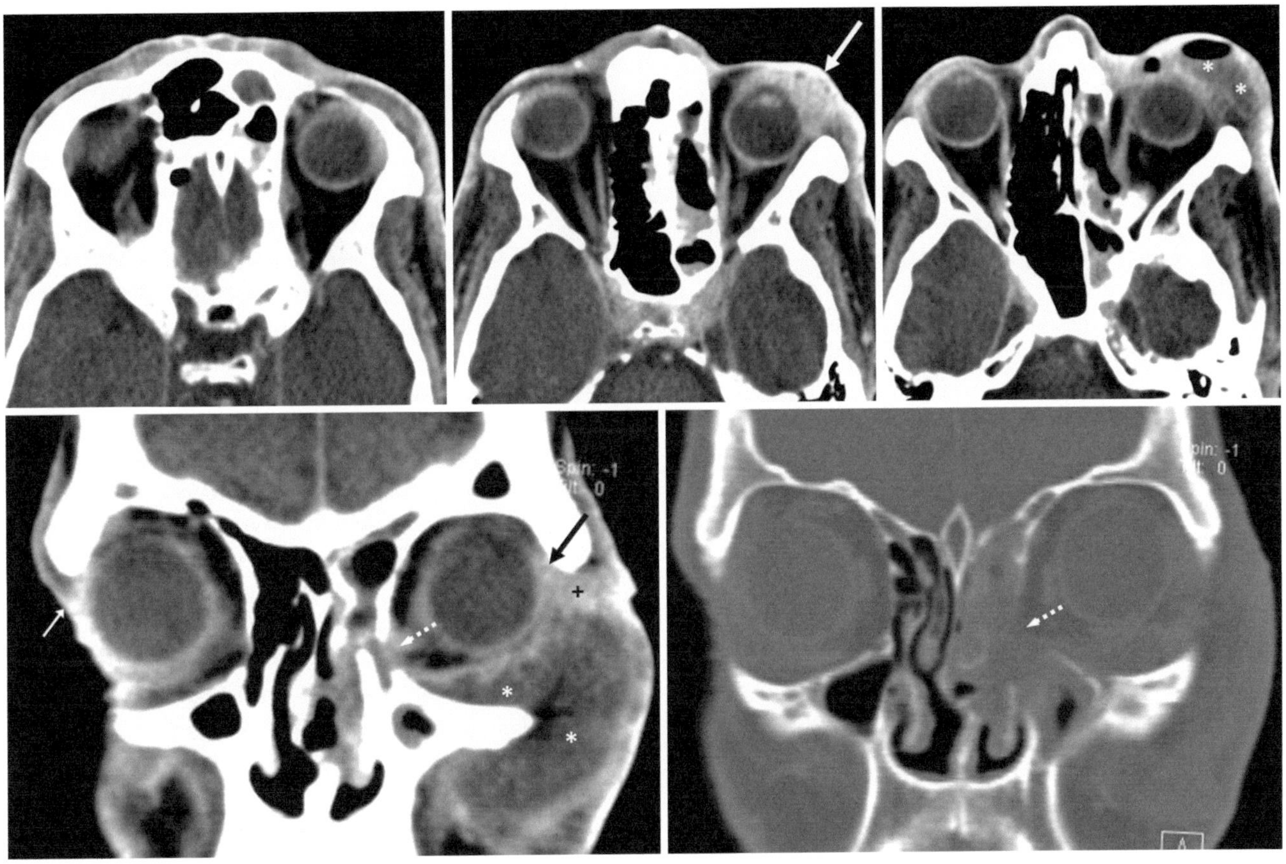

Fig. 3.37 Comparison case of lacrimal gland infection by orbital cellulitis and abscess. **Top row**: In a 47-year-old male, clinically evident left preseptal cellulitis was refractory to therapy and extended into the lateral orbital extraconal space on serial axial CECT images. Note the enlarged/infected lacrimal gland (*arrow, middle*) and preseptal abscess with air-fluid level (*asterisks, right*). **Bottom row**: CECT coronal reformats with soft-tissue (*left*) and bone (*right*) windows demonstrate that the abscess (*asterisks, left*) extended into the inferior orbital extraconal space as well; the enhancing phlegmonous tract (*plus sign, left*) leading to the infected lacrimal gland (*arrow, left*) is also demonstrated. The CECT bone window (*right*) was able to depict the left medial orbital wall/lamina papyracea defect (*dotted arrows*) that was the source of the orbital infection from sinusitis (not from preseptal cellulitis as clinically suspected). Note the normal right lacrimal gland (*thin arrow, left*)

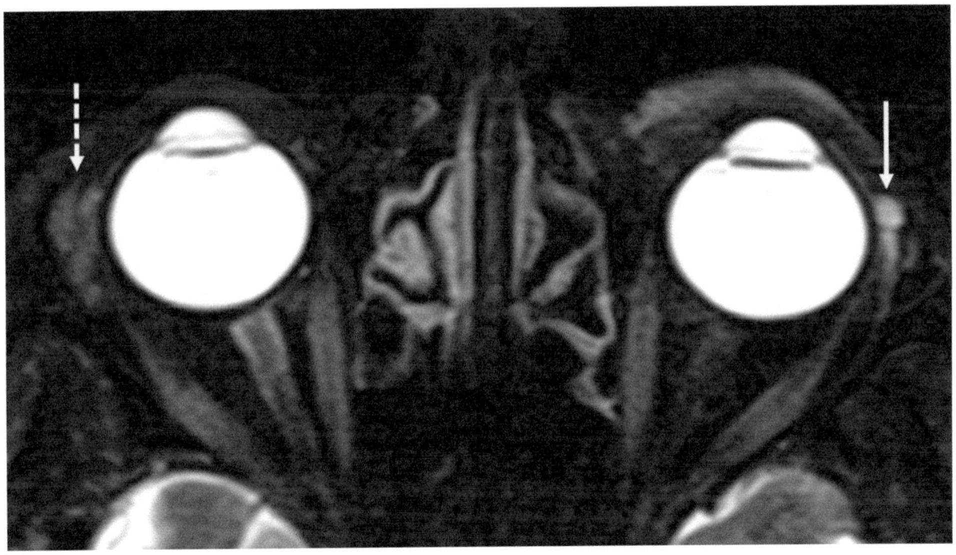

Fig. 3.38 Axial FS-SET2WI of an 80-year-old male with an incidentally noted small well-circumscribed cystic T2 hyperintense focus centered in the left lacrimal gland (*solid arrow*), being consistent with a lacrimal gland cyst. Note the normal right lacrimal gland (*dashed arrow*) for comparison

3.9 Nasolacrimal Duct

3.9.1 Opacification/Aeration and Size/Morphology

Tears that are produced by the secretory lacrimal system track medially across the surfaces of the globe and eyelids into the medial canthus, where outflow occurs via the lacrimal drainage apparatus. Tears descend from the lacrimal sac through the *nasolacrimal duct* into the nasal cavity, where they exit via the inferior nasal meatus just below the inferior nasal turbinate.

The lacrimal sac is contiguous with the nasolacrimal duct on conventional cross-sectional imaging, but it may be identified using bony landmarks located in the lacrimal fossa bounded anteriorly by the anterior lacrimal crest of the maxilla and posteriorly by the posterior lacrimal crest of the lacrimal bone. Either aeration or opacification of the nasolacrimal sac/duct complex may be seen in normal asymptomatic patients. Opacification is more commonly seen, occurring in up to 70% of patients, although this predominance may be related to supine positioning during scanning. Opacification of the nasolacrimal duct appears as nonspecific soft-tissue density on CT. On MRI, normal opacification demonstrates near fluid bright T2 hyperintense signal, whereas low to intermediate T2 signal suggests complex debris or tumor.

The nasolacrimal ducts are symmetric structures with a parallel course and shape, varying from oval to round. Because of the posterior slope of the bony canal, the anteroposterior diameter of the canal can be exaggerated in the axial plane. The normal minimal diameter of the nasolacrimal canal ranges from 1.5 to 6.3 mm (mean 3.5 mm). It has been postulated that narrowing of the osseous nasolacrimal canal may contribute to impaired tear drainage, although patients with symptomatic epiphora demonstrate bony canal diameters within the normal range. The nasolacrimal canal diameter does not vary significantly with age, race, or gender. However, an increase in nasolacrimal canal length proportional to height results in larger nasolacrimal canal volumes in males relative to females. Asymmetric enlargement and remodeling of the nasolacrimal canal is not typical and should raise suspicion of an underlying mass or obstructive process (Figs. 3.39, 3.40, and 3.41).

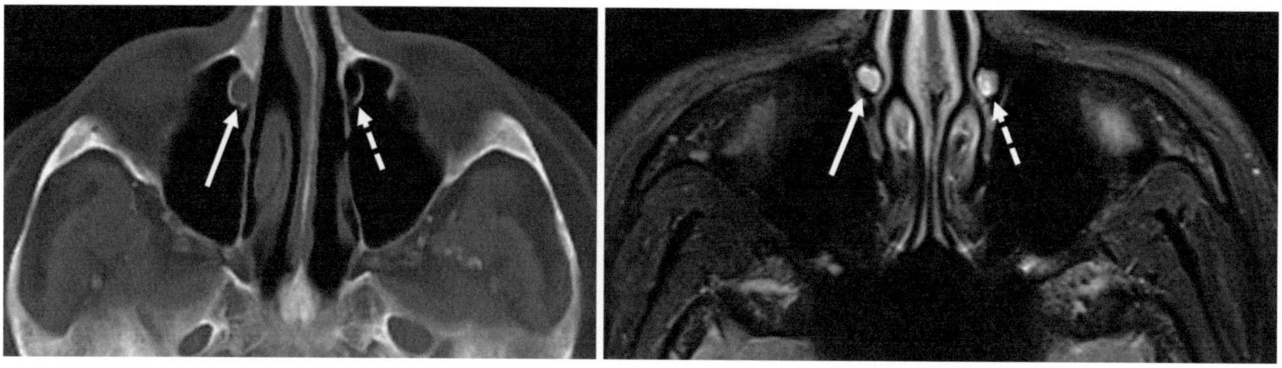

Fig. 3.39 In a 40-year-old male with a suspected stroke, axial NECT (*left*) demonstrates normal opacification of the right nasolacrimal duct (*arrows*) and aeration of the left nasolacrimal duct (*dashed arrows*). Axial FS-SET2WI MRI (*right*) performed later the same day demonstrates near-fluid T2 bright signal filling and opacifying the nasolacrimal ducts both on the right (*arrows*) and left (*dashed arrows*) sides. This case demonstrates how the nasolacrimal duct can normally be variably filled with air or fluid

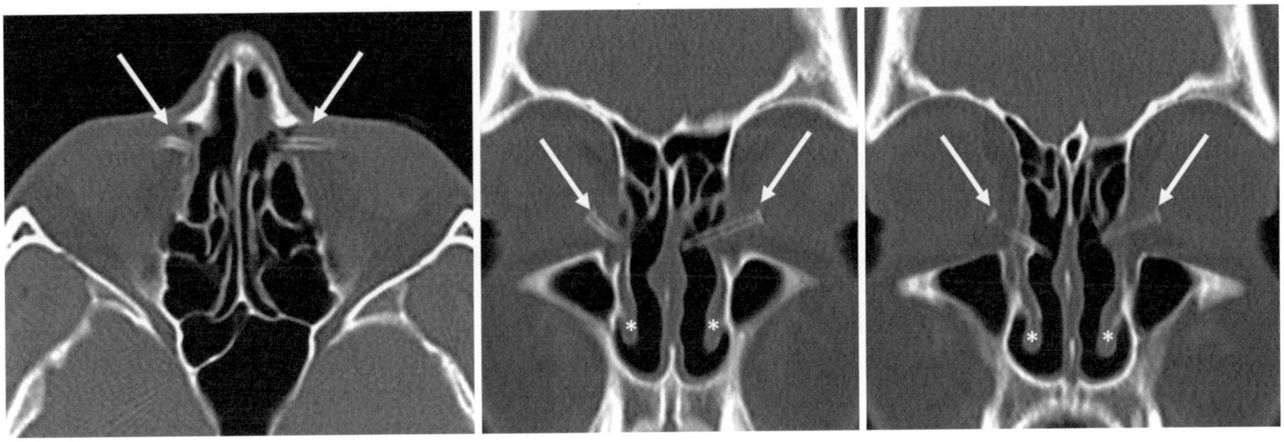

Fig. 3.40 Nasolacrimal duct stents/drains (*arrows*) are present bilaterally on NECT in a 34-year-old female with headaches and a feeling of orbital pressure, as shown on axial (*left*) and coronal (*middle, right*) reformats. Note that while the nasolacrimal ducts normally drain *below* the inferior turbinates (*asterisks*), the stents in this patient drain *above* the level of the inferior turbinates, since such surgically placed stents are intended to drain above the level of obstruction

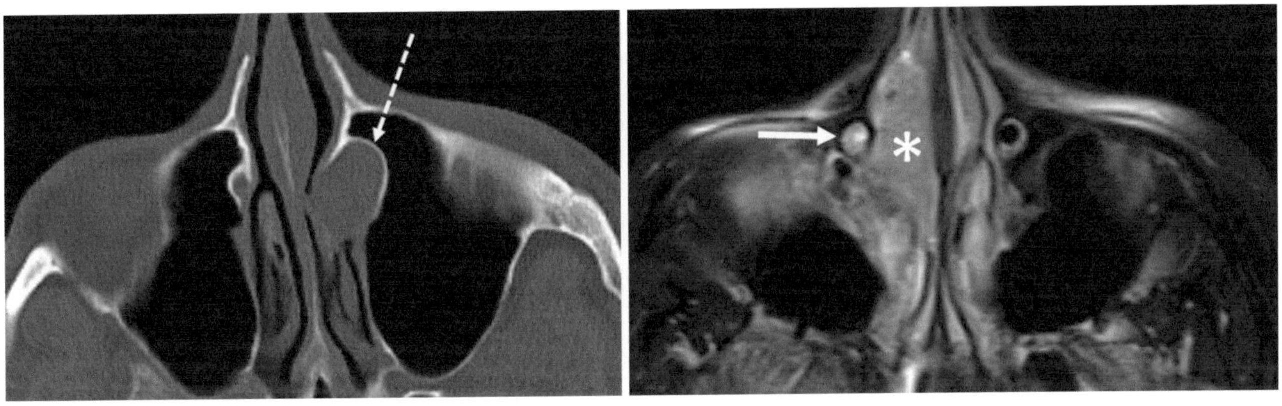

Fig. 3.41 Comparison cases of two different patients with nasolacrimal duct neoplasms. **Left**: An axial NECT image of a 75-year-old male with primary oncocytoma of the left nasolacrimal duct, resulting in expansion with bony remodeling of the left nasolacrimal canal (*dashed arrow*). **Right**: On an axial FS-SET2WI MRI of a 70-year-old female with a right nasal cavity intermediate-grade adenocarcinoma, there is an intermediate T2 signal mass within the right nasal cavity (*asterisk*) that infiltrates and results in partial circumferential filling of the right nasolacrimal duct (*arrow*). There is also a small degree of preserved T2-bright signal within the right nasolacrimal duct with central opacification, where such central opacification can also be seen in normal ducts

3.10 Orbital Artifacts

3.10.1 Incomplete Fat Suppression

As a result of the preponderance of background fat within the orbit, fat-suppression (FS) techniques are commonly employed and often necessary for the detection of orbital pathology on MR imaging. The orbit is a challenging anatomic region for fat-suppression because of susceptibility artifact from the air-tissue interface formed with the adjacent paranasal sinuses and its relatively close proximity to dental restorations within the oral cavity. When FS fails or is incomplete, it results in the appearance of increased T2 signal or enhancement; depending on the distribution, this may mimic pathology. Incomplete fat suppression is most commonly seen at the margins of the orbit, although it can be asymmetric and extend throughout the orbital fat. FS techniques most predisposed to susceptibility artifact are CHESS and SPIR. Dixon, STIR, and SPAIR are least sensitive to field inhomogeneity.

3.10.2 Ocular Motion Artifact

Stemming from voluntary and involuntary ocular movements, ghosting artifact is often present in the phase encoding direction, typically the left to right dimension of axial and coronal images through the orbits.

3.10.3 Truncation Artifact

Truncation artifact (Gibbs phenomenon) occurs if too few phase-encoding steps are used, resulting in wavy bands or an indistinct appearance at the margins of the globe. Truncation artifact tends to occur at the margins of the globe as a result of the abrupt fluid-soft tissue interface. The artifact is exacerbated using fast Fourier transform acquisition techniques such as T2-HASTE (half-Fourier acquisition single-shot turbo spin-echo).

3.10.4 Metallic Susceptibility Artifact from Adjacent Facial Hardware or Orbital Foreign Body

Facial reconstruction hardware, screws, prostheses, or dental restorations can cause large swaths of metallic susceptibility artifact that can variably obscure the entire orbit, or on the other end of the spectrum they can cause milder artifacts such as increased noise or incomplete FS. Regarding foreign bodies, although intraocular, intraorbital, or intracranial metal are considered contraindications to MRI and screening questionnaires are filled out by patients prior to undergoing MRI, forgotten or unknown exposures with resultant small intraorbital foreign bodies may be present, albeit a relatively rare phenomenon. If an orbital metallic foreign body is suspected during an MR acquisition, the scan should be aborted immediately at first detection (Figs. 3.42, 3.43, and 3.44).

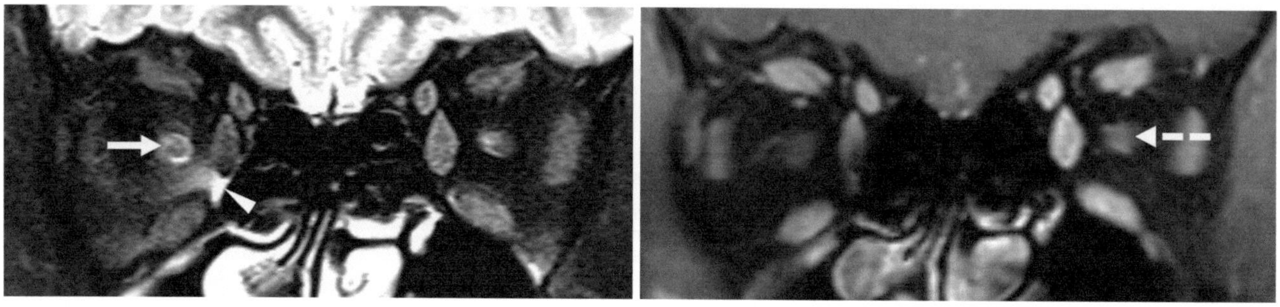

Fig. 3.42 Coronal FS-SET2WI using chemical FS technique (*left*) of a 17-year-old male with suspected left optic neuritis demonstrates a small region of incomplete FS in the inferonasal aspect of the right orbit (*arrowhead*); this results in the artefactual appearance of asymmetric T2-hyperintense signal within the right optic nerve (*arrow*), mimicking edema from optic neuritis. Coronal postcontrast FS-SET1WI (*right*) obtained using the fat-water separation technique from the same examination demonstrates uniform FS throughout both orbits and true enhancement of the *left* optic nerve (*dashed arrow*), consistent with the patient's clinical presentation. This case demonstrates how incomplete/inhomogeneous FS can simulate orbital or optic pathology

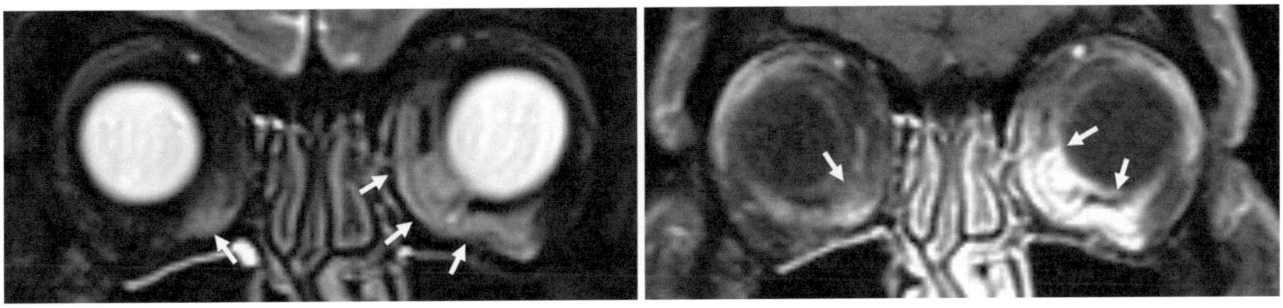

Fig. 3.43 Coronal FS-SET2WI (*left*) and FS-SET1WI (*right*) through both orbits in a 58-year-old male demonstrate incomplete FS of the inferonasal aspect of both orbits adjacent to the pneumatized paranasal sinuses (*arrows*), left greater than right, simulating the T2 hyperintense signal and enhancement of an inflammatory/infiltrative pathologic orbital process. However, this patient lacked such symptoms. Hence, as in this patient, incomplete FS can mimic orbital pathology

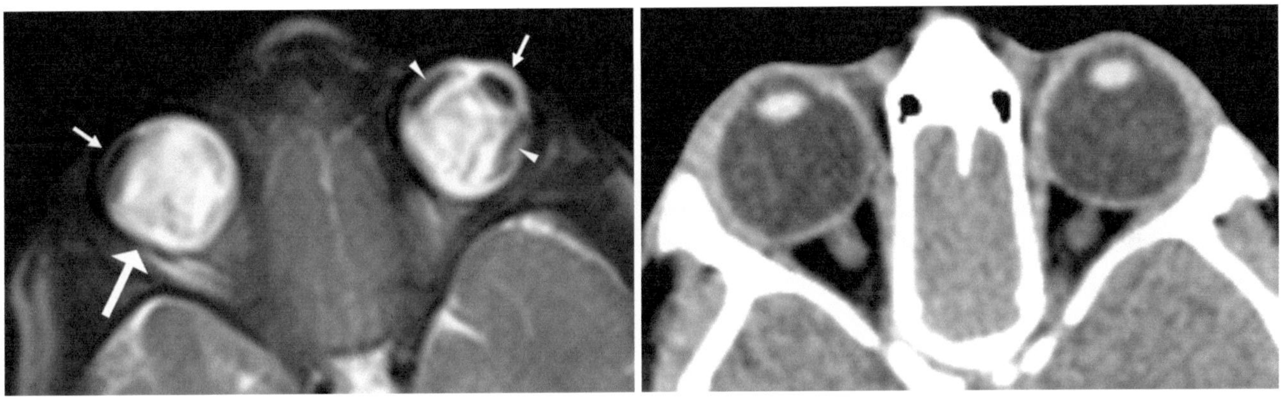

Fig. 3.44 A 4-year-old male with suspected ventriculoperitioneal shunt malfunction. Ocular motion was present on axial HASTE-T2WI MRI (*left*) despite a rapid brain imaging technique, which results in artefactual exotropia (*tiny arrows*), an appearance of a flattened contour abnormality of the wall of the globe (*fat arrow*), and heterogeneous vitreous contents (*arrowheads*). These findings were not evident on an axial NECT (*right*) performed later the same day. This case demonstrates how truncation artifact from quick brain imaging can simulate orbital pathology

Suggested Reading

Adam CR, Shields CL, Gutman J, Kim HJ, Hayek B, Shore JW, et al. Dilated superior ophthalmic vein: clinical and radiographic features of 113 cases. Ophthal Plast Reconstr Surg. 2018;34:68–73.

Agid R, Farb RI, Willinsky RA, Mikulis DJ, Tomlinson G. Idiopathic intracranial hypertension: the validity of cross-sectional neuroimaging signs. Neuroradiology. 2006;48:521–7.

Al-Haddad CE, Sebaaly MG, Tutunji RN, Mehanna CJ, Saaybi SR, Khamis AM, et al. Optic nerve measurement on MRI in the pediatric population: normative values and correlations. Am J Neuroradiol. 2018;39:369–74.

Amano Y, Amano M, Kumazaki T. Normal contrast enhancement of extraocular muscles: fat-suppressed MR findings. Am J Neuroradiol. 1997;18:161–4.

Anzai Y, Lufkin RB, Jabour BA, Hanafee WN. Fat-suppression failure artifacts simulating pathology on frequency-selective fat-suppression MR images of the head and neck. Am J Neuroradiol. 1992;13:879–84.

Armstrong GT, Localio AR, Feygin T, Bilaniuk L, Phillips PC, Fisher MJ, et al. Defining optic nerve tortuosity. Am J Neuroradiol. 2007;28:666–71.

Benson J, Nascene D, Truwit C, McKinney AM. Septo-optic dysplasia: assessment of associated findings with special attention to the olfactory sulci and tracts. Clin Neuroradiol. 2018; https://doi.org/10.1007/s00062-018-0687-z. [Epub ahead of print]

Bingham CM, Castro A, Realini T, Nguyen J, Hogg JP, Sivak-Callcott JA. Calculated CT volumes of lacrimal glands in normal caucasian orbits. Ophthal Plast Reconstr Surg. 2013;29:157–9.

Boegel KH, Tyan AE, Iyer VR, Rykken JB, McKinney AM. Utility of coronal contrast-enhanced fat-suppressed FLAIR in the evaluation of optic neuropathy and atrophy. Eur J Radiol Open. 2017;28(4):13–8.

Buch K, Nadgir RN, Tannenbaum AD, Ozonoff A, Fujita A, Sakai O. Clinical significance of trochlear calcifications in the orbit. Am J Neuroradiol. 2014;35:573–7.

Cheung N, McNab AA. Venous anatomy of the orbit. Invest Ophthalmol Vis Sci. 2003;44:988–95.

Czyz CN, Bacon TS, Stacey AW, Cahill EN, Costin BR, Karanfilov BI, et al. Nasolacrimal system aeration on computed tomographic imaging: effects of patient positioning and scan orientation. Clin Ophthalmol. 2015;9:469–73.

Janssen AG, Mansour K, Bos JJ, Castelijns JA. Diameter of the bony lacrimal canal: normal values and values related to nasolacrimal duct obstruction: assessment with CT. Am J Neuroradiol. 2001;22:845–50.

Degnan AJ, Levy LM. Pseudotumor cerebri: brief review of clinical syndrome and imaging findings. Am J Neuroradiol. 2011;32:1986–93.

Del Grande F, Santini F, Herzka DA, Aro MR, Dean CW, Gold GE, et al. Fat-suppression techniques for 3-T MR imaging of the musculoskeletal system. Radiographics. 2014;34:217–33.

Dijkstal JM, Bothun ED, Harrison AR, Lee M. Normal exophthalmometry measurements in a United States pediatric population. Ophthal Plast Reconstr Surg. 2012;28:54–6.

Dunsky IL. Normative data for hertel exophthalmometry in a normal adult black population. Optom Vis Sci. 1992;69:562–4.

Erie JC. Rising cataract surgery rates: demand and supply. Ophthalmology. 2014;121:2–4.

Gaddikeri S, Mossa-Basha M, Andre JB, Hippe DS, Anzai Y. Optimal fat suppression in head and neck MRI: comparison of multipoint Dixon with 2 different fat-suppression techniques, spectral presaturation and inversion recovery, and STIR. Am J Neuroradiol. 2018;39:362–8.

Garcia-Rojas L, Adame-Ocampo G, Alexanderson E, Tovilla-Canales JL. 18-Fluorodeoxyglucose uptake by positron emission tomography in extraocular muscles of patients with and without Graves' ophthalmology. J Ophthalmol. 2013;2013:529187.

Geeraerts T, Newcombe VF, Coles JP, Abate MG, Perkes IE, Hutchinson PJ, et al. Use of T2-weighted magnetic resonance imaging of the optic nerve sheath to detect raised intracranial pressure. Crit Care. 2008;12:R114.

Gordon RN, Slamovits TL, Rosenbaum PS, Bello J. Calcified scleral plaques imaged on orbital computed tomography. Am J Ophthalmol. 1999;127:461–3.

Gufler H, Preiss M, Koesling S. Visibility of sutures of the orbit and periorbital region using multidetector computed tomography. Korean J Radiol. 2014;15:802–9.

Harris MA, Realini T, Hogg JP, Sivak-Callcott JA. CT dimensions of the lacrimal gland in Graves orbitopathy. Ophthal Plast Reconstr Surg. 2012;28:69–72.

Hart BL, Spar JA, Orrison WW Jr. Calcification of the trochlear apparatus of the orbit: CT appearance and association with diabetes and age. Am J Roentgenol. 1992;159:1291–4.

Herrick RC, Hayman LA, Taber KH, Diaz-Marchan PJ, Kuo MD. Artifacts and pitfalls in MR imaging of the orbit: a clinical review. Radiographics. 1997;17:707–72.

Huh HD, Kim JH, Kim SJ, Yoo JM, Seo SW. The change of lacrimal gland volume in Korean patients with thyroid-associated ophthalmopathy. Korean J Ophthalmol. 2016;30:319–25.

Goldenberg-Cohen N, Naftaliev E, Millmond SH, Segev Y, Reider-Groswasser I. Ophthalmic artery calcification in a patient with renal failure. Neuroradiology. 2001;43:1005–6.

Ji J, Shimony J, Gao F, DiMario FJ Jr, Ramsby G, Greenstein R. Optic nerve tortuosity in children with neurofibromatosis type 1. Pediatr Radiol. 2013;43:1336–43.

Kaissar G, Kim JH, Bravo S, Sze G. Histologic basis for increased extraocular muscle enhancement in gadolinium-enhanced MR imaging. Radiology. 1991;179:541–2.

Karim S, Clark RA, Poukens V, Demer JL. Demonstration of systematic variation in human intraorbital optic nerve size by quantitative magnetic resonance imaging and histology. Invest Ophthalmol Vis Sci. 2004;45:1047–51.

Khanna RK, Pham CJ, Malik GM, Spickler EM, Mehta B, Rosenblum ML. Bilateral superior ophthalmic vein enlargement associated with diffuse cerebral swelling. Report of 11 cases. J Neurosurg. 1997;86:893–7.

Ko SJ, Nasseri F, Mohan S. Imaging of the postoperative orbit. Neuroimaging Clin N Am. 2015;25:457–76.

Ko SJ, Kim YJ. Incidence of calcification of the trochlear apparatus in the orbit. Korean J Ophthalmol. 2010;24:1–3.

Learned KO, Nasseri F, Mohan S. Imaging of the postoperative orbit. Neuroimaging Clin N Am. 2015;25:457–76.

Lenzi R, Casani AP, Sellari-Franceschini S. Ectopic intraorbital lacrimal ductal cyst: a case report. Orbit. 2012;31:350–1.

Lirng JF, Fuh JL, Wu ZA, Wang SJ. Diameter of the superior ophthalmic vein in relation to intracranial pressure. Am J Neuroradiol. 2003;24:700–3.

Lorber M, Vidić B. Measurements of lacrimal glands from cadavers, with descriptions of typical glands and three gross variants. Orbit. 2009;28:137–46.

McAlinden C. An overview of thyroid eye disease. Eye Vis (Lond). 2014;1:9.

McKinney AM. Pediatric skull: normal pediatric sutures on computed tomography; Sutures: fronto-ethmoidal, spheno-ethmoidal, fronto-sphenoidal, zygomatico-sphenoidal, and zygomatico-frontal sutures; Zygomatico-frontal and spheno-ethmoidal sutures versus fractures. In: AM MK, editor. Atlas of normal imaging variations of the brain, skull, and craniocervical vasculature. Cham: Springer; 2017a. p. 749, 761–4.

McKinney AM. Vasculature. Emissary veins, vascular-containing foramina, and vascular channels through the orbital roof simulating fracture. In: AM MK, editor. Atlas of normal imaging variations of the brain, skull, and craniocervical vasculature. Cham: Springer; 2017b. p. 859–62.

McKinney AM, Lohman BD, Sarikaya B, Benson M, Lee MS, Benson MT. Accuracy of routine fat-suppressed FLAIR and diffusion-weighted images in detecting clinically evident acute optic neuritis. Acta Radiol. 2013;54:455–61.

Mohan S, Hegde A, Tchoyoson Lim CC. Lacrimal glands: size does matter! Middle East Afr J Ophthalmol. 2011;18:328–30.

Murray JL, Hayman LA, Tang RA, Schiffman JS. Incidental asymptomatic orbital calcifications. J Neuroophthalmol. 1995;15:203–8.

Nair G, Kim M, Nagaoka T, Olson DE, Thulé PM, Pardue MT, et al. Effects of common anesthetics on eye movement and electroretinogram. Doc Ophthalmol. 2011;122:163–76.

Nakamura S, Okochi K, Murata Y, Shibuya H, Kurabayashi T. [18F] Fluorodeoxyglucose-PET/CT differentiation between physiological and pathological accumulations in head and neck. Nucl Med Commun. 2009;30:498–503.

Nakamoto Y, Tatsumi M, Hammoud D, Cohade C, Osman MM, Wahl RL. Normal FDG distribution patterns in the head and neck: PET/CT evaluation. Radiology. 2005;234:879–85.

Ozgen A, Ariyurek M. Normative measurements of orbital structures using CT. Am J Roentgenol. 1998;170:1093–6.

Ozgen A, Aydingoz U. Normative measurements of orbital structures using MRI. J Comput Assist Tomogr. 2000;24:493–6.

Ozgonul C, Uysal Y, Ayyildiz O, Kucukevcilioglu M. Clinical features and management of dacryops. Orbit. 2018;4:1–4.

Ramey NA, Hoang JK, Richard MJ. Multidetector CT of nasolacrimal canal morphology: normal variation by age, gender, and race. Ophthal Plast Reconstr Surg. 2013;29:475–80.

Rootman DB. Orbital decompression for thyroid eye disease. Surv Ophthalmol. 2018;63:86–104.

Rowe F, VIS group UK. The profile of strabismus in stroke survivors. Eye (Lond). 2010;24:682–5.

Russell EJ, Czervionke L, Huckman M, Daniels D, McLachlan D. CT of the inferomedial orbit and the lacrimal drainage apparatus: normal and pathologic anatomy. Am J Roentgenol. 1985;145:1147–54.

Shofty B, Ben-Sira L, Constantini S, Freedman S, Kesler A. Optic nerve sheath diameter on MR imaging: establishment of norms and comparison of pediatric patients with idiopathic intracranial hypertension with healthy controls. Am J Neuroradiol. 2012;33:366–9.

Smith EV, Gragoudas ES, Kolodny NH, D'Amico DJ. Magnetic resonance imaging: an emerging technique for the diagnosis of ocular disorders. Int Ophthalmol. 1990;14:119–24.

Tamboli DA, Harris MA, Hogg JP, Realini T, Sivak-Callcott JA. Computed tomography dimensions of the lacrimal gland in normal Caucasian orbits. Ophthal Plast Reconstr Surg. 2011;27:453–6.

Taoka T, Iwasaki S, Uchida H, Fukusumi A, Kichikawa K, Nakagawa H, et al. Enhancement pattern of normal extraocular muscles in dynamic contrast-enhanced MR imaging with fat suppression. Acta Radiol. 2000;41:211–6.

Tsutsumi S, Nakamura M, Tabuchi T, Yasumoto Y. The superior ophthalmic vein: delineation with high-resolution magnetic resonance imaging. Surg Radiol Anat. 2015;37:75–80.

Ueno H, Ariji E, Izumi M, Uetani M, Hayashi K, Nakamura T. MR imaging of the lacrimal gland. Age-related and gender-dependent changes in size and structure. Acta Radiol. 1996;37:714–9.

Watanabe A, Kinouchi H, Horikoshi T, Uchida M, Ishigame K. Effect of intracranial pressure on the diameter of the optic nerve sheath. J Neurosurg. 2008;109:255–8.

Yazici Z, Yazici B, Parlak M, Tuncel E, Ertürk H. Treatment of nasolacrimal duct obstruction with polyurethane stent placement: long-term results. Am J Roentgenol. 2002;179:491–4.

Zincirkeser S, Sahin E, Halac M, Sager S. Standardized uptake values of normal organs on 18F-fluorodeoxyglucose positron emission tomography and computed tomography imaging. J Int Med Res. 2007;35:231–6.

4 Neck Soft Tissue Variants

4.1 Introduction, Technique, and Basic Anatomy

There are multiple developmental variations of soft-tissue neck structures that can be detected on computed tomography (CT), magnetic resonance imaging (MRI), and 18 fluro-deoxy-glucose position emission tomography (FDG-PET). These need to be recognized and differentiated from actual pathologies. There can also be benign lesions involving the soft tissue neck that are caught incidentally while the study is obtained to evaluate other pathologies. Being aware of these variations and certain common benign lesions is quite important. If such variants or "don't touch lesions" are diagnosed correctly, this can prevent unnecessary patient anxiety, possible invasive procedures, and potential complications. For example, being knowledgeable about the common FDG-PET findings of brown fat activation-related FDG uptake in certain parts of the body prevents misdiagnosis of disease progression and possibly unnecessary biopsies.

Regarding CT techniques, for evaluation of the neck soft tissues, ideally CT images are acquired following intravenous contrast administration. Typically, helically-acquired images are reconstructed in the axial, coronal, and sagittal planes for interpretation. The field of view should include from the aortic arch up to the level of the skull base, and the entire mandible and nose should be included within the field of view. However, certain techniques can better reveal pathology based on the location of the suspected lesion. For example, regarding *oral cavity* lesions, the "puffed cheek" technique can better evaluate the oral tongue and buccal mucosa lesions. For evaluation of the cause of vocal cord paralysis, the field of view should be extended caudally to include the subaortic region so that the entire length of the left recurrent laryngeal nerve can be evaluated. For patients with extensive dental amalgam, gantry tilt can be obtained for an attempt to eliminate the streak artifact from the amalgam, which may preclude oral cavity evaluation. If the area of interest is in the supraclavicular region, the contrast administration should be administered via the contralateral arm to avoid intense streak artifact from venous contrast.

Regarding MRI, for optimal neck evaluation axial T1-weighted imaging (SET1WI) *without* fat suppression (FS) is one of the most important sequences, as most pathologies are easily visible on the background of hyperintense (T1-bright) fat. Axial FS-T2-weighted imaging (SET2WI) *with* FS and postgadolinium axial FS-SET1WI are other necessary sequences. Axial diffusion weighted imaging (DWI) has also been shown to have value in certain neck pathologies, particularly certain malignancies. Additionally, coronal postgadolinium FS-SET1WI is valuable in evaluating for perineural spread of tumor.

Regarding FDG-PET imaging of the neck, it is critical to ensure that patients are kept in a dark, warm, and quiet environment during uptake time. Typically, warm blankets are provided to patients in an attempt to prevent any brown fat activation and resultant FDG uptake on PET imaging. Patients' arms should be held down along their bodies to minimize the attenuation of FDG uptake in the neck. It is critical that patients do not move between PET acquisition and CT acquisition in order to eliminate misregistration during the PET and CT fusion process. Attenuation-corrected PET data and CT should be interpreted hand-in-hand, with reference to "fused" images if needed. Uncorrected PET images should also be evaluated if there is suspicion of an over-correction artifact. Prior to the image interpretation session, all the available clinical information, including surgery and other types of therapy (for example, radiotherapy), should be gathered to prevent any interpretation errors. On PET imaging, nonmalignant FDG uptake is very commonly seen in a variety of neck structures, such as the extraocular muscles, tonsillar tissues, salivary tissues, brain parenchyma, certain neck muscles, reactive lymph nodes, tongue muscle, vocal cords, and so forth. Being aware of the normal distribution of FDG in the neck is mandatory in order to correctly diagnose such pathologic entities.

A. McKinney et al., *Atlas of Head/Neck and Spine Normal Imaging Variants*, https://doi.org/10.1007/978-3-319-95441-7_4

4.2 Tornwaldt Cyst (Pharyngeal Bursa)

Tornwaldt cyst or pharyngeal bursa is a benign developmental lesion within the midline nasopharynx, above the upper border of the superior constrictor muscle. This cyst represents the embryonic communication between the mesenteric notochord remnant and endodermal-derived nasopharyngeal mucosa. Its incidence has been reported to be in 4% of autopsy specimens and 0.2–5% on MRI examinations. These bursae can be seen in all age groups. Regarding their size, they typically range from 2 to 20 mm. Occasionally, these cysts can be associated with a canalis basilaris medianus, which is a normal variant tubular defect in the skull base at the clivus present in 1–3% of adults. (Note: there is debate as to whether when these occur together it is truly considered a Tornwaldt cyst.) While typically it is a "don't touch lesion" since most patients are symptom-free, rarely inflammation or even an abscess may develop within the cyst. Various mechanisms that cause occlusion of the cyst orifice (usually due to iatrogenic trauma) can result in the development of Tornwaldt disease, which includes nasal discharge, occipital headaches, halitosis, and an unpleasant taste in the mouth.

On CT, Tornwaldt cysts appear hypo- or isodense, while on MRI the cyst usually exhibits an internally high signal on T1-weighted imaging (SET1WI), and fluid attenuation inversion recovery (FLAIR) images. The cyst does not enhance with gadolinium contrast. The differential diagnosis of Tornwaldt cyst is adenoid retention cysts. Retention cysts are small (<5 mm) and often occur with multiplicity (Figs. 4.1 and 4.2).

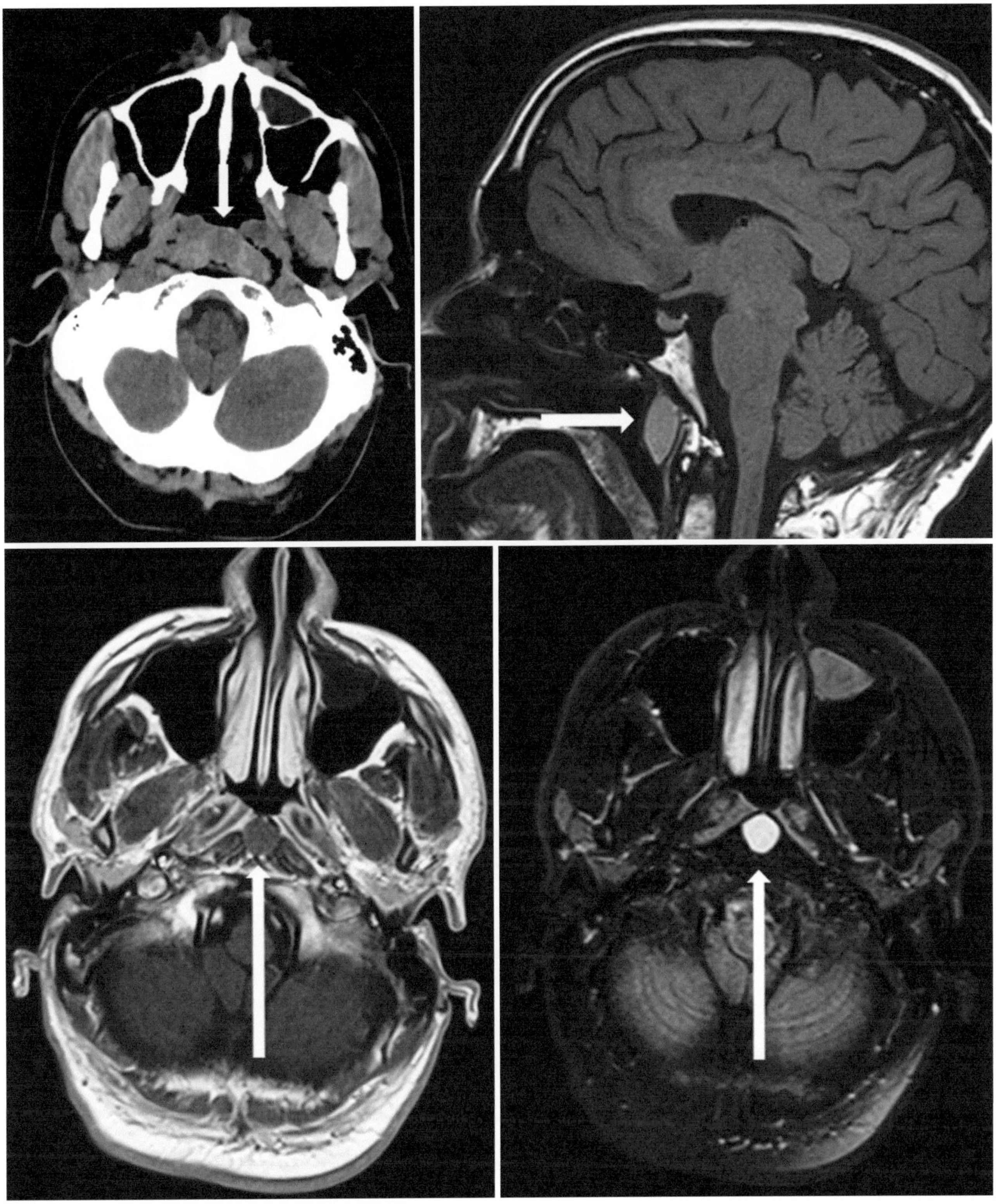

Fig. 4.1 A 40-year-old male with a Tornwaldt cyst visualized in the posterior nasopharynx midline. On NECT (*upper left*), the cyst (*arrow*) demonstrates isodensity with the prevertebral muscles. On noncontrast sagittal SET1WI (*upper right*), the well-marginated cyst (*arrow*) demonstrates slight hyperintensity compared with the brain parenchyma. On postgadolinium T1-weighted sequence (*bottom left*), there is no enhancement of the cyst (*arrow*). On FLAIR MRI (*bottom right*), the cyst has hyperintense signal (*arrow*)

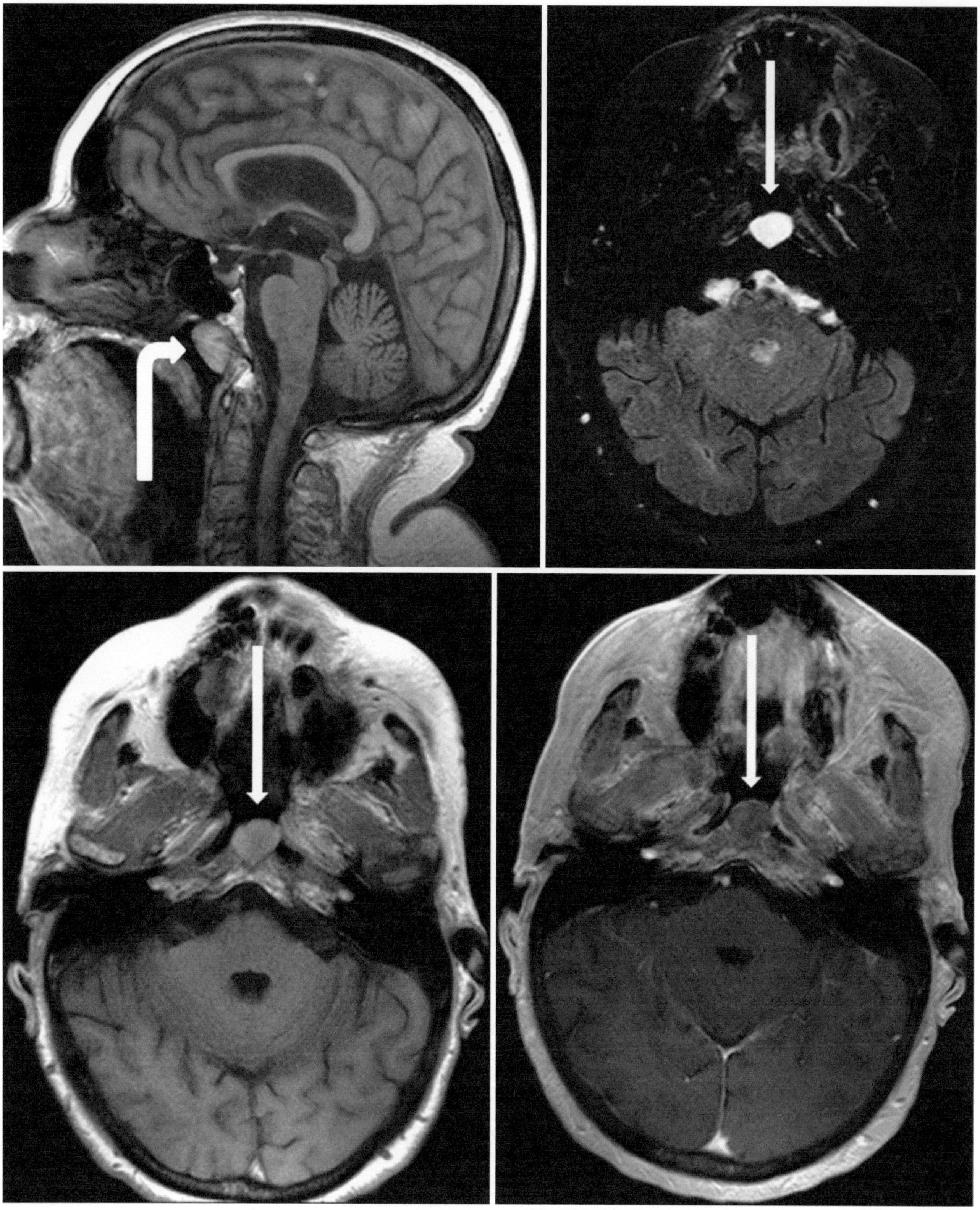

Fig. 4.2 An 89-year-old woman presenting with a facial mass. Sagittal noncontrast SET1WI (*upper left*) shows a midline hyperintense lesion along the nasopharyngeal mucosa and protruding into the lumen of the nasopharynx (*curved arrow*). Axial FLAIR (*upper right*), noncontrast SET1W1 (*bottom left*) and postcontrast SET1WI (*bottom right*) sequences show T1- and FLAIR- hyperintense signal but nonenhancement within the cyst (*arrows*). The signal characteristics, typical location at the midline, and the nasopharynx level are diagnostic of a Tornwaldt cyst

4.3 Adenoidal Retention Cyst

Benign occlusion of the adenoid crypts may lead to the formation of *retention cysts* within the adenoids, which are encountered in up to 6% of individuals; they can be considered either normal variations or at least "don't touch lesions." The cysts are usually asymptomatic and located at or near the midline. If the cystic content is rich in protein, it may display high signal on T1WI MRI. These cysts do not enhance with gadolinium. Their presence within the adenoids, their rhomboidal shape, and their typical MR appearance usually make them easily recognizable (Fig. 4.3).

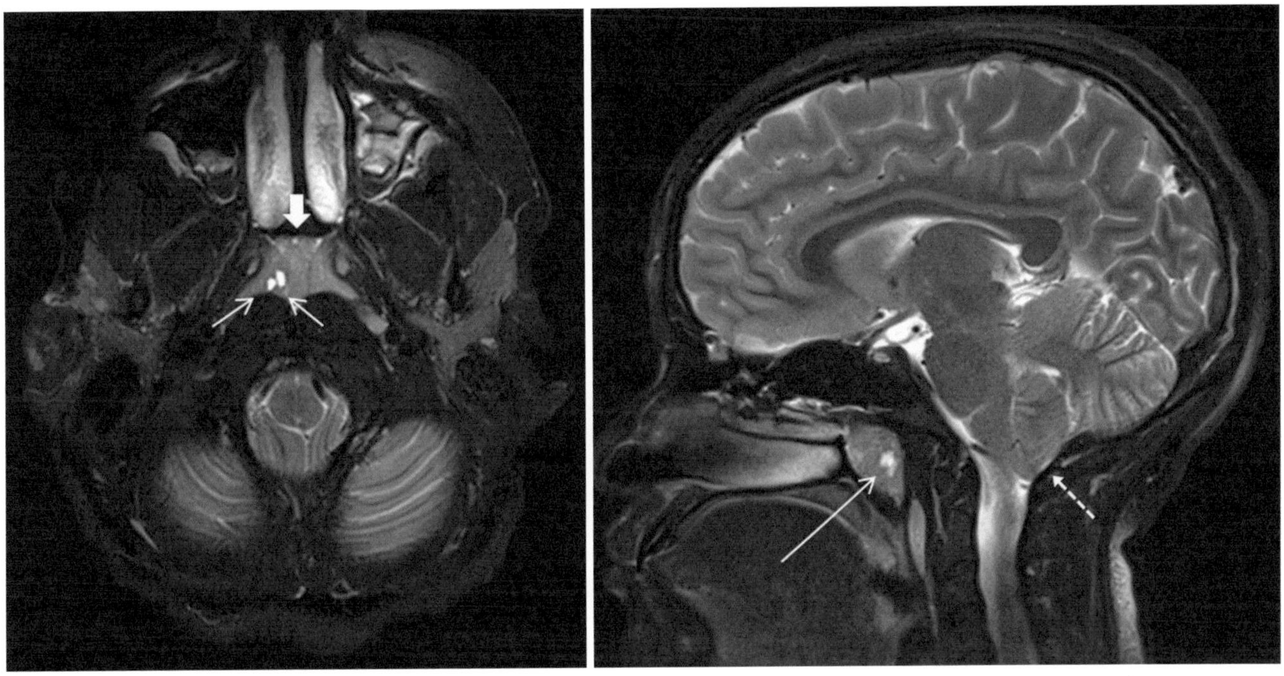

Fig. 4.3 A 14-year-old girl with known Chiari 1 malformation. Axial (*left*) and sagittal (*right*) fat suppression-SET2WI sequences demonstrate prominent nasopharyngeal adenoids (*short thick arrow, left*). There are a couple of small cystic lesions within the adenoidal tissue (*thin arrows*) situated to the right of the midline. Since there is more than one, their localization at the right of midline and their being embedded within the adenoidal tissue solidify the diagnosis of retention cysts. Also, note mild cerebellar tonsillar ectopia (*dashed arrow, right*), the reason for the examination

4.4 Lingual Tonsillar Hypertrophy

The most common cause of *lingual tonsillar enlargement or hypertrophy* is compensatory enlargement following tonsillectomy. Other causes include chronic infection, human immunodeficiency virus positivity, irritation from smoking and gastroesophageal reflux, and immunosuppressant drugs. Malignancies such as lymphoma and leukemia should also be excluded. Lingual tonsillar hypertrophy in adults is often asymptomatic. It can, however, present with symptoms, including throat pain, dysphagia, voice changes, a foreign body sensation, coughing and choking, and obstructive sleep apnea. While typically a "don't touch" lesion, lingual tonsillar hypertrophy is occasionally of clinical significance owing to the potential for difficulty it causes in a patient receiving anesthesia, since it has the potential to cause fatal airway obstruction in cases of prominent enlargement. Treatment is considered only if it is symptomatic or contributing to airway obstruction (Fig. 4.4).

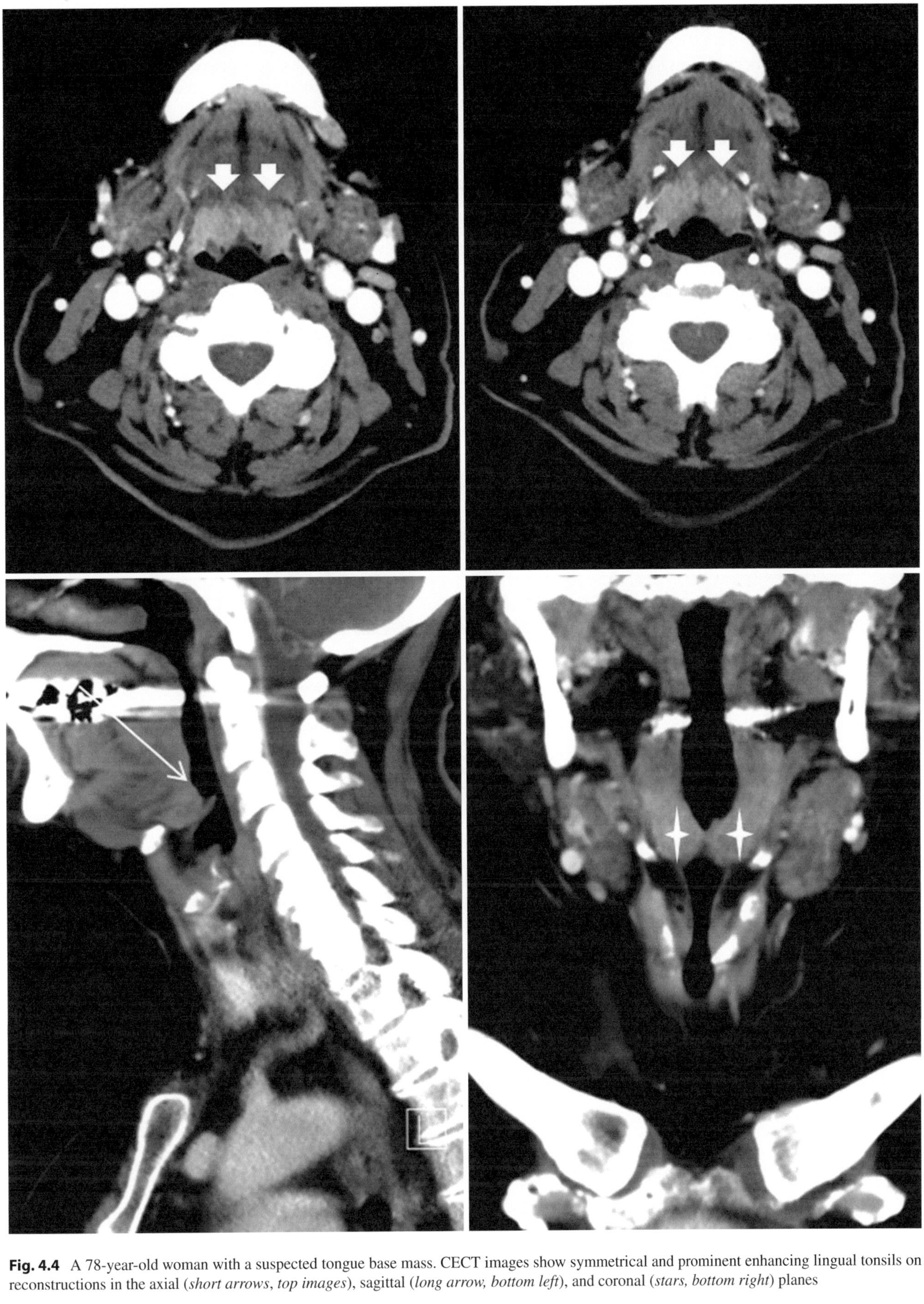

Fig. 4.4 A 78-year-old woman with a suspected tongue base mass. CECT images show symmetrical and prominent enhancing lingual tonsils on reconstructions in the axial (*short arrows, top images*), sagittal (*long arrow, bottom left*), and coronal (*stars, bottom right*) planes

4.5 Vallecular Cyst

Laryngeal cysts can occur in any part of the larynx but are more frequent in supraglottic locations such as the epiglottis and vallecula. The prevalence of each location varies in different studies. Laryngeal cysts represent a rare entity, about 5% of benign laryngeal lesions, with no gender predilection. These are typically "don't touch lesions" found in patients with nonspecific symptoms or who are asymptomatic. If they are large in size, patients can develop laryngeal stridor or dyspnea. Different forms of treatment have been described for large laryngeal cysts such as aspiration, marsupialization with laser ablation, and complete excision. Recurrence of the cyst is directly related to the maintenance of remnants of the cyst wall.

On CT, these cysts are well-defined, fluid dense, nonenhancing, and rounded. On MRI, they are also well-defined, have fluid signal, and are nonenhancing. Included in the differential diagnosis are laryngeal oncocytic papillary cystadenoma and thyroglossal duct cyst of the tongue base (Fig. 4.5).

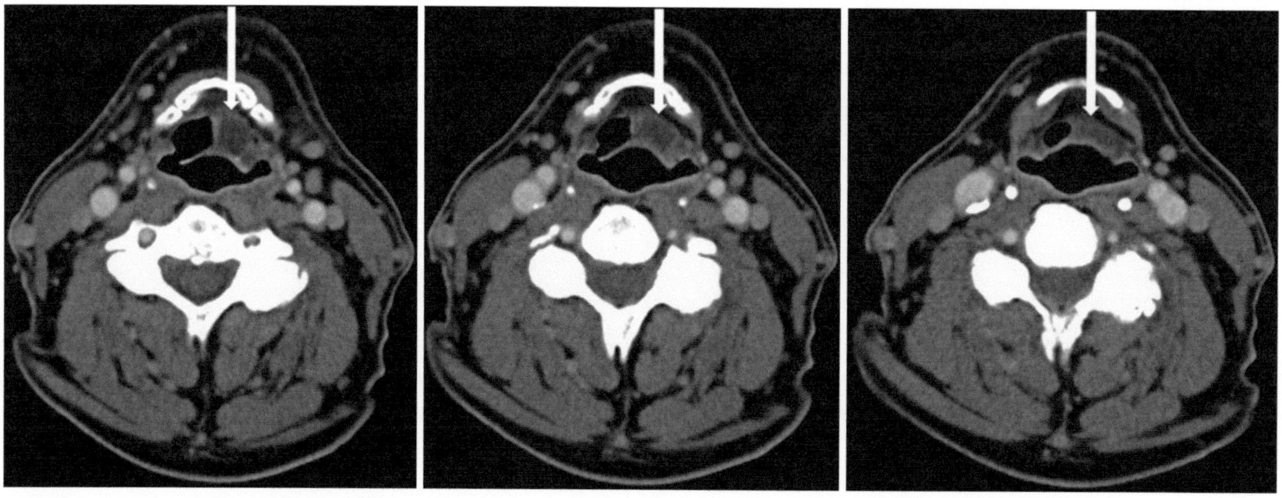

Fig. 4.5 A 62-year-old male with a parotid mass. Multiple axial CECT images through the neck show asymmetry of the valleculae, being more prominent on the left side. On the left side there is a low attenuation (fluid density) focus, suggestive of a vallecular cyst (*arrows*)

4.6 Laryngocele

Laryngoceles refer to dilatations of the laryngeal ventricle saccule located in the paraglottic space of the supraglottis. On imaging, these lesions are generally characterized as well-defined, thin-walled, and fluid or air-filled cystic lesions of the paraglottic space. The communication with the laryngeal ventricle is not always identified, and an extra laryngeal extension through the thyrohyoid membrane may or may not be present. When small, these "don't touch lesions" are usually asymptomatic and incidentally discovered upon imaging the neck for other reasons. Symptoms vary accordingly to the size and extent of the lesion and may include a sore throat, dysphagia, stridor, neck lump, and/or airway obstruction. Laryngoceles are usually acquired rather than congenital. They are lined by pseudostratified, columnar, ciliated epithelium. Occasional areas of stratified squamous epithelium +/− submucosal serous and mucous glands may be present.

Three laryngocele subtypes are described as follows:

(a) Internal (or "simple"): the dilated ventricular saccule is confined to the paralaryngeal space (~40%);
(b) External: the saccule herniates through the thyrohyoid membrane, and the superficial portion is dilated (~25%);
(c) Mixed: with dilated internal and external components (~45%).

Raised intralaryngeal pressure secondary to excessive cough, playing woodwind/brass instruments, glass blowing, and an obstructing lesion (e.g., tumor) can result in acquired laryngoceles. The finding of a laryngocele should prompt a search for an underlying laryngeal carcinoma obstructing the orifice of the laryngeal ventricle, although this is only present in a minority of laryngoceles. A secondary laryngocele is the term for when a tumor causes a laryngocele.

Attenuation characteristics on CT may vary, depending on the laryngocele content (e.g., air, fluid, mucus). On MRI, the characteristics are typically T1WI: low signal; T2WI: high signal; postcontrast T1WI: absent-to-minimal linear peripheral enhancement. If thick enhancing walls are present, a pyolaryngocele (a secondary infection of a laryngocele) should be considered (Figs. 4.6, 4.7, and 4.8).

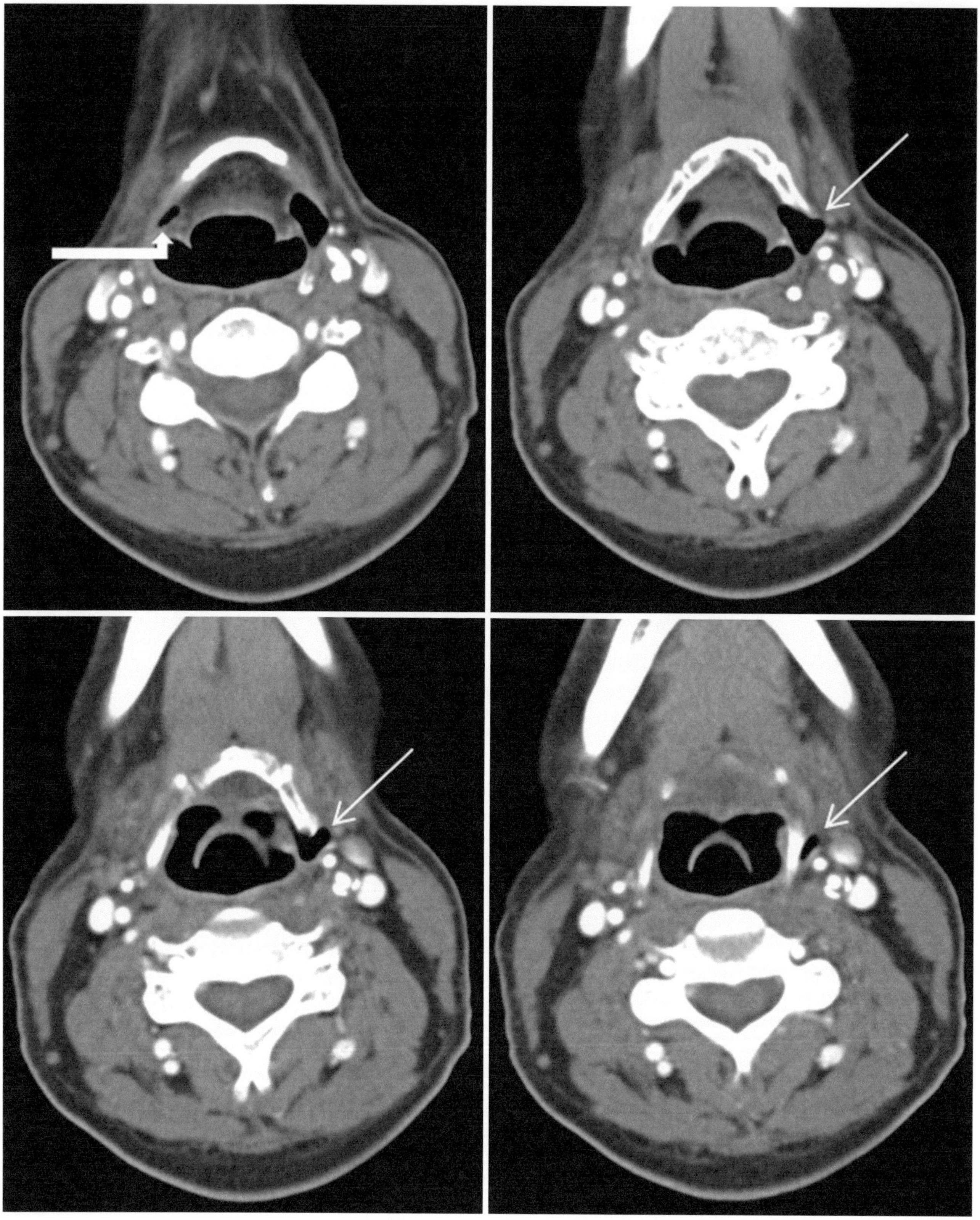

Fig. 4.6 A 54-year-old male with a history of tonsillar squamous cell cancer. Multiple postcontrast axial CT slices demonstrate air-filled pockets in the bilateral paralaryngeal fat at the supraglottic larynx level, which are larger on the left. The *upper left image* shows a small right internal laryngocele (*arrow*). On the patient's left side, there is also a component extending through the thyrohyoid ligament laterally (*arrows* in *upper right, bottom right,* and *bottom left images*). Thus, there is an internal laryngocele on the right and a mixed laryngocele on the left

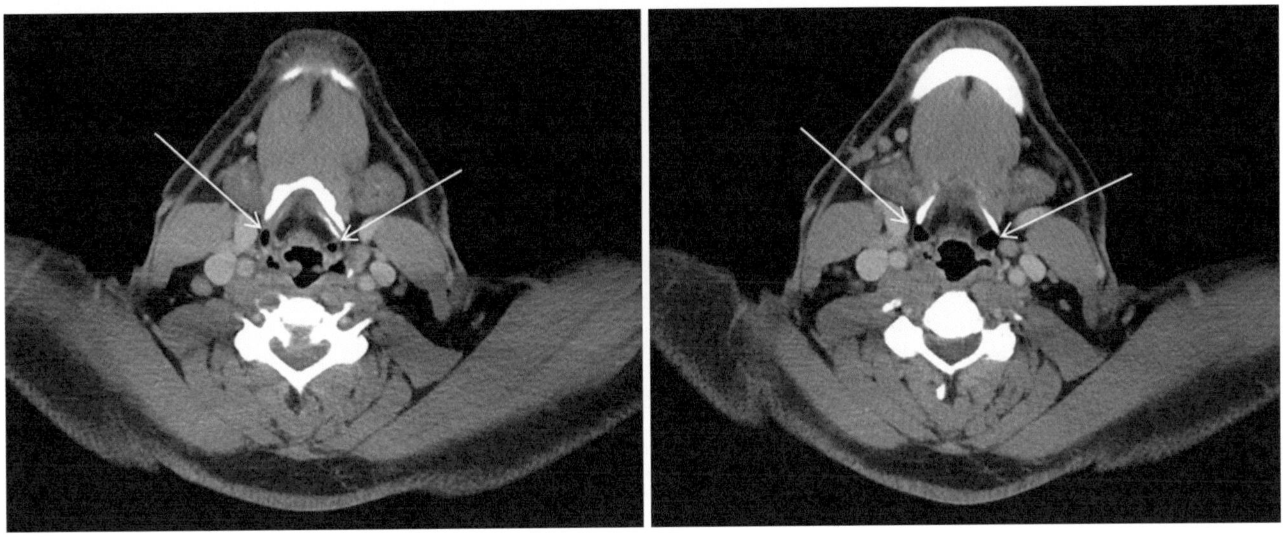

Fig. 4.7 A 54-year-old male with throat pain. The air-filled pockets are confined to paralaryngeal fat; thus, these are consistent with small bilateral internal laryngoceles (*arrows*)

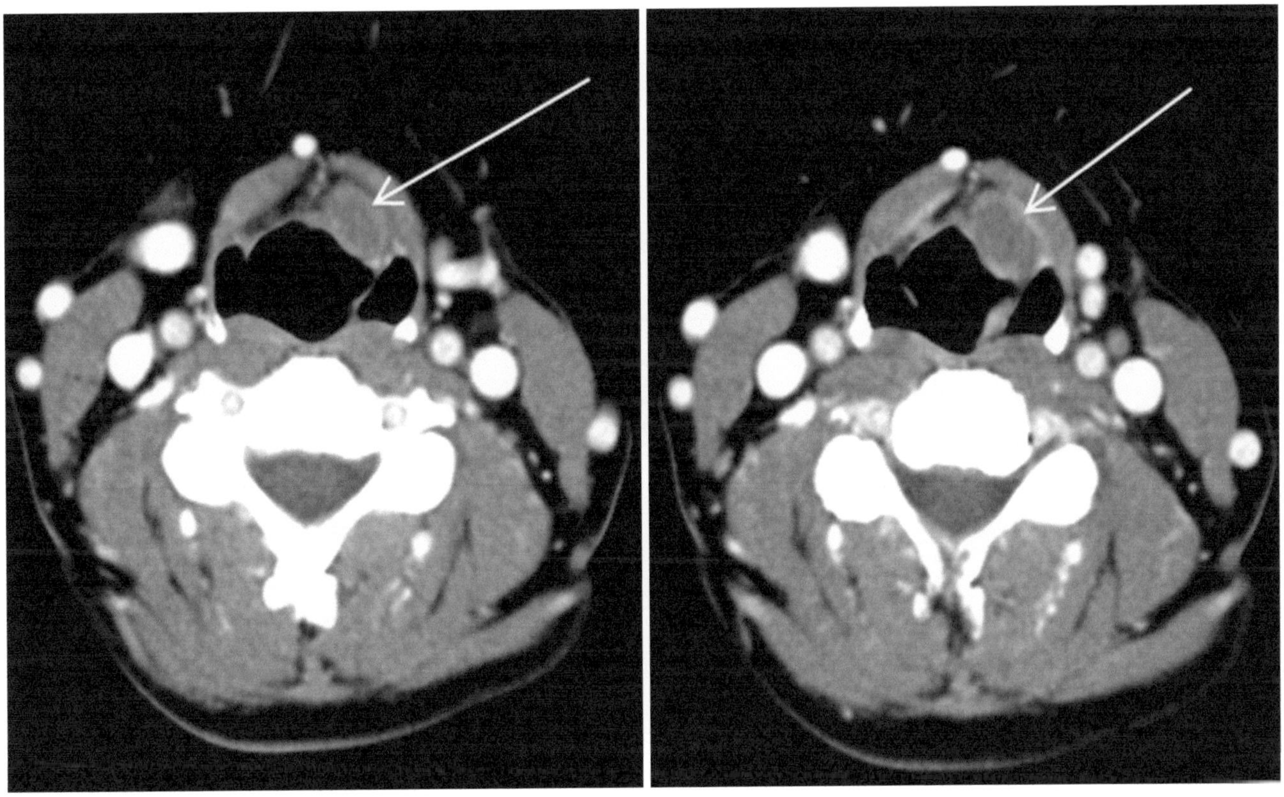

Fig. 4.8 Comparison case of small cell cancer. A 56-year-old female with hoarseness. Axial postcontrast CT (CECT) images demonstrate a lesion within the left supraglottic paralaryngeal submucosa; the lesion is well-defined with a hypodense center and has a thin enhancing rim (*arrows*). The lesion mimics a benign proteinaceous or infectious content filled laryngocele, that is, a pyolaryngocele. However, histopathologic examination of this lesion showed it to be a small cell tumor with neuroendocrine features

4.7 Parapharyngeal Space Lipoma

The parapharyngeal space (PPS) is a critical anatomic space to identify in the neck as it is surrounded by several other important spaces. Parapharyngeal space tumors account for 0.5–0.8% of head and neck tumors. The PPS is anatomically akin to an inverted pyramid with the skull base at the bottom and the apex at the greater cornu of the hyoid bone. The styloid process divides it into the anterior prestyloid and posterior poststyloid compartments. The prestyloid compartment is a potential space that may contain salivary tissue from either the deep lobe of the parotid or accessory salivary tissue and lymph nodes. The poststyloid or neurovascular compartment contains the internal carotid artery, internal jugular vein, IX, X, and XI cranial nerves, and the cervical sympathetic chain. Nearly 13% of lipomatous tumors occur in the head and neck, making them the most common benign mesenchymal tumors. In the PPS, however, they account for just 1–2% and are usually restricted to either the prestyloid or poststyloid compartment.

While usually initially asymptomatic, *PPS lipomas* produce a bulge in the lateral oropharyngeal wall, resulting in medial prolapse of the ipsilateral tonsil once they reach a size of about 3.0 cm, since the PPS is limited by unyielding bony structures. Meanwhile, tumors are free to expand medially. Other clinical features of PPS lipomas include swelling below the angle of the mandible, dysphagia caused by mass effect, respiratory distress, and obstructive sleep apnea. Also, eustachian tube obstruction may result in serous otitis media and conductive hearing loss. Features of malignant disease (as opposed to typically incidental lipomas) include compression of lower cranial nerves resulting in hoarseness, tongue deviation, Horner syndrome, and trismus due to infiltration of the medial pterygoid musculature.

The evaluation of tumors within the PPS poses a significant challenge. Fine needle aspiration cytology (FNAC) of these deep-seated and "difficult to assess" lesions can be arduous and are often inconclusive. However, imaging modalities such as CT and MRI are often diagnostic of benign versus malignant lesions, where the smaller, asymptomatic lipomas (<2 cm size) can be considered "don't touch lesions." Benign PPS lipomas appear as typically homogeneous, nonenhancing low-density areas on CT, with high signal intensity on SET1WI and SET2WI. In addition, FS-SET1WI sequences obtained provide better contrast with the surrounding soft tissue. If they are large and symptomatic, PPS lipomas can be treated surgically. The surgical approach depends on the size, vascularity, and the compartment of the PPS involved. The transcervical approach, with retraction or removal of the submandibular gland, is the most popular approach to the PPS and is suitable for tumors as large as 8 cm (Fig. 4.9).

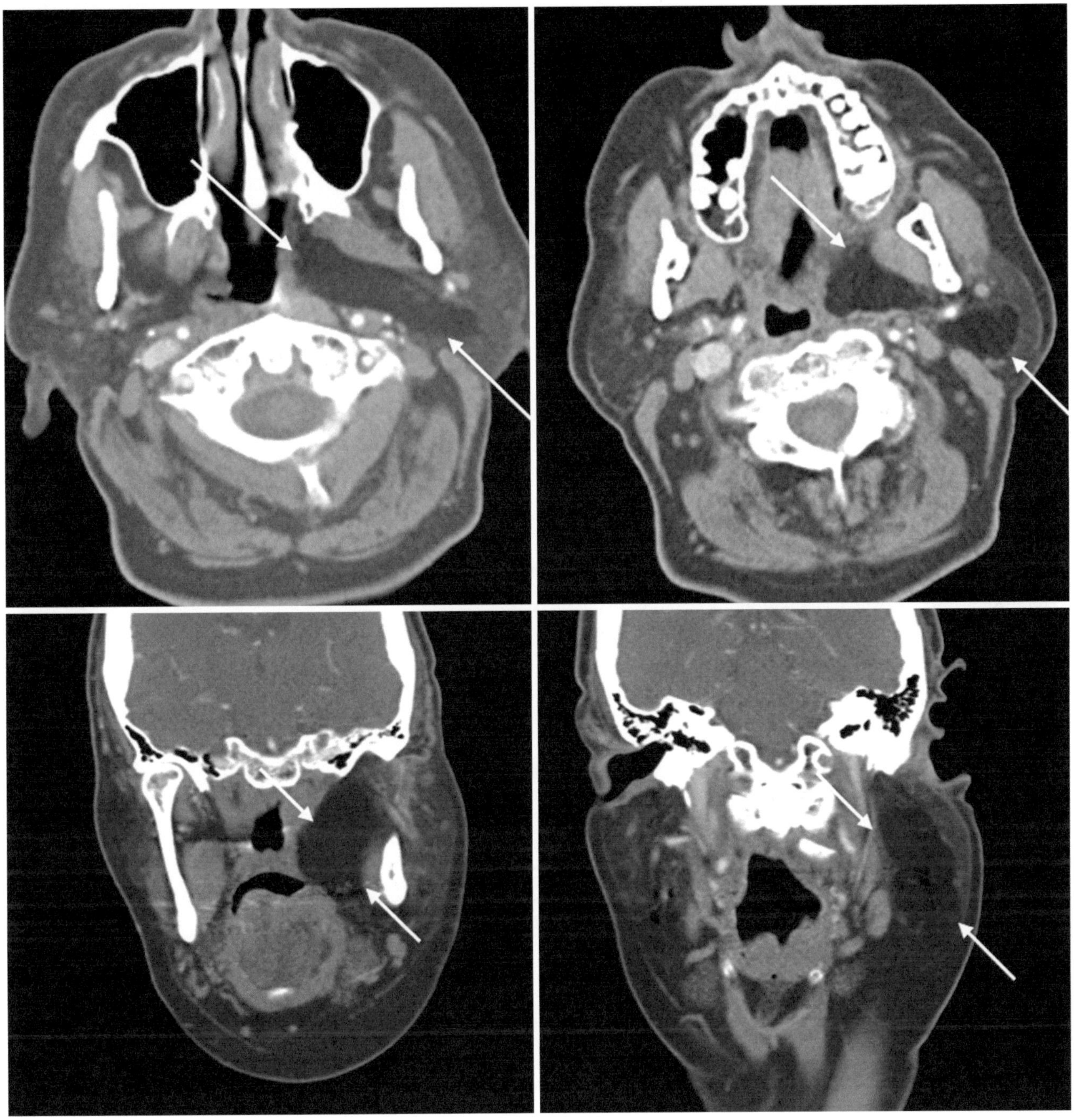

Fig. 4.9 A 73-year-old woman with a thyroid goiter and a parapharyngeal lipoma (*between arrows in each image*). Postcontrast axial (*top row*) and coronal (*bottom row*) CECT images demonstrate a large area of asymmetric fat density lesion (*between arrows in each image*) within the left parapharyngeal space. The lesion displaces the deep lobe of the left parotid gland laterally and displaces the left lateral nasopharyngeal wall medially (*top left*), resulting in mild airway narrowing. While these are usually "don't touch" lesions when smaller (<2–3 cm size), larger lesions such as this causing adjacent mass effect may necessitate surgical removal

4.8 Medial Retropharyngeal Lymph Nodes in Children

The retropharyngeal space is the potential space surrounded by the buccopharyngeal fascia anteriorly and the alar fascia posteriorly. The contents of the retropharyngeal space include fibro-fatty tissue, blood vessels, and lymph nodes. The presence of retropharyngeal lymph nodes was first described by Rouviere in 1938. Retropharyngeal lymph nodes are classified into medial and lateral groups. Lateral retropharyngeal lymph nodes are located just medial to the carotid sheath in the lateral aspect of the retropharyngeal space. They are immediately anterior to the lateral margins of the longus colli and longus capitis muscles. *Medial retropharyngeal lymph nodes* are located near the midline immediately anterior to the prevertebral musculature. The appearance of retropharyngeal nodes should not be considered abnormal in and of itself. As per a study by Costa et al. (2011), lateral retropharyngeal lymph nodes are very common, occurring in about 91–97.3% of the population to varying degrees and sizes. When present, lateral retropharyngeal lymph nodes are typically bilateral and located at the skull base (down to the C1 or C1–2 level). Medial retropharyngeal lymph nodes (median size, 3.5–5.1 mm) are less common than lateral retropharyngeal lymph nodes (median size, 5.5–6.8 mm based on multiple studies) but are not rare. According to the aforementioned study results, such medial nodes occurred in 17–21.3% of the children who did not have obstructive sleep apnea. They can be normal (i.e., "don't touch" nodes) but are prominent in reactive states, particularly in children with underlying viral infections. When medial retropharyngeal lymph nodes are present, they are more commonly unilateral than bilateral and are usually located inferiorly at the C2 to C3 level. These are far less visualized in adults.

Regarding pathology, there may be no well-defined criteria to call a medial or lateral retropharyngeal lymph node abnormal. There are some general rules: if it is larger than 1 cm in an adult or with a necrotic center at any size (particularly in the presence of primary head and neck malignancy), it might be a metastatic node. If the node shows markedly disproportionate enlargement in a child (>2 cm), this occasionally can be seen in leukemia or lymphoma. Rarely, vascular malformations such as hemangiomas, cystic hygromas (venolymphatic malformations), or arteriovenous malformations can be present in this region as well (Figs. 4.10 and 4.11).

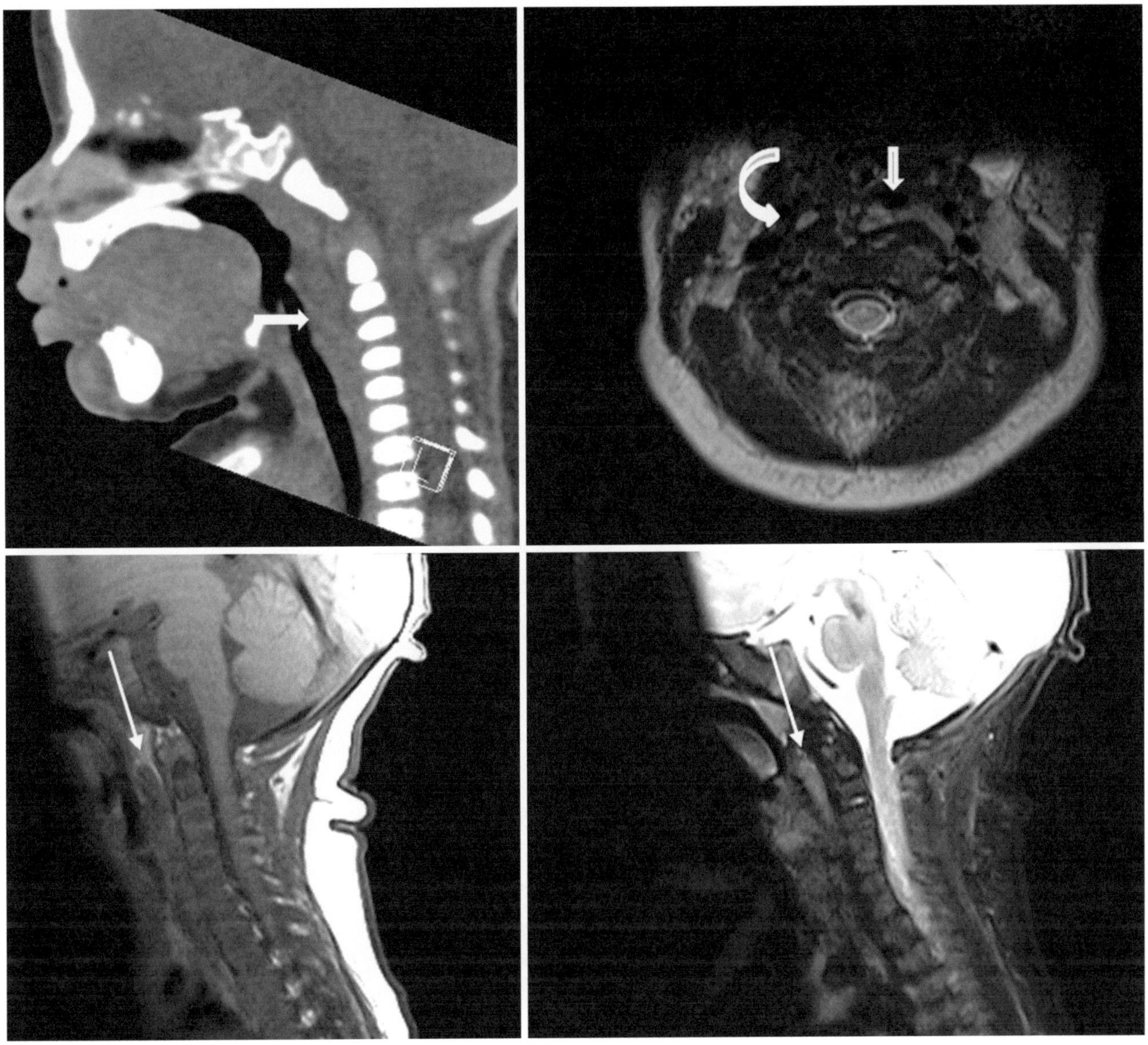

Fig. 4.10 A 3-month-old infant hospitalized for trauma and mandibular fracture, where enlarged retropharyngeal nodes simulate prevertebral swelling. Sagittal reconstruction of a cervical spine NECT (*upper left*) shows an enlarged prevertebral space, raising the suspicion for prevertebral edema (*short thick arrow*). On MRI with axial SET2WI (*upper right*), there is an intermediate signal within the medial retropharyngeal node extending laterally (*short arrow*), also with a smaller right lateral retropharyngeal node (*curved arrow*). On sagittal SET1WI (*bottom left*) and SET2WI (*bottom right*) images, there is a prominent T1-hypointense and T2-intermediate signal node within the retropharyngeal space (*arrows*), which is likely at least in part what mimicked the prevertebral edema on NECT

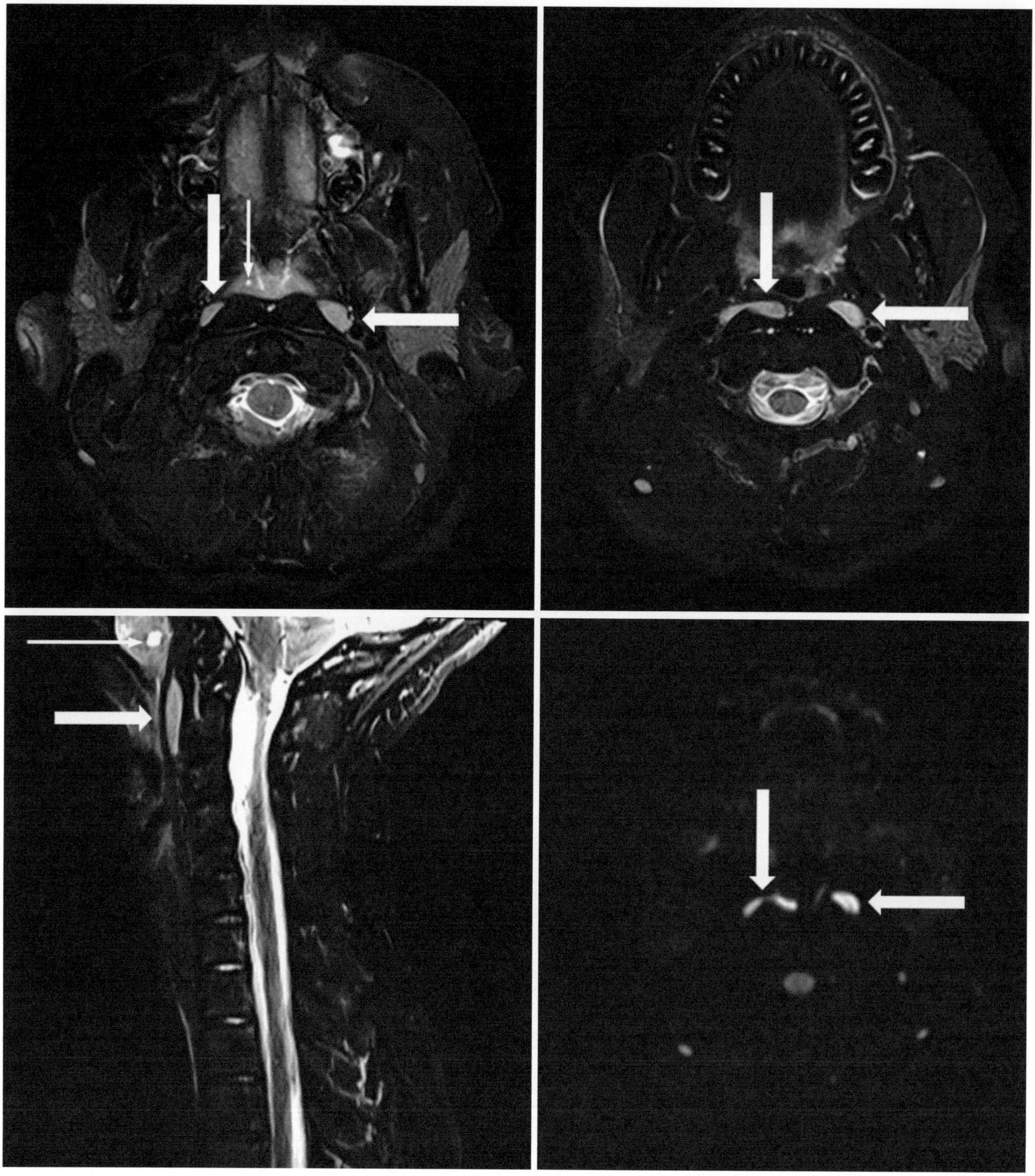

Fig. 4.11 Comparison cases of reactive nodes and adenoidal retention cysts. A 14-year-old female with Chiari 1 malformation. On axial SET2WI (*upper right* and *upper left*), sagittal SET2WI (*bottom left*), and axial diffusion-weighted MRI (*bottom right*), there are right medial and left lateral retropharyngeal nodes (*arrows* in each image). These are reactive nodes from concomitant known viral infection. Incidentally, there are also adenoidal retention cysts (*tiny arrows*) on axial and sagittal SET2WI (*upper left* and *bottom left images, respectively*)

4.9 Pterygoid Venous Plexus Asymmetry

The pterygoid venous plexus has a wide range of sizes in normal individuals and is present in most individuals to varying degrees. It lies within and around the pterygoid muscles in the medial masticator space. The venous plexus can be asymmetric in size as a normal variant. An *asymmetric pterygoid venous plexus* can mimic an enhancing or infiltrative mass, such as a carcinoma, an infection (such as a phlegmon), or a benign parotid pleomorphic adenoma (of the deep lobe) (Figs. 4.12 and 4.13).

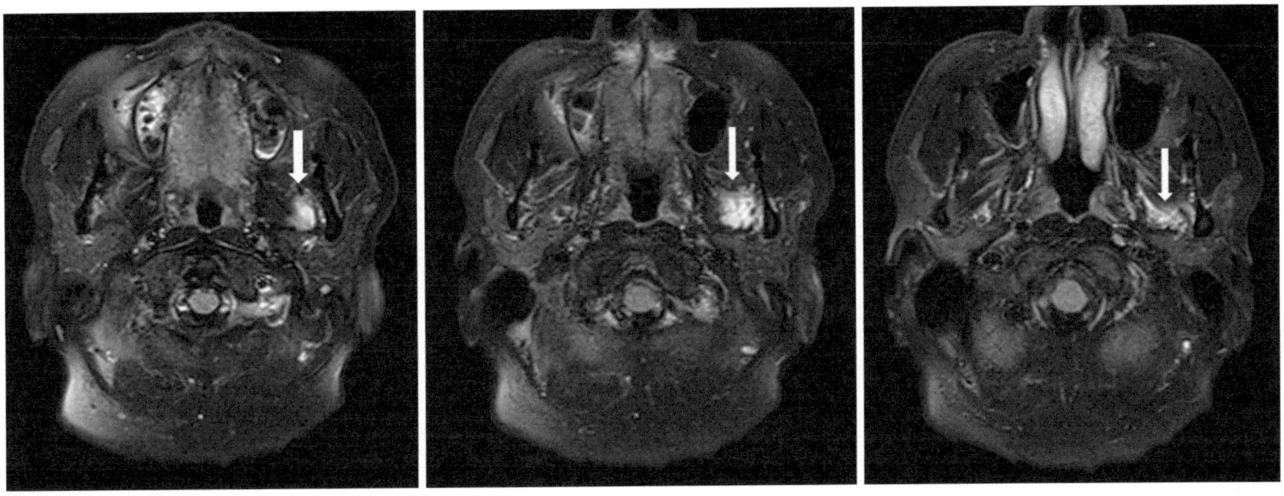

Fig. 4.12 A 50-year-old male patient with headache. Multiple postgadolinium MRI axial FLAIR images at the skull base level demonstrated asymmetrical appearances of the masticator space. On the left there is increased signal along the lateral aspect of the pterygoid muscles (*arrows*), mimicking a neoplasm. However, this is a typical location and appearance of a normal variant prominent pterygoid venous plexus

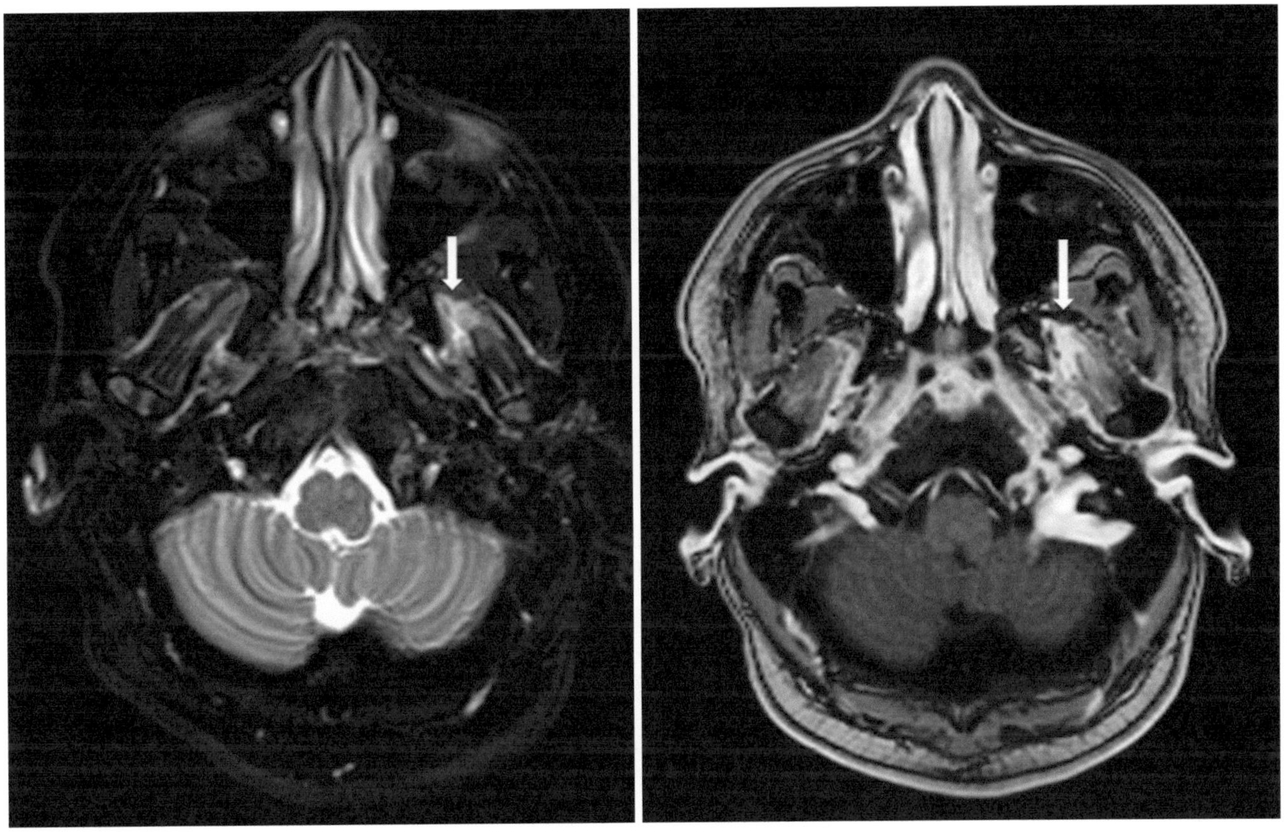

Fig. 4.13 A 56-year-old woman with a history of osteosarcoma. Axial fat suppressed-SET2WI (*left*) and postcontrast axial SET1WI (*right*) images demonstrate asymmetric T2 hyperintensity and contrast enhancement along the medial aspect of the left lateral pterygoid muscle (*arrows*), simulating recurrent neoplasm. However, there was no mass-like appearance. Hence, this was a case of a normal, asymmetric venous plexus that had been present on prior examinations (*not shown*)

4.10 Denervation Atrophy of Masticator Muscles and Asymmetric Masticator Uptake on PET-CT

In the acute phase of denervation, the affected muscles of the neck (whether in the floor of the mouth, neck, or tongue base) may be mistaken for tumor infiltration as they enlarge and enhance. This is typically a "don't touch lesion." The sparing of the muscle ligaments is an important clue to the true diagnosis. In late denervation, *muscular atrophy* can be mistaken for a tumor (due to asymmetric normal muscle bulk) on the contralateral side. In particular, following surgery or radiation therapy, such avid enhancement can simulate a recurrent carcinoma near the operative site.

Asymmetric muscular uptake on PET-CT can be a normal variant that is present for a variety of reasons that are noncancerous. These are typically attributable to unilateral or asymmetric muscular contractions. Such asymmetric muscle uptake can be visualized in nearly any musculature of the head and neck, including the muscles of mastication, the tongue base, the floor of mouth, the strap muscles, the sternocleidomastoid, the muscles of facial expression, and even the muscles of vocalization, to name a few (Figs. 4.14 and 4.15).

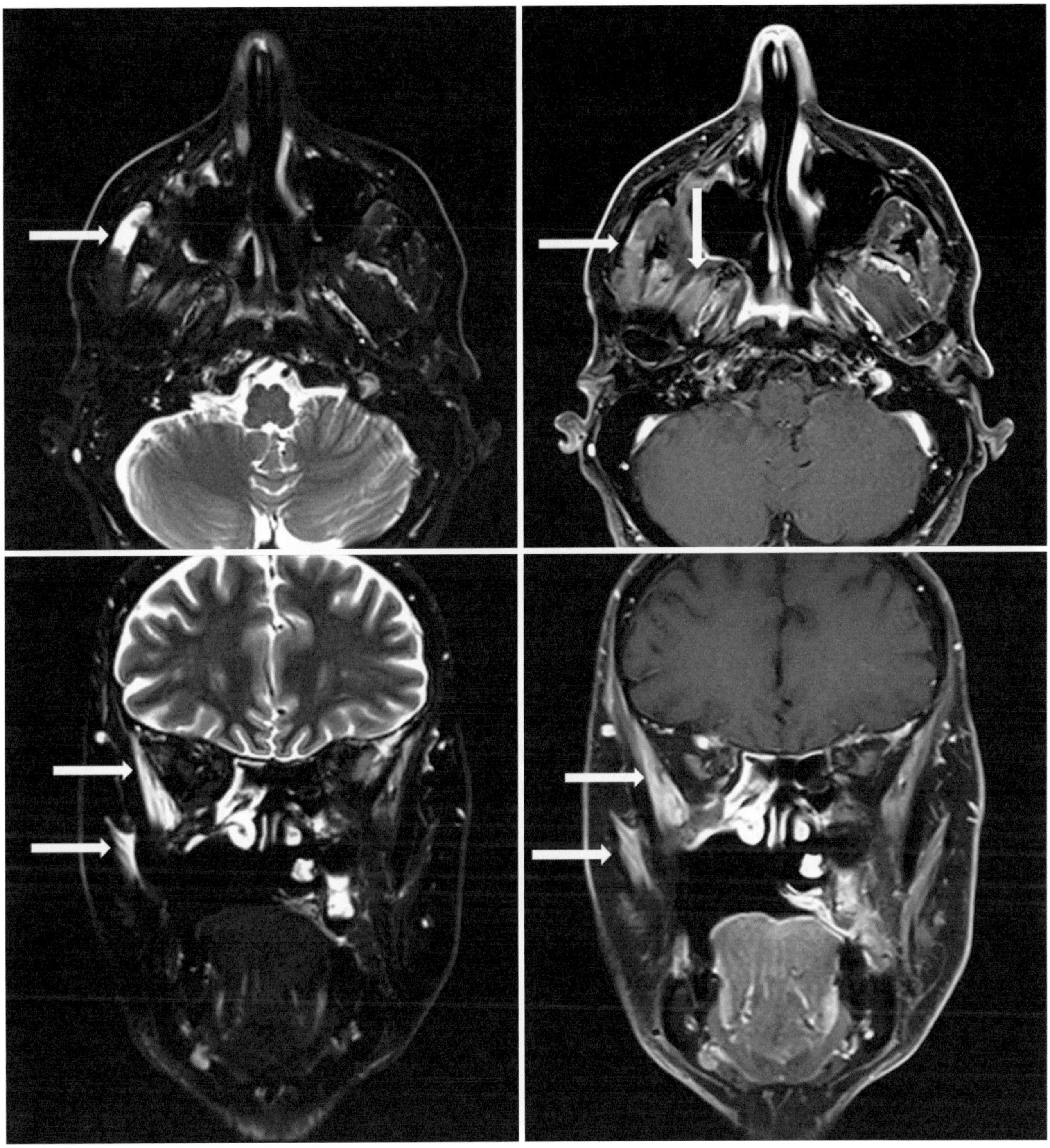

Fig. 4.14 A 62-year-old male with a history of right maxillary sinus adenoid cystic carcinoma; status was post treatment with both surgery and radiation therapy. On MRI, axial and coronal SET2WI (*upper left* and *bottom left*) demonstrate hyperintensity, and axial and coronal post-contrast fat suppression-SET1WI (*upper right* and *bottom right*) show abnormal enhancement of the right temporalis, pterygoid, and perhaps masseter muscles (*arrows*). The signal abnormalities extend along the muscle fibers without being mass-like, making them unlikely to be malignant. This is a case of denervation atrophy (a "don't touch lesion") that can show enhancement in the acute and subacute stages

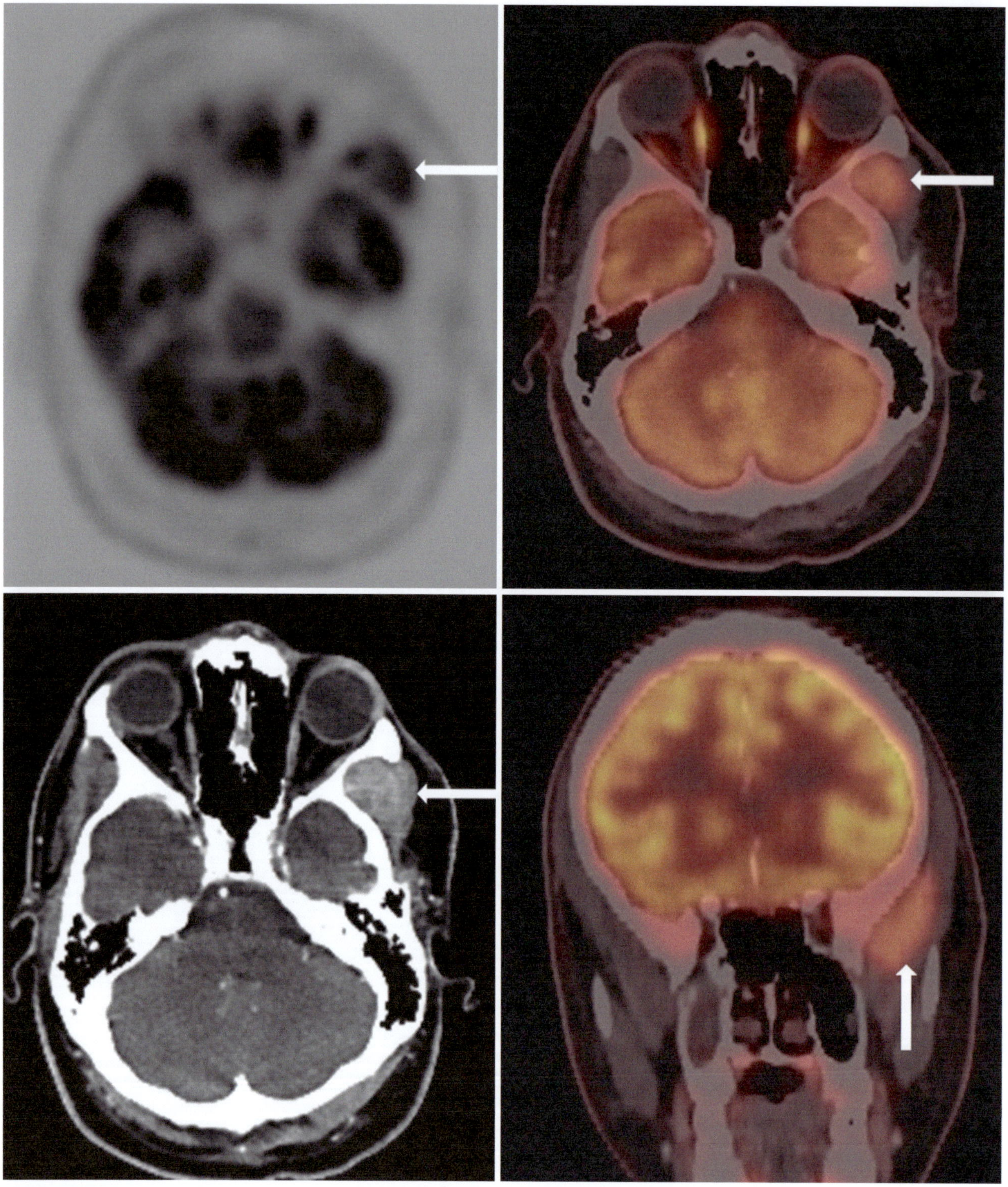

Fig. 4.15 Comparison case of granulocytic sarcoma within musculature. This patient is a 23- year-old male with a history of leukemia, status post-chemotherapy treatment. FDG PET-CT images including attenuation-corrected PET (*upper left*), axial fused PET-CT (*upper right*), coronal fused PET-CT (*bottom right*), and axial CECT (*bottom left*) images are shown. On axial and coronal fused images; there is asymmetric FDG uptake of the left suprazygomatic temporalis muscle (*arrows*). Asymmetrical muscle FDG uptake is a common finding on PET images, usually being a benign finding and present owing to asymmetrical muscular contraction on that side for various noncancerous reasons. When uptake is caused by benign muscular contraction, the FDG uptake pattern typically follows the expected muscular orientation. In this patient, there is a rather roundish appearance of the uptake on PET and fused images (*arrows*). On the CECT image (*bottom left*), there is indeed a subtly enhancing mass centered in this muscle (*arrows*). This is a pathology-proven granulocytic sarcoma. This case demonstrates that although one should be aware of common variant findings in the neck, it is important to also be observant of any findings that would be suspicious for underlying actual pathology

4.11 Hypoglossal Denervation and Hemiglossal Atrophy

Extensive fatty replacement of the affected hemitongue with loss of normal tongue muscle volume and prolapse of the affected hemitongue into the oropharynx owing to loss of normal tongue muscle tone are the findings seen in the chronic phase of the *hypoglossal denervation*. In an earlier (acute, subacute) phase there may be edema-like T2 prolongation and enhancement. This "don't touch lesion" is of importance because the prolapsed tissue can displace posteriorly and cause asymmetry (and appear as enlargement) of the oropharynx and tongue base on the side of fatty replacement, and thus simulate recurrent tongue cancer (Fig. 4.16).

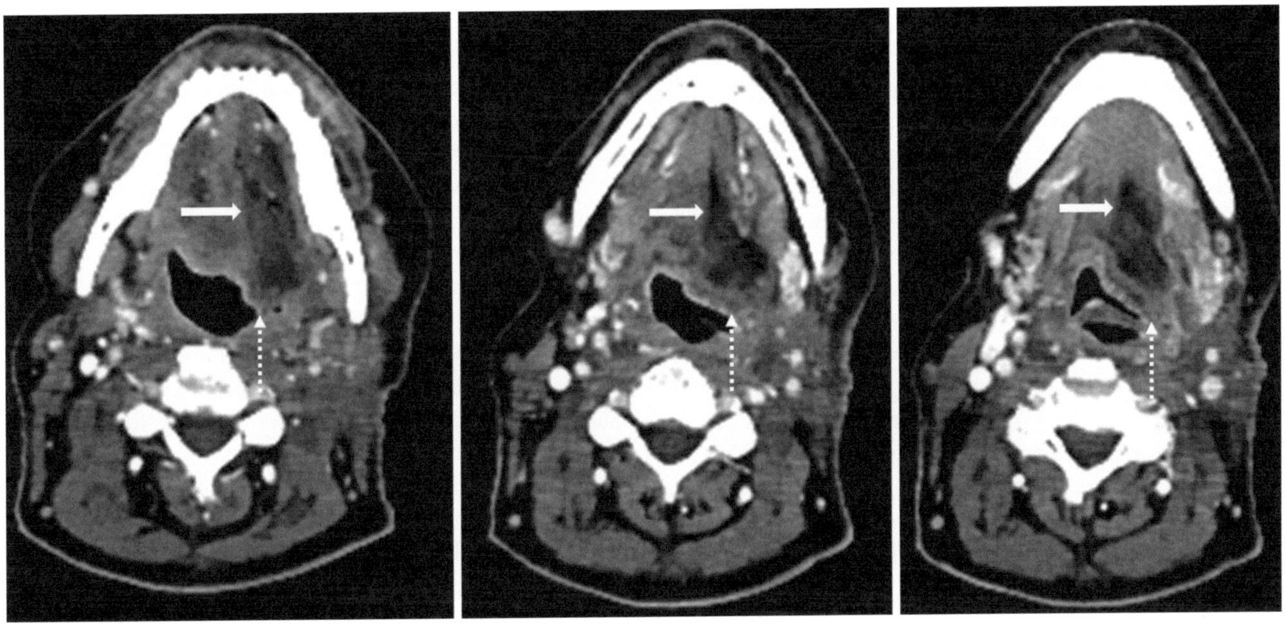

Fig. 4.16 In a 68-year-old male status post treatment for left-sided skull base metastasis, serial axial CECT images demonstrate an asymmetrically larger left hemitongue with posterior prolapse of the left tongue base (*dotted arrows*). This mimics a mass involving the left hemi-tongue; however, the fatty density change of the left hemi-tongue (*thick arrows*) suggests that there is fatty replacement and pseudohypertrophy of the left hemi-tongue, which are typical findings for ipsilateral hypoglossal denervation, a "don't touch lesion"

4.12 Retropharyngeal Carotid Artery (If Bilateral: "Kissing Carotid Arteries")

The carotid arteries may follow a more medial (retropharyngeal) course than normal. Various theories have been proposed regarding the cause of *retropharyngeal carotid arteries*, typically being the internal carotid artery (ICA) rather than the common carotid artery (CCA), which is a normal variation. Congenital alterations of the normal anatomy and increasing tortuosity of the arteries with progressing age have both been suggested as possible causes. In addition to increasing age, atherosclerosis and hypertension have also been linked to abnormalities of the carotid arteries, including tortuosity, kinking, and coiling.

A recent study by Lukins et al. (2015) evaluated the position of the internal carotid arteries on cervical spine MRI. In that study, retropharyngeal carotid arteries (defined by these authors as medial to the uncovertebral joint) were present in 2.6% of patients. Their results demonstrated that a change in the position of the carotid artery from lateral to retropharyngeal or vice-versa is not an uncommon phenomenon, occurring in 6.3% of their patients. That study also did not demonstrate a definite correlation between the degree of atherosclerosis and the degree of carotid deviation. The findings of that and other studies would suggest that the phenomenon of retropharyngeal carotid arteries is a dynamic one and could represent one or a combination of numerous possible causes, including pharyngeal contraction phase, respiratory phase, head/neck positioning, laxity or defects developmentally in the cervical fascial layers, or position relative to the stylohyoid ligament (or other ligaments).

This normal variation can be identified on nonenhanced (noncontrast) CT (NECT), contrast-enhanced CT (CECT), neck CT, neck MRI or magnetic resonance angiography (MRA), or even on a sinus CT as well as on other imaging examinations. It is perhaps best confirmed on CECT (filling with vascular contrast) or on noncontrast SET2WI MRI (due to the T2-dark flow void posterior to the pharyngeal mucosa). On a neck CT or MRI, is important to identify its location relative to any mucosal lesion or lymphadenopathy and to note whether it is the CCA or ICA, given the possibility of iatrogenic injury if a procedure is warranted to biopsy or remove such a mucosal or nodal lesion.

Thus, the clinical implications of this "don't touch" anatomic variant mainly include potential procedural complications (i.e., iatrogenic complications). Specifically, such possible complications include potentially lethal hemorrhage from injury to the internal carotid artery during surgical procedures involving the pharynx, including tonsillectomy, peritonsillar abscess drainage, and transoral tumor resection. A catastrophic complication could be ligation of the ICA to control hemorrhage, which could result in hemiplegia. Another example is during a transoral approach for blocking of the glossopharyngeal nerve, where there may be inadvertent arterial puncture or injection of local anesthetic into the retropharyngeal ICA. Additionally, there is a risk of injury to and resultant hemorrhage from the retropharyngeal ICA during tracheal intubation. Finally, a questionable association of import is that the retropharyngeal carotid artery has also been implicated as a potential contributing factor to obstructive sleep apnea, a disorder that can alter the pharyngeal anatomy. (Note: further discussion and figure examples are also provided in an associated earlier text: McKinney A. Retropharyngeal internal carotid artery. In: McKinney A. *Atlas of normal imaging variations of the brain, skull, and craniocervical vasculature*. Cham, Switzerland: Springer International Publishing; 2017. p. 1017–20) (Fig. 4.17).

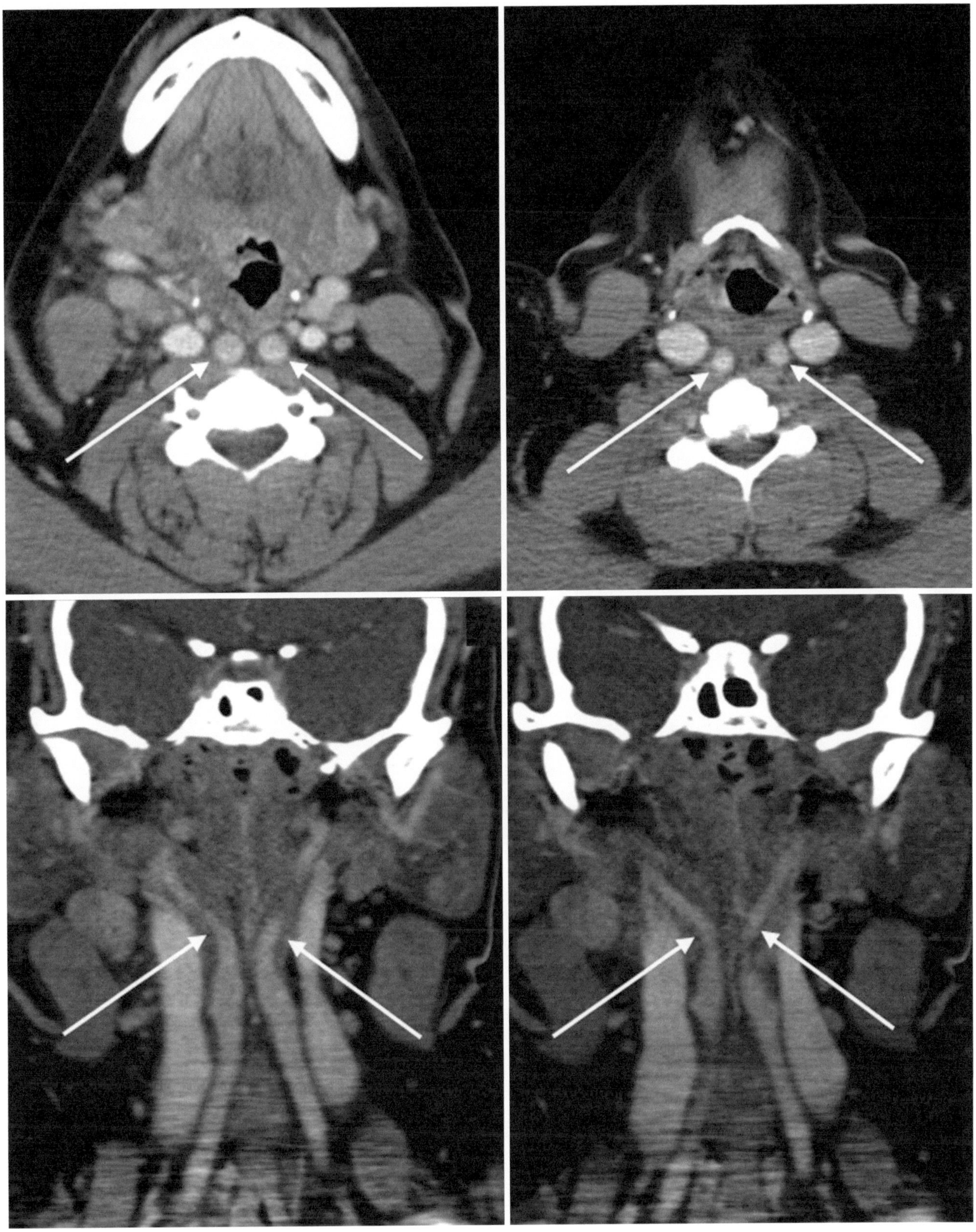

Fig. 4.17 A 35-year-old female suspected to have a neck abscess. Postcontrast axial (*top row*) and coronal (*bottom row*) CECT images demonstrate the retropharyngeal course of the proximal cervical internal carotid arteries bilaterally (*arrows*), a normal variant

4.13 Thyroid Lipoma

An *adenolipoma of the thyroid gland* (also known as a *thyrolipoma* or a *thyroid hamartoma*) is a rare, fat-containing lesion of the thyroid. These benign lesions are usually well encapsulated and are composed of varying degrees of follicular thyroid tissue (thyroid adenoma) and mature adipose tissue; the amount of fat can vary markedly (from 10% to 90%). Since this lesion has no malignant potential and rarely enlarges, it is considered a "don't touch lesion" (Fig. 4.18).

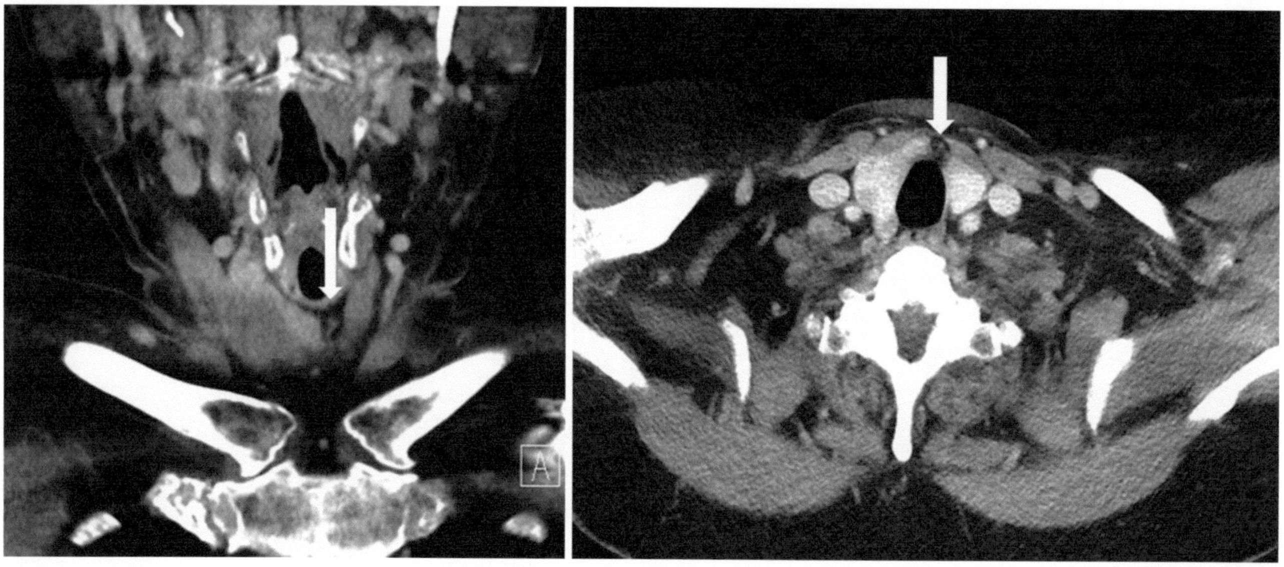

Fig. 4.18 A 78-year-old female patient with a known parotid mass. A CECT obtained to evaluate for a parotid lesion (negative) incidentally demonstrated a hypodense (fat density) focus within the isthmus/left thyroid lobe junction (*arrows*). This is an incidental benign thyroid lipoma

4.14 Thyroid Cartilage Lipoma

Tumors of the laryngeal skeleton are rare and account for less than 1% of laryngeal neoplasms. The most common entities are chondromas and chondrosarcomas. Besides these, amyloidomas, aneurysmal bone cysts, giant cell tumors, aggressive osteoblastomas, osteosarcomas, and plasma cell tumors have all been described in the literature. *Thyroid cartilage lipoma* is a rare but benign lesion and is typically detected incidentally. It is usually readily diagnosed by the visualization of fat density and fat signal characteristics on CT and MRI. Thus, this is a "don't touch" variant that is usually not confused with a malignant neoplasm, although occasionally it could be confused with a thyroid nodule (and thus undergo biopsy) if one does not observe the characteristic fatty characteristics on imaging or does not recognize the true anatomic location (Fig. 4.19).

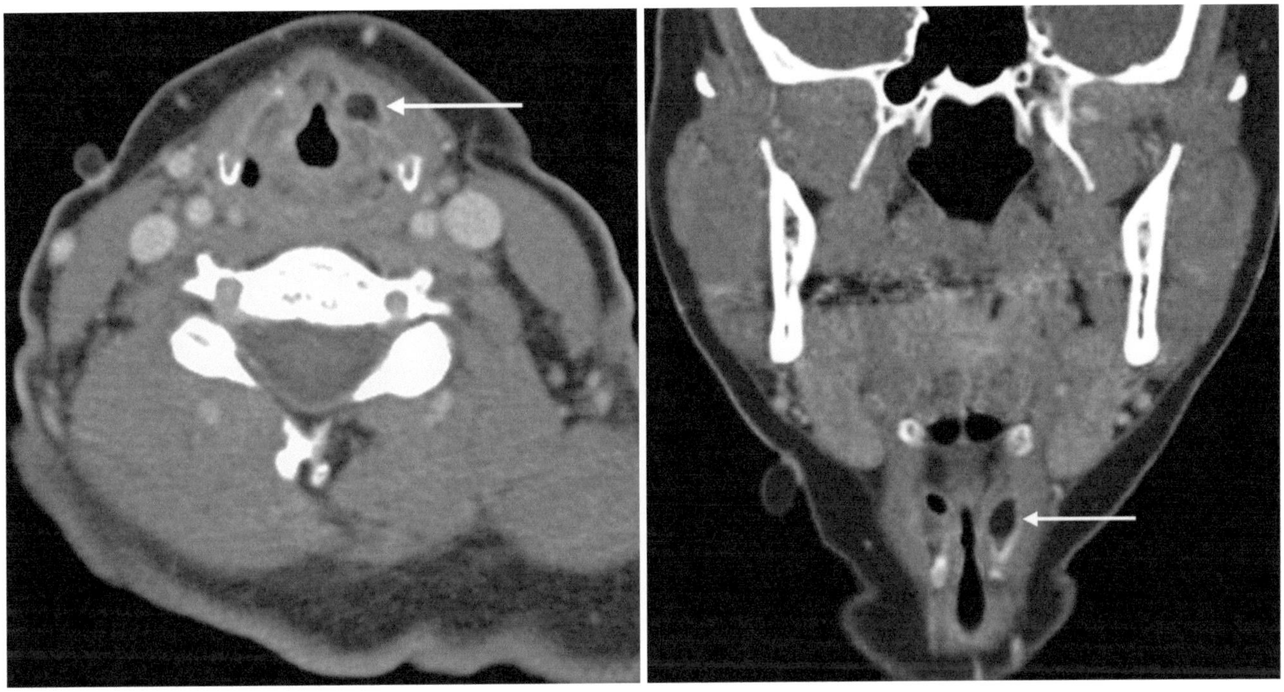

Fig. 4.19 A 54-year-old male with a neck mass. Axial (*left*) and coronal (*right*) CECT images demonstrate asymmetry of the thyroid cartilage. There is focal fat deposition within the left thyroid cartilage (*arrows*), representing a thyroid cartilage lipoma, an incidental benign "don't touch" finding

4.15 Thyroglossal Duct Cyst

Thyroglossal duct cysts (TGDCs) are found along the path of the embryonic thyroglossal duct, which can lie anywhere along the development path of the thyroid beginning in the fetal oropharynx with eventual descent down through the tongue, hyoid, and anterior strap musculature to its ultimate position. TGDCs are the most common thyroglossal duct lesions and likely the most common congenital cystic neck lesion, where 20% to 25% is suprahyoid in location. They have a generic cystic appearance, typically being well-circumscribed and homogeneous low density/high T2-signal on MRI with a very thin rim of enhancement on postcontrast T1WI but occasionally with thin septa or lobulations. As with most neck cysts, the attenuation of TGDCs is usually hypodense (between 0 and 20 HU) at CT, with high T2 signal and intermediate T1 signal at MR imaging. The fluid within the lesion can at times appear complex, either being proteinaceous or hemorrhagic, which cause the lesion to have higher attenuation on CT and a brighter signal on T1WI MRI. These cysts are most often "don't touch lesions" that are smaller (<2 cm size) and initially simple and well-circumscribed, but occasionally they become complex lesions that are infected or hemorrhagic; in such complicated TGDCs, the cyst appears heterogeneous and complex with profuse surrounding soft-tissue edema. Rarely, another complication of these cysts is the development of malignancy, which has been reported to occur in about 1–2%. TGDCs may need to be distinguished from other cystic lesions when a component closely associated with the hyoid bone is discovered, such as cystic lymph nodes, abscess, or necrotic metastasis, but with a characteristic location and appearance. In the uncommon scenario in which these are quite large or complex, they can also mimic a plunging ranula (from the enlarged sublingual or submandibular gland) or rarely a complex branchial cleft cyst if both are quite large and extensive. In such uncommon cases where a TGDC must be excised, the Sistrunk procedure is most commonly employed; this procedure is based on earlier embryologic studies of the thyroid gland's developmental tract, which involves resection of the body of the hyoid bone (Fig. 4.20).

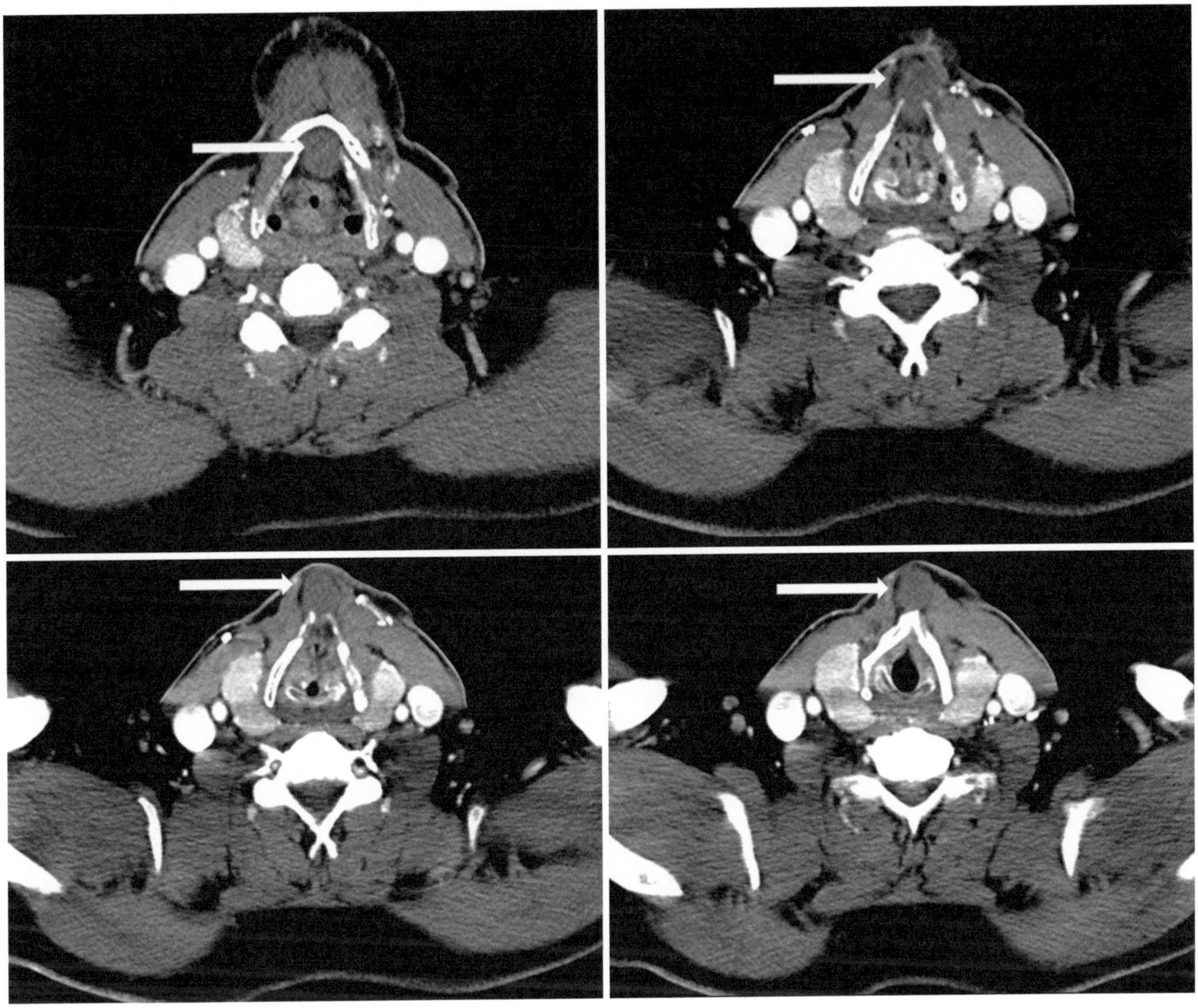

Fig. 4.20 A 55-year-old male with floor of the mouth cancer. Multiple axial neck CECT images of the neck demonstrate a well-defined midline fluid density lesion in the anterior neck, below the level of the hyoid bone (*arrows*), with no associated enhancement. This is a typical location and appearance of a thyroglossal duct cyst, which is a benign developmental variant

4.16 Ectopic Thyroid

Ectopic thyroid glands are found along the path of the thyroglossal duct, which involutes in most adults but is found between the foramen cecum (located at the midline posterior tongue) and the thyroid gland during development. The duct passes through the posterior root of the tongue before reaching the hyoid bone. In the suprahyoid neck, the thyroglossal duct is found along the midline, although it diverges laterally within the infrahyoid neck. On NECT ectopic thyroids are mildly hyperdense relative to other nonbony structures (due to iodine content), while on contrast-enhanced CT (CECT), they are hyperattenuating relative to muscle owing to (a) the thyroidal tissue's iodine content, as well as (b) avid contrast enhancement. At MR imaging, they are usually solid in appearance, mildly T1-hyperintense or isointense (relative to musculature), and they are avidly enhancing. High iodine-123 (^{123}I) and technetium-99m-uptake on radiotracer studies are typical and very specific. Approximately 90% of ectopic thyroids are found within the tongue ("lingual thyroid"). The remaining 10% can be visualized anywhere along the expected path of the thyroglossal duct. In 75% of patients with ectopic thyroid, the ectopic thyroid represents the only functioning thyroid tissue; thus, as this is typically a "don't touch" variant, if there is consideration of resection, it is important to establish if there is normally functioning thyroid tissue elsewhere prior to surgery. As with other thyroid tissue, these lesions can undergo cancerous and goiterous transformation (in approximately 3% of cases) (Fig. 4.21).

Fig. 4.21 Three separate patients with different locations of ectopic thyroidal tissue. **Top row**: A 6-year-old female with questioned respiratory difficulties and a possible "tongue mass" on clinical examination was found to have ectopic "lingual thyroid" tissue (*arrows*) at the posterior tongue base on a CECT in coronal (*left*) and axial (*middle*) reformats; no thyroidal tissue was noted within the expected normal location of the thyroid on an axial image through the level of the thyroid cartilage (*right*). **Middle row**: A different 25-year-old female presenting with a palpated midline neck mass underwent axial CECT images (*left and right images*), which demonstrated a corresponding midline hyperdense focus of ectopic thyroid tissue situated beneath the external marker (*arrows*) and slightly below the normal thyroid gland level, where the patient did not have thyroid tissue at the expected axial level on the CT scan (*not shown*). **Bottom row**: Another 43-year-old female felt a neck lump on the right side of her neck, where a hyperdense focus (*arrows*) was noted on axial (*left*) and sagittal (*right*) CECT images underlying the skin marker; the focus was overlying the right thyroid cartilage and was subsequently biopsied and proved to be an aberrant location of ectopic thyroidal tissue. Note the normal location of thyroidal tissue posteriorly and inferiorly (*asterisk, right*)

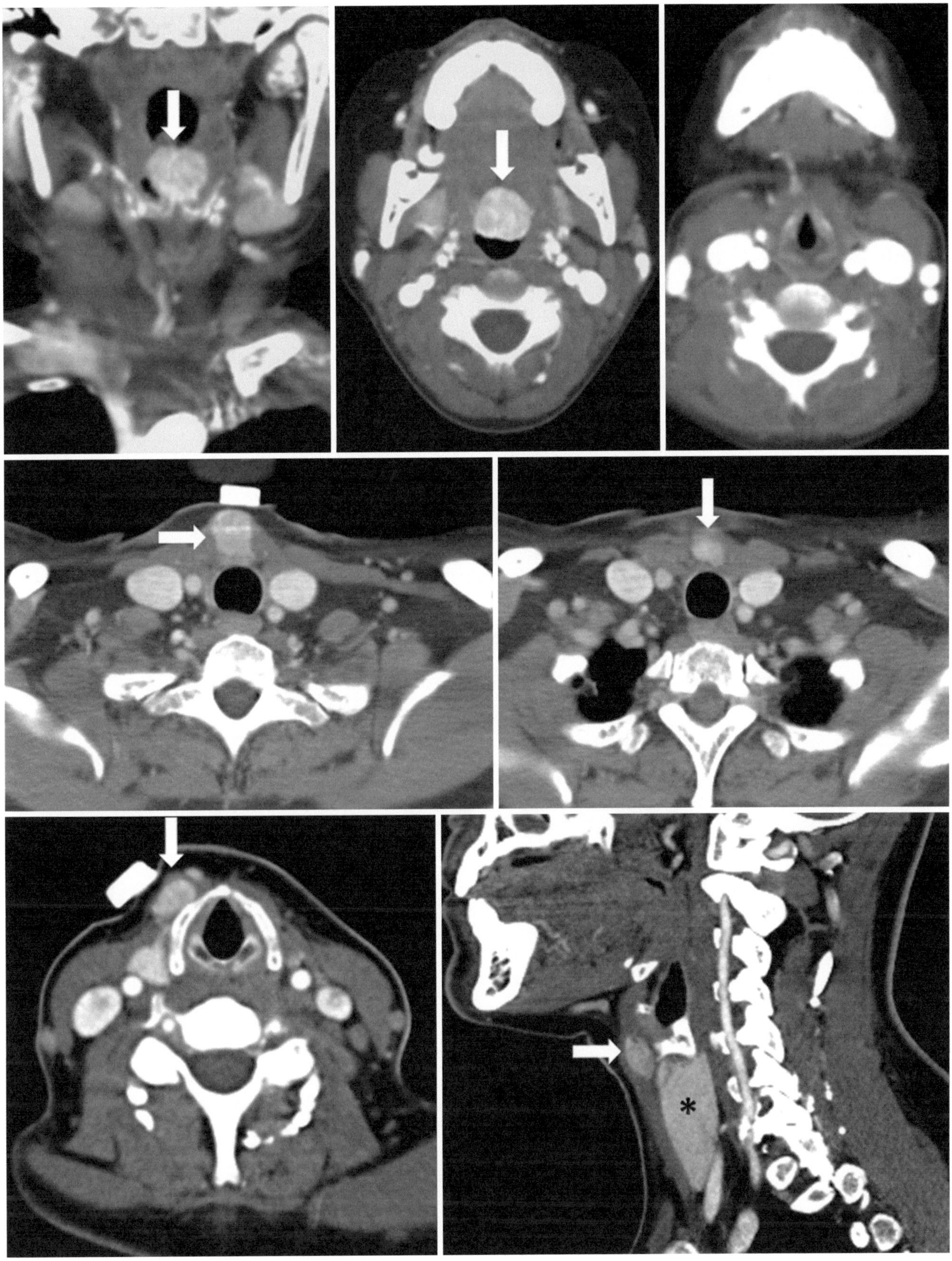

4.17 Thyroid Isthmus Agenesis

The right and left lobes of the thyroid gland are connected by the thyroid isthmus. The isthmus lies at the level of the second and third tracheal rings, although often it can be situated higher or sometimes lower, as its size varies greatly. The isthmus measures an average of approximately 1.25 cm in both the craniocaudal and transverse dimensions. However, the isthmus may occasionally be absent. The incidence of *agenesis of the thyroid isthmus* has been reported to vary from 5% to 10%. The basic mechanism can be attributed to anomalous embryologic development, while the literature suggests that chromosome 22 plays a major role (Fig. 4.22).

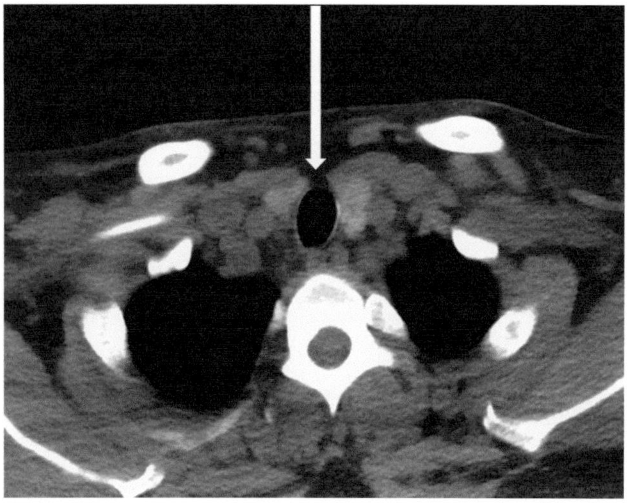

Fig. 4.22 The patient was a 32-year-old male with occasional swallowing difficulty. A single axial postcontrast neck CECT image showed normal size and homogeneous density of the right and left thyroid lobes, with the thyroid gland overall being located at the expected level. However, no thyroid isthmus was visualized, which can be a normal developmental variation

4.18 Thyroid Lobe Asymmetry and Agenesis

Asymmetry in the size of the thyroid lobes is common and normal in healthy individuals. It has even been reported that the right thyroid lobe is more often significantly larger than the left lobe! An interesting description in the literature by Ying et al. is that the handedness may be associated with the asymmetry of the thyroid size, in that right-handed subjects had a significantly larger right lobe size than left-handers but not vice versa, as handedness did not affect the volume of the left lobe; there was no significant difference found in the left lobe volume between right and left handers.

Thyroid lobe agenesis is much rarer, being estimated to occur in approximately 0.2% of the population, and it is often asymptomatic. About 80% of the time the agenesis is left-sided and may occur with or without thyroid isthmus agenesis. This normal variant is more common in females (Fig 4.23).

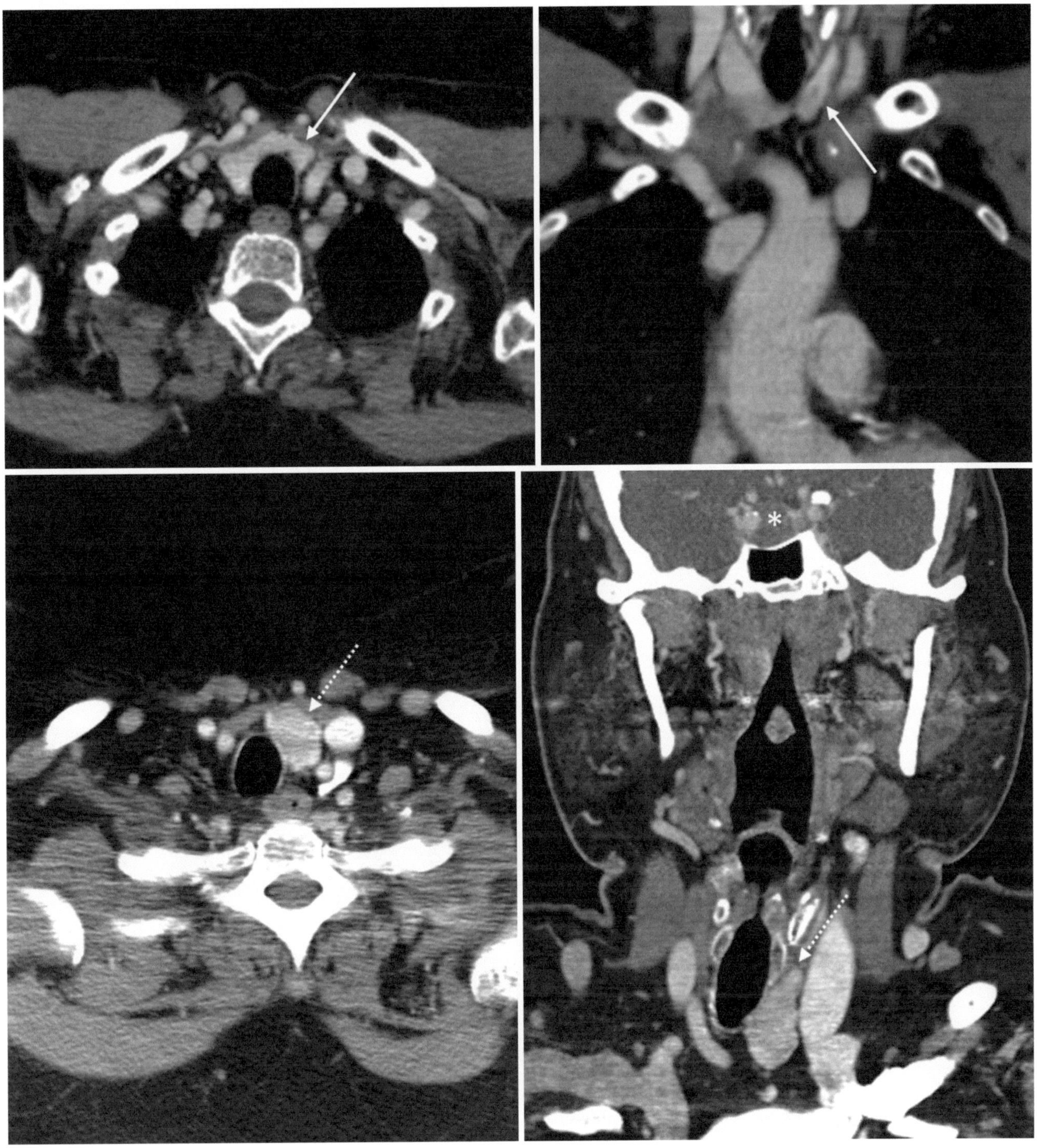

Fig. 4.23 Thyroid lobe asymmetry and agenesis in two separate patients. **Top row**: A 71-year- old female with breast cancer underwent CECT, where axial (*left*) and coronal (*right*) reconstructed images from a chest CT show asymmetry in the sizes of the thyroid lobe; the left lobe (*arrows*) is smaller than the right, a normal anatomical variation. **Bottom row**: A 59-year-old female evaluated for a pituitary mass (*asterisk, right*) had only a left thyroid lobe (*dotted arrows*), with absence-agenesis of the right thyroid lobe (no history of surgery) on axial (*left*) and coronal (*right*) reconstructions from the CECT

4.19 Pyramidal Lobe of Thyroid

The *thyroid pyramidal lobe* is a normal variant. It is visualized as a third thyroid lobe and is variably present in 10% to 30% of the population. It is likely related to a remnant of the thyroglossal duct. It usually arises from the isthmus upward along the midline, or alternatively is it shifted toward the left of neck. Also, it is usually located anterior to the thyroid cartilage. Notably, the pyramidal lobe is normal thyroidal tissue that can be involved in any parenchymal disease that diffusely involves the thyroid gland, such as thyroiditis or lymphoma (Fig. 4.24).

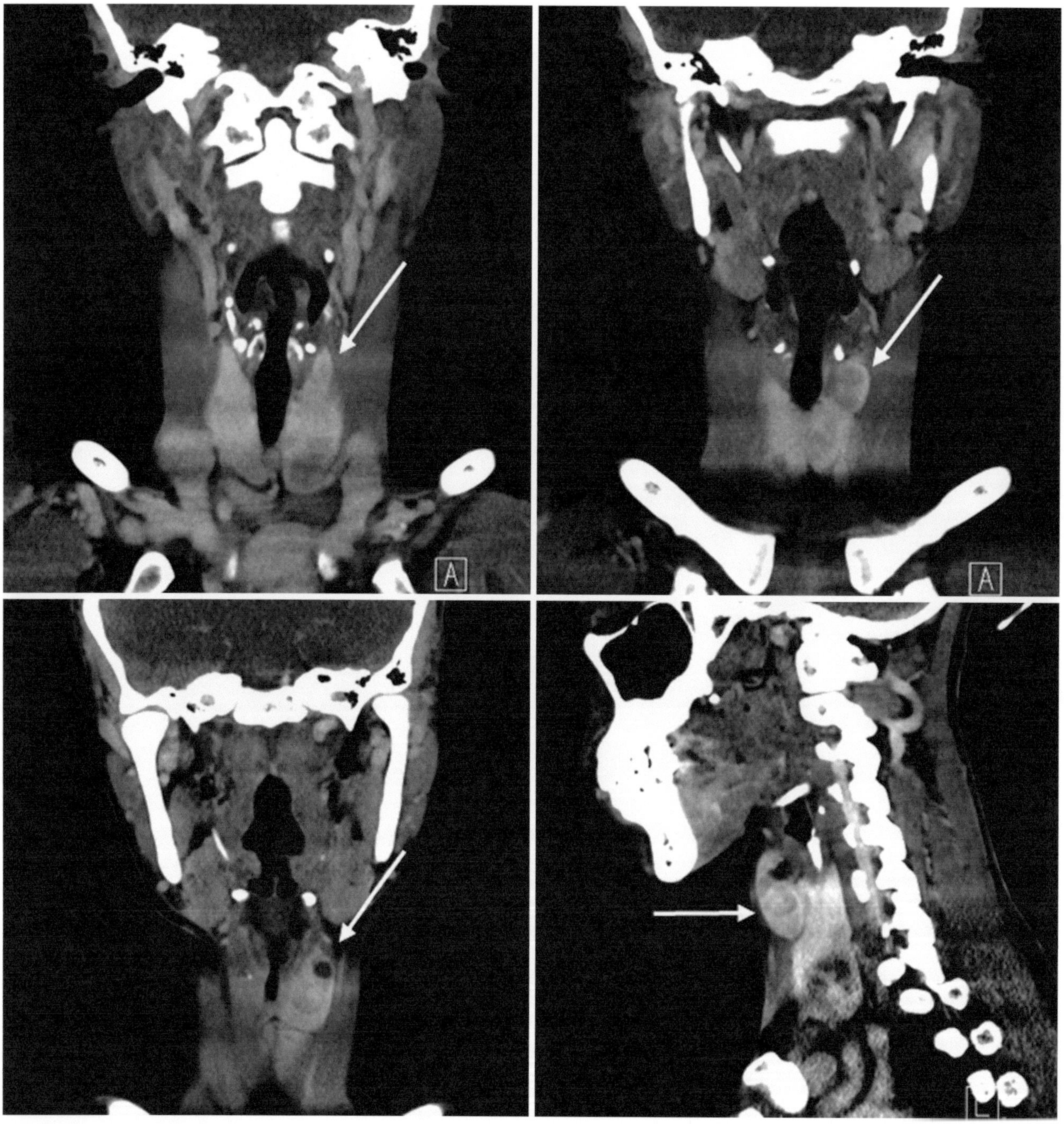

Fig. 4.24 A 36-year-old female with a multinodular goiter. Postcontrast coronal (*top left, top right,* and *bottom left images*) and sagittal (*bottom right*) images reconstructed from a CECT demonstrate a nodular and diffusely enlarged thyroid gland. Note the nodular-like and finger-like appearance extending from the superior aspect of the left thyroid lobe cranially along the left lateral aspect of the cricoid cartilage, which represents a nodule (*arrows*) that occurs within a normal variant pyramidal lobe

4.20 Submandibular Gland Agenesis (Unilateral)

The salivary glands arise as buds from the epithelial lining of the oral cavity. These primordial buds grow and extend into the underlying mesenchymal tissue as a solid core of cells. The parotid glands appear during the fourth week of gestation in the angle between the maxillary process and the mandibular arch. The submandibular glands appear in the sixth week, and the sublingual glands arise during the ninth week between the tongue and the mandibular arch.

Congenital absence of the salivary glands is infrequent and more often involves multiple major salivary glands. *Isolated unilateral major salivary gland aplasia* is a rare entity with only a few cases reported of this variant in the literature to date. The aplasia is likely caused by arrest in organogenesis, but the exact etiology is unknown.

Salivary gland aplasia may be associated with first branchial arch defects in the Treacher-Collins syndrome (mandibulofacial dysostosis) or orbital abnormalities like lacrimal hypoplasia, canalicular atresia, and absence of the lacrimal puncta. Absence of salivary glands may also be seen as part of the lacrimoauriculodentodigital syndrome that is characterized by hypoplasia, aplasia, or atresia of the lacrimal system, deafness and ear malformations, and dental and digital anomalies.

The clinical picture of patients with salivary gland aplasia is variable. They may be asymptomatic or may complain of dry mouth, have difficulty chewing and swallowing, and have an increased incidence of dental caries, which is thought to be caused by reduction of the protective effect of saliva within the oral cavity.

Salivary gland aplasia can be diagnosed with a variety of imaging techniques, which include CT, MR imaging, sonography, sialography, or nuclear medicine (technetium Tc99m-pertechnetate) studies. Radiologists should be familiar with this "don't touch" variant and its imaging findings to prevent unnecessary biopsy of this benign condition (i.e., prevent biopsying the normal side which may seem asymmetric to the patient or palpating clinician) (Figs. 4.25 and 4.26).

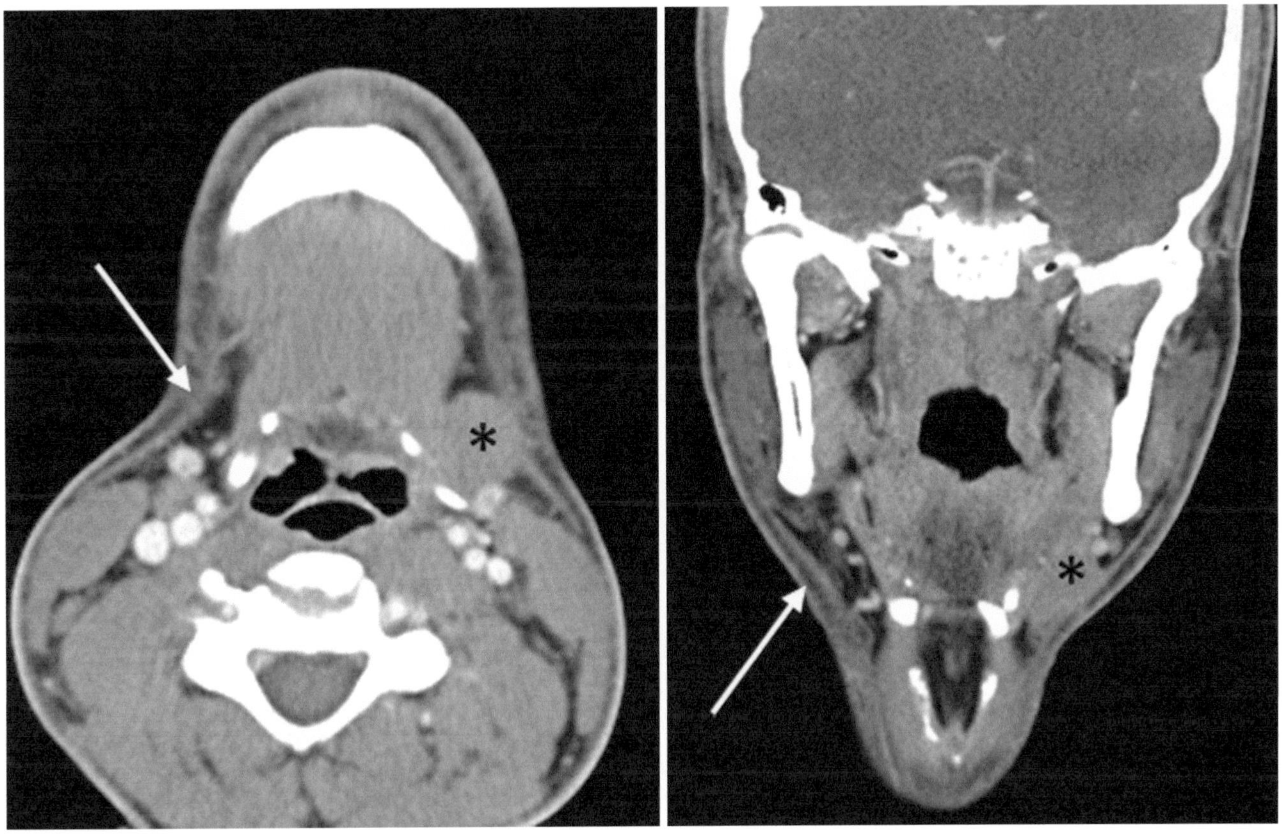

Fig. 4.25 A 22-year-old male presented with left-sided neck swelling. Axial (*left*) and coronal (*right*) reconstructions of a CECT demonstrate an absent right submandibular gland within the right submandibular fossa (*arrows*). The normal left submandibular gland was falsely palpated and thought to be a neck mass (*asterisks*) due to the submandibular asymmetry between sides

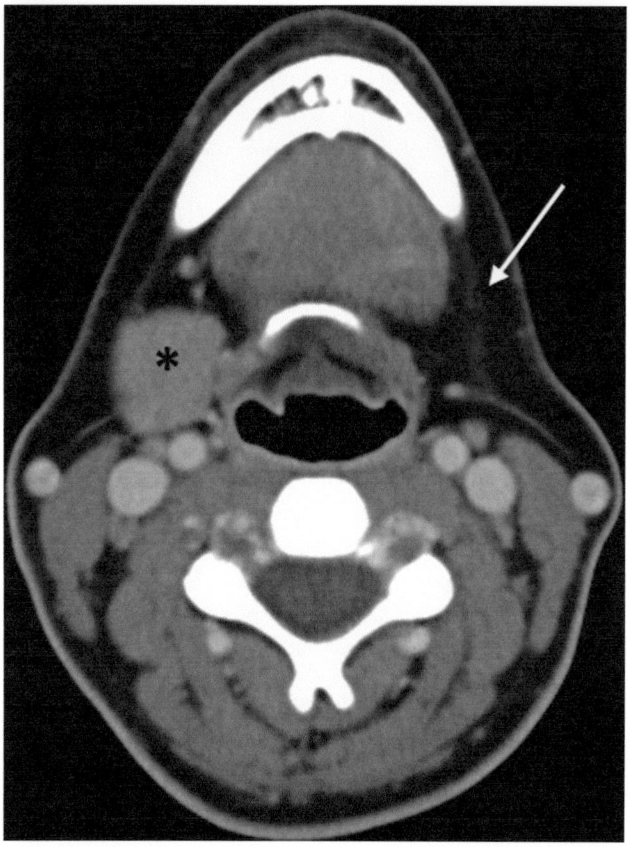

Fig. 4.26 A 35-year-old female presented with fullness in the right side of the neck. An axial CECT image showed a normal right submandibular gland (*asterisk*) with an absent left submandibular gland (*arrow*), an anatomical variation

4.21 Sublingual Gland Hypertrophy

The sublingual glands are salivary glands that lie in the floor of the mouth anterior to the submandibular glands. They may be hypertrophied when the ipsilateral submandibular gland is hypoplastic or aplastic, which is a "don't touch" variant. There also can be normal asymmetry in size, another normal variant (Figs. 4.27 and 4.28).

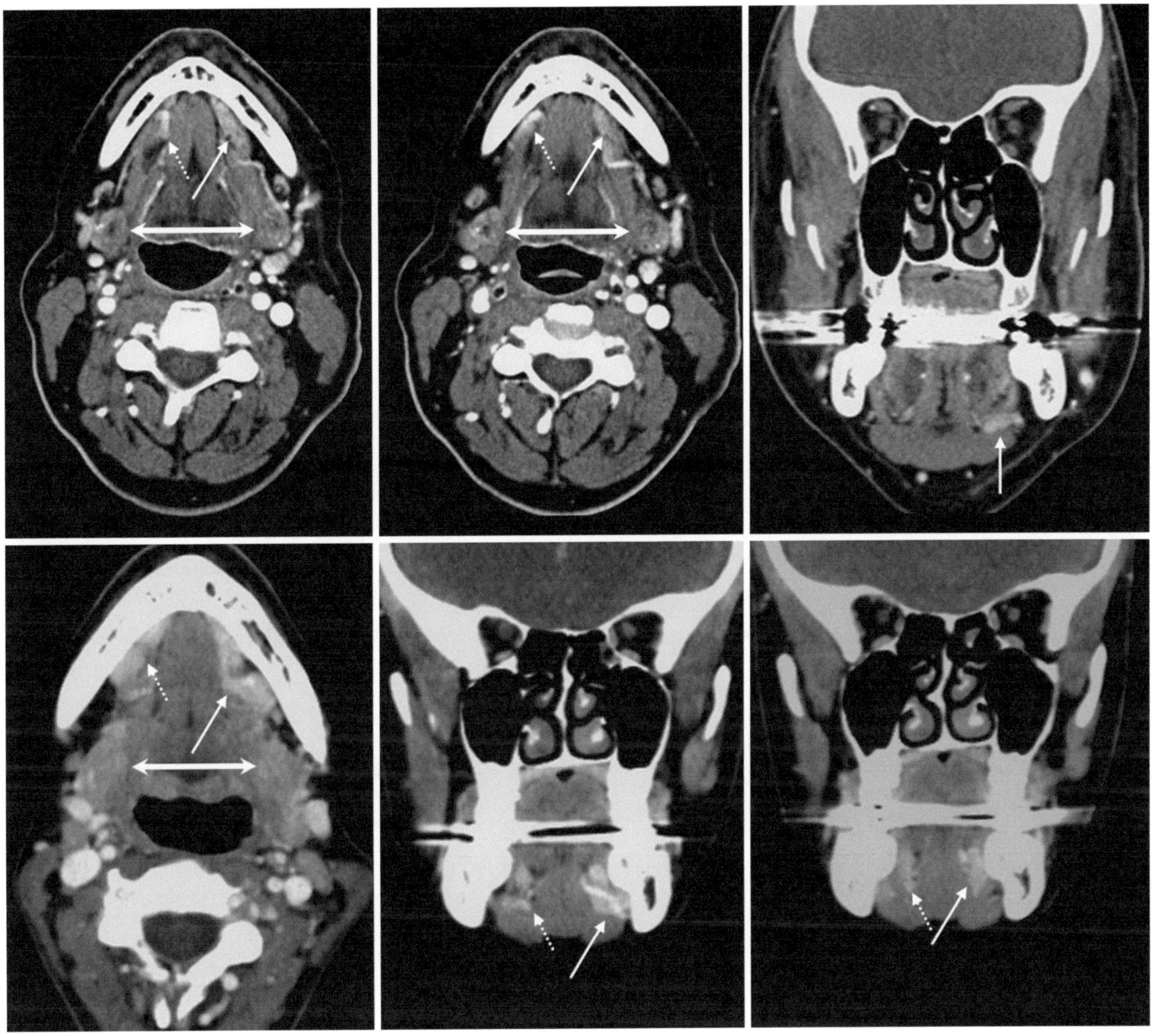

Fig. 4.27 Sublingual radiation-related enhancement and hypertrophy in two separate patients. **Top row**: In a 60-year-old male with tonsillar cancer (post-radiation), the submandibular glands (*double arrows*) are severely atrophied bilaterally, accounting for the appearance of sublingual gland enhancement-mild hypertrophy that is present on the patient's left side (*arrows*) more than the right side (*dotted arrows*), as demonstrated on CECT axial (*left, middle*) and coronal (*right*) reconstructions. **Bottom row**: In a different 37-year-old female patient who clinically had dysfunction of the parotid (*not shown*) and submandibular glands (*double arrows*), a CECT was negative for abnormalities in those aforementioned glands. However, axial (*left*) and coronal (*middle, right*) reformats demonstrate that the left sublingual gland is moderately hypertrophied and enhancing (*arrows*), while the right is also hypertrophied to a lesser degree (*dotted arrows*). In both patients, such sublingual gland hypertrophy and enhancement is a "don't touch" finding and should not be mistaken for a neoplasm at the floor of mouth or tongue base

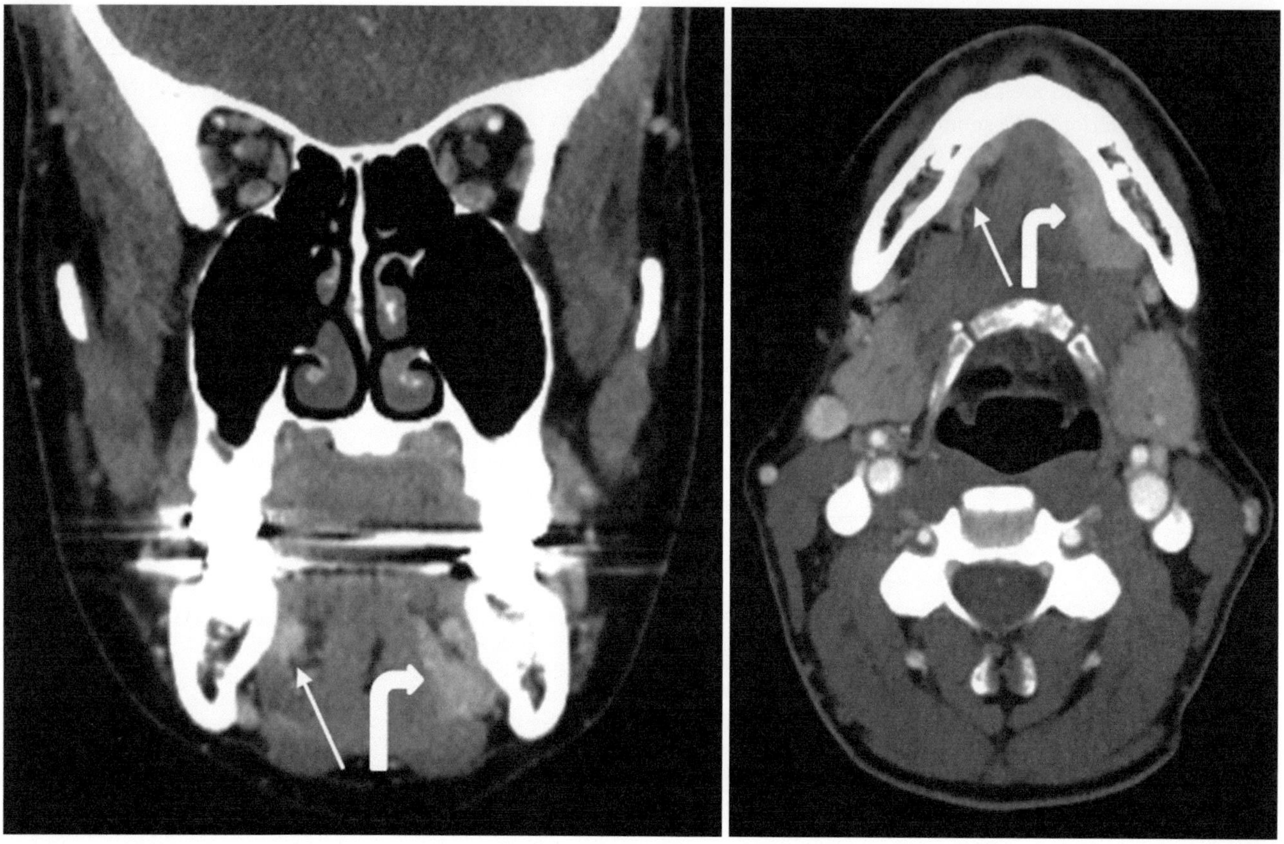

Fig. 4.28 A 53-year-old female with throat and ear pain. On a CECT with coronal (*left*) and axial (*right*) reconstructions, there is an asymmetrical appearance of the sublingual space. Larger enhancing sublingual glandular tissue is seen on the left side of the floor of the mouth (*curved arrows*), a normal variation. Note the smaller and more typical size of the enhancing sublingual glandular tissue on the right side (*straight arrows*)

4.22 Parotid Gland Fatty Replacement: Unilateral and Bilateral

Unilateral fatty replacement of parotid gland tissue is a common finding in previously irradiated patients having head and neck primary malignancies. Irradiation to one side of the face/neck results in atrophy and fatty replacement of the parotid gland that is in the field of radiation. The contralateral asymmetric larger gland (normal gland) should not be mistaken for an abnormality. This can also arise from chronic sialadenitis. Thus, a unilateral fatty parotid gland may not be "normal" but is typically a "don't touch lesion," while bilateral fatty parotid glands can arise from irradiation as well but can also arise from multiple possible underlying comorbidities.

Bilateral fatty replacement of parotid gland tissue with an atrophic decrease in size is also a "don't touch lesion" but suggests an underlying pathologic process in most patients; however, occasionally it can occur to a milder degree with advanced age (>70 years). It is important to note that the parotid gland parenchyma is subject to changes in local or systemic conditions. Notably, these glands can overall be decreased in size (atrophied) but can also be increased in size (hypertrophied). Some systemic conditions that may have diffuse and bilateral fatty parotid infiltration (with or without an atrophic decrease in size) include hypertriglyceridemia (fat infiltration within the parotid without inflammatory activity), a decrease in ovarian hormones after ovariectomy, Sjögren syndrome (can have premature fat deposition within the parotid glands and parenchyma heterogeneity rather than diffuse fatty infiltration), or other diseases causing bilateral chronic sialadenitis, human immunodeficiency virus (HIV, fatty infiltration with lymphocytes, lymphoepithelial cysts, or adenopathy), and alcoholism or diabetes (the latter two etiologies perhaps occur because of a reduction in the rate of fat tissue metabolism of the stroma). Also, as stated above, age-related fatty replacement may occur from declining secretory abilities of the parotid glands and not be related to a pathologic process; as such, studies in rats have shown increased lipids and degeneration of secretory granules with increasing age.

As mentioned in the previous topic, radiation therapy can cause unilateral or bilateral fatty replacement following therapy, depending on the field of radiation treatment. Radiation sialadenitis can also occur following the radioactive iodine (I^{131}) treatment of thyroid carcinoma because of the unique ability of the salivary glands to concentrate iodine. The parotid glands are affected more than other major salivary glands, with transient bilateral parotid swelling occurring usually within 1 day of iodine ingestion; this usually resolves spontaneously within a week. While the diagnosis can be made purely on clinical grounds and imaging is usually not required, a long-term follow up imaging examination (often obtained for other indications) may demonstrate a bilateral small size of the parotid glands from progressive and chronic atrophy with fatty replacement (Figs. 4.29 and 4.30).

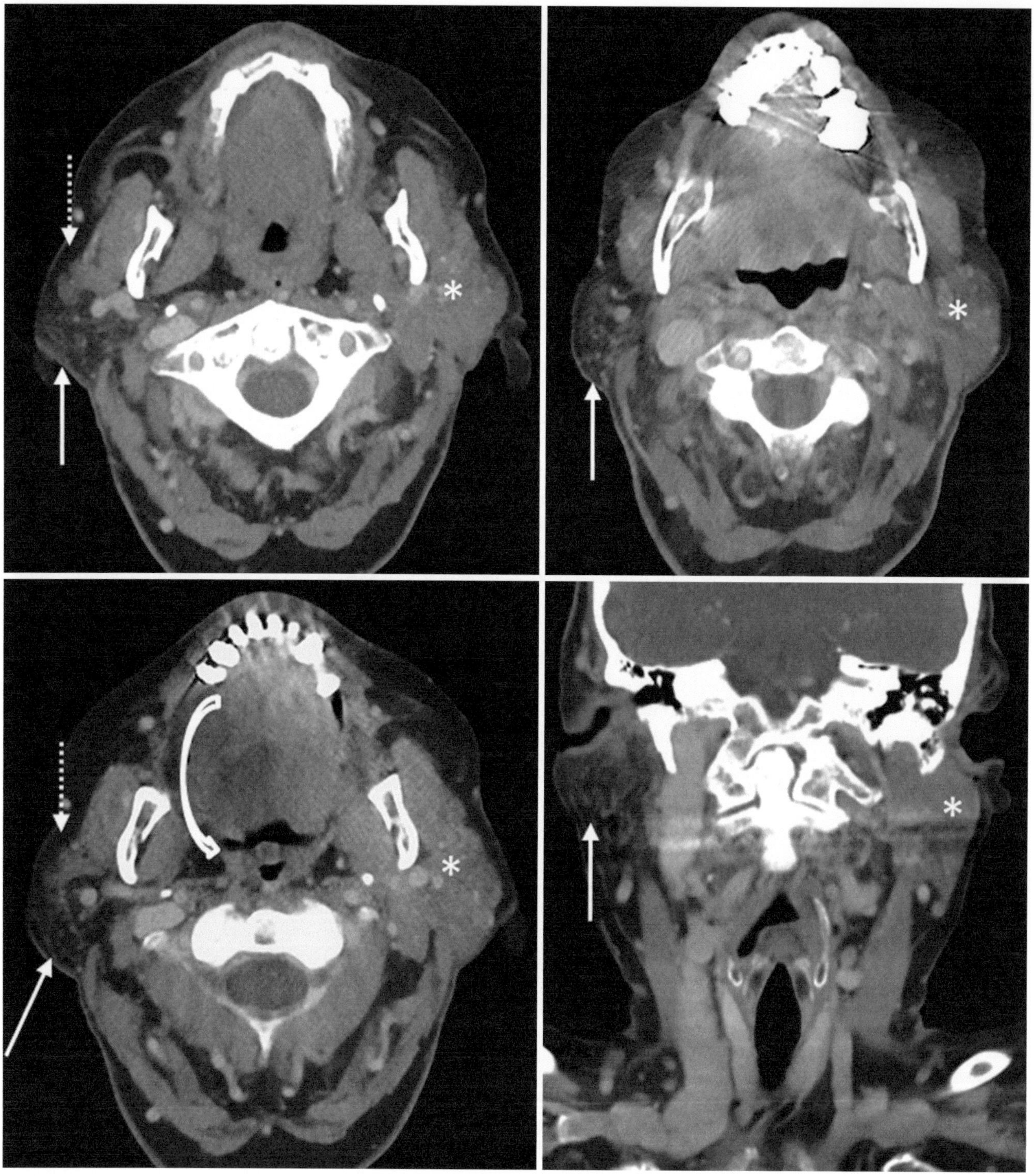

Fig. 4.29 A 78-year-old female with neck pain. Multiple axial CECT images (*top row* and *bottom left*) and a coronal CECT image (*bottom right*) together demonstrate asymmetry of the parotid glands, the left being greater in size and denser than the right gland (*arrows*). There is a mostly fatty replaced right parotid gland (*arrows*), with some residual parotid tissue visible anteriorly (*dotted arrows*, *top left* and *bottom left*). There is compensatory hypertrophy of the left parotid gland (*asterisks*). The fat density component or the residual glandular tissue seen anteriorly can potentially be mistaken for a mass. Notably, as in this patient, the parotid glands can be entirely or partially replaced by fatty tissue

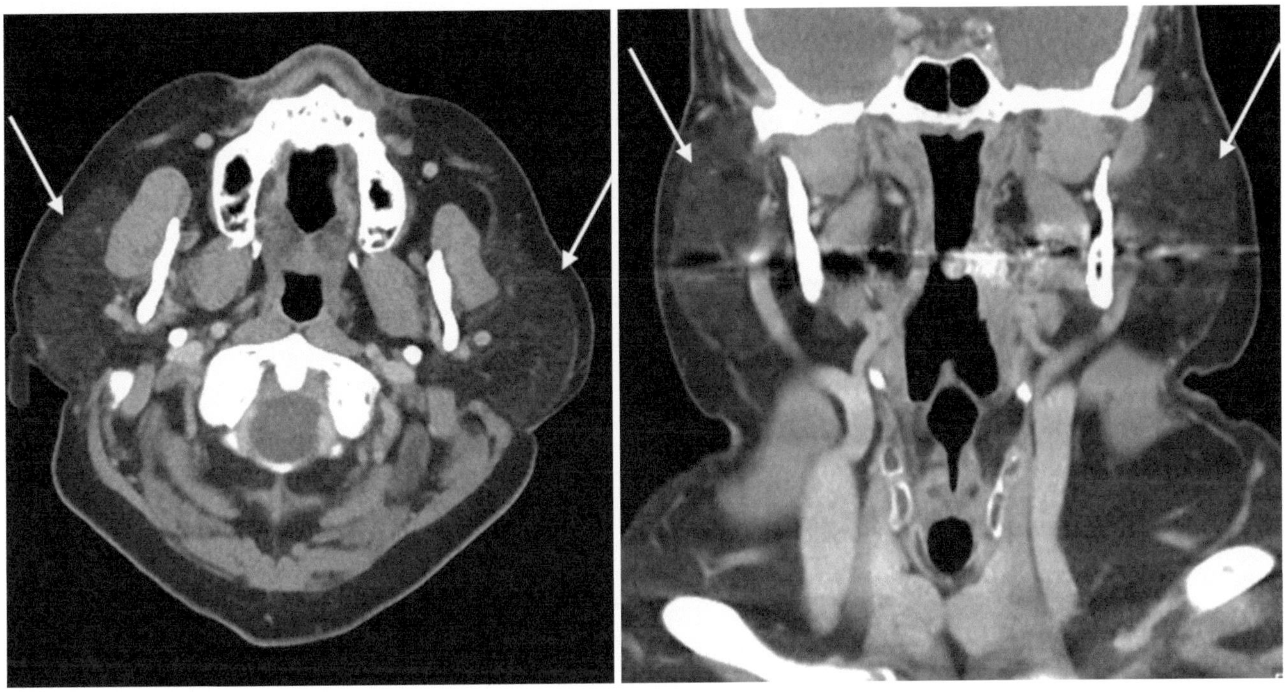

Fig. 4.30 A 65-year-old male presents with bilateral facial fullness. Axial (*left*) and coronal (*right*) CECT images demonstrate symmetrically enlarged parotid glands, with diffuse low density (*arrows*). The glands each measure an attenuation (density) of about −50 HU, suggestive of fat density. Thus there are bilateral fatty, hypertrophied parotid glands of uncertain etiology in this patient

4.23 Accessory Parotid Gland

The prominent or *asymmetric accessory lobe of the parotid gland* can mimic a mass when asymmetrically enlarged on one side, but it is a normal variation present in about 20% to 30% of normal patients. The accessory lobe has the same density or signal and enhancement pattern as the remainder of the parotid gland on CT or MR imaging. The accessory component may be continuous with the main parotid gland, or there may be a discontinuous gap between this component and the main body of glandular parotid tissue (Figs. 4.31 and 4.32).

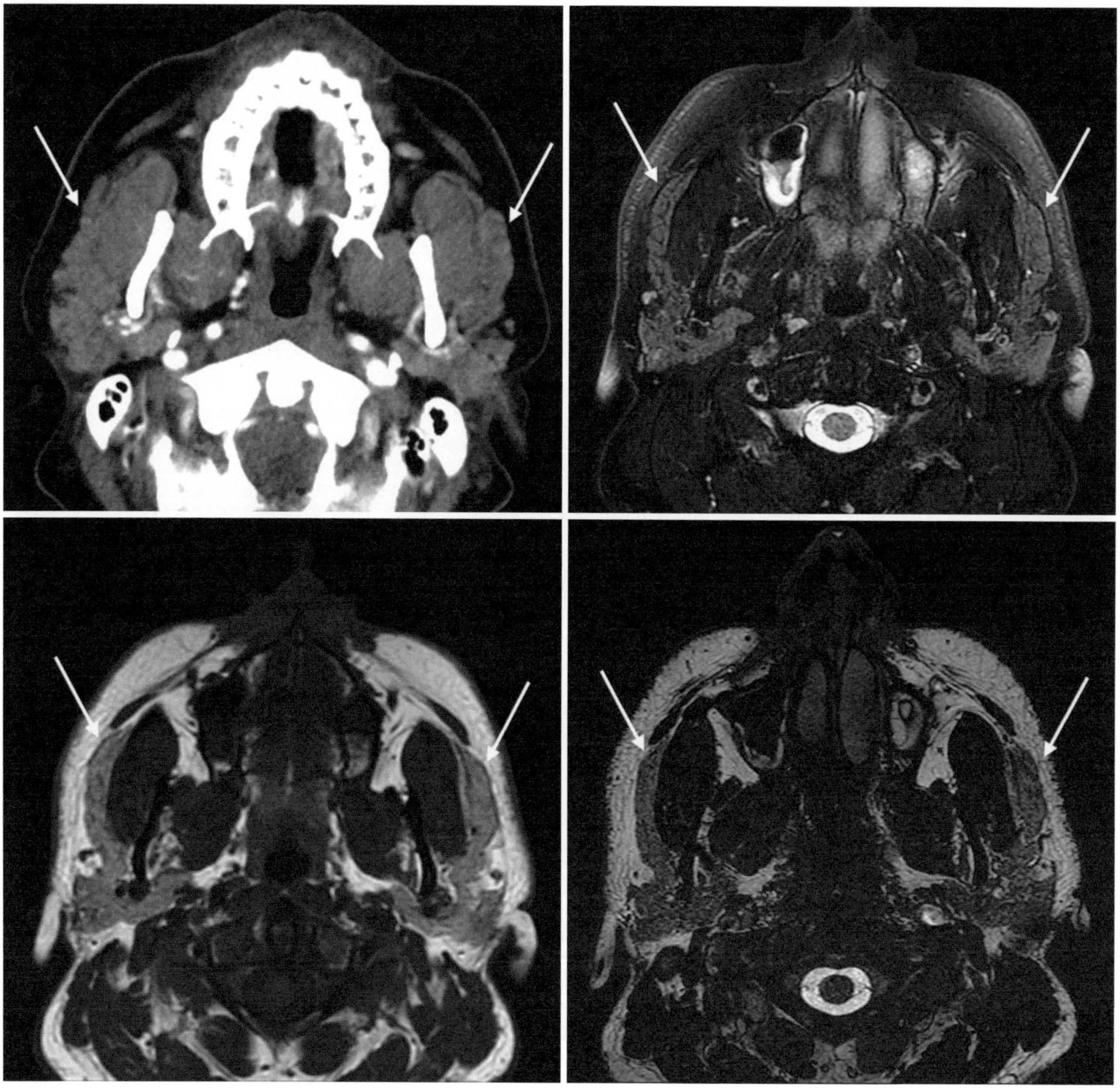

Fig. 4.31 A 40-year-old male with ethmoid sinus squamous cell cancer. On axial CECT (*upper left*), axial SET2WI (*upper right*), axial SET1WI (*bottom right*) and axial FIESTA (a balanced-echo type of T2WI to accentuate fluid, *bottom right*) MR images, there is bilateral symmetrical soft tissue signal (*arrows*) extending from the main parotid glands anteriorly superficial to the masseter muscles on both sides. The density and signal intensity of these soft tissues are identical to the density and signal intensity of the main parotid glands. Thus, as these are in continuity with the parotid glands, they represent bilateral accessory parotid glands, a normal variation

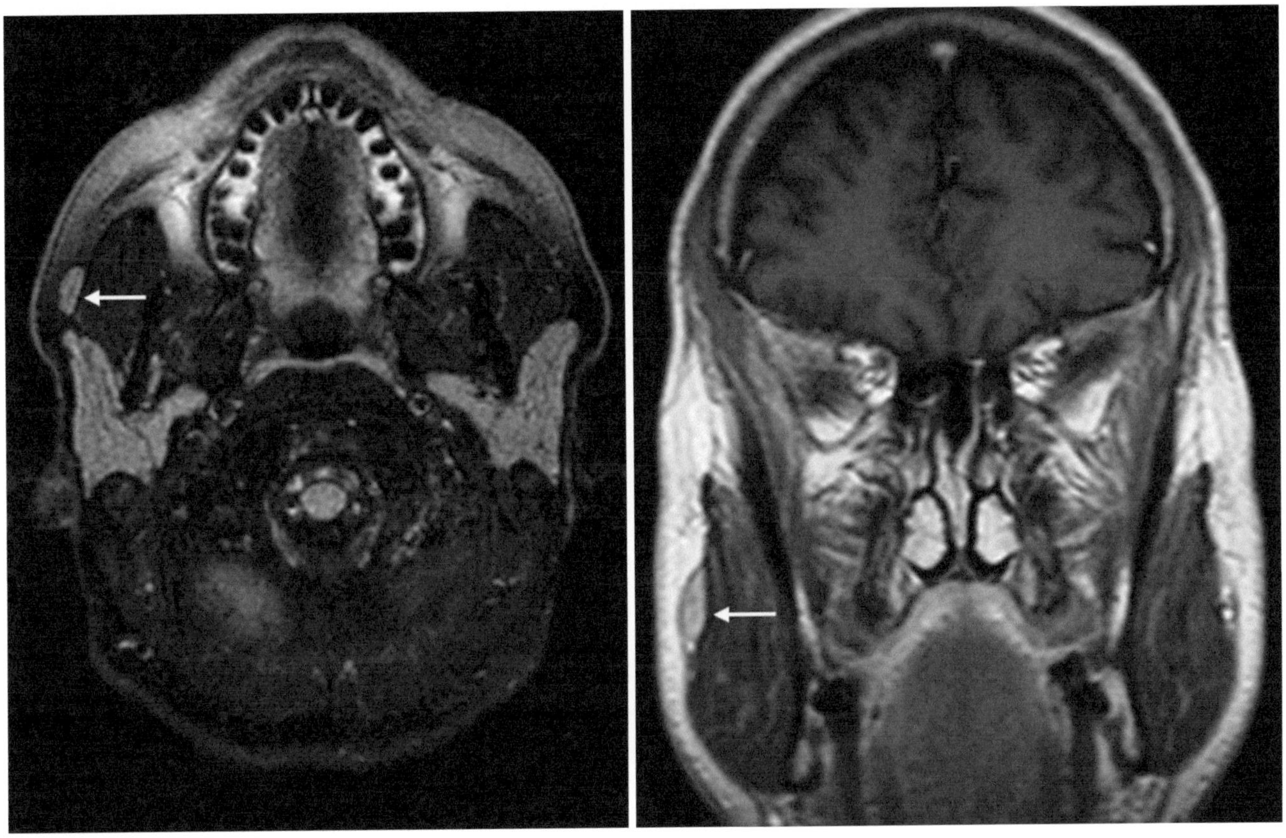

Fig. 4.32 A 42-year-old male with a history of seizures. An axial FLAIR MR image at the skull base level (*left*) demonstrates a normal left parotid gland. On the patient's right side, anterior to the parotid gland but discontinuous from it, there is a small similar signal accessory parotid tissue (*arrows*) located lateral to the masseter muscle. On a coronal postcontrast SET1WI (*right*), there is an asymmetrical nodular focus lateral to the right masseter muscle (*arrows*) representing the same small accessory parotid tissue that was seen on the FLAIR image. This normal variation can be mistaken for a mass if not carefully evaluated on each sequence and in every plane

4.24 Pneumoparotid

Pneumoparotid has been described in patients who generate increased intraoral pressures, whether from playing wind instruments, during coughing, or if undergoing dental work. It often presents as unilateral or bilateral facial swelling over the parotid region. The swelling may be painless or tender, and it may be associated with warmth and erythema. There is crepitus on palpation of the gland in 50% of patients; frothy saliva or air bubbles may be seen emanating from the Stensen duct during massage of the gland. Plain radiographs may show air in the soft tissues and may even outline the course of the main parotid duct. Sialography and/or ultrasound may also demonstrate air bubbles within the duct. NECT or CECT elegantly depicts air within both the duct and the gland (Fig. 4.33).

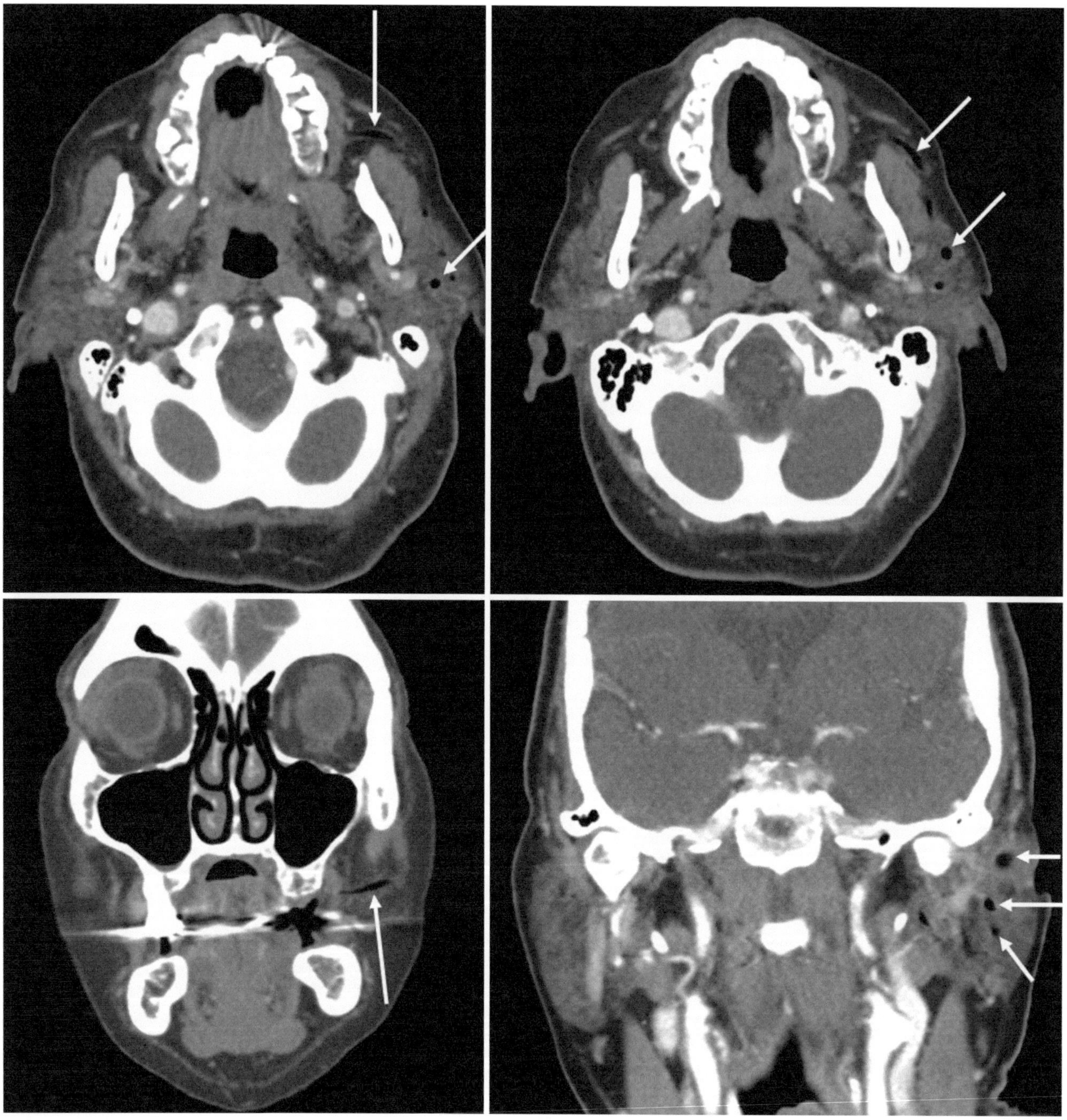

Fig. 4.33 A 69-year-old female with tonsillar cancer. Axial (*top row*) and coronal (*bottom row*) CECT reconstructions show multiple foci of air (*arrows*) within the left parotid gland superficial lobe, also with air extending along the left Stensen duct, consistent with pneumoparotid

4.25 Thymic Hyperplasia

The thymus is a lymphatic organ that plays a vital role in the development and maturation of the immune system during childhood, specifically regarding T cells (which are instrumental in regulating cellular immunity) and B cells (which are instrumental in regulating humoral immunity). The thymus is sensitive to stressors on the body, such as infection, neoplasm, surgery, and chemotherapy. It may respond with rapid atrophy but can later regain its original size or become larger. It is disproportionately larger in infants but gradually becomes replaced by fat and involutes throughout maturation. It is usually much smaller or barely visible in adults. Nevertheless, the thymus maintains its ability to grow back at any time and at any age.

Its variations in size and shape continue to be a source of misinterpretation. Unfortunately, these misinterpretations may result in unnecessary percutaneous or open biopsies, total thymectomies, and irradiation. Examples of thymic variants are ectopic and accessory thymic tissue, which may occur anywhere along the path of descent (the thymopharyngeal duct) as the result of failure of descent, sequestration, or failure to involute. Such ectopic or accessory thymic tissue may be found in the vicinity of the superior vena cava, brachiocephalic vessels, or aorta. Rarely, it may be found in the posterior mediastinum or even in the dermis. Ectopic thymic tissue may also simulate a neck neoplasm, which can be mistaken for a pathologic process.

Thymic morphology varies greatly, even in the same age group. For instance, in young adults, it is typically bilobed and "V-shaped," with two small processes extending into the neck; however, it can also be unilobed, trilobed, or shaped like an "X" or inverted "V." The size and weight of the thymus vary as well; it can weigh from 5 to 50 g throughout a person's life, with a slight increase during the first decade of life followed by a gradual decrease thereafter. The weight of the thymus as a percentage of total body mass is greatest at or near the time of birth. As children grow older and their immune systems mature, the thymus undergoes physiologic involution. Ultimately, it becomes replaced by fat, yet maintains its original configuration.

In addition to being aware of the normal and varying appearances in children and occasionally adults, thymic hyperplasia can lead to the waxing and waning of size that can cause consternation. *Hyperplasia of the thymus* can be divided into two distinct types: true hyperplasia and lymphoid (follicular) hyperplasia. True hyperplasia is characterized by an increase in the size and weight of the thymus, with preservation of its organized microscopic features. Although the thymus retains its normal shape, it more commonly loses its distinct bilobed appearance and instead appears oval. Clinically, patients with true thymic hyperplasia can be divided into three groups: those without a related preexisting condition; those recovering from a recent stress event such as corticosteroid therapy for pneumonia, radiation therapy, chemotherapy, surgery, or burns; and those with other disorders such as hyperthyroidism, sarcoidosis, or red blood cell aplasia.

The diagnostic challenge in patients with a known neoplasm is to distinguish thymic hyperplasia from recurrent or metastatic tumors. Thymic "rebound" hyperplasia is a "don't touch" phenomenon that typically shows diffuse enlargement, a fine mixture of fat and lymphoid tissue, a smooth contour, and normal vessels. In contrast, pathologic thymic neoplasia (e.g., thymoma) is usually associated with a nodular contour and frequently contains necrotic or calcified foci. There are heterogeneous features seen on US, CT, or MR imaging, with contrast enhancement being a particularly distinguishing feature for hyperplasia. Regarding the other type of thymic hyperplasia, thymic lymphoid hyperplasia, it is characterized by the presence of a hyperplastic lymphoid germinal center within the thymic medulla, being associated with lymphocytic and plasma cell infiltration. Unlike true hyperplasia, lymphoid hyperplasia may occur with or without thymic enlargement and is commonly associated with autoimmune diseases such as myasthenia gravis, thyrotoxicosis, connective tissue disease, and sometimes in the early stages of human immunodeficiency virus (HIV) infection. Although thymic lymphoid hyperplasia usually appears as a normal thymus on conventional radiography, on CT it may appear normal (45% of cases), enlarged (35%), or as a focal thymic mass (20%).

Given the variability in shape and size of the thymus, a familiarity with the broad spectrum of imaging appearances of the normal thymus will help radiologists minimize the number of invasive procedures. As mentioned previously, it is paramount not only to be aware of the normal prominence of the thymus in children but also the normal variability in size in adults. Also of concern are possible locations of ectopic thymus and other normal variants of the thymus or "don't touch" appearances, such as thymic hyperplasia. Again, the differential diagnosis of these variants is typically head/neck cancer, lymphoma, metastatic lymph node, thymoma, or thyroid mass, to name a few (Figs. 4.34 and 4.35).

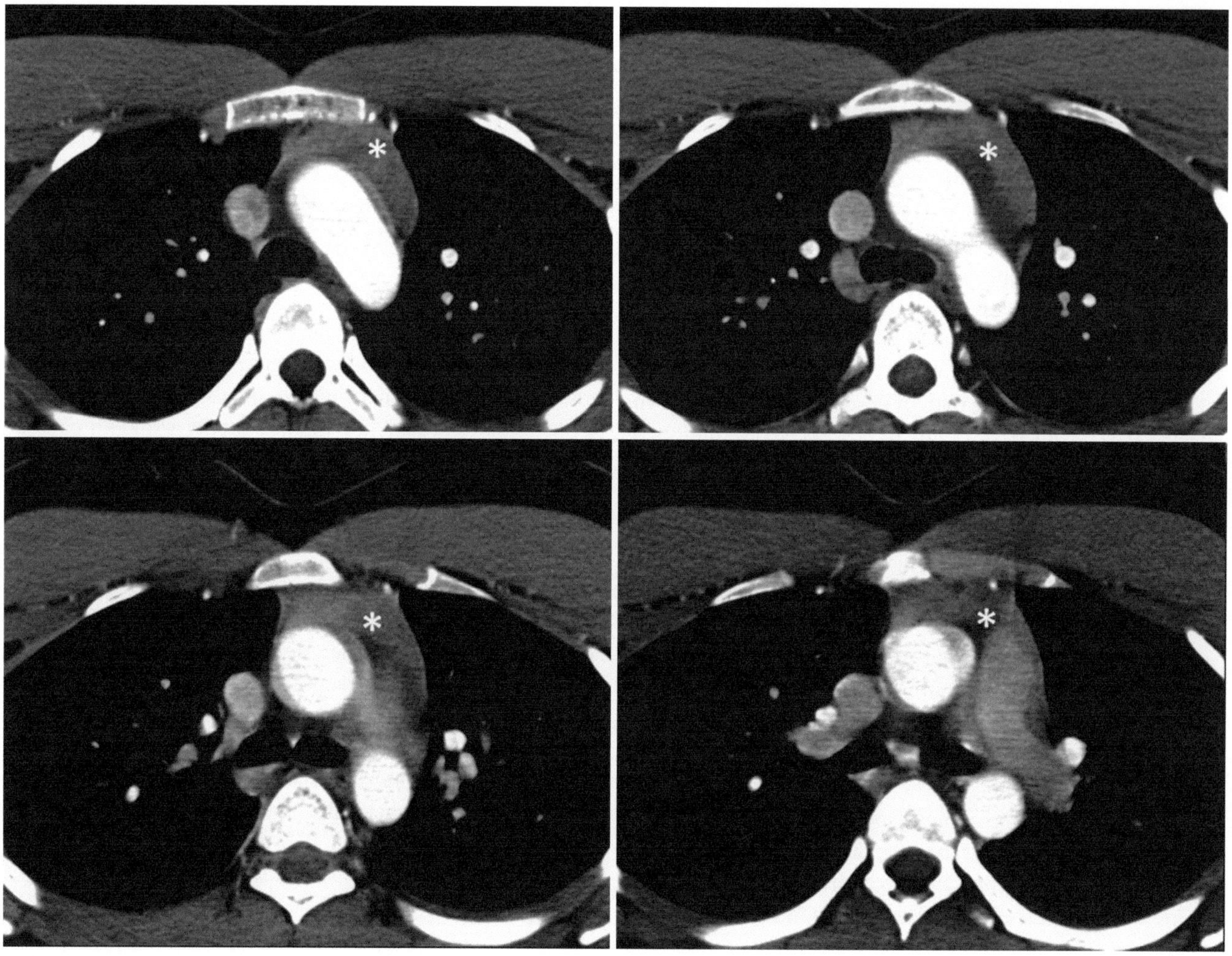

Fig. 4.34 A 24-year-old male presented with a left-sided neck mass. Multiple axial postcontrast axial CECT images demonstrated the crescentic shape of a soft-tissue density within the anterior mediastinum (*asterisks*), which is consistent with benign residual or reactive thymic tissue, considered either a normal variant or a "don't touch" lesion

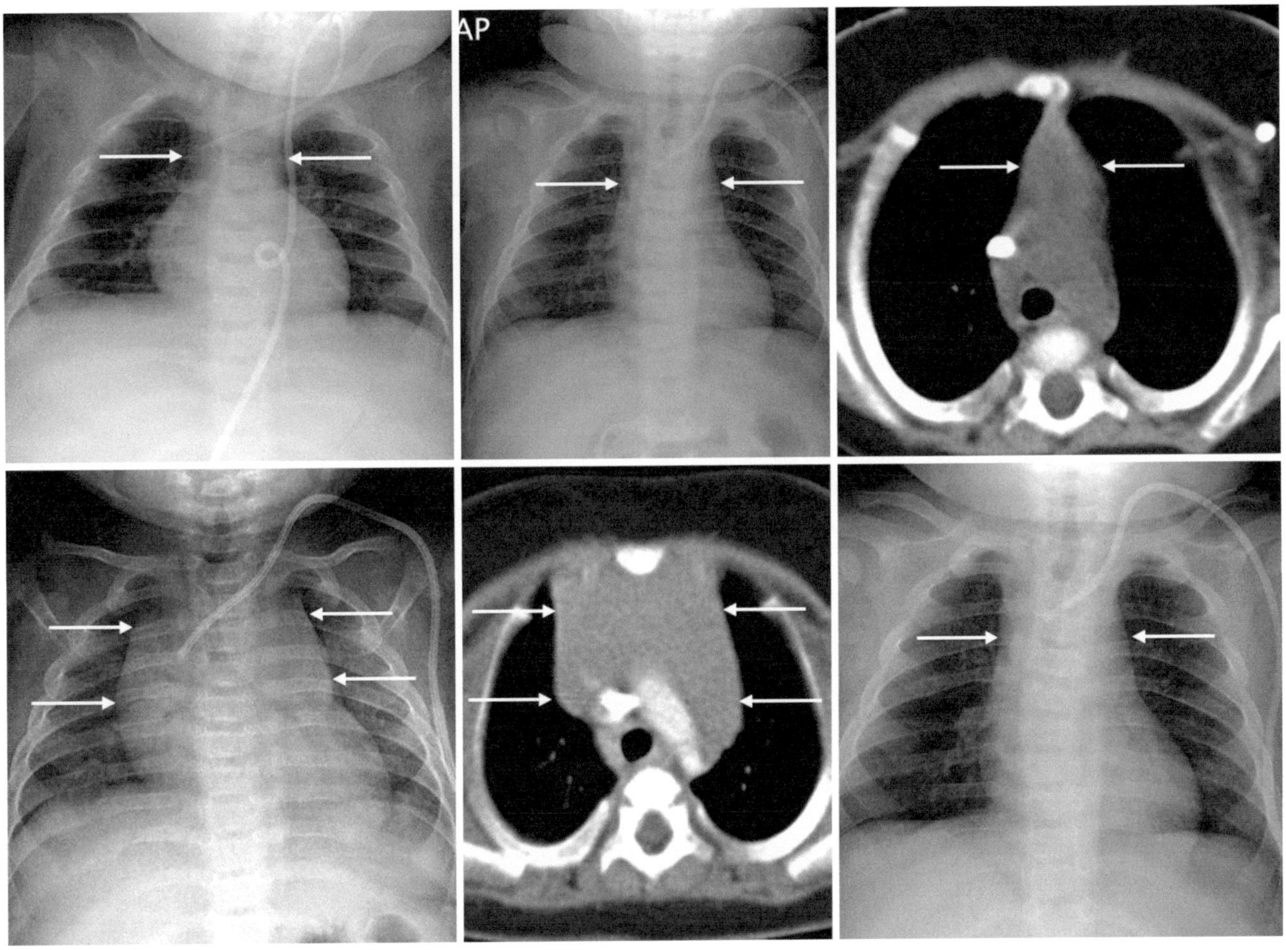

Fig. 4.35 A 1-year-old male with an initially normal thymus, followed by thymic rebound after hematopoetic stem cell transplantation (HSCT) for an uncommon disorder (hemophagocytic lymphohistiocytosis). **Top row**: Initially, a screening chest x-ray (CXR) at 4 months of age (*not shown*) was normal, while also being normal prior to HSCT at 7 months (*left*) and 8 months (*middle*) as well, with a normal thymic outline (outlined by *arrows*); also, pre-HSCT imaging by NECT at 8 months of age (*right*) depicts normal thymic tissue (*arrows*) in an infant. **Bottom row**: One day after HSCT, a CXR at 12 months of age (*left*) shows marked enlargement of the thymus (outlined by *arrows*, perhaps quadrupled in size), confirmed on a CECT 1 day later (*middle*) and suggestive of thymic rebound; this thymic enlargement resolved by 14 months of age on CXR (*right*). Thus, the smooth contour of the enlargement without nodularity, lack of vascular involvement, and the eventual tapering size of the thymus following HSCT are consistent with thymic rebound, which has been described in the literature to occur after both HSCT and chemotherapy in both adults and children, typically due to acute systemic stress

4.26 Elongated Styloid Process or Calcified Stylohyoid Ligament (Eagle Syndrome)

The styloid process is a thin, cylindrical, bony projection, measuring 25 mm in average length, and it is derived from the second branchial arch (Reichert cartilage). Reichert cartilage can be divided into four segments based on its embryonic origin from the second branchial arch, where the first segment/origin is in the tympanic portion of the temporal bone (posterior to the mastoid apex), the second segment becomes the distal styloid process, the third segment is the stylohyoid ligament, and the fourth segment/distal edge is the lesser cornu of the hyoid bone. Calcification/ossification can occur anywhere along this pathway but typically is more prominent at the more cranial portions. An *elongated styloid process and calcified styloid-stylohyoid ligament* may be part of a condition known as the *Eagle syndrome or stylohyoid syndrome*, as the associated facial pain syndrome was described by Eagle in 1937; much earlier, Marchetti described the elongated styloid process related to stylohyoid ligament ossification in the year 1652. Eagle classified this syndrome into two types: classic type and carotid artery type. The first type relates to nerve compression by the elongated/calcified/ossified styloid and may present with symptoms of foreign body sensation, referred ear pain, dysphagia, or difficulty swallowing. This type is thought to be caused by varying degrees of impingement of cranial nerves V, VII, IX, or X. The second type has vascular-related symptoms (typically carotid but less commonly jugular-related) and may present with symptoms such as headaches, pain in the temporal or maxillary branches, and other neurologic symptoms; rarely, even carotid artery compression (as confirmed on CTA) can induce ischemia caused by the patient turning his or her head to the side of the elongated/calcified styloid process!

About 4% of the population has an elongated styloid process, but only 4% of this subgroup has symptoms. These are usually (but not always) bilateral. Thus, in the vast majority of patients, an elongated or calcified styloid process is much more likely to be a normal variation. Some have proposed criteria to call an elongated/ossified styloid as abnormal (i.e., suspicious for Eagle syndrome) when: it is longer than 3 cm, there is compression of the vasculature (best confirmed on CECT or CT angiography), and there are cranial nerve or other neurologic-related symptoms (Figs. 4.36 and 4.37).

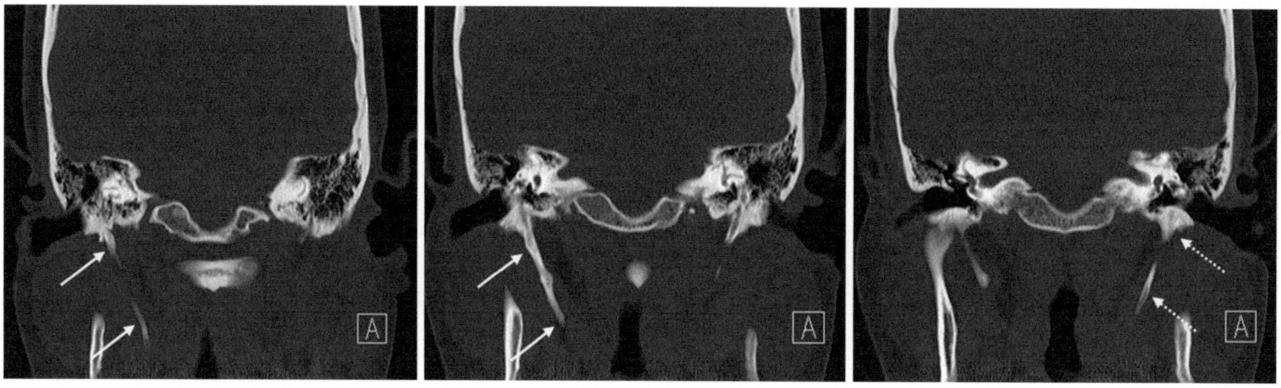

Fig. 4.36 A 50-year-old female with a known history of thyroid eye disease had incidental and asymptomatic bilateral elongation of the styloid processes on serial coronal NECT images in bone algorithm windows; this was more prominent on the patient's right side (just over 3 cm length, *arrows*) as compared to the left side (*dotted arrows*). Although over 3 cm in length on the right, this was considered a normal variation as there was no compression of adjacent vascular structures on axial imaging (*not shown*), and the patient clinically lacked cranial nerve symptoms or symptoms from vascular compression related to this finding

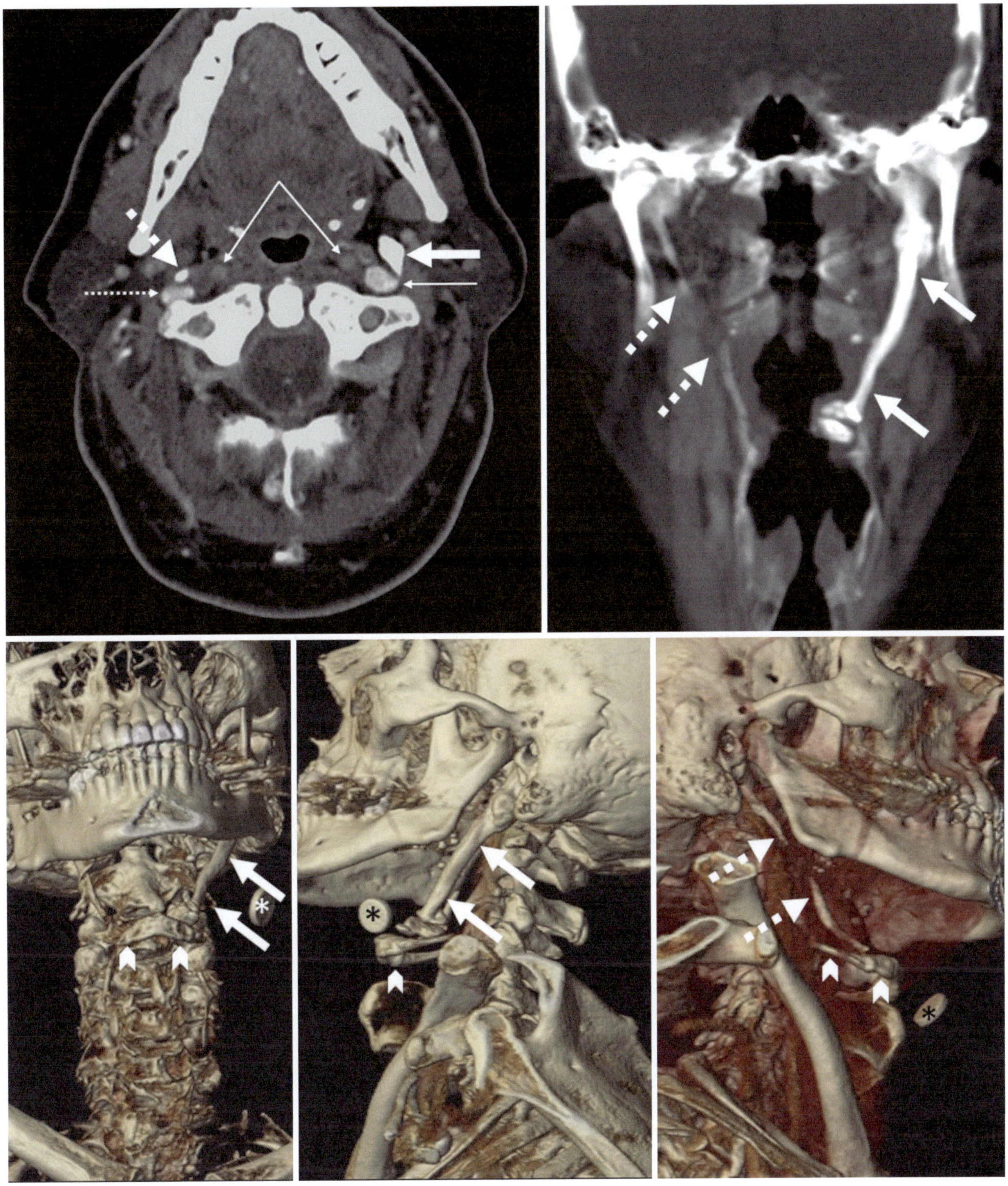

Fig. 4.37 A 50-year-old female with symptomatic styloid ossification (Eagle syndrome). The patient had intermittent left-sided neck pain and dysphagia, and the clinician had palpated a left-sided neck mass. **Top row**: On CECT axial 3-mm thickness (*left*) and a reconstructed coronal 18-mm-thick multiplanar reformat slab (*right*), the styloid processes were elongated and severely calcified bilaterally, the left side (*thick arrows*) more than the right (*thick dotted arrows*); note the lack of compression of the internal carotid arteries (*double arrows*) in the neutral position, while only the right internal jugular vein is compressed (*thin dotted arrow, left*), but not the left internal jugular (*thin arrow, left*). **Bottom row**: Three-dimensional volume-rendered reconstruction in the anteroposterior (AP) (*left*), left lateral (*middle*), and right lateral (*right*) planes demonstrate that the 8-cm-long left styloid process (*thick arrows*) is completely ossified down to and fused with the hyoid bone (*chevrons*), which is below the rounded skin marker (*asterisks*), while the right styloid is also elongated but discontinuous (*thick dotted arrows*). An interesting point is that although the patient was presumably symptomatic on the left side from Eagle syndrome causing the left-sided dysphagia and pain, and the palpated lesion was later confirmed to be the severely elongated-ossified left styloid process, there was no vascular compression, further demonstrating that the degree of vascular compression (incidentally present on the contralateral right side) does not always correlate with the presence of symptoms

4.27 Brown Fat on FDG-PET

Brown adipose tissue (BAT, also called "brown fat") functions as a thermogenic organ by producing heat to maintain body temperature in many mammals, especially in the young. It is involved in nonshivering thermogenesis and in diet-induced thermogenesis, and is noted incidentally in about 4–6% of patients who undergo Fluorodeoxyglucose (FDG) PET-CT. This phenomenon is more prevalent in patients with lower weight and body mass index, and in females (6.0–7.5%) as compared to males (2.7–3.1%); this is significantly more prevalent within the winter months (3.9–7.2%) as compared to the summer (2.5%).

Fluorodeoxyglucose (FDG) uptake in hypermetabolic BAT can be confused with nodal uptake, leading to false-positive results that mimic neoplasm or nodal metastases. It not only can lead to false-positive findings but also can decrease the sensitivity of the tumor uptake by decreasing the pool of FDG availability. BAT is richly innervated by the sympathetic nervous system predominantly expressing β_3-adrenergic receptor, while glucose accumulation of brown fat is increased by sympathetic stimulation. Brown fat uptake can be noted in the neck, shoulder, paravertebral, supraclavicular, mediastinum, perirenal, and perigastric regions. PET-CT allows the verification that BAT uptake (standardized uptake value max = 1.9–20) foci have no corresponding anatomic soft-tissue mass detectable by CT scanning. Rather, the FDG-avid foci are shown to be fused into tissues having fat density, and the corresponding Hounsfield unit (HU) densities are within the reported fat-density range (−150 to −50).

The intensity and standardized uptake value on PET are not reliable tools for differentiating "don't touch" BAT/brown fat from neoplasm. Several pharmacologic methods have been tried to reduce FDG uptake by hypermetabolic BAT, such as the use of medications such as propranolol and fentanyl. Among the nonpharmacologic approaches, the use of a high-fat, very low-carbohydrate, protein-permitted diet and warming of the patient can be useful approaches to significantly reduce the frequency of BAT hypermetabolism. None of these approaches has been consistently reliable, and most of them involve pharmacologic intervention, which is especially undesirable in the pediatric population. Notably, nicotine has been found to increase the uptake of hypermetabolic BAT (Figs. 4.38 and 4.39).

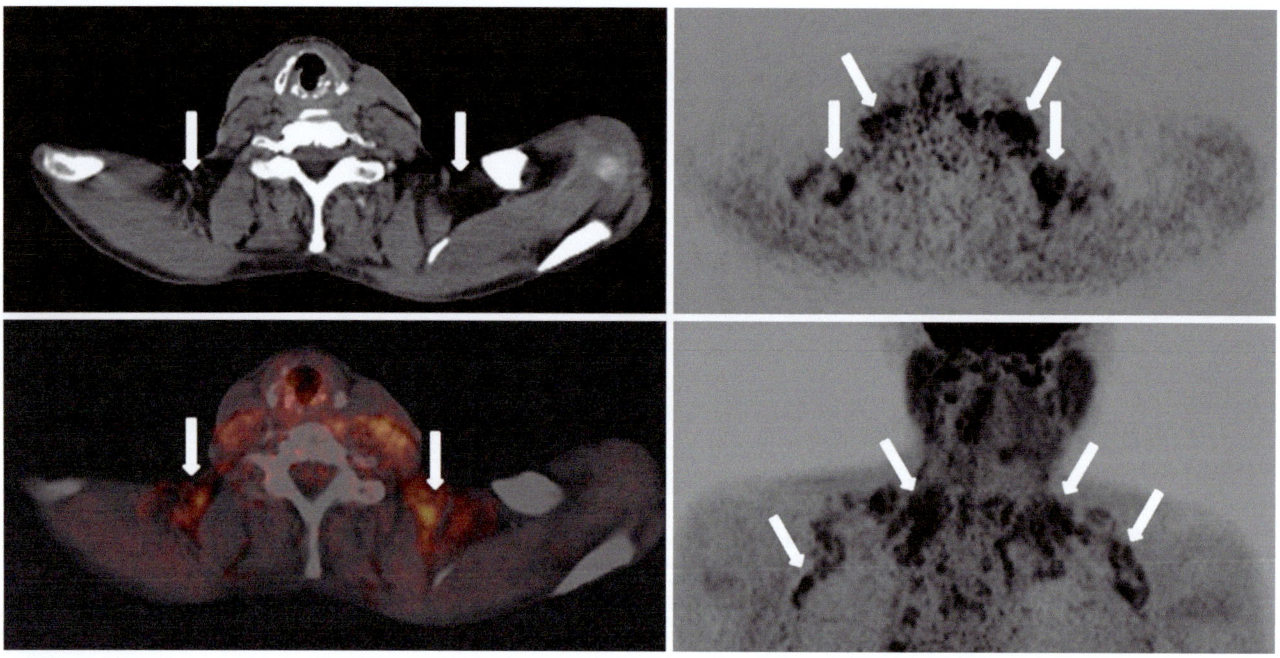

Fig. 4.38 A 47-year-old female with breast cancer. Attenuation corrected PET (*upper right*), fused PET-CT (*bottom left*), and maximum intensity projection (*bottom right*) images demonstrate bilateral multiple areas of FDG uptake in bilateral supraclavicular and infraclavicular regions as well as at the thoracic inlet (*arrows*). On routine NECT (*upper left*), within the posterior triangles there is no mass identified on either side, but there is normal fat density visualized (*arrows*). Thus, when correlating the routine NECT images with the fused PET-CT images, the elevated diffuse uptake within the supraclavicular regions bilaterally is from benign brown fat uptake, a common finding on PET images and a "don't touch" appearance

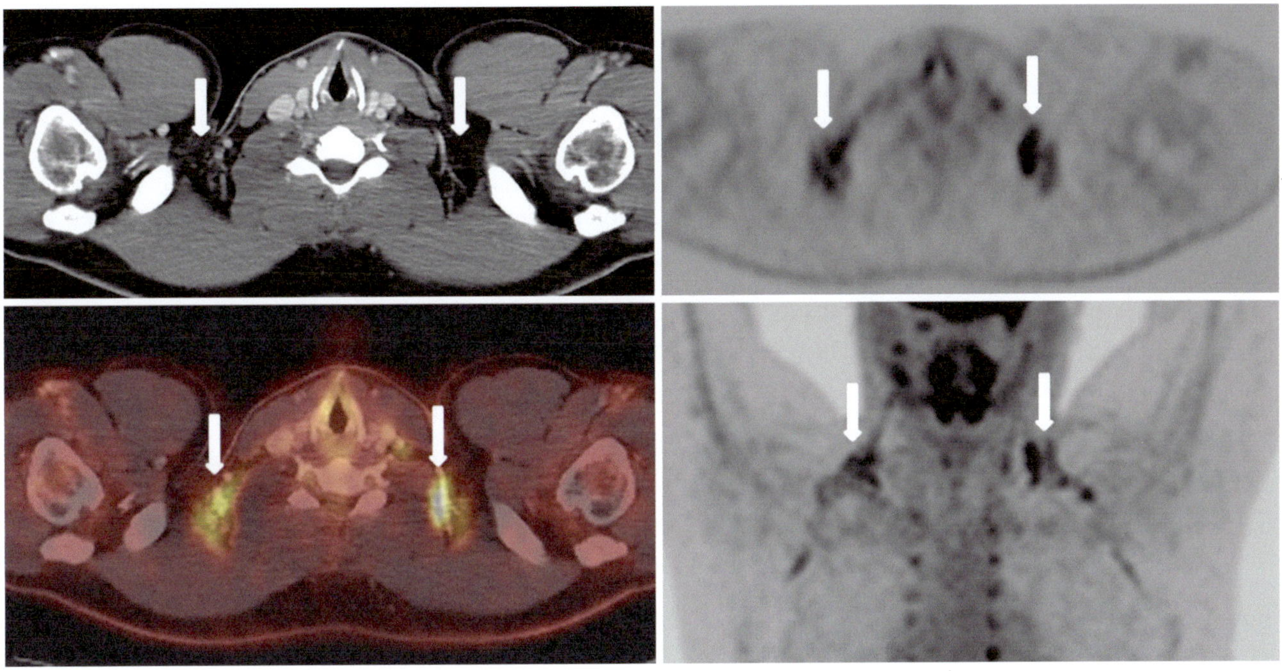

Fig. 4.39 A 65-year-old male with lymphoma. Attenuation corrected PET (*upper right*), fused PET-CT (*bottom left*), and maximum intensity projection (*bottom right*) images demonstrate bilateral multiple areas of FDG uptake more focally within the supraclavicular regions (*arrows*), simulating bilaterally hypermetabolic masses on PET. However, on routine NECT (*upper left*), within the posterior triangles there is no mass identified on either side, while there is normal fat density visualized (*arrows*); this is a typical "don't touch" appearance of brown fat

4.28 Vocal Cord FDG Uptake

It is well recognized that talking during the FDG uptake phase will cause *bilateral symmetric vocal cord radiotracer uptake*. Another muscle that can appear as a focal area of FDG uptake is the cricopharyngeus muscle. Coughing during the uptake phase produces FDG activity in the pharyngeal constrictor muscles as well as in the vocal cords. Pronounced uptake in these muscles can interfere with interpretation of PET scans in any patient, but especially in patients with head and neck malignancies, thyroid cancer, or lymphoma, in whom it can be very difficult to distinguish physiologic muscle "don't touch" uptake from pathologic uptake.

Asymmetric vocal cord uptake following injury to the recurrent laryngeal nerve can be seen. This "don't touch" phenomenon represents altered physiologic or hyperphysiologic uptake by compensation of the contralateral vocal cord during phonation. Asymmetric FDG uptake within a single vocal cord can mimic malignancy, especially at PET, if direct anatomic correlation is not available (Fig. 4.40).

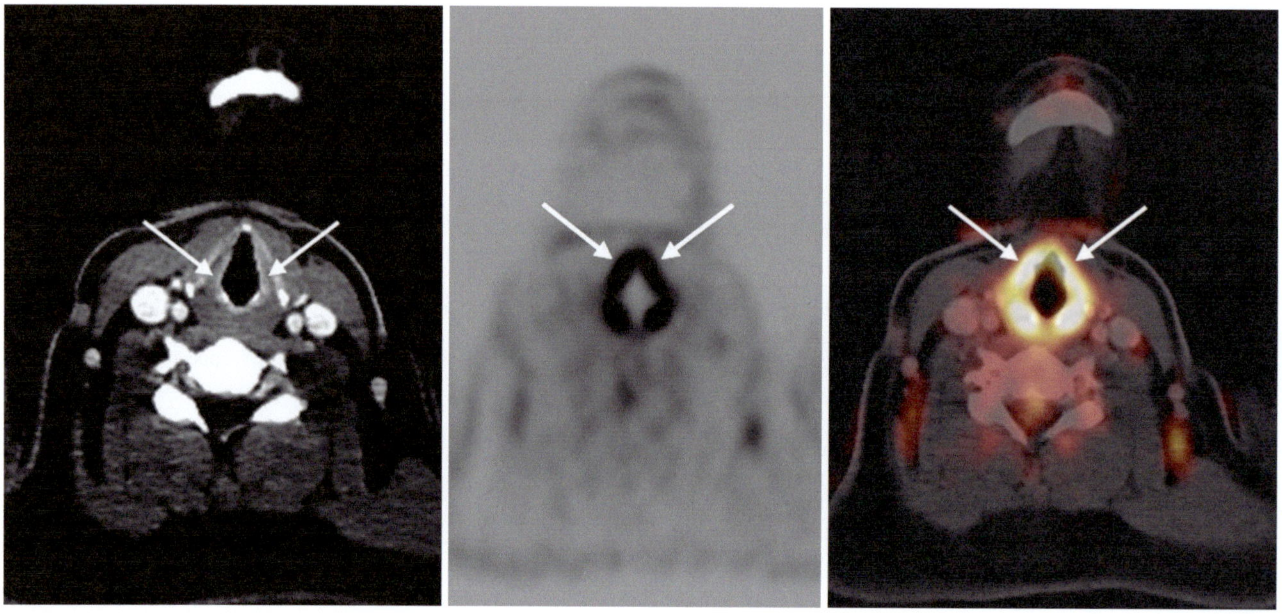

Fig. 4.40 A 32-year-old male with melanoma. Fused PET-CT (*left*) and attenuation-corrected PET (*right*) images demonstrate symmetrical FDG uptake of the true vocal cords (*arrows*). This is a common normal finding on FDG-PET caused by patient phonation following injection of the radiotracer (i.e., during the time of FDG uptake)

4.29 Lymphoid Tissue FDG Uptake

There are many lymphatic structures in the head and neck, including the Waldeyer ring (adenoids, palatine tonsils, and lingual tonsils), lymph nodes, and lymphatic channels. *Physiologic FDG uptake of lymphoid tissue* can be visualized in any lymphatic structure in the head and neck, at least in part due to FDG accumulation within macrophages and lymphocytes. The interpretation is straightforward in most cases, especially when there is symmetric uptake. However, malignancy or lymphoid hyperplasia may have a similar symmetrical appearance.

Uptake in Waldeyer ring can often be asymmetrical, even from benign conditions such as infection or inflammation; this is a "don't touch" appearance. Malignancy will usually manifest as asymmetrical FDG uptake as well, with or without significant anatomic abnormalities (Fig. 4.41).

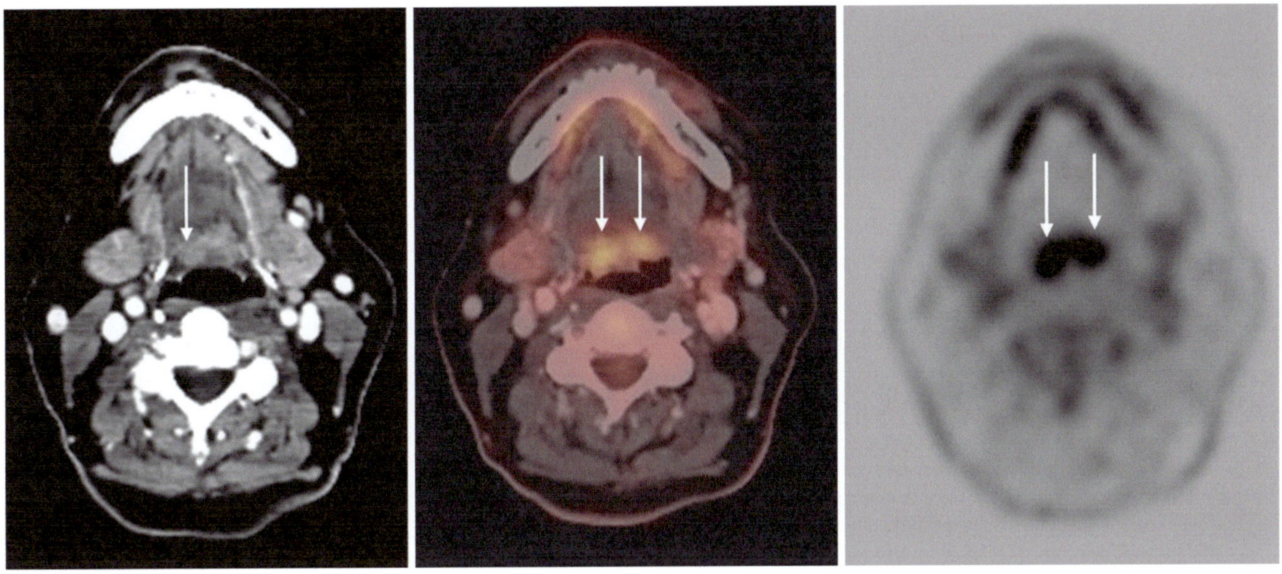

Fig. 4.41 A 57-year-old female with cervical cancer. FDG-PET images through the neck show prominent lingual tonsils on CECT (*left*) filling the vallecula on both sides, the right side more than the left (*arrows*). On fused PET-CT (*middle*) and attenuation-corrected PET (*right*) images, there is bilaterally increased FDG uptake of these slightly enlarged tonsillar tissues (*arrows*). Tonsillar FDG uptake is one cause of physiologic distribution of FDG uptake

Suggested Reading

Abdullah BJJ, Liam CK, Kaur H, Mathew KM. Parapharyngeal space lipoma causing sleep apnea. Br J Radiol. 1997;70:1063–5.
Arekapudi SR, Varma DR. Lingual thyroid. Pediatr Radiol. 2007;37:940.
Chakraborty D. Patterns of brown fat uptake of 18F-fluorodeoxyglucose in positron emission tomography/computed tomography scan. Indian J Nucl Med. 2015;30:320–2.
Chandra RK, Maddalozzo J, Kovarik P. Histological characterization of the thyroglossal tract: implications for surgical management. Laryngoscope. 2001;111:1002–5.
Chuang WC, Short JH, McKinney AM, Anker L, Knoll B, McKinney ZJ. Reversible left hemispheric ischemia secondary to carotid compression in Eagle syndrome: surgical and CT angiographic correlation. Am J Neuroradiol. 2007;28:143–5.
Costa NS, Salisbury SR, Donnelly LF. Retropharyngeal lymph nodes in children: a common imaging finding and potential source of misinterpretation. Am J Roentgenol. 2011;196:W433–7.
Cronin CG, Prakash P, Daniels GH, Boland GW, Kalra MK, Halpern EF, et al. Brown fat at PET/CT: correlation with patient characteristics. Radiology. 2012;263:836–42.
Cypess AM, Lehman S, Williams G, Tal I, Rodman D, Goldfine AB, et al. Identification and importance of brown adipose tissue in adult humans. N Engl J Med. 2009;360:1509–17.
Demirpolat G, Guney B, Savas R, Tuncay G, Alper H, Sener RN. Radiologic and cytologic findings in a case of thyrolipoma. Am J Neuroradiol. 2002;23:1640–1.
DeSanto LW, Devine KD, Weiland LH. Cysts of the larynx-classification. Laryngoscope. 1970;80:145–76.
Frommer J. The human accessory parotid gland: its incidence, nature, and significance. Oral Surg Oral Med Oral Pathol. 1977;43:671–6.
Fuentes R, Saravia D, Garay I, Ottone N. Asymptomatic bilateral calcified stylohyoid ligaments detection by panoramic radiography and cone beam computerized tomography. Biomed Res. 2016;27:4.
Giovanni B, De Stefani A, Balasso P, Sergio Mazzoleni S, Gracco A. Elongated styloid process: an epidemiological study on digital panoramic radiographs. J Clin Exp Dent. 2017;9:e1446–52.
Glazer HS, Mauro MA, Aronberg DJ, Lee JK, Johnston DE, Sagel S. Computed tomography of laryngoceles. Am J Roentgenol. 1983;140:549–52.
Hara M, McAdams HP, Vredenburgh JJ, Herndon JE, Patz EF Jr. Thymic hyperplasia after high-dose chemotherapy and autologous stem cell transplantation: incidence and significance in patients with breast cancer. Am J Roentgenol. 1999;173:1341–4.
Harnsberger HR, Wiggins RH, Hudgins P, Davidson C. Diagnostic imaging: head and neck. Salt Lake City: Amirsys; 2004. p. 6–7, 14–5, 22–3, 38–41, 50–3.
Heller MT, Meltzer CC, Fukui MB, Rosen CA, Chander S, Martinelli MA, et al. Super-physiologic FDG uptake in the non-paralyzed vocal cord: resolution of a false-positive PET result with combined PET-CT imaging. Clin Positron Imaging. 2000;3:207–11.
Ikushima I, Korogi Y, Makita O, Komohara Y, Kawano H, Yamura M, et al. MR imaging of Tornwaldt's cysts. Am J Roentgenol. 1999;172:1663–5.
Izumi M, Eguchi K, Nakamura H, Nagataki S, Nakamura T. Premature fat deposition in the salivary glands associated with Sjogren syndrome: MR and CT evidence. Am J Neuroradiol. 1997;18:951–8.
Kadivar M, Kheirkhah Rahimabad P, Salarinejad S. Prominent cold nodule in multinodular goiter revealed to be thyrolipoma: a case report. Iran J Pathol. 2016;11:456–9.
Karabay N, Comlekci A, Canda MS, Firat Bayraktar F, Degirmen B. Thyroid hemiagenesis with multinodular goiter: a case report and review of the literature. Endocrine J. 2003;50:409–13.
Kiesler K, Friedrich G, Beham A, Ebner F, Gugatschka M, Ebner F, Gugatschka M. First report of intralaminar tumorlike lipomatous lesions of the thyroid cartilage. J Voice. 2011;25:487–9.
Kostakoglu L, Wong JC, Barrington SF, Cronin BF, Dynes AM, Maisey M. Speech-related visualization of laryngeal muscles with fluorine-18-FDG. J Nucl Med. 1996;37:1771–3.
Lohman BD, Sarikaya B, McKinney AM, Hadi M. Not the typical Tornwaldt's cyst this time? A nasopharyngeal cyst associated with canalis basilaris medianus. Br J Radiol. 2011;84:e169–71.
Lukins DE, Pilati S, Escott EJ. The moving carotid artery: a retrospective review of the retropharyngeal carotid artery and the incidence of positional changes on serial studies. Am J Neuroradiol. 2016;37:336–41.
Madani G, Beale T. Inflammatory conditions of the salivary glands. Semin Ultrasound CT MRI. 2006;27:440–51.
Mancuso AA, Harnsberger HR, Muraki AS, Stevens MH. Computed tomography of cervical and retropharyngeal lymph nodes: normal anatomy, variations of normal, and applications in staging head and neck cancer. Part 1. Normal anatomy. Radiology. 1983;148:709–14.
Mandel L, Surattanont F. Bilateral parotid swelling: a review. Oral Surg Oral Med Oral Pathol Oral Radiol Endod. 2002;93:221–7.
Marcucci C, Thomas P, Sewell DA. Retropharyngeal carotid artery: an important anatomic variation for the anesthesiologist. Anesthesiology. 2009;111:454–5.
Matthews TW, Dardick I. Morphological alterations of salivary gland parenchyma in chronic sialadenitis. J Otolaryngol. 1988;17:385–94.
McKinney AM. Canalis basilaris medianus. Atlas of normal imaging variations of the brain, skull, and craniocervical vasculature. Cham: Springer; 2017. p. 797–800.
McKinney AM. Retropharyngeal internal carotid artery. Atlas of normal imaging variations of the brain, skull, and craniocervical vasculature. Cham: Springer; 2017. p. 1017–20.
Merlo C, Bohl L, Carda C, Gómez de Ferrari ME, Carranza M. Parotid sialosis: morphometrical analysis of the glandular parenchyma and stroma among diabetic and alcoholic patients. J Oral Pathol Med. 2010;39:10–5.
Nasseri F, Eftekhari F. Clinical and radiologic review of the normal and abnormal thymus: pearls and pitfalls. Radiographics. 2010;30:413–28.
Oiki H, Murata K. Fatty degeneration of the parotid gland after ovariectomy. Nihon Jibiinkoka Gakkai Kaiho. 2000;103:539–46.
Ovassapian A, Glassenberg R, Randel G, Mesnick PS, Klafta JM. The unexpected difficult airway and lingual tonsil hyperplasia: a case series and a review of the literature. Anesthesiology. 2002;97:124–32.
Practical Head and Neck Ultrasound. Greenwich medical media. Oxford: Oxford University Press; 2000.
Rouviere H. Anatomy of the human lymphatic system. Ann Arbor: Edward Brothers; 1938. p. 3–28.
Russo CP, Smoker WRK, Weissman JL. MR appearance of trigeminal and hypoglossal motor denervation. Am J Neuroradiol. 1997;18:1375–83.
Sekiya K, Watanabe M, Nadgir RN, Buch K, Flower EN, Kaneda T, et al. Nasopharyngeal cystic lesions: Tornwaldt and mucous retention cysts of the nasopharynx: findings on MR imaging. J Comput Assist Tomogr. 2014;38:9–13.
Sheikh JS, Sharma M, Kunath A, Fritz DA, Glueck CJ, Hess EV. Reversible parotid enlargement and pseudo-Sjögren's syndrome secondary to hypertriglyceridemia. J Rheumatol. 1996;23:1288–91.
Sheikhi M, Jalalian F, Rashidipoor R, Mosavat F. Plunging ranula of the submandibular area. Dent Res J. 2011;8:S114–8.
Shiraishi H, Oiki H, Murata K. Fatty degeneration of the parotid gland after ovariectomy. Nihon Jibiinkoka Gakkai Kaiho. 2000;103:539–46.

Shreve PD, Anzai Y, Wahl RL. Pitfalls in oncologic diagnosis with FDG PET imaging: physiologic and benign variants. RadioGraphics. 1999;19:61–77.

Smith JC, Snyderman CH, Kassam AB. Giant parapharyngeal space lipoma: case report and surgical approach. Skull Base. 2002;12:215–20.

Som PM, Brandwein MS. Salivary glands: anatomy and pathology. In: Som P, Curtin H, editors. Head and neck imaging, vol. 2. 4th ed. St. Louis: Mosby; 2000. p. 2005–33.

Srinivasan A, Moyer JS, Mukherji SK. Unilateral submandibular gland aplasia associated with ipsilateral sublingual gland hypertrophy. Am J Neuroradiol. 2006;27:2214–21.

Thomson JA. The normal thyroid scan. Lancet. 1966;2:308–9.

Tiwari PK, Baxi M, Baxi J, Koirala D. Right-sided hemiagenesis of the thyroid lobe and isthmus: a case report. Indian J Radiol Imaging. 2008;18:313–5.

Toh H, Kodama J, Fukuda J, Rittman B, Mackenzie I. Incidence and histology of human accessory parotid glands. Anat Rec. 1993;236:586–90.

Ulku CH, Uyar Y. Parapharyngeal lipoma extending to skull base: a case report and review of the literature. Skull Base. 2004;12:121–5.

Vázquez-Chávez C, Acevedo-Rivera K, Sartorius C, Espinosa-Said L. Thyroid hemiagenesis: report of 3 cases and review of the literature. Gac Med Mex. 1989;125:395–9.

Wiener JD, Roos P. Thyroid asymmetry. Br Med J. 1968;3:312–3.

Yaman H, Durmaz A, Arslan HH, Ozcan A, Karahatay S, Gerek M. Thyroglossal duct cysts: evaluation and treatment of 49 cases. B-ENT. 2011;7:267–71.

Ying M, Yung D. Asymmetry of thyroid lobe volume in normal Chinese subjects: association with handedness and position of esophagus. Anatomical Record. 2009;292:169–74.

Zander DA, Smoker WR. Imaging of ectopic thyroid tissue and thyroglossal duct cysts. Radiographics. 2014;34:37–50.

5 Temporal Bone Variants

5.1 Introduction

Temporal bone imaging has a well-deserved reputation as being one of the more challenging aspects of radiology. To paraphrase a neurotology colleague, an amazing amount of intricate anatomy is packed into a very small box. Furthermore, the pathology affecting these structures can be very subtle and affect minute areas. Understanding the myriad appearances of normal structures in unusual places or of unexpected size is quite important. Frequently, these variations are of no consequence but occasionally a similar structure of a comparable size and location that is asymptomatic in one person may be problematic in another.

Nonenhanced computed tomography (NECT) has long been the primary modality for imaging of the temporal bones. For the purposes of high-resolution temporal bone CT (HRCT), a slice thickness of 0.75 mm or less is important to visualize difficult to perceive structures such as the modiolus and osseous spiral lamina in the apex of the cochlea in a child with sensorineural hearing loss. To detect subtle pathologic entities, the HRCT images must have sufficient signal to noise to detect subtle hypodensity of the otic capsule in patients with otosclerosis/otospongiosis, or the subtle hyperdensity of the cochleae or semicircular canals in patients with labyrinthitis ossificans. Also, thin reconstructions outside of the typical axial, sagittal, and coronal planes (planes that are mainstays in the remainder of neuroradiology), such as the planes of Stenver and Poschl, are important to evaluate for the many "third window phenomenon" possibilities, particularly dehiscence of the semicircular canals.

Once mostly an adjunct to NECT and HRCT, temporal bone MRI has become ever more important in recent years. Heavily T2-weighted three-dimensional (3D T2WI) images are useful to diagnose cochlear nerve hypoplasia or aplasia, detect fibrosing labyrinthitis before the development of ossification, and can detect basement membrane displacement in the incomplete partition type II deformity. Diffusion-weighted imaging (DWI) can confirm or deny the presence of cholesteatoma. Combined with newer techniques such as the intratympanic injection of gadolinium, MRI can theoretically improve the diagnostic confidence in conditions that have been traditionally difficult to diagnose, such as Ménière disease.

Many structures in the temporal bone exhibit considerable variability in size. As the literature progresses from case reports to larger series, normative size values of many of these structures in the temporal bone have been determined. However, many studies continue to suffer from selection bias, such as in children, who are usually not imaged if they are asymptomatic. Many (if not most) studies are retrospective, and often patients who seek out temporal bone imaging suffer from tinnitus, hearing loss, or dizziness. Therefore, it can be difficult to determine whether or not a variant should be considered truly "normal" or merely "usually asymptomatic." This chapter attempts to clarify many of these topics.

5.2 Internal Auditory Canals: Bulbous or Asymmetric, Small Canals, and Crista Falciformis

5.2.1 Bulbous or Prominent Internal Auditory Canals (IACs)

A mildly enlarged, "bulbous" appearance of the internal auditory canals (IACs) is a normal variant that has been described more than 40 years ago on cisternography/myelography, and it can be noted on routine NECT or noncontrast routine MRI. This may be unilateral or bilateral and may simulate an extra-axial mass such as a schwannoma, which can expand the porus acousticus of the IAC as the mass enlarges. The frequency of this uncommon variant has not been described, but anecdotally it appears to occur in less than 1% of the population (unpublished data). The vast

A. McKinney et al., *Atlas of Head/Neck and Spine Normal Imaging Variants*, https://doi.org/10.1007/978-3-319-95441-7_5

majority of cases are asymptomatic, whether unilateral or bilateral, but since benign tumors such as schwannomas can occasionally present in asymptomatic patients who have not yet had dedicated testing, postcontrast spin-echo T1-weighted imaging (SET1WI) MRI can confirm that no mass is present in questionable cases. While an asymmetric, or bulbous, IAC is a normal variant, there are a few rare syndromes that may lead to dilation/enlargement of the IACs as well as the subarachnoid spaces in other locations, such as X-linked causes of deafness and Usher syndrome. Hence, a quick check for enlargement of the subarachnoid spaces in the Meckel cave and around the cranial nerves as they enter/exit the skull base as well as review for other findings on HRCT of the temporal bones can exclude such rare entities. Such patients typically have sensorineural hearing loss as well and moderate to marked enlargement of the IACs (greater in degree than normal bulbous IACs), which are other clues to their not being a normal variation in such syndromic patients.

5.2.2 Small Internal Auditory Canals (IACs)

Some size variability of the IACs can be expected in a small minority of patients. In a 2012 study by Erkoç et al. of nearly 4000 adults with normal hearing, the mean anteroposterior (AP) diameter of the IAC was 5.9 mm (SD 0.25 mm). Diffusely hypoplastic IACs are strongly associated with hypoplasia or absence of the cochlear division of the vestibulocochlear nerve (CN VIII), with the expected AP diameter of the IAC in children normally being greater than 2 mm. However, a possibly benign narrowing of the medial opening of the IAC, also called the internal auditory meatus or porus acusticus, is not uncommon in adults. Osteomas, exostoses, or bony overgrowth of the internal auditory meatus is not rare, although the precise incidence is not known since much of the literature consists of anecdotal reports. Bony overgrowth about the IAC meatus appears to have a female predominance, although it is not as strong as the 9:1 female-to-male ratio seen with the benign entity hyperostosis frontalis interna. While overgrowth of the IAC meatus is usually discovered incidentally and proves unchanged on follow-up imaging, some patients are rarely symptomatic. Auditory, vestibular, and facial nerve symptoms are possible with severe IAC meatus narrowing, but a review for other causes of symptomatology should be performed; cases have been described of improvement in vestibular symptoms and tinnitus following IAC decompression for severe narrowing.

5.2.3 Crista Falciformis

The crista falciformis is a transverse/horizontal bridge that separates the IAC into the superior and inferior segments, while the Bill bar is a vertical bony ridge that separates the superior compartment of the IAC into anterior and posterior segments. Together these form four quadrants that contain the facial nerve in the anterosuperior quadrant, the cochlear nerve in the anteroinferior quadrant, and the superior and inferior segments of the vestibular nerve in the corresponding posterior quadrants (these can be visible on sagittal high-resolution spin-echo T2-weighted imaging [SET2WI] or balanced-echo imaging through the IAC). The importance of knowing this anatomy is that the bony ridge of the crista falciformis can be variably visible on HRCT along the medial edge of the IAC, a normal variation that can even extend more medially in various patients. While it is typically not visible on MRI (as bone is dark on most sequences), it can be seen occasionally. Notably, the crista is increasingly visible as one increases the coronal obliquity of the reconstruction plane (i.e., as one approaches the true coronal plane of reconstruction) (Figs. 5.1, 5.2, 5.3, 5.4, 5.5, 5.6, 5.7, and 5.8).

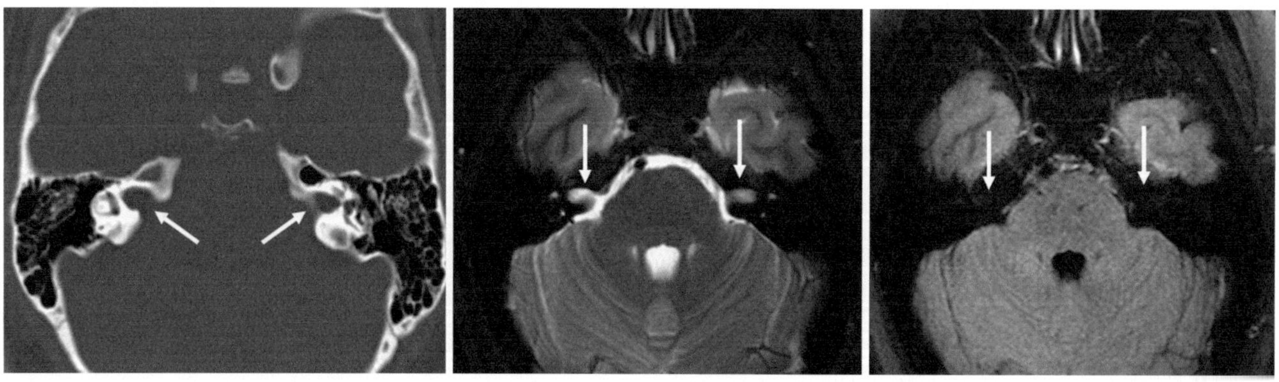

Fig. 5.1 A 24-year-old male underwent an otherwise negative head NECT for headaches, which noted bilateral prominent ("bulbous") IACs (*arrows*) on axial NECT (*left*). A 1.5T MRI with axial SET2WI (*middle*) and postcontrast SET1WI (*not shown*) confirmed that these were normal variant prominent IACs (*arrows*) and that no mass/schwannoma was present. The fluid/CSF signal within the IACs suppressed on FLAIR (*right*), whereas masses within the IACs also would not completely suppress as with the CSF signal

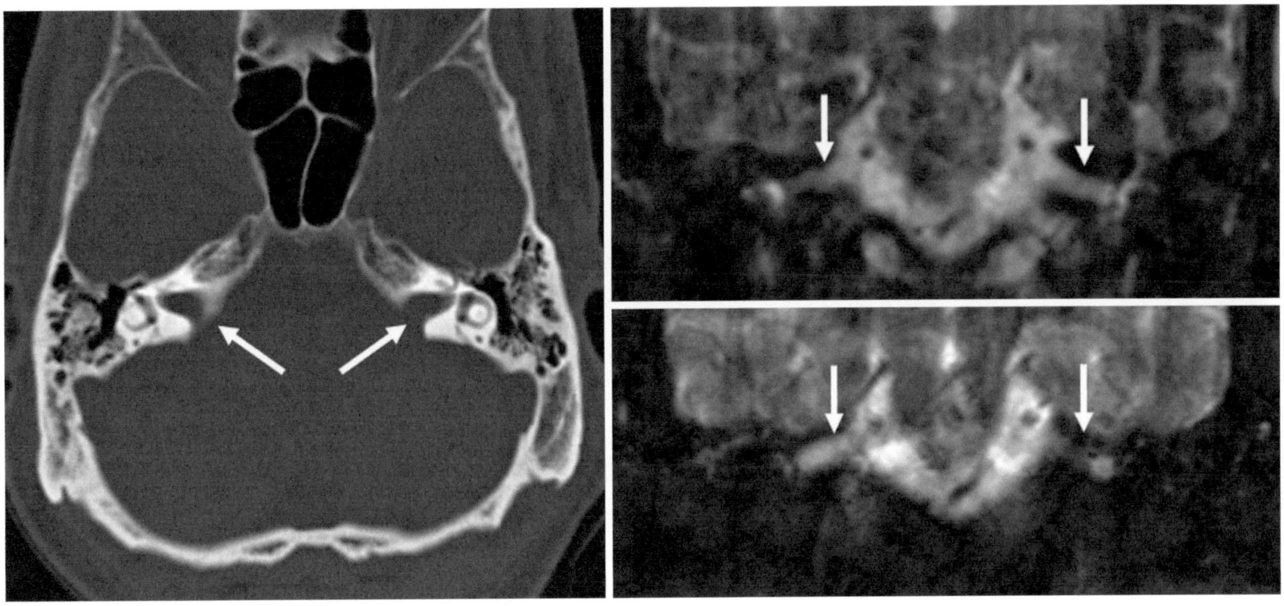

Fig. 5.2 In a 60-year-old male with altered mental status (negative examination), axial NECT (*left*) demonstrated prominent and slightly bulbous IACs bilaterally (*arrows*). On 1.5T coronal SET2WI (*right, top and bottom images*), there was moderate motion throughout the MRI examination, but the normal variant bulbous/prominent IACs were confirmed, and lacking any mass

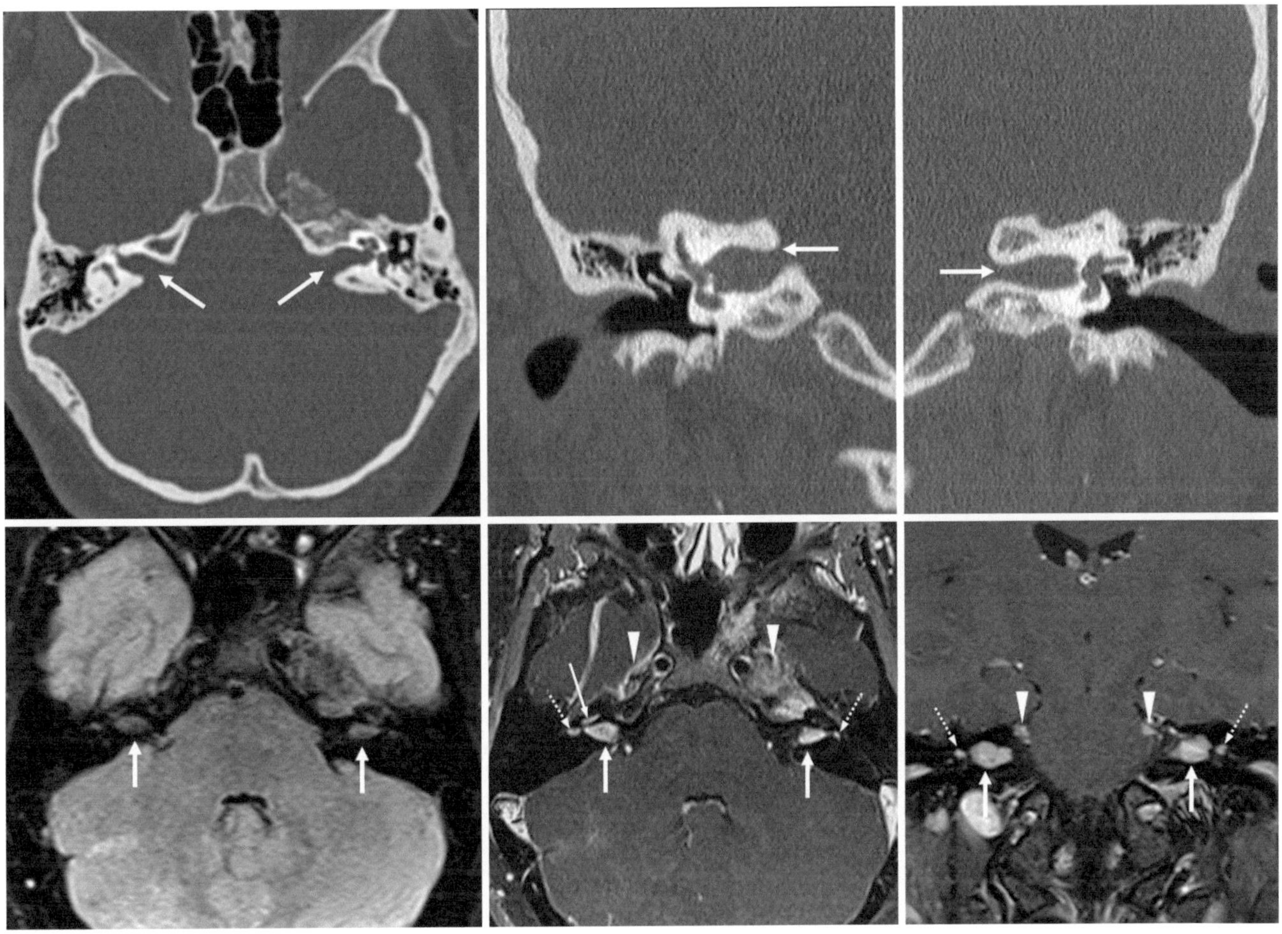

Fig. 5.3 Comparison case of enlarged IACs in neurofibromatosis type 2 (NF-2). Top row: In a 16-year-old female with NF-2, there was bilateral bulbous enlargement of the IACs (*arrows*) on axial NECT (*left*), with coronal reformats of the right (*middle*) and left (*right*) sides. **Bottom row:** On 3T MRI, there was nonsuppression of the CSF signal on noncontrast axial FLAIR (*left*), suggesting IAC masses bilaterally (*arrows*). Postcontrast SET1WI in the axial (*middle*) and coronal (*right*) planes confirmed the bilateral IAC schwannomas of NF-2 (*arrows*) as well as tiny bilateral cochlear schwannomas (*thin arrows*), facial nerve schwannomas (*thin dotted arrows*), and cranial nerve V schwannomas that also involve Meckel cave (*arrowheads*)

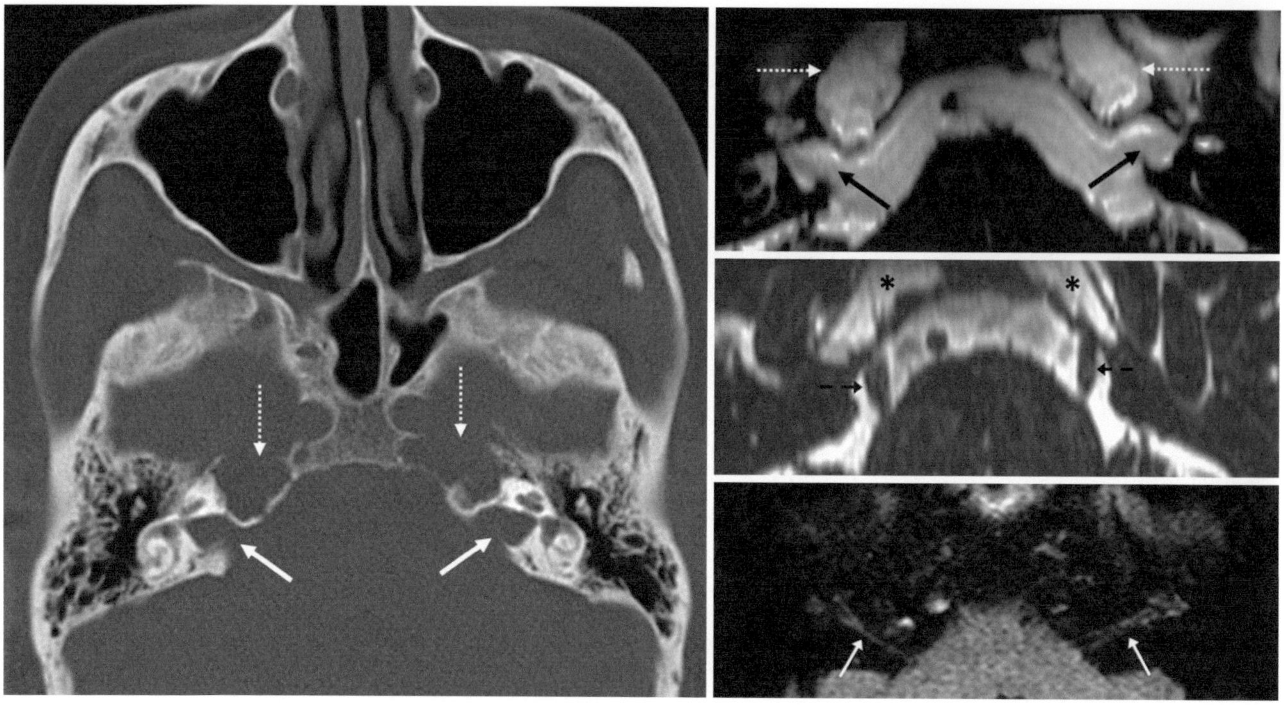

Fig. 5.4 **Comparison case of enlarged IACs in Usher syndrome.** In a 58-year-old male with congenital Usher syndrome, moderately prominent, bulbous IACs (*arrows*) were present bilaterally on axial NECT (*left*). Also note abnormal petrous apex cephaloceles (*dotted arrows*), which suggest abnormal enlargement of the subarachnoid spaces. On 1.5T axial SET2WI MRI (*right top and middle images*), the IACs (*black arrows, right top image*) are confirmed to be moderately enlarged as a result of subarachnoid space enlargement (and thus are not masses), which are contiguous with the aforementioned petrous apex cephaloceles (*dotted arrows, right top image*). There is also enlargement of Meckel caves (*asterisks, right middle image*), which cranial nerve V (*black dashed arrows*) passes into. On axial FLAIR MRI (*right bottom image*), the cranial nerves VII and VIII (*tiny arrows*) are visualized after CSF suppression, also confirming that the IAC enlargement was due to CSF subarachnoid space enlargement

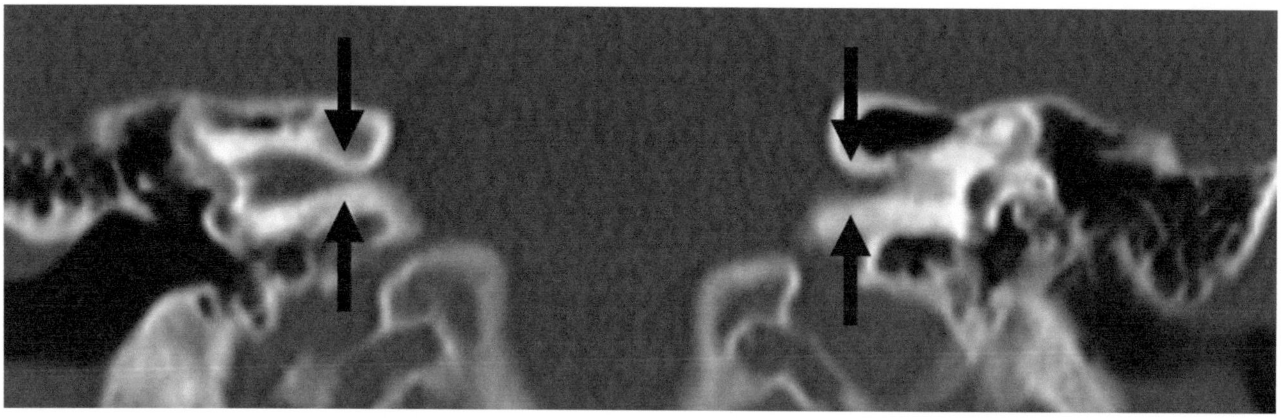

Fig. 5.5 In a 5-year-old male with normal hearing, small IACs are noted (*arrows*) on corona 0.9-mm thickness HRCT images of both sides. Three-dimensional SET2WI (*not shown*) did not demonstrate hypoplasia of the facial or vestibular nerves. Rarely, the IACs may be small in people with normal hearing, and if MRI with three-dimensional reconstructions of the nerves confirms that no cranial nerve VII or VIII hypoplasia is present, this can be considered a normal variation

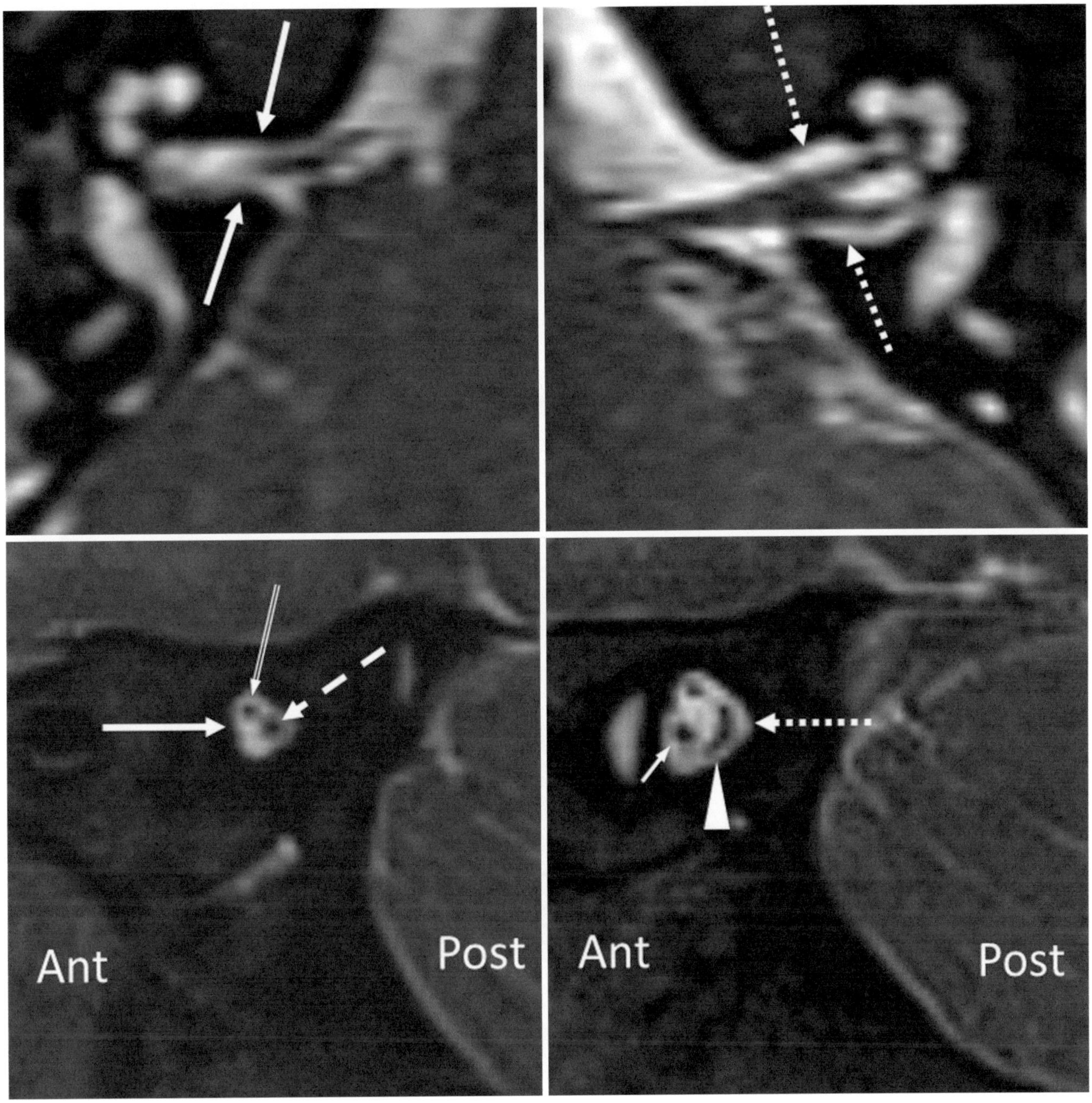

Fig. 5.6 Comparison case of unilateral small internal auditory canal (IAC) caused by hypoplasia. The patient was a 1-year-old male with right-sided deafness and normal left-sided hearing. An MRI with three-dimensional SET2WI images in the axial (*top row*) and oblique sagittal (*bottom row*) planes show a small right IAC (*arrows*) and a normal left IAC (*dotted arrows*). With similar magnification, the right IAC (*arrows, bottom left*) is markedly smaller than on the left side (*dotted arrow, bottom right*). A normal left cochlear nerve (*tiny arrow*) and inferior segment of the vestibular nerve (*arrowhead*) are seen on the left side (*bottom right image*). In the *bottom left* image, note the absence of both the right cochlear and right inferior vestibular division on the right, which should be in the anteroinferior and posteroinferior portions of the canal, respectively; the right facial nerve (*beveled arrow*) and superior division of the right vestibular nerve (*dashed arrow*) are both present and normal

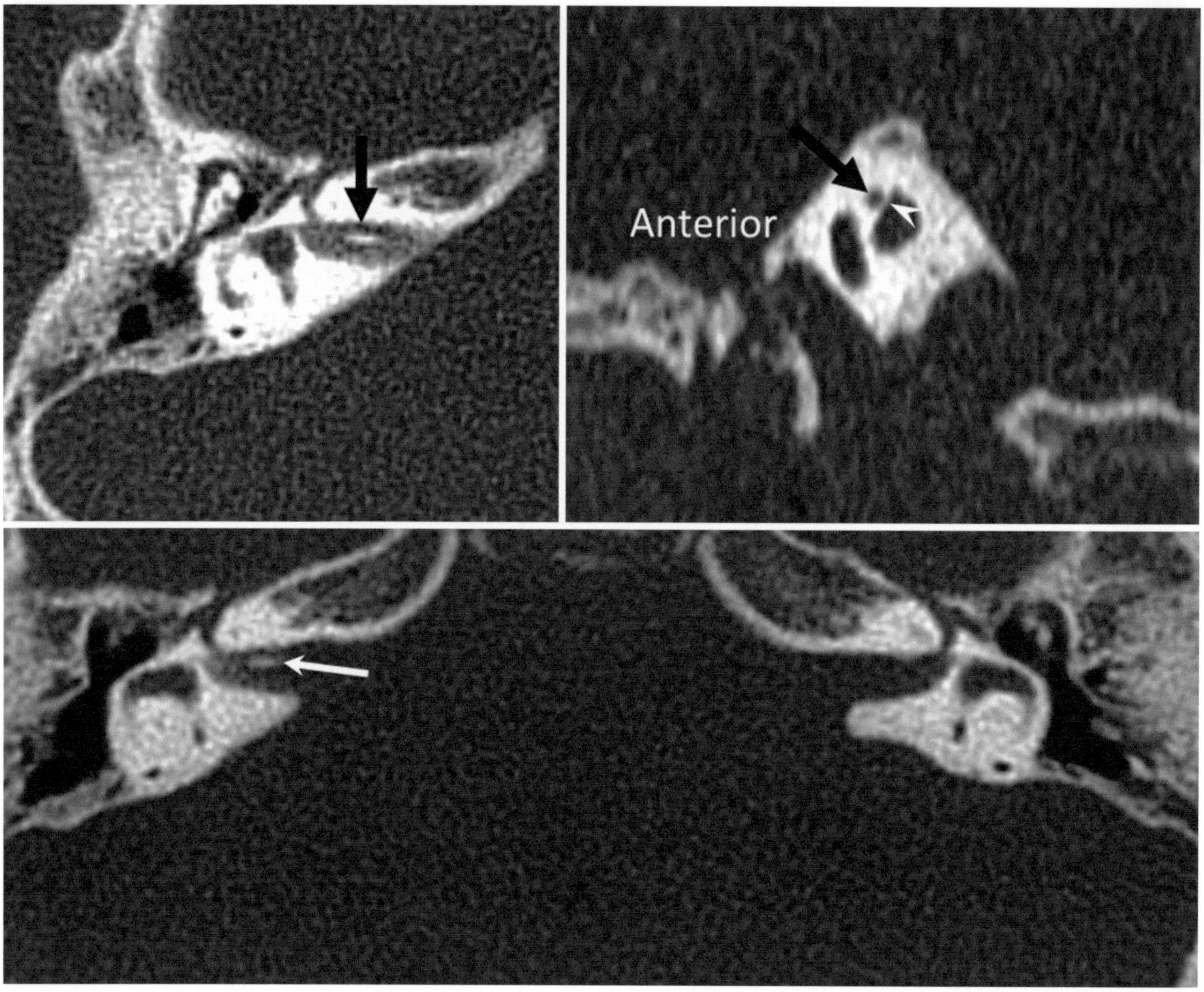

Fig. 5.7 In a 6-year-old boy with conductive hearing loss and recent bilateral tympanostomy tube placement, a HRCT 0.6-mm thickness axial image of the right side (*top left*) and a sagittal reconstruction of the left side (*top right*) demonstrate a short segment canal (*black arrows*) within the right IAC that contains the facial nerve. There is an accessory bone (*arrowhead, top right*) that separates the facial nerve from the remainder of the IAC. Note the normal axial appearance of the left IAC for comparison on an axial NECT image that shows both sides simultaneously (*bottom*)

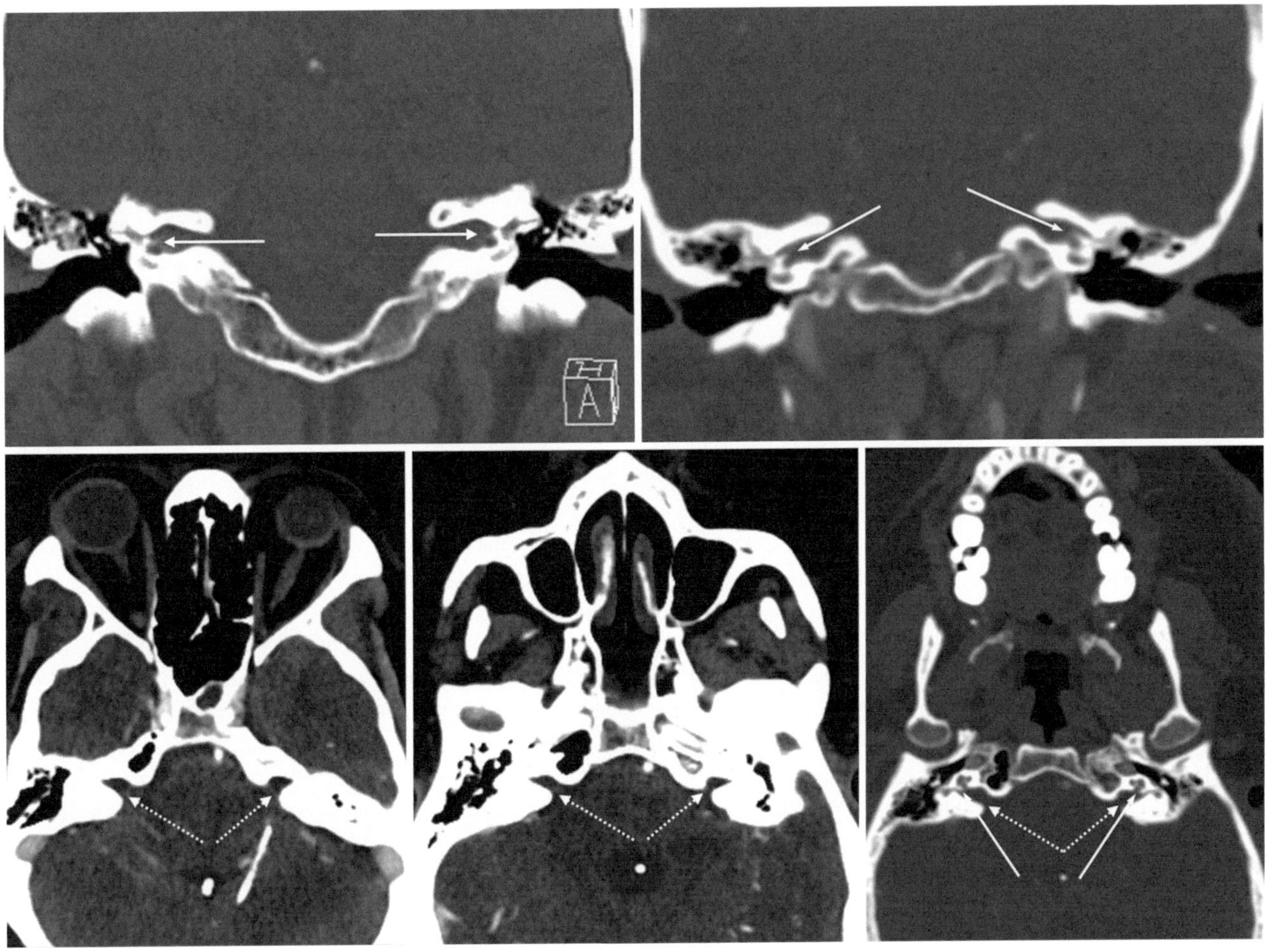

Fig. 5.8 Crista falciformis in two patients and the effect of angulation on its visibility. **Top left:** In a 65-year-old male to rule out stroke a negative NECT scan shows a barely visible crista falciformis bilaterally (*arrows*) on coronal 1-mm thickness reconstructions. **Top right:** In another patient, a 25-year-old female with Moya-Moya syndrome had incidental prominence of the crista falciformis bilaterally on a 1-mm thickness coronal reconstruction. **Bottom row:** In that same 25-year-old patient as the *top right* image, axial images with increasing obliquity in the coronal plane demonstrate that the cristae come into view (*arrow, bottom right*) within the IACs (*dotted arrows*) with increasing coronal obliquity of the axial slice reconstruction plane

5.3 Cochlear Variants: Osseous Spiral Lamina, Cochlear Cleft, Noise, Canals, and Aqueduct

5.3.1 Osseous Spiral Lamina

Within the cochlea, the osseous spiral lamina is a thin, linear hyperdense shelf of bone that projects outward from the bony modiolus, segmenting the turns of the cochlea into two chambers, the scala tympani toward the base, and the scala vestibuli toward the apex. This thin band of bone should roughly separate each turn in half, but the osseous spiral lamina does not reach the outer walls of the cochlea. Like the cochlea itself, the spiral lamina makes approximately 2.5 turns. At the apex of the cochlea, the spiral lamina terminates at the helicotrema, where the scala tympani and scala vestibuli can communicate with one another. As CT detector technology improves, this formerly undetectable structure is infrequently visible and should not be mistaken for pathologic calcification from a prior infection, such as labyrinthitis ossificans. Notably, absence of the spiral lamina at the cochlear apex and poor distinction of the middle and apical turns of the cochlea are termed incomplete partition type II (IP-II). In addition, displacement of the osseous spiral lamina toward the base of the cochlea away from its typical midline position (with a measurement of the outer spiral lamina to the top of the scala vestibuli greater than 1.2 mm) has recently been shown on MRI to be highly suggestive of IP-II. To discern normal, mild hyperdensity of the osseous spiral lamina from labyrinthitis ossificans, a helpful sign is to note a regular, smooth contour and number of turns of the cochlea, while in labyrinthitis ossificans, the calcified/ossified cochleae and semicircular canals may be irregular, multifocal, narrowed, and obscured.

5.3.2 Cochlear Cleft

The otic capsule refers to the cochlea, vestibule, and semicircular canals and the dense bone that encompasses them, also known as the bony labyrinth. This portion of the temporal bone is typically homogeneously hyperdense throughout life. In young children, however, a small area of slightly lower density can be seen lateral to the middle/apical turn junction near the fissula ante fenestram. This normal variant usually appears as a thin curvilinear band that appears slightly larger in the coronal plane than the axial plane and has been referred to as the "cochlear cleft." Chadwell et al. studied 200 pediatric temporal bones by CT and found an overall incidence of the cochlear cleft to be about 41%; interestingly, in the youngest age group (under 4 years old) the incidence was 62%, which dropped to 19% in the 10–19-year-old group. It is speculated that the cochlear cleft may represent a region of the otic capsule at a boundary between the outer periosteal layers and the enchondral layer. The decreasing incidence of the cochlear cleft with increasing age suggests that this area, which is initially hypodense, ossifies over time and is no longer recognizable. This normal variant "cleft" may mimic true disease such as fenestral ostospongiosis (otosclerosis), but otospongiosis-otosclerosis usually occurs in older patients within the fissula ante fenestram itself.

5.3.3 Cochlear Hypoattenuation from Noise and Quantum Mottle

Proper NECT imaging often requires a prudent balancing act between signal-to-noise and radiation dose to obtain adequate imaging, particularly for HRCT of the temporal bone. As voxel size and slice thickness decrease, correspondingly fewer photons travel through each voxel. For HRCT of the temporal bone, the typical slice and recommended thicknesses are usually less than 1 mm. As such, varying pixel densities can impart a "grainy" look referred to as quantum mottle (artifact from noise). In certain locations in the temporal bone, a cluster of apparent hypodense pixels may mimic pathology. In particular, hypodensity at the fissula ante fenestram must be carefully evaluated, since such hypoattenuating artifact from quantum mottle can simulate pathology such as early fenestral otosclerosis. When present, the hypodensity in otosclerosis/otospongiosis is usually more homogeneous and less speckled than the hypodensity seen with quantum mottle artifact.

5.3.4 Cochlear Aqueduct: Normal Size and Appearance

The imaging appearance of the cochlear aqueduct (CA) has been studied several times over the decades but has not garnered the research or clinical interest that the vestibular aqueduct has. The CA is a funnel-shaped channel through the temporal bone, connecting the perilymph of the cochlea with the cerebrospinal fluid (CSF). The CA is largest medially, tapering as it travels superiorly and laterally to insert on the cochlea just anterior to the round window. Several studies have described the variability in sizes of the medial opening of the CA, ranging from 0 to 11 mm with a mean of 4.5 mm. The tapering laterally is often so pronounced that the lateral portion through the otic capsule can only be visualized in 56% of temporal bones. In a 1993 study by Jackler and Hwang, the lateral portion of the CA did not exceed 2 mm in any case. It is important to recognize the expected size variability of the CA, particularly medially, and that it may be normal for the CA to be barely visible. There have been some reports of smaller CAs being associated with Ménière disease, but further study will be needed as this is preliminary and debatable. In summary, the CA is quite variable in size and is not always easily seen, and when small and thin it can be mistaken for a pathologic temporal bone fracture if one is unfamiliar with the normal variation in size of this structure.

5.3.5 Cochlear Nerve Canal: Normal Size and Appearance

The cochlear nerve canal (also known as the cochlear aperture) is the canal through the otic capsule transmitting the cochlear division of the vestibulocochlear nerve from the anterior inferior internal auditory canal into the base of the cochlea. A diameter measurement at the narrowest portion of less than 1.5 mm is strongly associated with sensorineural hearing loss, usually caused by a hypoplastic or absent cochlear nerve. Not surprisingly, the finding of a small cochlear nerve canal is more strongly associated with cochlear nerve hypoplasia than a small internal auditory canal. As a caution, a normal-sized cochlear nerve canal does not always equate to a normal cochlear nerve, and MRI is an important adjunct to temporal bone CT in the evaluation of pediatric deafness. Thus, it is important to be aware of the normal sizes of the cochlear aperture, where mild prominence or asymmetry can be normal, but there is a threshold that is too small and should raise the question of cochlear nerve hypoplasia-aplasia (Figs. 5.9, 5.10, 5.11, 5.12, 5.13, 5.14, and 5.15).

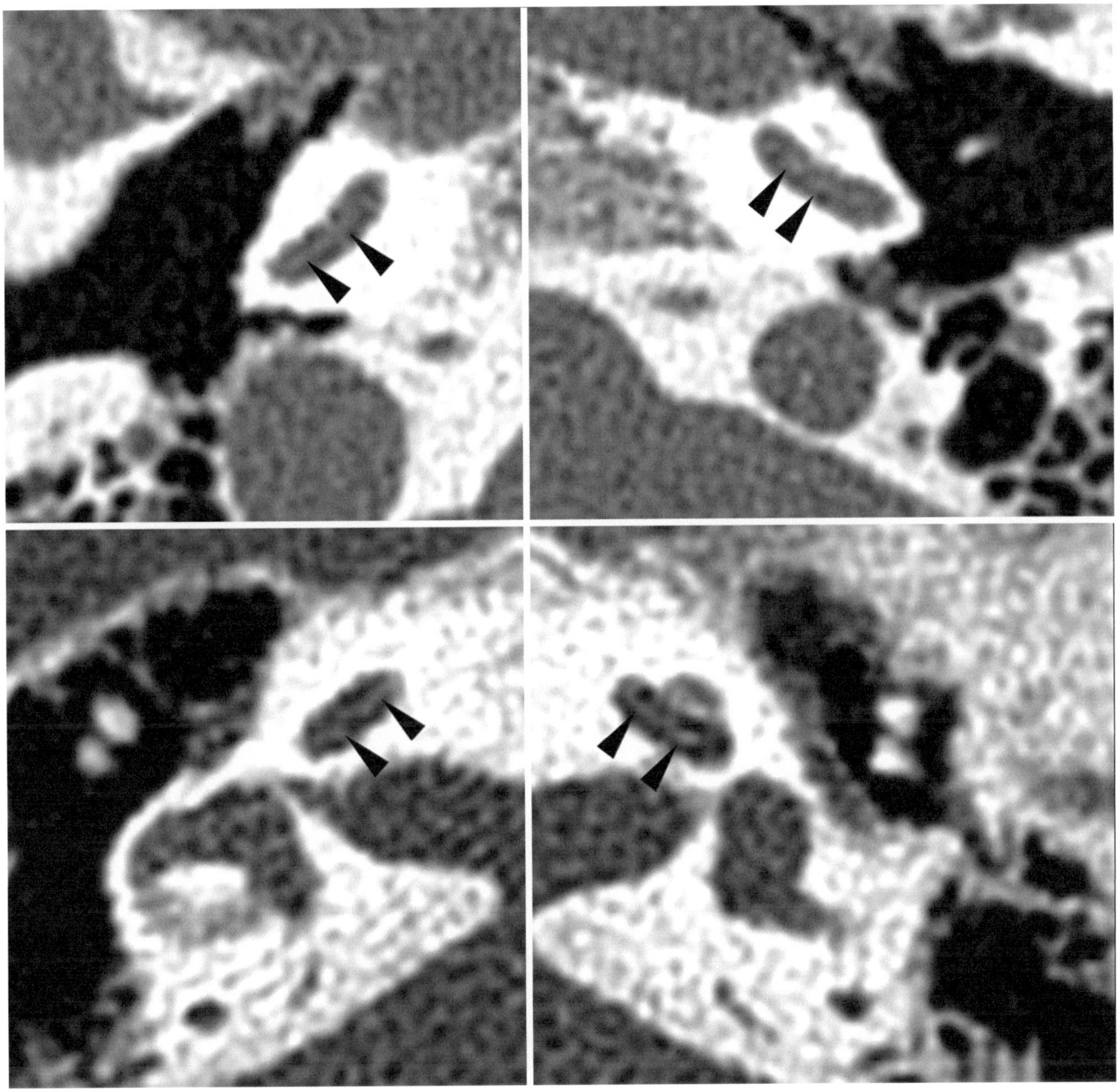

Fig. 5.9 Normal osseous spiral laminae of the cochleae in two different patients. **Top row:** In a 30-year-old male with dizziness (no hearing deficits), a thin curvilinear band of hyperdensity denotes the normal osseous laminae (*arrowheads*) in the basal turns of the cochleae. **Bottom row:** In a 58-year-old female with a prior tympanostomy tube placement for recurrent otitis media, there are normal hyperdense osseous spiral laminae in the cochlear middle turns (*arrowheads*). Both cases demonstrate how the normally dense osseous laminae can simulate the sequelae of chronic inflammation/infection, such as labyrinthitis ossificans; however, labyrinthitis ossificans causes narrowing of the cochlear turns and semicircular canals, which are not present in these two patients

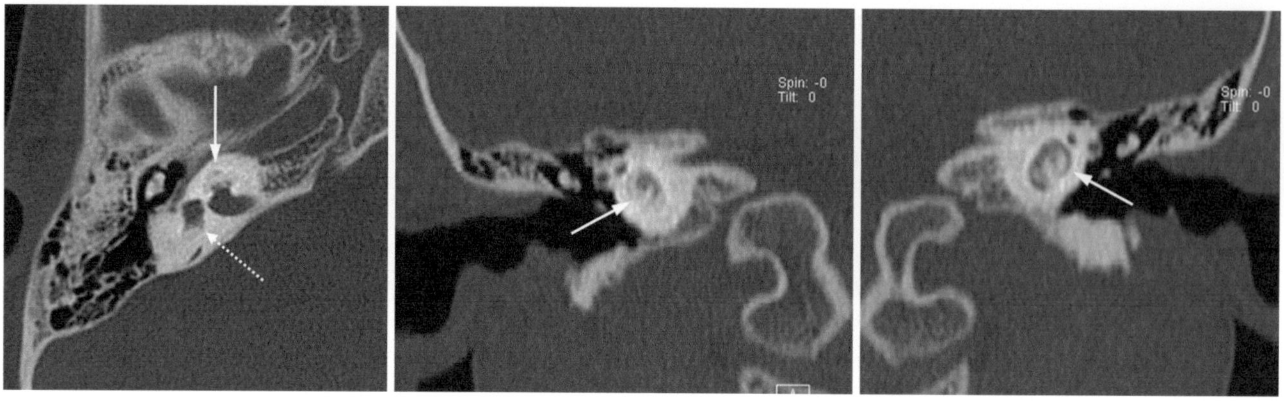

Fig. 5.10 Comparison case of labyrinthitis ossificans. In an 8-year-old male with sensorineural hearing loss, NECT with axial (*left*) HRCT reconstruction (0.6-mm thickness) of the right side demonstrates that both the cochlea (*arrows*) and the vestibular structures (*dotted arrows*) are heavily calcified, consistent with the sequela of inflammation from labyrinthitis ossificans. Similar findings are noted on coronal HRCT reformats of the right (*middle*) and left sides (*right image*), where the cochleae are quite calcified bilaterally (*arrows*)

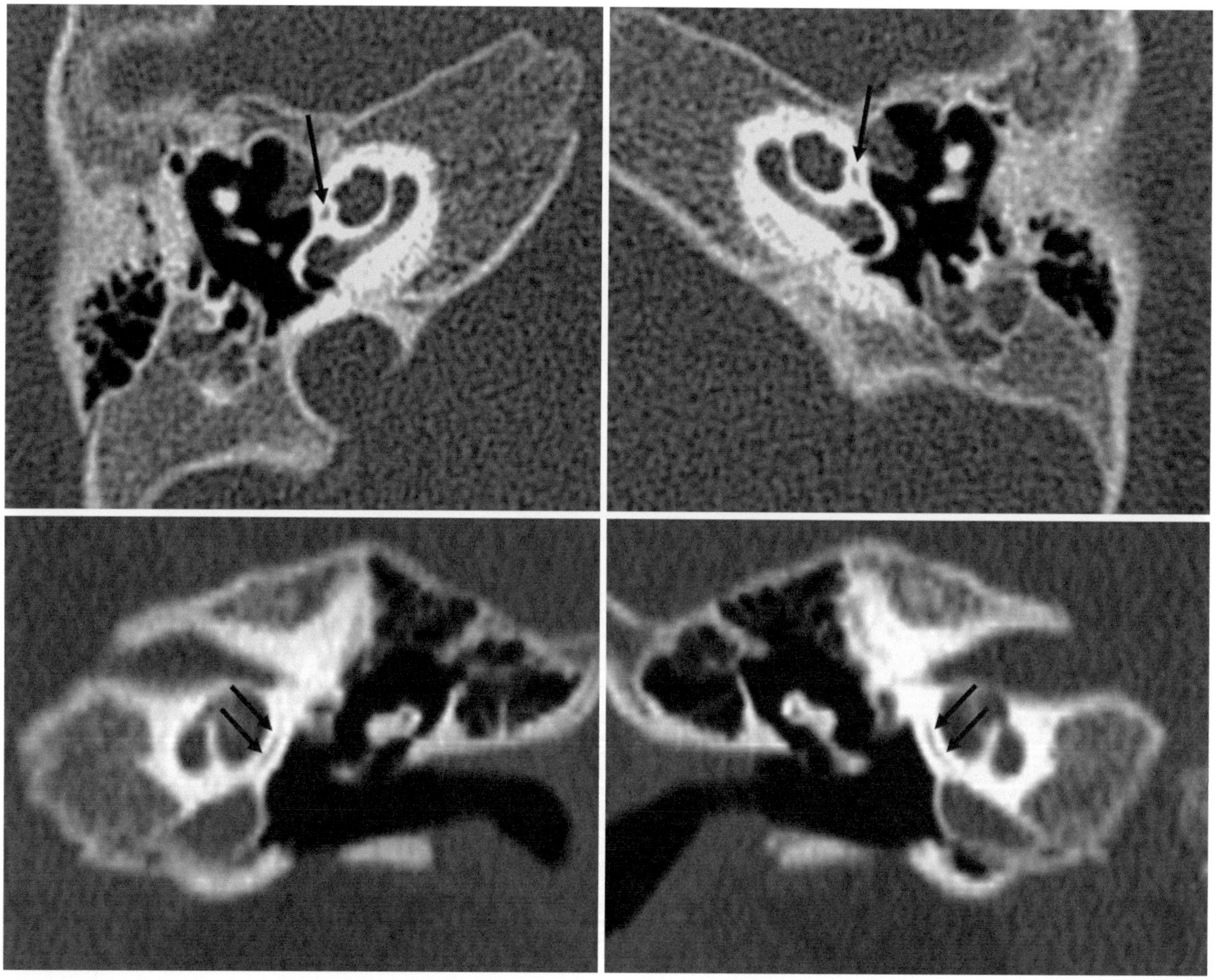

Fig. 5.11 In a 14-month-old male on HRCT 0.6-mm axial images (*top row*) symmetric, focal lucencies (*arrows*) are noted medial to the cochleae, which appear punctate near the middle/apical turn junction. On coronal reconstructed images (*bottom row*), these lucencies appear as thin, curvilinear bands (*arrows*) on each side. Note that these normal infantile pericochlear lucencies ("clefts") do not extend to the lateral cortex, as would be expected with abnormal resorption in the entity fenestral otosclerosis

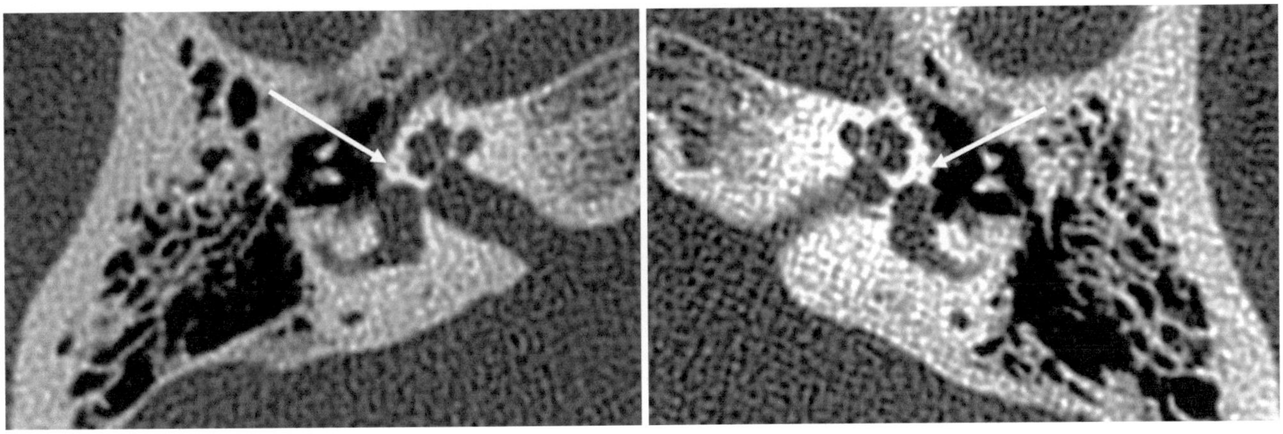

Fig. 5.12 In a 58-year-old female with dizziness, punctate areas of decrease density (*arrows*) are noted within the otic capsule medial to the cochleae bilaterally on an otherwise negative HRCT with 0.6-mm thickness axial images. These hypodense foci are caused by noise (quantum mottle) and should not be mistaken for fenestral otosclerosis

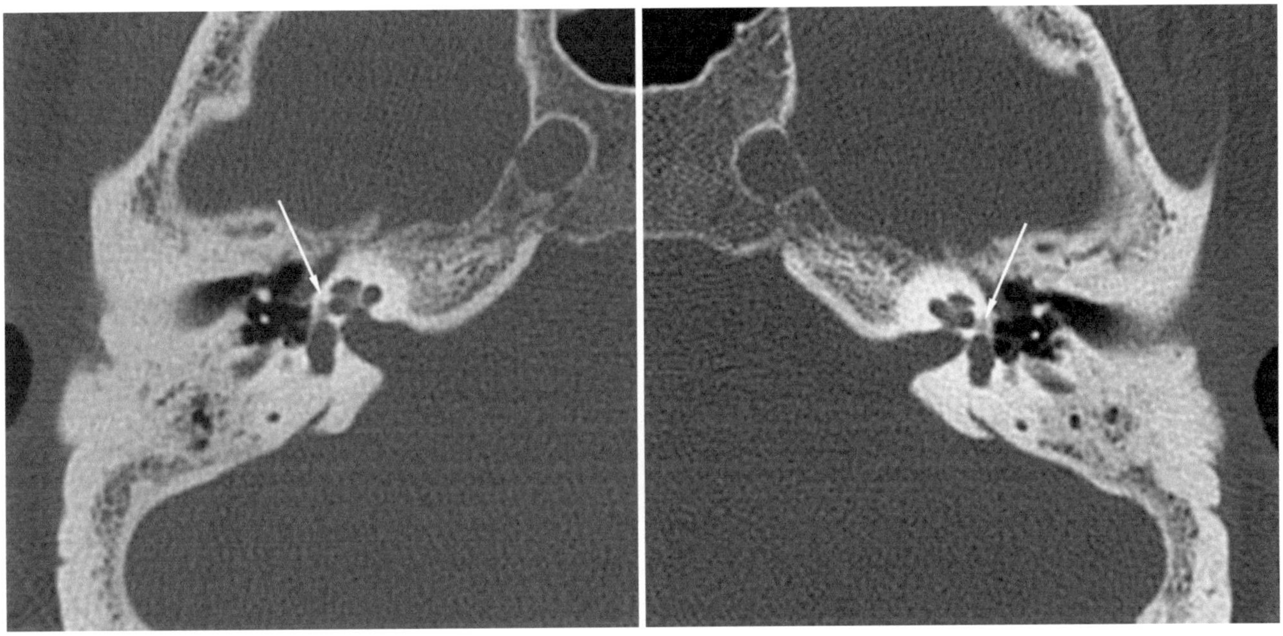

Fig. 5.13 Comparison case of fenestral otospongiosis. In a 39-year-old male with bilateral hearing loss, subtle lucency is noted of the fissula ante fenestram bilaterally (*arrows*), situated posterior to the cochlear promontory; this is consistent with early fenestral otospongiosis

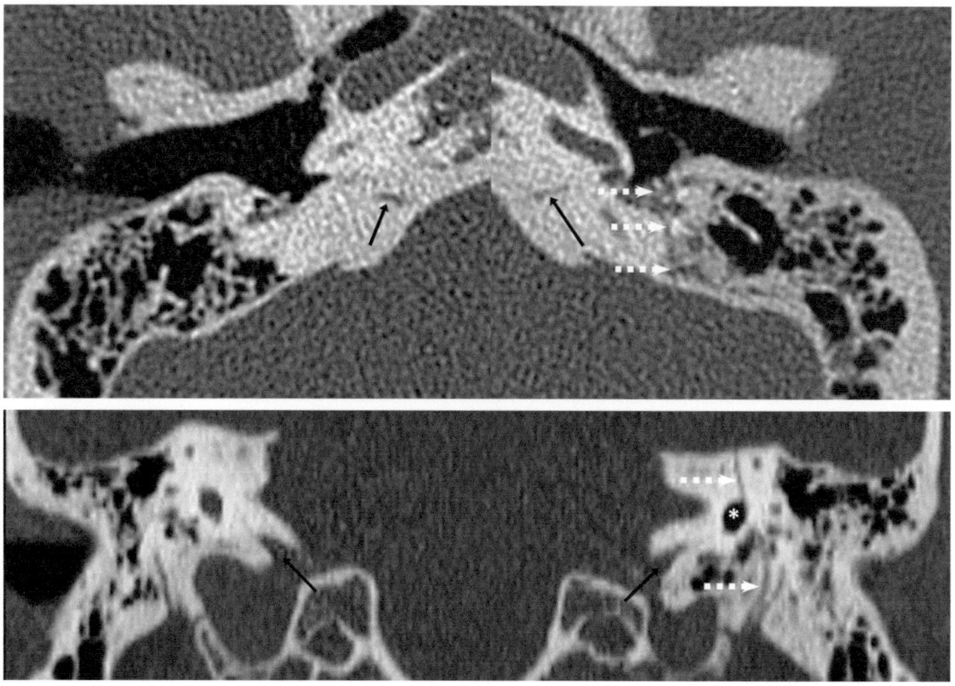

Fig. 5.14 Normal small, difficult to visualize cochlear aqueducts in a 33-year-old male with dizziness, left hearing loss, and left facial nerve paralysis after an altercation in which he suffered a transverse fracture of the left petrous temporal bone. **Top row:** Note the normal, small cochlear nerve canals (*black arrows*) on HRCT 0.6-mm thickness axial reconstructions, and the left-sided transverse petrous fracture (*dotted arrows*). **Bottom row:** Note the oblique course of the small cochlear nerve canals (*black arrows*) on the reconstructed coronal images, appearing oblique beginning inferior to the internal auditory canals, and tapering as the canals ascend toward the junction of the basal turn of the cochlea with the vestibule; this appearance should not be mistaken for a fracture. An actual transverse fracture (*dotted arrows, right*) extends through the vestibule and causes pneumolabyrinth (*asterisk*), also extending through the apex of the cochlea and the labyrinthine segment of the facial canal (*not shown*)

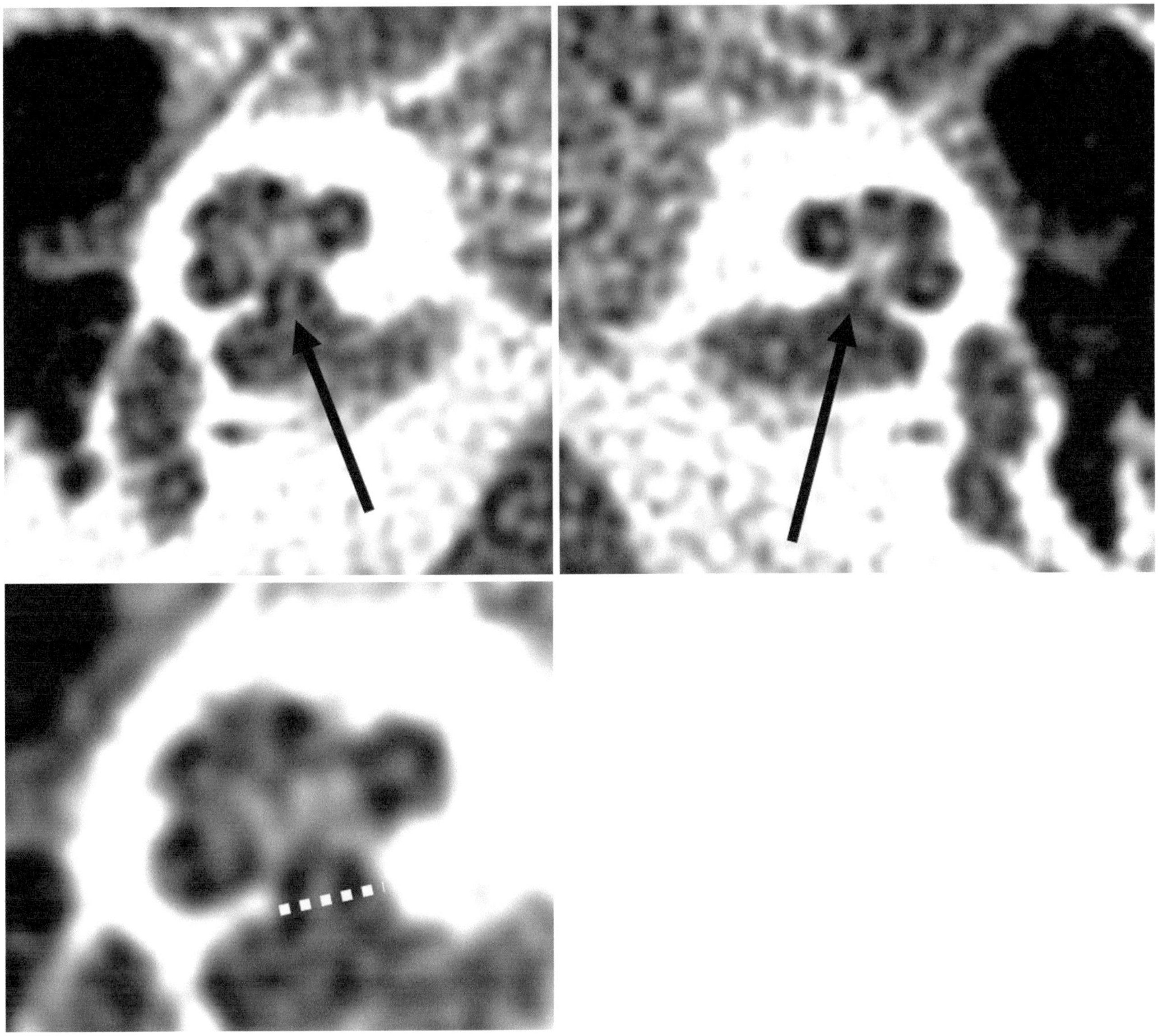

Fig. 5.15 Example of normal and abnormal cochlear nerve canal diameters in the same patient. In a 10-year-old boy with left-sided deafness and normal right hearing, on HRCT 0.6-mm thickness axial images note the normal cochlear nerve canal (2.0 mm diameter) on the right side (*top left*) and a smaller cochlear nerve canal (0.8 mm diameter) on the left side (*top right*); both cochlear canals are denoted by the *black arrows*. Measurements less than 1.4 mm are strongly associated with hypoplastic or absent cochlear nerves. A magnified axial image (*bottom left*) shows the measurement plane for the diameter of the normal right side

5.4 Semicircular Canal Variants: Crura Relative to Thin Apices of Semicircular Canals

The sizes of the semicircular canals that have typically been described in the anatomic literature have not been traditionally described as diameters but rather as based functionally on their degree of radial curvature and ratio of the canal plane area to streamline length. However, for radiologic purposes, particularly on HRCT, there may be asymmetry in size (whether "diameter/caliber," "height," or "width") of semicircular canals (SCCs) relative to each other, between the proximal and distal crura of the SCCs, and relative to the apices of each SCC. Notably however, the SCCs should be symmetric with the same canal on the opposite side. For example, the anterior/superior SCC tends to be thinner (smaller caliber) than the other two canals, while the posterior SCC tends to have a slightly greater "height" and "width" of the overall loop relative to the lateral SCC. Also, it is important to note that unlike the brain and other organs in the body, the size of the SCCs remains relatively constant from childhood (around 5–7 years) to the elderly years. Finally, the three SCCs may be slightly larger in males relative to females, a finding in the literature of as yet unknown significance.

A potential source of confusion may arise when evaluating the anterior/superior SCC, where the apex of the SCC may appear slightly smaller in diameter than the proximal or distal crura (joining point to the vestibule or common crus). This normal variant may simulate disease, such as labyrinthitis ossificans (a remote sequela of inflammation or infection), which causes calcification/ossification of the inner ear. A normal variant thin SCC apex may be distinguished from labyrinthitis ossificans in that there is no membranous ossification in this variant, while in labyrinthitis ossificans there is ossification of vestibular or cochlear structures that can either be diffuse, multifocal, or irregular. It is recommended that the anterior/superior SCC on Poschl view (an oblique coronal view to maximize the full view of the superior SCC) be viewed on HRCT or HRMRI to distinguish this variant. Notably, such thinning at the apex of the SCC can be noted on any of the SCCs but seems to be most notable at the apex of the anterior/superior SCC on dedicated Poschl HRCT reconstructions. This normal variant apparent "thinning" can be exacerbated on T2WI high resolution MRI, perhaps caused by an artifact from adjacent mastoid bone or gas (Fig. 5.16).

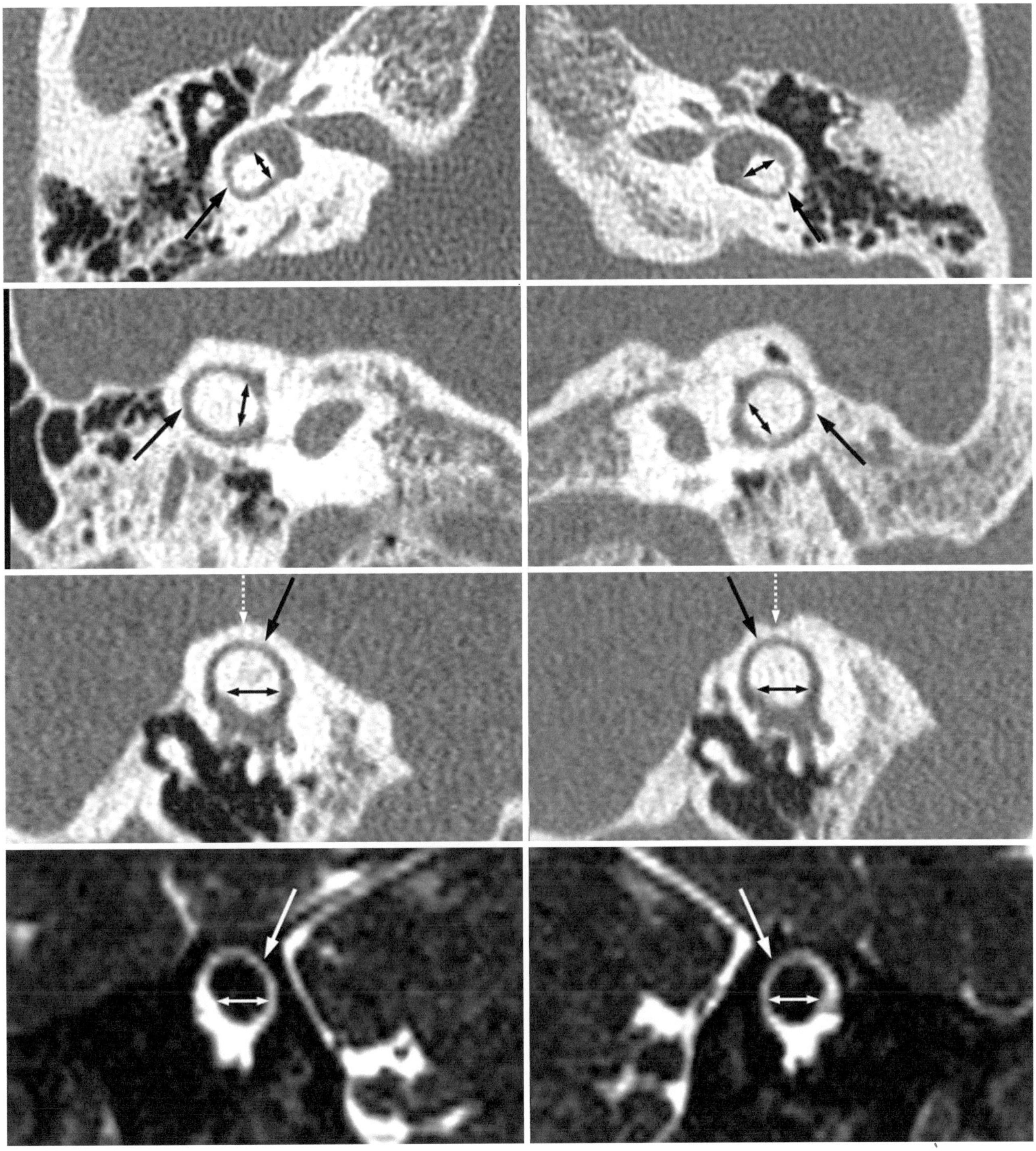

Fig. 5.16 In a 20-year-old female with a HRCT for conductive (not sensorineural) hearing loss, normal variant smaller diameter of the apices (*arrows* in each image) of each of the three SCCs is illustrated relative to their proximal and distal crura (*double arrows* in each). The left column of images is the patient's right side, while the right column is the patient's left side. **Top row:** On axial images profiling the horizontal-lateral SCC, the apices (*arrows*) of the SCC on each side appear thinner relative to the proximal and distal crura (*double arrows*). **Second row:** On oblique coronal images aligned along the plane of the petrous apex profiling the posterior SCC, similarly the apices (*arrows*) of each posterior SCC appear thinner relative to the proximal and distal crura (*double arrows*). **Third row:** On oblique coronal (Poschl view) images profiling the anterior/superior SCCs, the apices also appear smaller in caliber; note the normal thickness of the bone overlying each SCC, the arcuate eminence (*dotted arrows*), an area to evaluate for dehiscence potentially causing "third-window" phenomena. **Bottom row:** HRMRI T2WI Poschl views depict similar findings as in the third row, where the apices (*arrows*) of each SCC appear thinner relative to the proximal and distal crura (*double arrows*). This case also demonstrates that while there is normal variation thinning of the apices relative to the crura, the findings should be symmetric with the corresponding SCC on the opposite side. Also, note the differences in overall height and width of the three SCCs relative to each other: the posterior SCC tends to have the overall widest/longest loop, the lateral/horizontal SCC the shortest, while the anterior/superior SCC tends to be the thinnest in caliber/diameter

5.4.1 Vestibular Aqueduct: Normal Size and Appearance

The vestibular aqueduct (VA) connects the endolymphatic sac to the vestibule (serving as a conduit between the inner ear and cranial vault and carrying endolymph); the endolymphatic duct runs within the VA. Regarding the size of the VA, there are several methods of measuring it. A smaller than average VA is considered a normal variant, but an enlarged VA (EVA) is usually pathologic. EVA is one of the most common abnormalities identified in children with sensorineural hearing loss. This is particularly true in those with non–syndromic hearing loss, in whom up to 32% are found to have EVA. When present, EVA is usually bilateral, occurring in 55–94% of affected children, but it can be unilateral as well. While the type of hearing loss is typically sensorineural, there may be a conductive component, potentially due to the "third window" effect of the EVA. The relationship of the degree of the VA enlargement to the severity of hearing loss has been controversial, with some authors reporting a correlation, while others report no association. A 2018 study by Song et al. found hearing loss in 90.2% of EVA ears; of those ears, purely sensorineural hearing loss was found in 92%, with mixed hearing loss in 4.8%, and conductive hearing loss in 2.4%; dizziness was found in 63.6%.

An accepted method of VA measurement is to measure the AP diameter of the aqueduct at its midportion, where quantitatively it should measure less than 1.5 mm, and qualitatively it should be smaller than the adjacent limb of the posterior semicircular canal. An enlarged vestibular aqueduct may be an isolated finding but is frequently seen with Incomplete Partition type 2 and Pendred syndrome. A small VA is typically not present (and is more commonly related to suboptimal slice selection plane), but if present may be associated with Ménière disease, which is typically a clinical diagnosis. However, the exact cause and specific HRMRI diagnostic criteria of Ménière are still being debated. Hence, in summary, it is normal to have a small VA in patients without Ménière disease, but there is a maximum size threshold (1.5–2 mm) that raises the question of EVA syndrome (Figs. 5.17 and 5.18).

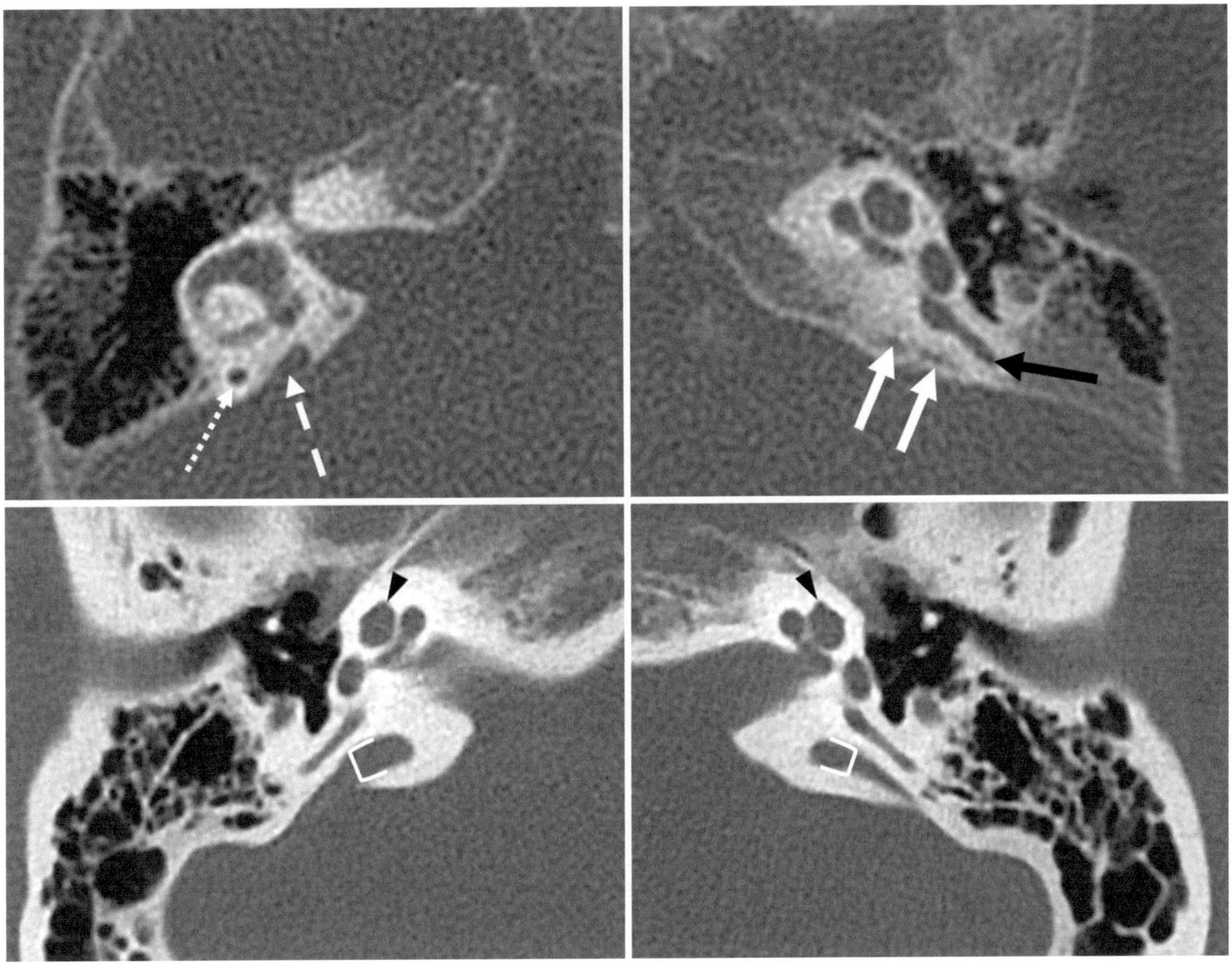

Fig. 5.17 **Comparison cases: Normal versus abnormal vestibular aqueduct sizes in two different patients with unilateral and bilateral vestibular aqueduct enlargement. Top row:** In a 6-month-old female with a failed newborn hearing screen of the right ear, axial HRCT shows a normal left vestibular aqueduct (diameter less than 1 mm, *arrows, right*) and an enlarged right vestibular aqueduct (diameter 2.6 mm, *dashed arrow, left*). Note that the abnormal right aqueduct (*dashed arrow, left*) is larger than the diameter of the adjacent crus of the posterior semicircular canal (*dotted arrow, left*), while the normal left vestibular aqueduct (*arrows, right*) is smaller than the adjacent posterior semicircular canal (*black arrow, right*) **Bottom row:** In a 51-year-old female with bilateral hearing loss since childhood, there are enlarged vestibular aqueducts bilaterally on axial HRCT, which are 2.9 mm on the right side (*bracket, left image*) and 2.5 mm on the left side (*bracket, right image*); the brackets delineate the plane of measurement of the diameter. Note the deficiency of the modiolus in and the poor distinction of the middle/apical turns of the cochlea (*black arrowheads in both images*), consistent with incomplete partition type 2. The combination of the poor definition of the middle and apical turns and an enlarged vestibular aqueduct has been termed the Mondini deformity

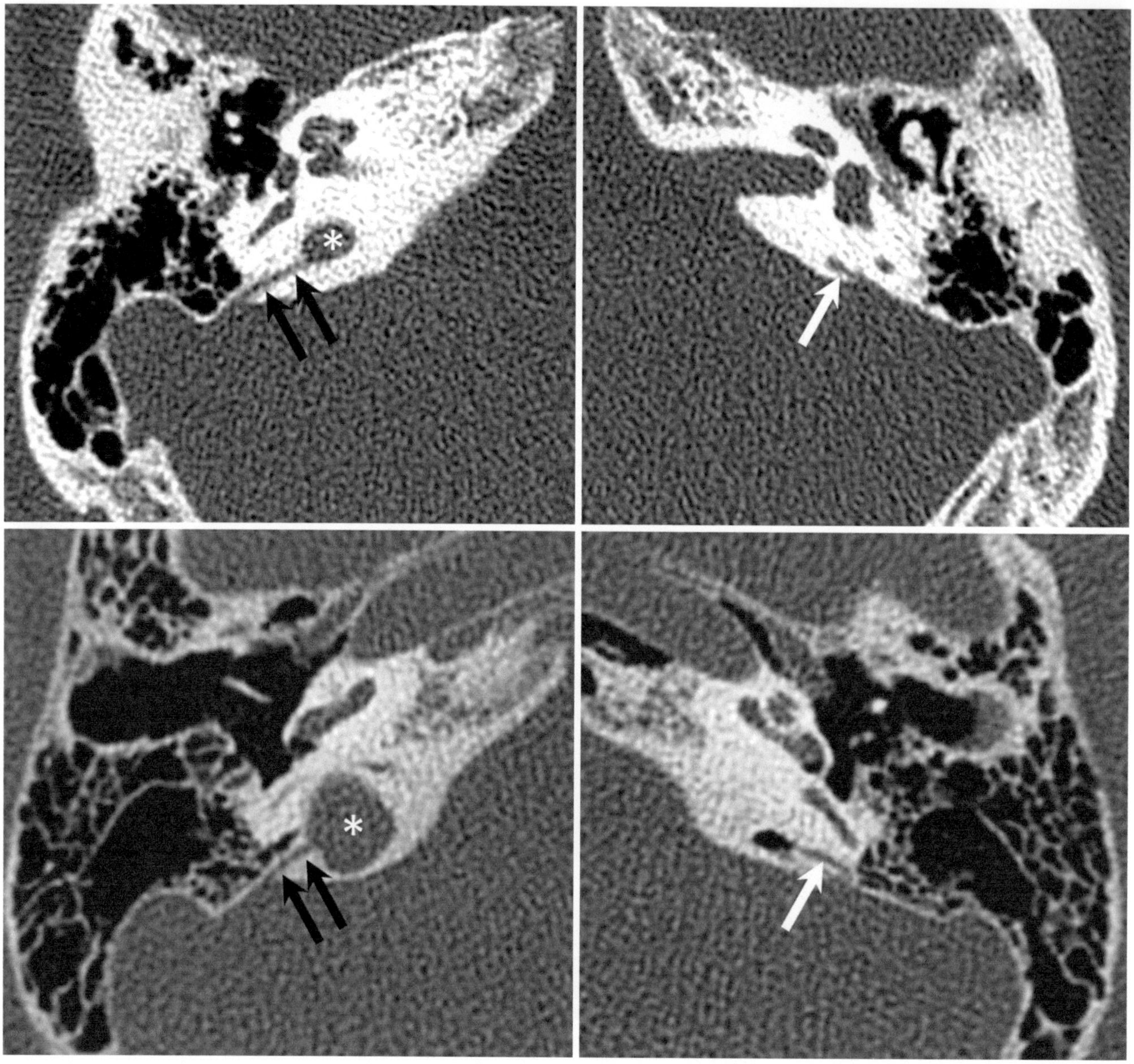

Fig. 5.18 Two different patients with jugular bulb diverticulum-dehiscence with the vestibular aqueduct. **Top row:** On axial 0.6-mm thickness HRCT images (otherwise negative) in a 21-year-old patient lacking hearing loss or balance issues, the right vestibular aqueduct (*double black arrows, left*) is in communication with a superiorly projecting diverticulum from the IJV (*asterisk*); the normal left vestibular aqueduct (*single white arrow, right*) is not in communication with the IJV. **Bottom row:** On axial 0.6-mm thickness HRCT images (otherwise negative) in a different 11-year-old patient with recurrent otitis media and a normal audiogram, the right vestibular aqueduct (*double black arrows*) is in communication with a superiorly projecting diverticulum from the IJV (*asterisk*), while the normal left vestibular aqueduct (*single white arrow*) does not communicate with the IJV. These cases are examples of what may be a normal variation but was traditionally thought to nearly always be abnormal

5.4.2 Subarcuate Canals

The subarcuate canal (also known as the petromastoid canal) connects the posterior fossa to the mastoid antrum and transmits the subarcuate artery (a branch of the anteroinferior cerebellar artery) in 80%, an accessory inferior cerebellar artery in 17%, and from the posterior inferior cerebellar artery in 3%. It is frequently seen curving across the posterior portion of the petrous temporal bone between the limbs of the superior semicircular canal. On HRCT, subarcuate canals have been described as being visualized as frequently as 95%; however, often very tiny subarcuate canals can be difficult to visualize, particularly without HRCT thin-section images. Enlarged subarcuate canals are considered normal variants and are more frequently seen in children with subarcuate canal diameters greater than 2 mm, being present in 22% of patients less than 5 years of age and 2.4% in children older than 5 years. While an enlarged subarcuate canal is considered a normal variant, it may theoretically provide a route for otomastoiditis to extend intracranially and can in theory be an important surgical consideration in the setting of temporal bone surgery (Figs. 5.19, 5.20, and 5.21).

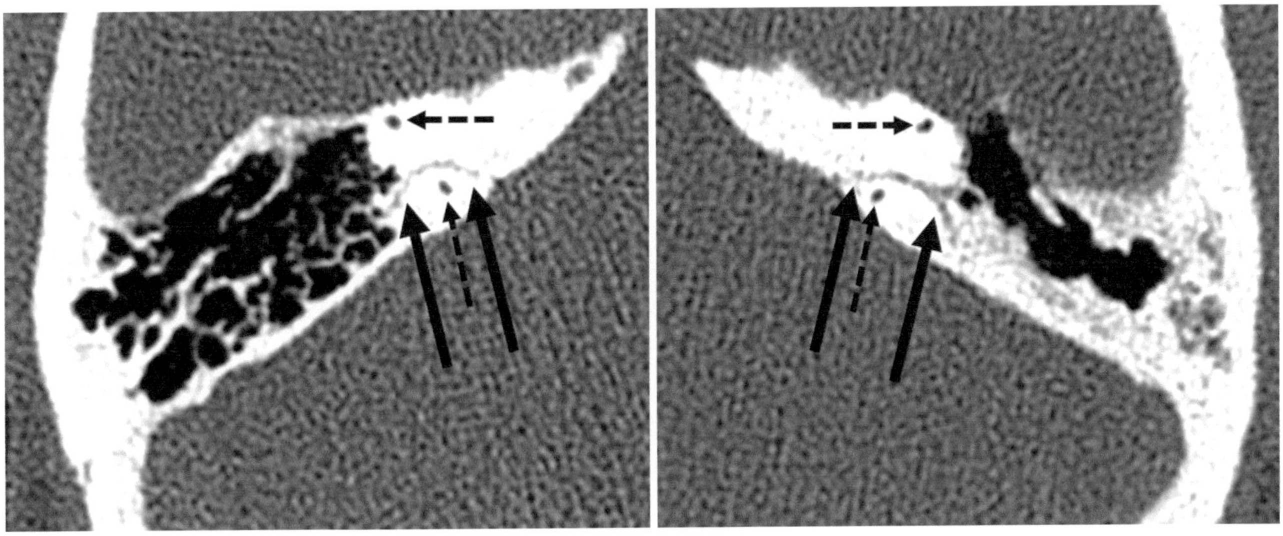

Fig. 5.19 In a 60-year-old female with recurrent left otitis (but no symptoms of balance, dizziness, or hearing loss), note the normal course of the subarcuate canals bilaterally (*arrows*), curving between the limbs of the superior semicircular canals (*dashed arrows*). The anterior and posterior crura of the superior semicircular canals appear as small circular structures on axial images (*dashed arrows*). This case demonstrates that normal variant subarcuate canals can be present bilaterally

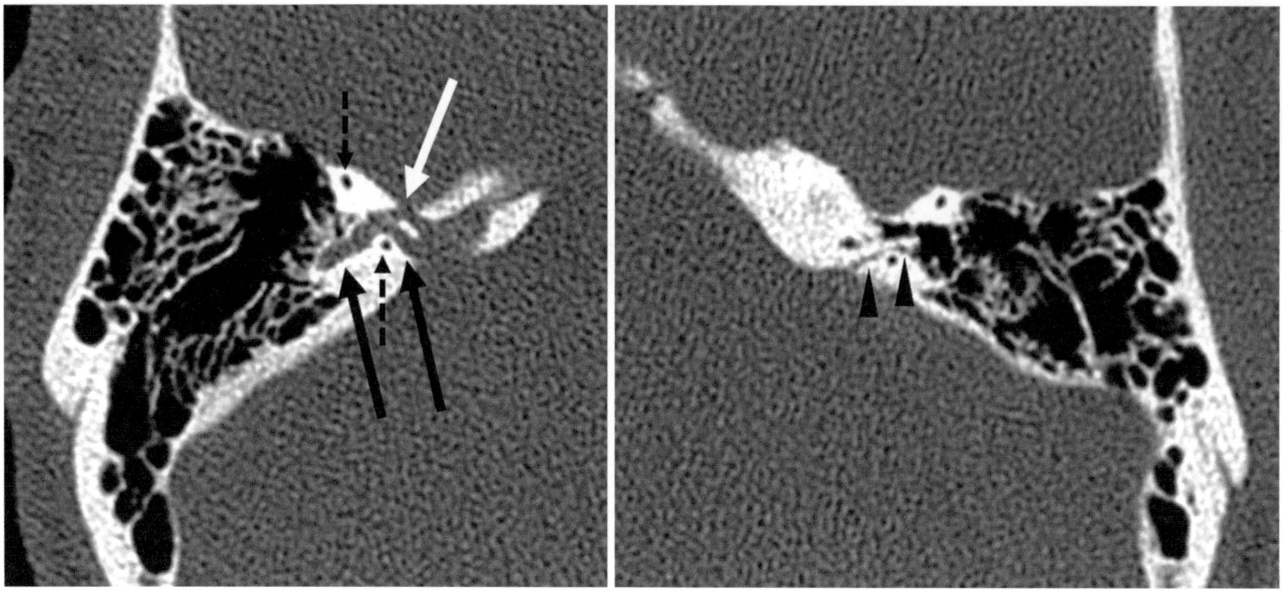

Fig. 5.20 In a 28-year-old male with dizziness (otherwise negative examination), axial 0.6-mm thickness HRCT images demonstrate an enlarged right subarcuate canal (*black arrows, left*) as well as an accessory subarcuate canal anteriorly (*white arrows, left*), while the left subarcuate canal is much smaller (*arrowheads, right*). Note the nearby limbs of the superior semicircular canals as well on the right side (*dashed arrows, left*). This case also demonstrates how there can be significant asymmetry or unilaterality of the normal subarcuate canals

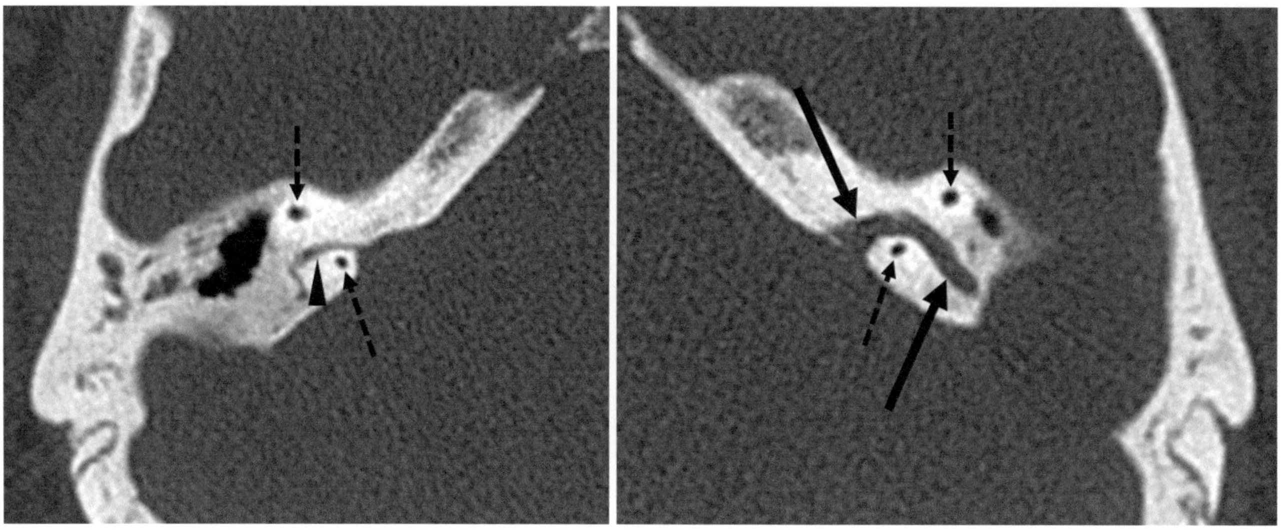

Fig. 5.21 In a 37-year-old male with Eustachian tube dysfunction (and chronic mastoiditis on NECT), there was an incidental markedly enlarged left subarcuate canal (*double black arrows, right*) with a much smaller canal on the right side (*arrowhead, left*) on axial HRCT images. Note the adjacent superior semicircular canals on both sides (*dashed arrows*). This case demonstrates the extreme degree to which a normal variant subarcuate canal can be enlarged

5.4.3 Superior Petrosal Sinus Variation in Course and Supply

The superior petrosal sinus (SPS) is a venous structure that connects the cavernous sinus to the transverse sinus, usually traveling in a shallow groove along the posterior petrous temporal ridge near the attachment of the tentorium cerebelli. The SPS is a highly constant and important venous pathway with relatively few anatomic variants. While many sources describe the superior petrosal sinus as receiving blood primarily from the ipsilateral cavernous sinus, an angiographic study found that the SPS filled in nearly 99% of vertebral artery injections and more than 5% of internal carotid artery injections. That study found that most of the angiographically determined flow was from the petrosal veins.

A deep SPS is best considered a normal variant unless it causes a dehiscence of the superior semicircular canal, which can be a "third window" anomaly. Absence of the superior petrosal sinus has been reported but appears to be uncommon, with the incidence unknown. However, preoperative recognition of absence of the SPS is important in order to preserve the remaining collateral circulation (Fig. 5.22).

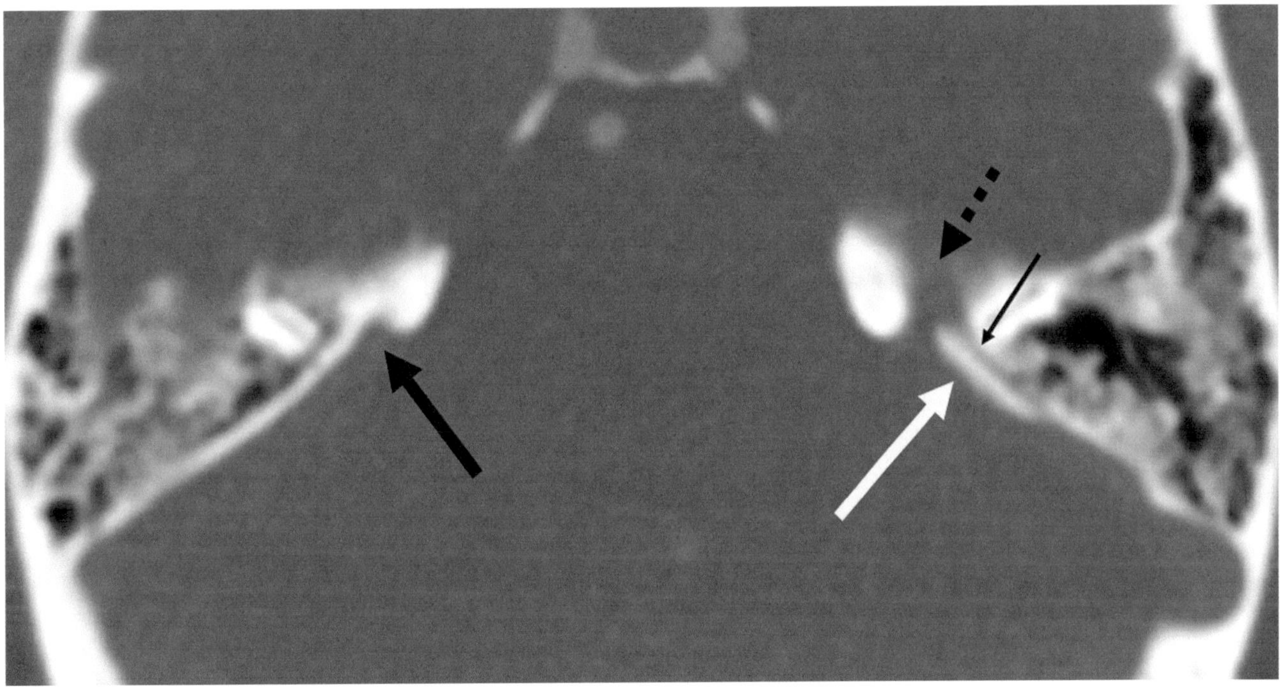

Fig. 5.22 In a 23-year-old woman who underwent a neck CECT for swallowing difficulty (negative study), axial bone window reformats demonstrate a normal variant superior left petrosal sinus (*thin black arrow, right*) coursing laterally toward a large variant accessory vein crossing the left petrous apex (*dotted arrow, right*); in this patient, the left superior petrosal vein lies within a deep trench in the temporal bone (*white arrow, right*). The typical anatomy is a shallow bony groove for the superior petrosal vein, which receives blood from the cavernous sinus and drains to the transverse sinus, as on the patient's right side (*large black arrow, left*)

5.4.4 Facial Nerve Canal Fallopian or Geniculate Segment Subarachnoid Space Enlargement

The facial nerve canal is generally only as wide as the facial nerve itself. Widening of the facial nerve canal can be the result of a neoplasm such as a schwannoma, a vascular process such as a venous malformation or hemangioma, or other pathologic enlargement of the facial nerve as can be seen with Charcot-Marie-Tooth syndrome. However, occasionally the CSF and the subarachnoid space may track along the labyrinthine segment of the facial nerve toward the geniculate ganglion, which can give the appearance of an enlarged facial nerve canal on CT. Studies have described this phenomenon as occurring in up to 12% of cadavers on light microscopy. As such SET2WI MRI can show the CSF signal intensity in such cases, and FLAIR images can null the fluid signal, confirming the benign nature of this anatomic variant. Rarely, if the facial nerve canal is extremely enlarged, anecdotal cases have been described that this causes CSF otorrhea, but typically this occurs only in the setting of concomitant disease (such as after surgery, trauma, or spontaneous intracranial hypertension). While gadolinium-based postcontrast SET1WI MRI can confirm that this is a normal variant and not a tumor, the lack of postcontrast imaging combined with subarachnoid space prominence of the fallopian/labyrinthine or geniculate segments of the facial nerve can simulate benign tumors such as schwannoma or meningioma, or focal mastoiditis. Heavily T2WI HRMRI, such as three-dimensional balanced-echo T2WI MRI with isotropic technique, can also discern this variant without using gadolinium contrast by distinguishing the nerve within the prominent CSF space surrounding it (Fig. 5.23).

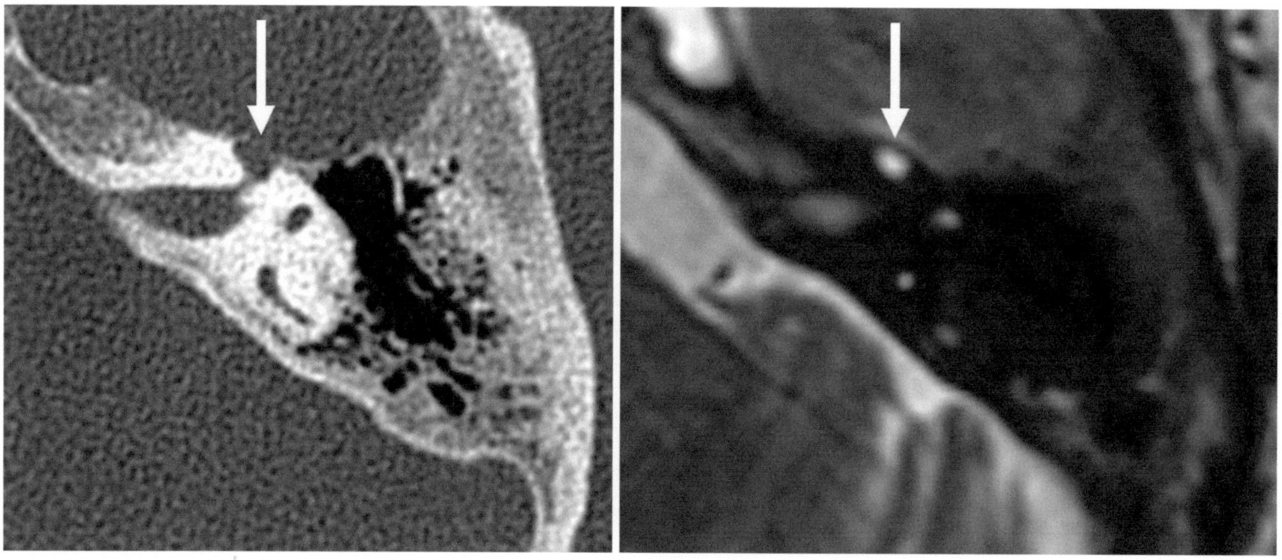

Fig. 5.23 In a 60-year-old female with dizziness, axial HRCT (*left*) shows an enlarged geniculate segment of the left facial nerve canal (*arrows*), simulating a facial nerve schwannoma of the geniculate ganglion. On a 1.5T axial SET2WI MRI (*right*), a CSF signal intensity focus is noted in that region of the geniculate ganglion (*arrows*), and that signal suppressed (darkened) on FLAIR images (*not shown*), thus confirming that it followed CSF signal. Hence, this is a collection of CSF along the facial nerve's geniculate segment caused by focal, normal prominence of the subarachnoid space surrounding the nerve. Of note, the patient had normal function of the facial nerve, and no abnormal enhancement was noted in that segment on postcontrast T1WI MRI (*not shown*). This demonstrates that on noncontrast CT (NECT), this variant may mimic tumor by enlarging the facial canal in the fallopian or geniculate segments

5.5 Ossicular and Middle Ear Ligamentous Normal Variants

5.5.1 Embryology and Development

Auditory signal/sounds from the external ear are delivered by vibration of the tympanic membrane to the three middle-ear ossicles (*malleus, incus, stapes*) and then to the inner ear via the stapes to the spiral, fluid-filled membranous labyrinth of the organ of Corti (within the cochlear duct). Embryologically, the tympanic membrane is derived from the first pharyngeal arch membrane, while the development of ossicles has been traditionally considered to be derived from separate origins of the cartilage of the first and second pharyngeal arches (hyoid arch) via a "dual-arch" hypothesis. However, recent evidence suggests that these may develop solely from the first arch. Regardless, on micro CT no mineralization is present within these ossicles at 17–19 weeks' gestation, but by 24 weeks, all three ossicles appear ossified, and the mineralization and ossification is complete by 35 weeks. Thus, congenital ossicular anomalies may develop in utero related to the ossicular chain but also may present with congenital conductive hearing loss much later in life as a result of delayed testing, concomitant infections, or inflammatory processes that exacerbate them. Therefore, an in-depth discussion of congenital ossicular anomalies that may lead to conductive hearing loss/dysfunction is too detailed to list here, and the reader is directed to an in-depth discussion of associations between such anomalies with external ear anomalies (most common) and inner ear anomalies between various syndromes. However, the most common of these symptomatic congenital ossicular anomalies is congenital stapes fixation, which may not be visible on HRCT, while a number of incidental, asymptomatic variants are present based on cadaver studies that are quite subtle and are on the magnitude of micrometers. Among the three ossicles, the stapes has the most "micro-variants," while the incus is considered the most stable (i.e., least variable). As the focus of this text is on normal imaging variants, we do not discuss such sub-millimeter variants but rather variants or normal appearances that may simulate pathology on HRCT.

5.5.2 Malleal Head "Notching" and Pseudo-Clefts from the Incudomallear Joint

As indicated above, the malleus is more variable in appearance than the incus. On micro CT at the sub-millimeter level the most common variants relate to relative curving or straightening of the manubrium of the handle of the malleus; these are usually not readily recognized on imaging and are of little clinical significance. More commonly recognized on standard HRCT imaging can be a simulated defect usually caused by too much or too little angulation on coronal or axial images. This is not as much of a normal variant as it is a pseudo-lesion related to the imaging plane reconstruction, in which the incudomallear joint (or "articulatio incudomallearis") is composed of the head of the malleus (or "caput mallei") that transmits movement to the body/corpus of the incus (or "corpus incudes") and then to the stapes. While the malleus and incus can appear as "ice cream on the cone" on standard axial HRCT, suboptimal angulation can bring the incudomallear joint into view to simulate a defect ("notch") within the malleal head. This pseudo-lesion can be confirmed by dedicated imaging in other planes or views, such as Stenver and Poschl views or reformatted axial and coronal planes.

5.5.3 Notch or Fenestration ("Hole") in the Incus

Extremely rare and perhaps not reported in the literature is a "notch" at times appearing as a "hole" in the incus in an otherwise normal patient in whom the remainder of the incus and the other two ossicles appear otherwise normal. It is uncertain if this is related to a partial duplication during development, as can occur with vascular and gut structures, or a defect in mineralization with subsequent pneumatization/aeration. In the absence of other associated external ear or inner ear anomalies, this is likely a normal variation but should be documented in a report since it may cause consternation with the referring neurotologist on review of HRCT imaging.

5.5.4 Suspensory Ligaments of the Middle Ear Ossicles

All patients have suspensory ligaments within the middle ear to support the ossicles, which include the anterior malleal, lateral malleal, superior malleal, and posterior incudal ligaments; these combine to conduct the vibrations of sound through the middle ear. However, the ability to visualize these ligaments on less than 1-mm thickness on HRCT varies with CT technique, patient motion, the patient's individual anatomy, the plane of reconstruction, and the presence of concomitant disease (e.g., debris within the middle ear). Of the above-mentioned ligaments, it has been described that the lateral malleal ligament is seen in the vast majority of patients on adequate HRCT (over 90%) and the anterior malleal ligament is visible in most (60–70%); the other above-named ligaments are visible in less than half of patients. Also, the tensor tympani tendon and the stapedius tendon are visible in the minority of cases. When they are normally mildly prominent, any of these above-mentioned ligaments or tendons may simulate disease, such as mild debris within the middle ear from otitis media, tympanosclerosis (simulating thickened, dense suspensory ligaments), a benign neoplasm such as a glomus tympanicum, or a tiny cholesteatoma. Notably, a benign inflammatory or neoplastic lesion such as a cholesteatoma should have bony erosions, while the glomus tympanicum also has a characteristic location. Finally, it can occasionally be difficult to differentiate normal variants and mildly prominent and slightly hyperdense suspensory ligaments from early tympanosclerosis in which there is thickening of the suspensory ligaments with suspected early calcification. Therefore, such cases of mild thickening of a suspensory ligament with questionable calcification may necessitate correlation with the clinical history and further planes of imaging to confirm (Figs. 5.24, 5.25, 5.26, 5.27, 5.28, 5.29, 5.30, 5.31, and 5.32).

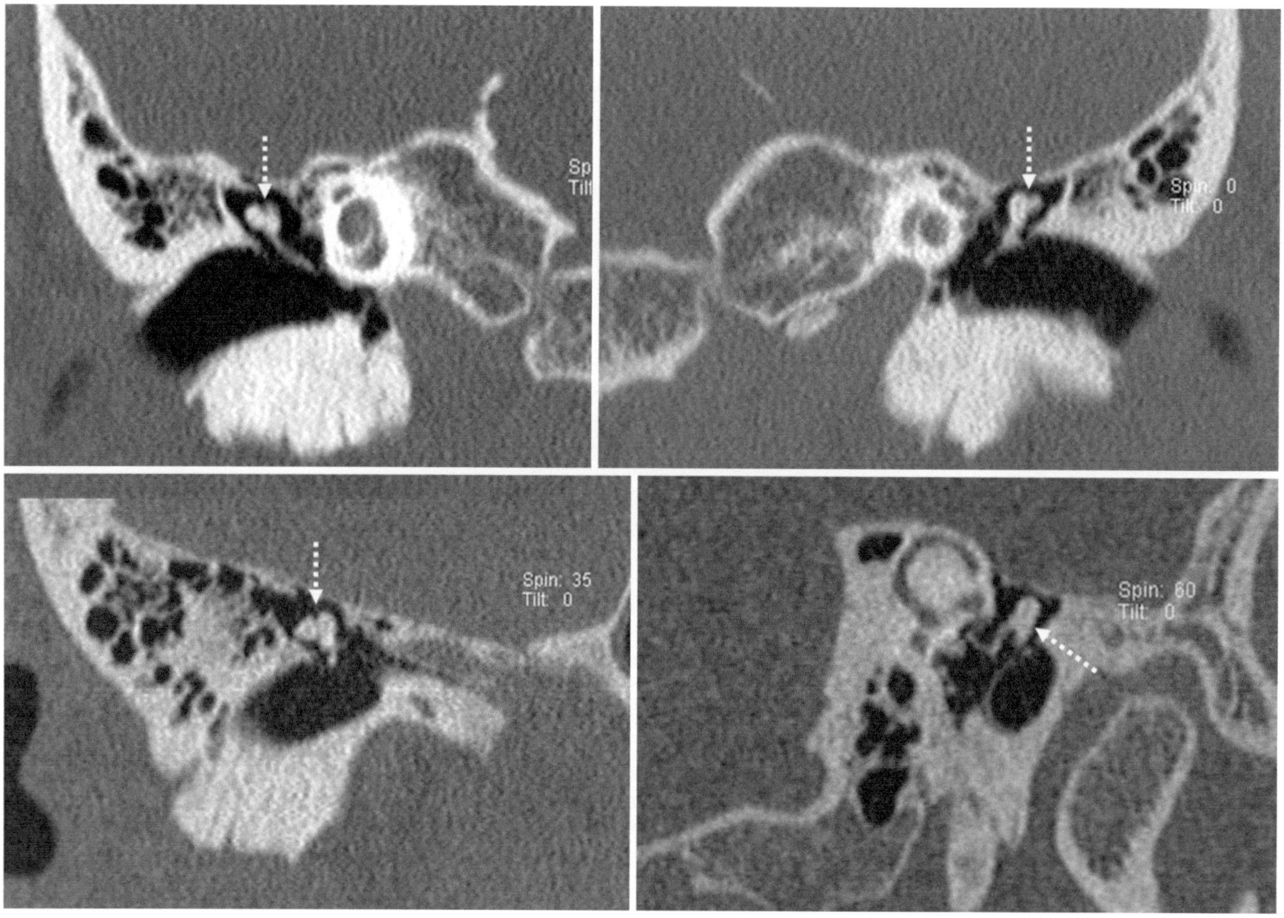

Fig. 5.24 In a 35-year-old male with a prior history of otitis media, the HRCT was normal, but a normal variant pseudo-cleft or notch is noted along the head of the malleus (*dotted arrows*); this artifact was caused by a partially visualized incudomallear joint on right-sided (*top left*) and left-sided (*top right*) coronal images; this was not visible on axial reconstructions (*not shown*). As this was suspected to represent the incudomallear joint, right-sided Stenver (*bottom left*) and left-sided Poschl (*bottom right*) reconstructions confirmed that this pseudo-defect or pseudo-cleft was actually the incudomallear joint. This patient did not have hearing loss

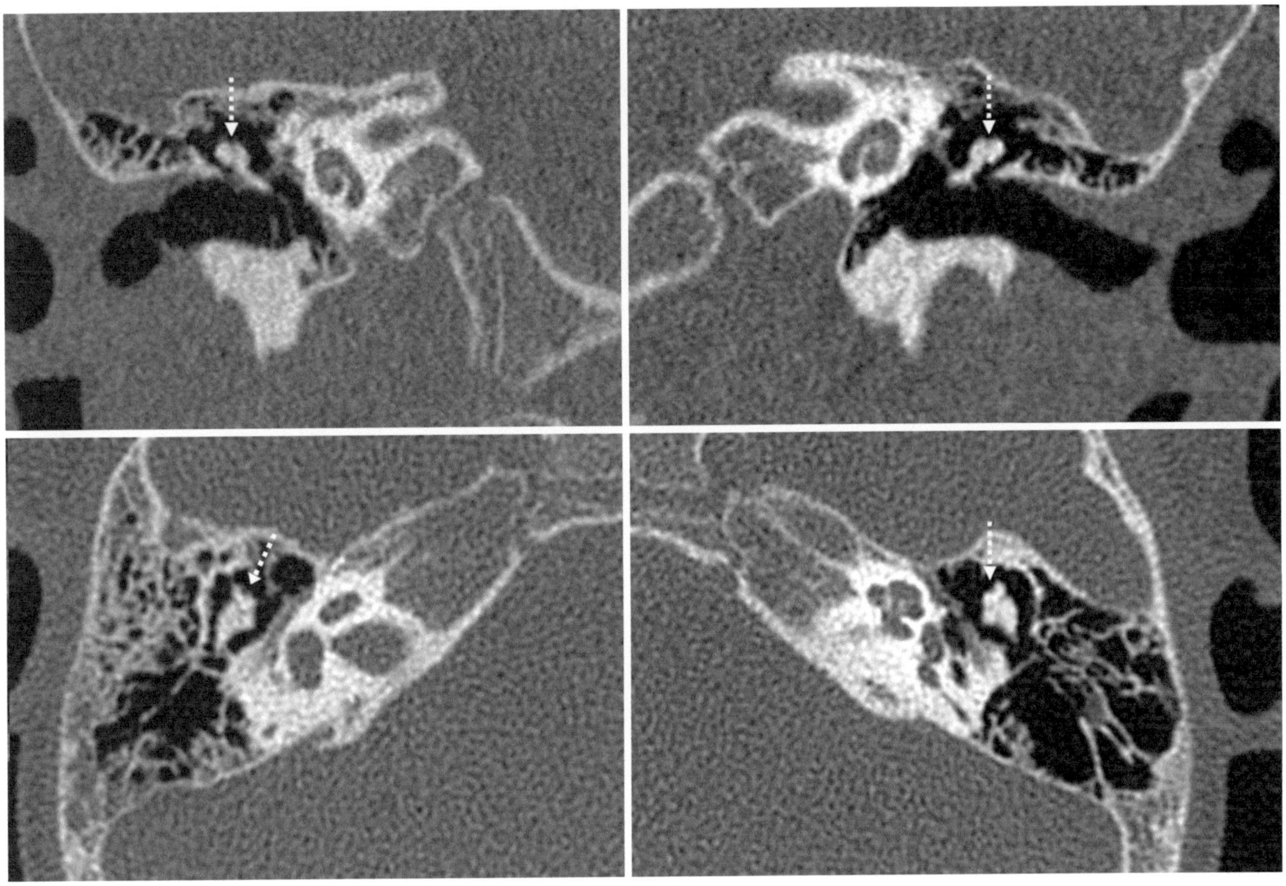

Fig. 5.25 In a 5-year-old male with development delay, a normal variant pseudo-cleft or notch is noted along the head of the malleus (*dotted arrows*). This artifact is caused by a partially visualized incudomallear joint on HRCT with right-sided coronal (*top left*), left-sided coronal (*top right*), right-sided axial (*bottom left*), and left-sided axial (*bottom right*) reconstructions. This patient did not have congenital hearing loss (rather he had a clinical history of only otitis media previously) and had only mild debris within the right mastoid air cells on HRCT

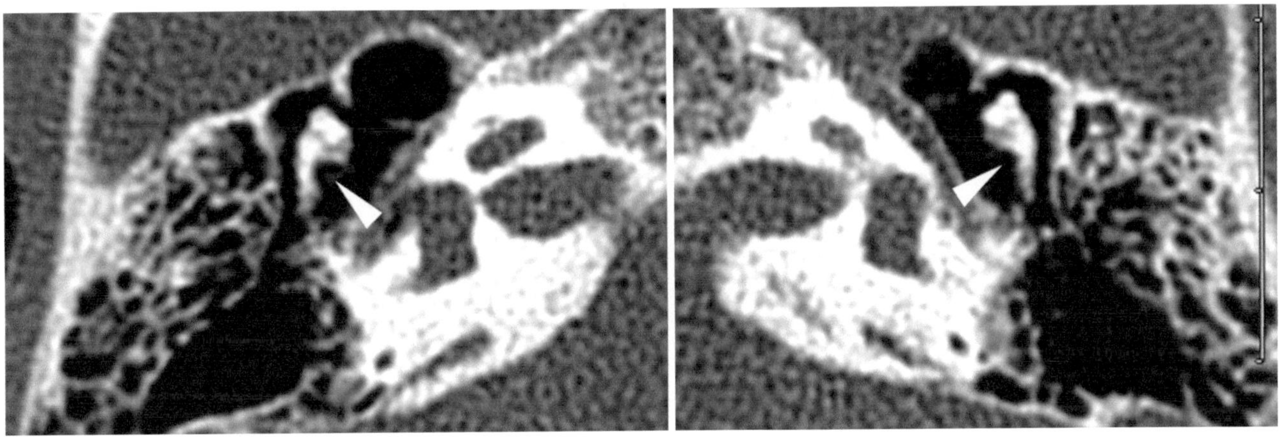

Fig. 5.26 In a 10-year-old boy with left-sided sensorineural hearing loss and normal hearing in the right ear, notch-shaped incus defects (*arrowheads*) were noted bilaterally on axial 0.7-mm thickness HRCT images, the right-sided defect being larger than the left. The sensorineural hearing loss was caused by an absent left cochlear nerve (*not shown*) and deemed unrelated

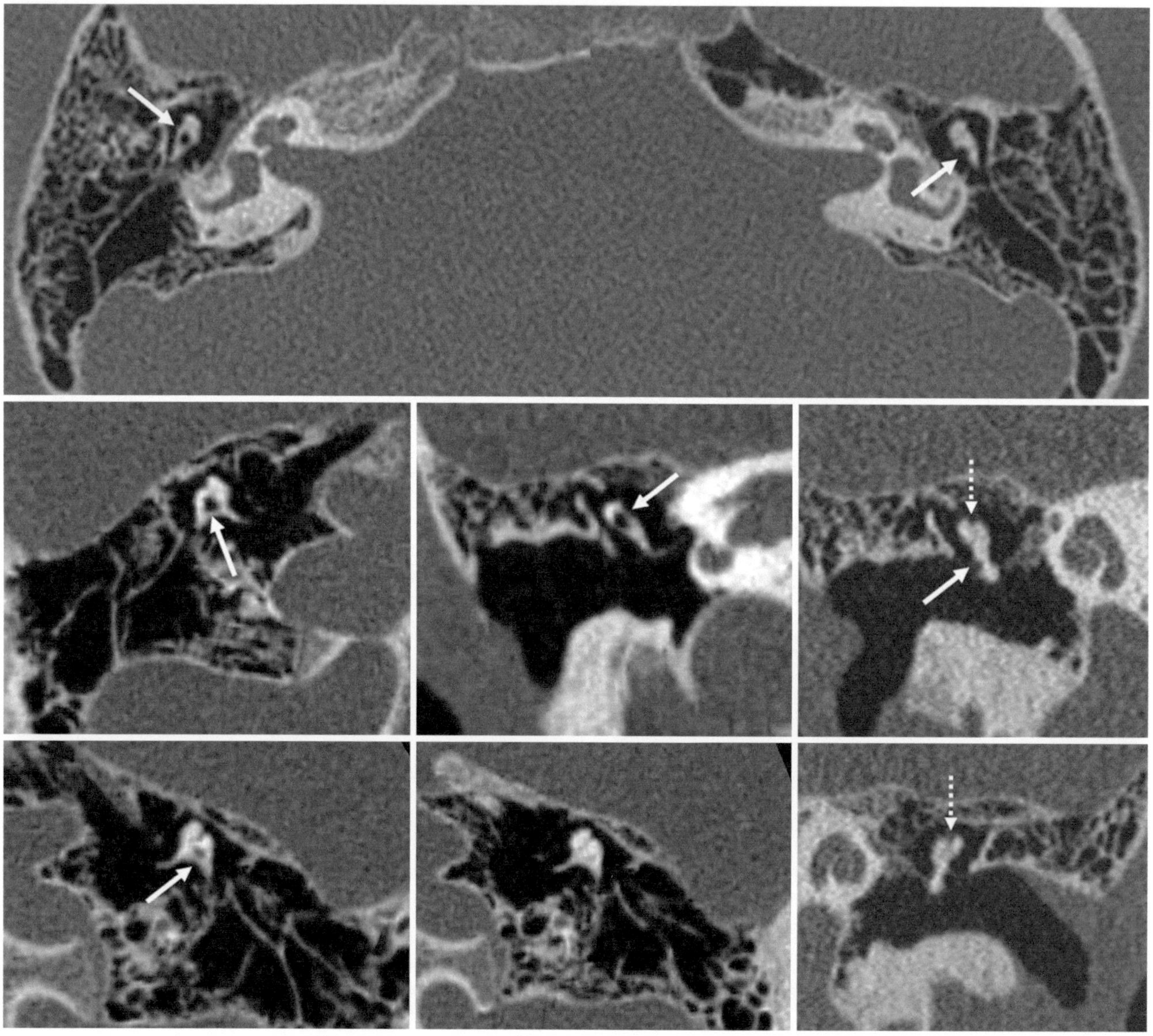

Fig. 5.27 The patient was an 11-year-old female with a history of right tympanic membrane inflammation (negative HRCT otherwise and no congenital hearing loss), without a history of prior ossicular or middle ear surgery. **Top row:** A 0.6-mm-thickness HRCT with axial reconstructions of the right (*left*) and left (*right*) sides depicted bilateral "holes" or notches reminiscent of fenestrations within the incus (*arrows*), being more prominent on the right side. **Middle row:** On further reconstructions of the right side, including reangulated axial (*left*) and coronal (*middle, right*) reformats, the "fenestration" of the incus (*arrows*) is better depicted and confirmed; note the variant pseudo-cleft around the mallear head (*dotted arrow, right*) caused by reangulation, bringing a portion of the incudomallear joint into view. **Bottom row:** On further reconstructions of the left side, including reangulated axial (*left, middle*) and coronal (*right*) reformats, the "notch" or "fenestration" of the incus that is smaller on this side is better depicted (*arrow, left*), while a normal variant mallear pseudo-cleft (*dotted arrow, right*) is also present on this side attributable to reangulation

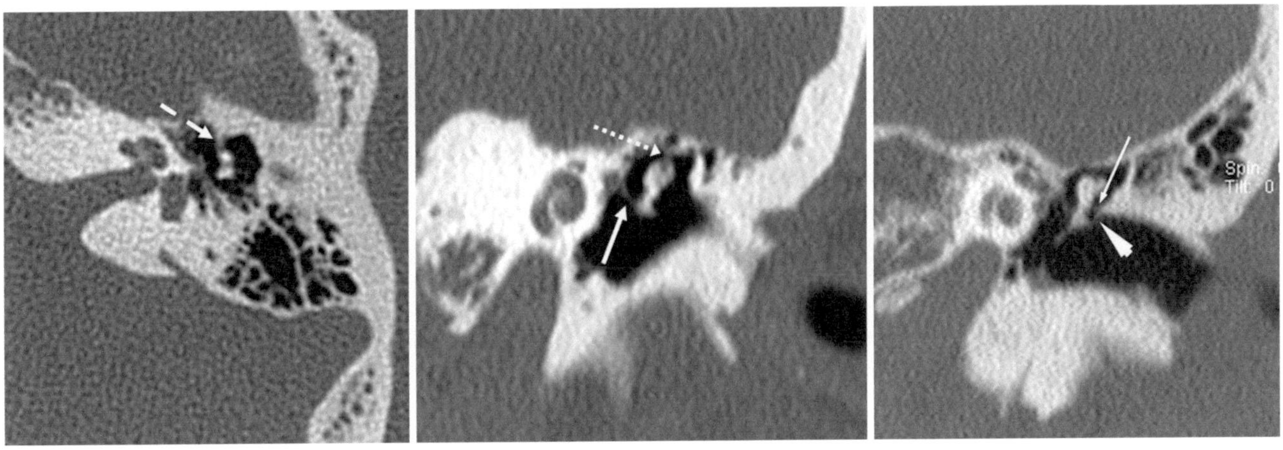

Fig. 5.28 HRCT 0.6-mm thickness images of typical suspensory ossicular ligaments in three different adult patients. **Left:** In a 35-year old male, the normal anterior malleal ligament (AML, *dashed arrow*) is identified on axial HRCT. **Middle:** In a 37-year-old female, the normal superior malleal ligament (SML, *dotted arrow)* is depicted on a coronal HRCT reformat as well as the normally prominent tensor tympani tendon *(arrow),* which is typically visible on HRCT. **Right:** In a 39-year-old male, the normal lateral malleal ligament (LML, *long thin arrow)* is noted and is almost imperceptible (often being difficult to visualize even on thin images from HRCT), as well as the normally thin tympanic membrane (*arrowhead*) projecting inferiorly from the scutum

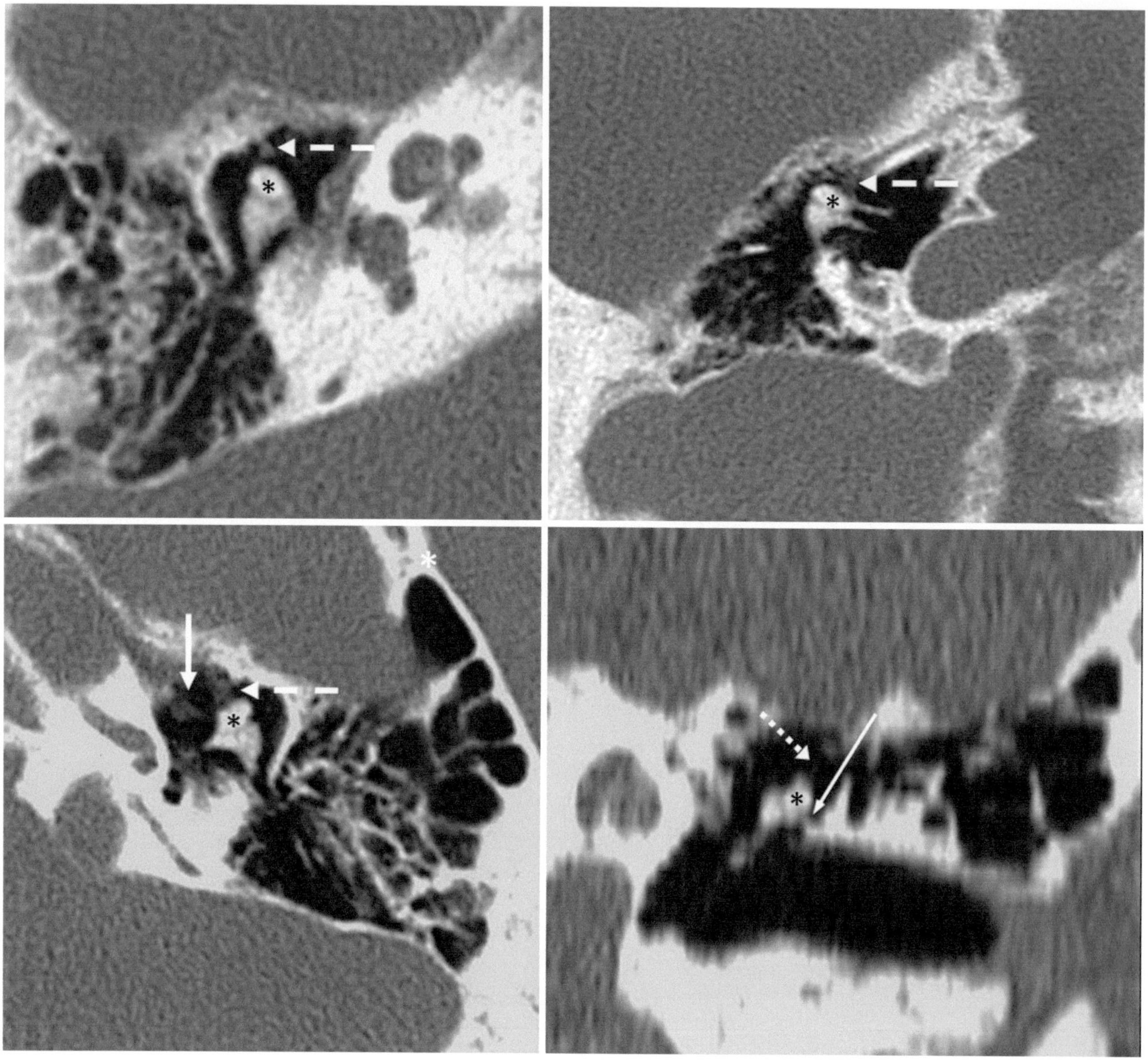

Fig. 5.29 HRCT in a 50-year-old male with right-sided hearing loss (interpreted as negative). **Top row:** On 0.6-mm thickness axial HRCT images of the right temporal bone, note the normal, slightly prominent anterior malleal ligament (AML, *dashed arrows*) attaching between the malleus (*asterisks*) and the anterior tympanic wall. **Bottom row:** On axial (*left*) and coronal (*right*) images of the left side, note an even more prominent but normal left AML (*dashed arrow, left*), tensor tympani tendon (*arrow, left*), and superior malleal ligament (SML, *dotted arrow, right*) attaching between the malleal head (*asterisks*) and the middle ear's roof/tegmen (; also note a tiny lateral malleal ligament (LML) attaching to the tympanic notch (*long thin arrow, right*). As the suspensory ligaments were more prominent on the side opposite the patient's side of hearing loss, these were deemed normal variations. On the *bottom left image*, this case also demonstrates how the tensor tympani tendon and ligaments (the AML in this case) can mimic middle ear debris/otitis

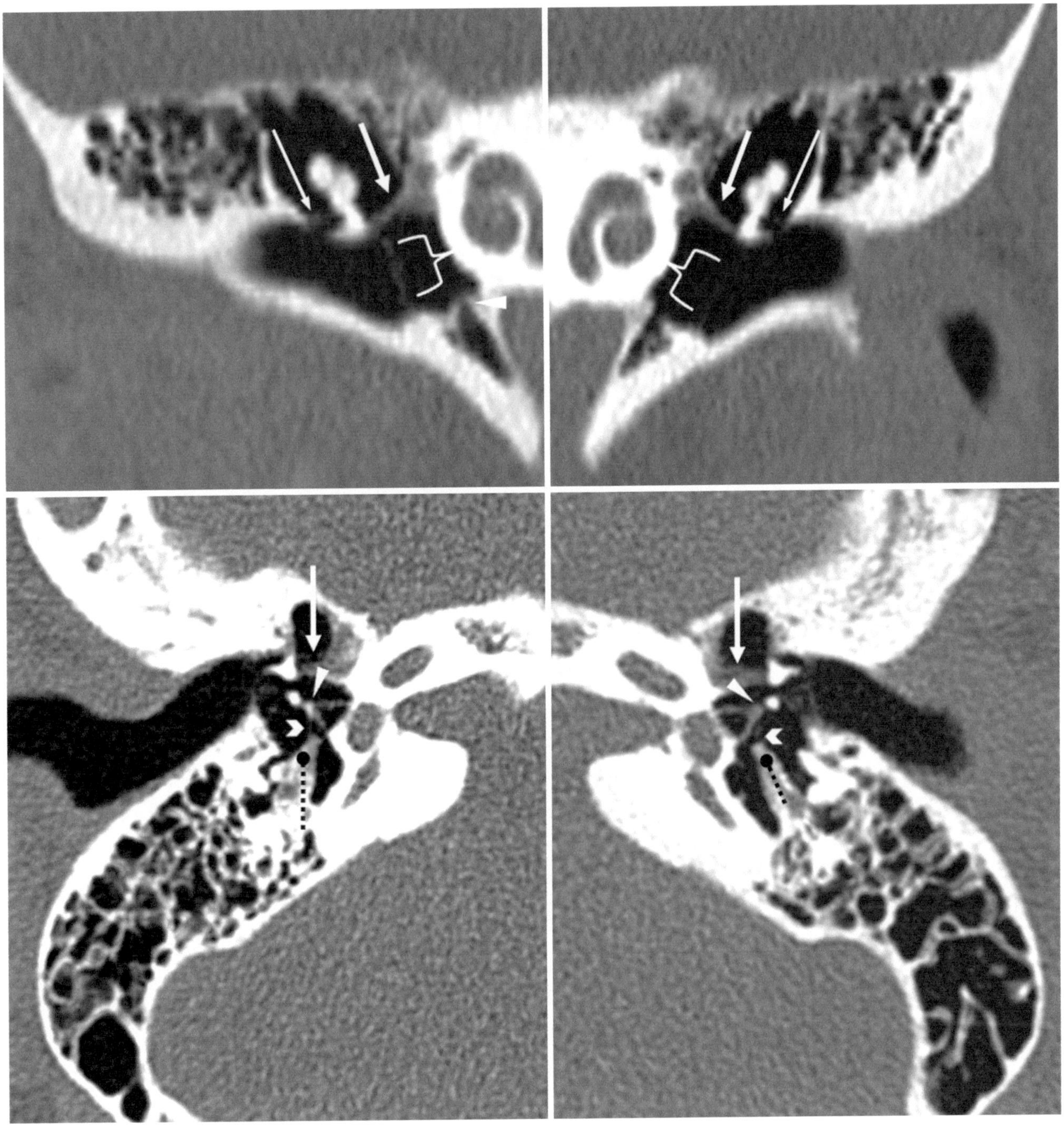

Fig. 5.30 HRCT 0.6-mm thickness images in a 19-year-old male who was 10 years post-cholesteatoma removal from the right ear (interpreted as negative). **Top row:** Coronal reconstructions demonstrate bilateral normal mild prominence of the tensor tympani tendon (*arrows*) and the very thin LML (*long thin arrows*) on coronal images of the right (*top left*) and left (*top right*) sides. Note the normal paper-thin tympanic membranes inferiorly on both sides (*brackets*). **Bottom row:** On axial images of the right (*bottom left*) and left (*bottom right*) sides, note the barely visible stapedius tendon on the right side (*chevron, being hardly visible on the left side*) connecting the pyramidal eminences (*circle tip arrows*) to the normal-appearing heads of the stapes (*arrowheads*) as well as the normally prominent tensor tympani tendons (*arrows*)

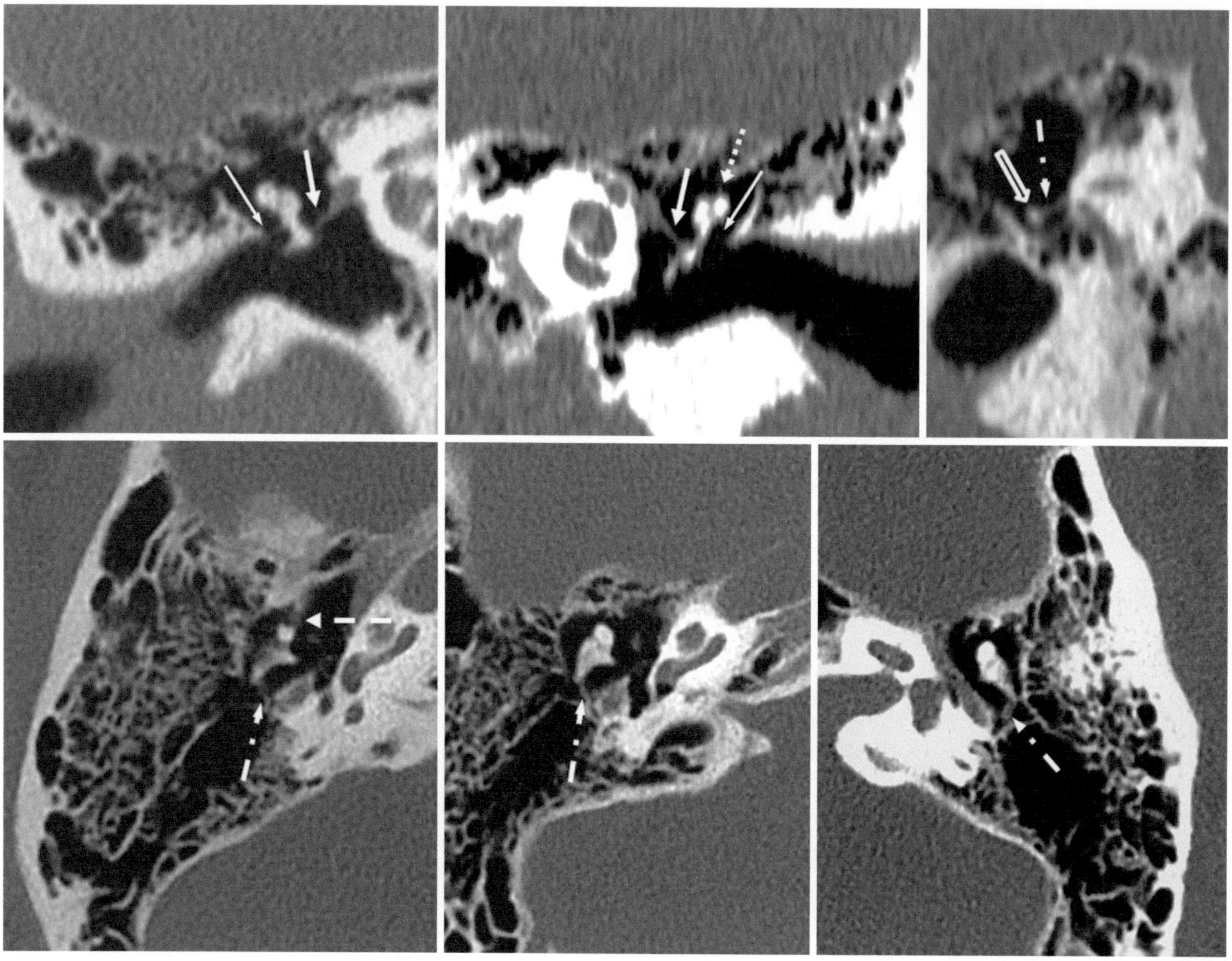

Fig. 5.31 HRCT 0.6-mm thickness images in a 63-year-old male with sensorineural (not conductive) hearing loss (interpreted as negative). **Top row:** Coronal reformats of the right side (*left*), left side (*middle*), and a sagittal reconstruction of the left side (*right*) depict a normal, barely visible LML (*long thin arrow, left*), bilateral mildly prominent tensor tympani tendons (*arrows*), and a mildly prominent left posterior incudal ligament (PIL, *dash-dot arrow, right*) that connects to the short process of the incus (*open arrow, right*); the SML is barely visible only on the left side (*dotted arrow, middle*). **Bottom row:** On axial images of the right (*left, middle*) and left (*right*) sides, note normal variant prominent PILs on each side (*dash-dot arrows*) as well as a prominent right AML (*dashed arrow, left*). Although prominent in this example (an uncommon variant), the PILs are normal because they are not calcified, and the patient did not test positive for conductive hearing loss

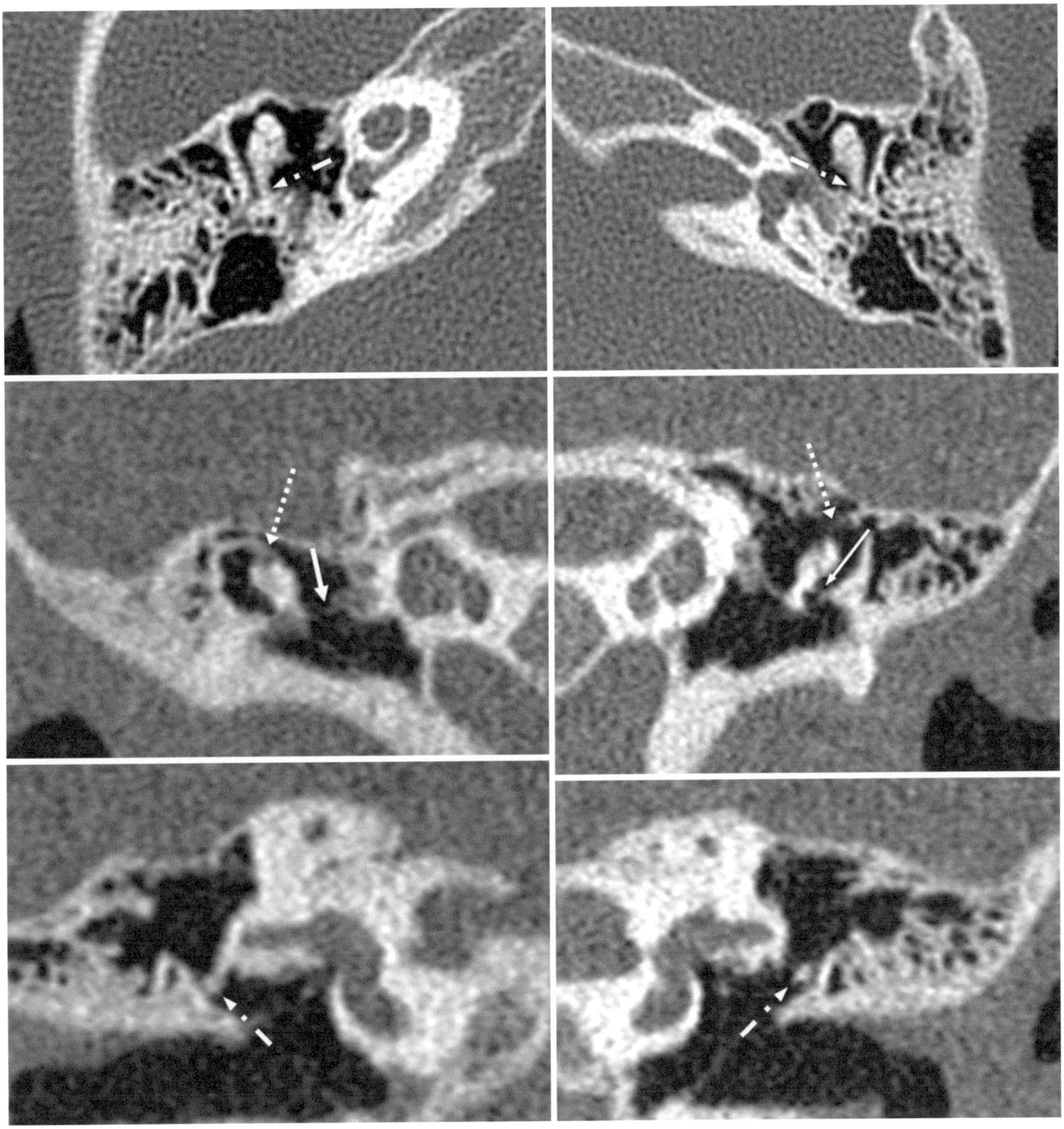

Fig. 5.32 **Comparison case of tympanosclerosis with incus short process fixation and SML sclerosis in a 4-year-old male with right-sided conductive hearing loss. Top row:** On axial HRCT 0.6-mm thickness images of the right side (*left*) and left side (*right*), there is calcification with fusion (*dash-dot arrow depicts site of fusion*) of the incus' short process to the posterolateral bony tympanic wall. **Middle row:** On coronal reformats through the ossicles on the right (*left*) and left (*right*) sides, the right SML is also quite thickened and partially calcified as compared to the normal left side (*dotted arrows on each side*); note the normal mildly prominent tensor tympani tendons on both sides (*arrows*) and a barely visible LML on the left side (*long arrow, right*). **Bottom row:** Coronal images slightly more posteriorly confirm that the short process of the right incus is fused to the posterior bony wall of the mesotympanum. Compare this to the normal left side, which has clear gas-density space surrounding the short process within the "fossa incudis" (*dash-dot arrows*)

5.6 Aberrant Internal Carotid Artery and Internal Carotid Artery Lateralization

The aberrant internal carotid artery (ICA) and lateralization of the ICA are perhaps related normal variants that should be distinguished, particularly prior to middle ear or temporal bone surgery, to prevent iatrogenic vascular injury. The aberrant ICA is thought to develop embryologically from a type of collateral network between the cervical and cranial vasculature caused by hypogenesis or agenesis of the first embryonic segment of the ICA. The incidence of the aberrant ICA is not entirely known, since various studies report that it occurs in less than 1% of the population, but it is often noted incidentally on CT or MRI. It can be reliably diagnosed even on NECT without contrast as a result of the characteristic findings and location of the aberrant vessel. The characteristic appearance is that of a hypoplastic ICA segment extending into the middle ear via an enlarged inferior tympanic canal. This ICA segment that traverses the middle ear has little or no bone covering it, which is why it is susceptible to iatrogenic injury in the setting of middle ear surgery if it is not recognized. This variant is typically unilateral, but can also be bilateral. Another name proposed for this variant is the "inferior tympano-caroticotympanic variant of the ICA." If it is not recognized on imaging, or if imaging is inadequate, in addition to the potential for surgical iatrogenic injury, it could mimic a middle ear inflammatory mass or tumor such as inflammatory debris from otitis, cholesteatoma, or glomus tumor (paraganglioma).

A lateralized ICA has less of an aberrant course than the aberrant ICA, since the ICA follows its normal position but simply extends further laterally (but not through the middle ear), due to focal dehiscence of the lateral wall of the bony carotid canal. Also, the inferior tympanic canaliculus is not prominent, as is the case with the aberrant ICA. This normal variant can be recognized and distinguished from the aberrant ICA because it is positioned more lateral to the cochlea than a normal ICA, and it can protrude (or is uncovered) partially in the anterior mesotympanum. This variant can also share part of a common foramen with the internal jugular vein owing to the carotid canal dehiscence. Thus, there still may be a surgical risk of iatrogenic injury if this variant is not recognized prior to middle ear or skull base surgery (Figs. 5.33 and 5.34).

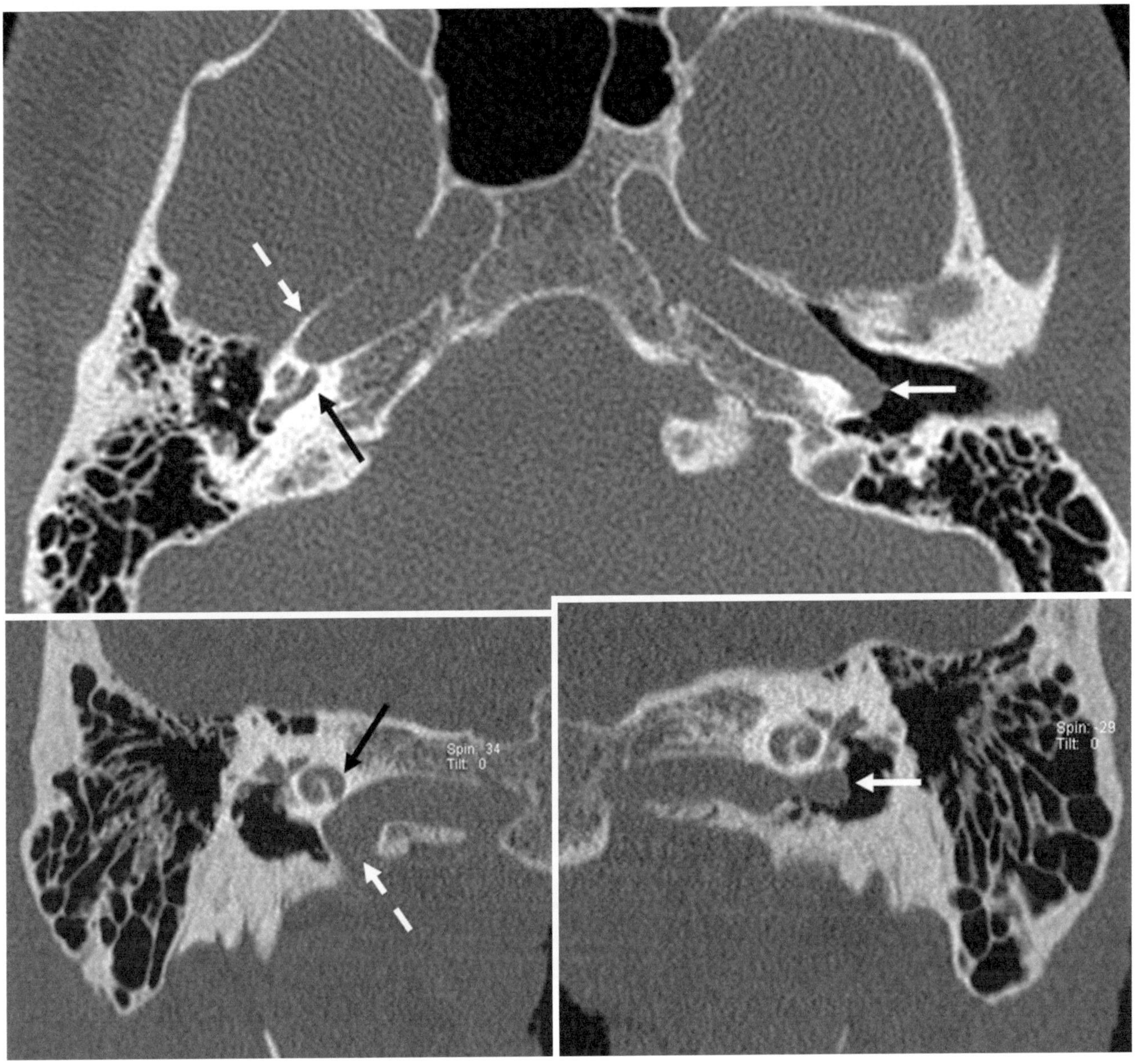

Fig. 5.33 In a 48-year-old male with left-sided conductive hearing loss, on 0.6 mm thickness HRCT there is an aberrant ICA (*white arrows*) located lateral to the normal position of the ICA as it extends through the left middle ear (*top right*), as noted on an axial NECT image of both sides and on coronal reconstructions of the right (*bottom left*) and left sides (*bottom right*). The more normal right ICA is visualized on axial and coronal NECT reformats (*dashed arrows, top left and bottom left*); this may actually be a slightly lateralized ICA (another normal variant), since the lateral edge of the ICA is just lateral to the medial edge of the basal turn of the cochlea (*black arrows*)

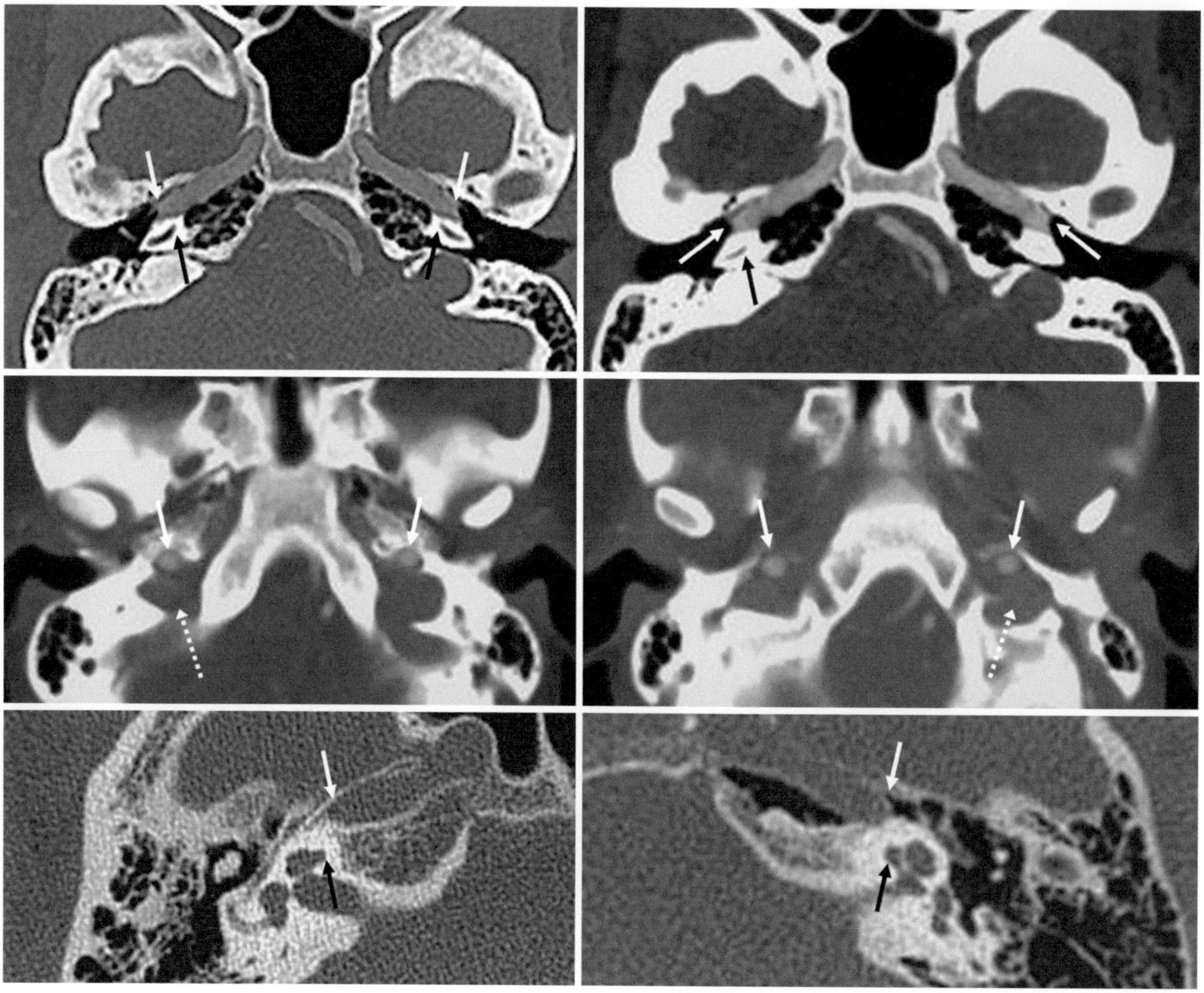

Fig. 5.34 Comparison of lateralized ICA's to normal ICA positions in different patients. **Top row:** In a 21-year-old male with a CT angiogram (CTA) obtained for a possible congenital vascular abnormality in the lower neck (negative examination), normal variant lateralized ICA's are identified bilaterally, where on axial bone (*left*) and soft tissue/vascular (*right*) windows, the lateral edge (*white arrows*) of the lateralized ICAs in the petrous segment are lateral to the medial edges of the basal turns of the cochlea (*black arrows*), a characteristic appearance of this variant. **Middle row:** On lower axial soft-tissue window images in this same patient, the ICAs (*white arrows*) share in the pars nervosa of the anterior portion of the jugular foramen, which also contains the internal jugular veins (*dotted arrows*). **Bottom row:** In two different patients with normal positions of the ICAs on the right (*left image*) and left sides (*right image*), comparisons are provided for the normal position of the ICA's most lateral edge of the petrous segments (*white arrows*) located medial relative to the medial edge of the basal turns of the cochleae (*black arrows*)

5.7 High-Riding Jugular, Jugular Diverticulum, and Jugular Dehiscence

The jugular bulb of the internal jugular vein (IJV) receives venous blood from the lateral venous sinuses and is highly variable in size and in position. A "high-riding" jugular bulb (HRJB) is the most frequent abnormality, with the term "high riding" being defined differently by various authors. A frequently quoted criterion is that the HRJB is situated at the level of the internal auditory canal (IAC). Although the right IJV is dominant (larger) in 70–80%, HRJB affects both sides equally. HRJB has an incidence of 4.5–8.5% and has an equal likelihood of being found in both males and females. The absence of jugular bulbs in early childhood is normal, and the portion of the jugular destined to become the jugular bulb is often referred to as the "jugular sinus" in infants. Some have not found a developed jugular bulb in children under 2 years of age; its development is thought to be influenced by changes in posture.

A jugular diverticulum is an outpouching from the jugular bulb that may lead to pulsatile tinnitus or alternatively may be asymptomatic. Jugular diverticula can also erode into the inner ear structures such as the vestibular aqueduct, facial nerve canal, or posterior semicircular canal. While initial studies found a correlation with such erosions and hearing loss or tinnitus, those studies were retrospective, and the correlations found in such studies may have been influenced by the enriched proportion of patients with coincident hearing loss and dizziness who undergo temporal bone imaging (i.e. selection bias). More recent and larger studies have found many patients with such communications with the jugular bulb to be asymptomatic. This is thought related to the phenomenon of jugular dehiscence (described in detail below), in which an extremely thin plate separates the jugular foramen and middle ear (a thin plate is found in up to 10–15% of the population). Notably, studies have noted an HRJB in about 3% to 10% of cases, and of those having a HRJB, 11–35% have dehiscence of the vestibular aqueduct into the HRJB, but the majority of such patients are asymptomatic. In larger studies, the association of the jugular bulb/VA communication with inner ear symptoms did not reach statistical significance. Hence, preliminary evidence suggests that a jugular bulb-VA dehiscence is more commonly an asymptomatic variant that can easily be detected by less than 1-mm thickness multiplanar HRCT, while a minority may have symptoms related to jugular dehiscence or diverticulum.

Of note is that the sigmoid plate refers to the bony wall separating the sigmoid sinus from the mastoid cavity. The term is also used to describe the bone separating the jugular bulb from the middle ear cavity. A defect in the sigmoid plate that allows the internal jugular vein to protrude into the middle ear is referred to as dehiscence of the internal jugular vein. Such a variant bulging vein into the middle ear or mastoid can cause pulsatile tinnitus or a visible retrotympanic mass and can mimic neoplastic or inflammatory processes such as paraganglioma or cholesteatoma. The lack of adjacent osseous erosions and the contiguity with the remainder of the jugular are important clues to the correct diagnosis.

Each of the above-mentioned jugular variants is typically easily discerned by less than 1-mm thickness on HRCT in multiple planes. Again, these variants can simulate disease such as glomus tumor, schwannoma, or cholesteatoma, particularly if the IJV is asymmetric, dehiscent, and protrudes into the middle ear. When necessary, postcontrast T1WI and even MR venography (MRV) can help confirm these jugular variants (Figs. 5.35 and 5.36).

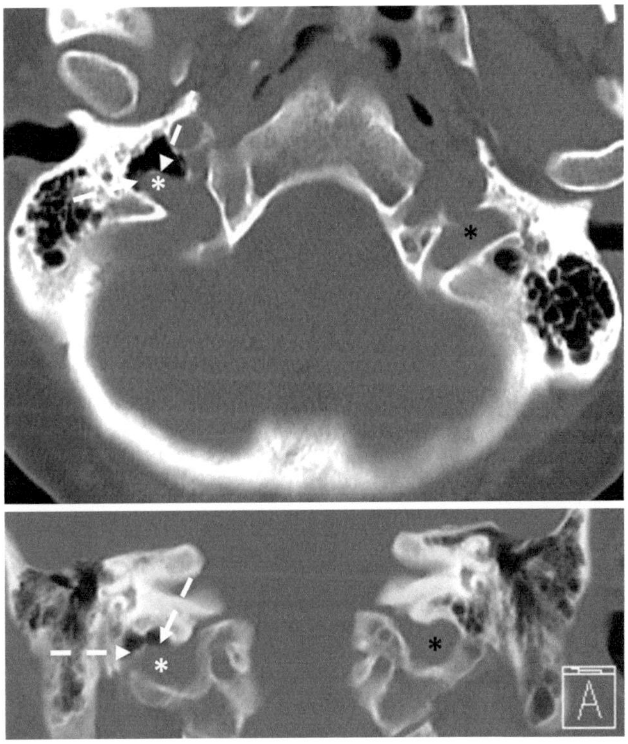

Fig. 5.35 In a 56 year-old female with headaches, a NECT of the head (negative examination) demonstrated an incidental projection of the right jugular bulb (*white asterisks*) into the aerated hypotympanum on axial images (*top*) and coronal reformats of the right (*bottom left*) and left (*bottom right*) sides. Two areas of dehiscence are seen laterally and anteromedially (*dashed arrows*). Note the normal left internal jugular vein (*black asterisks*), which lacks dehiscence. This case demonstrates how jugular dehiscence is most commonly an incidental "don't touch" lesion but is occasionally symptomatic

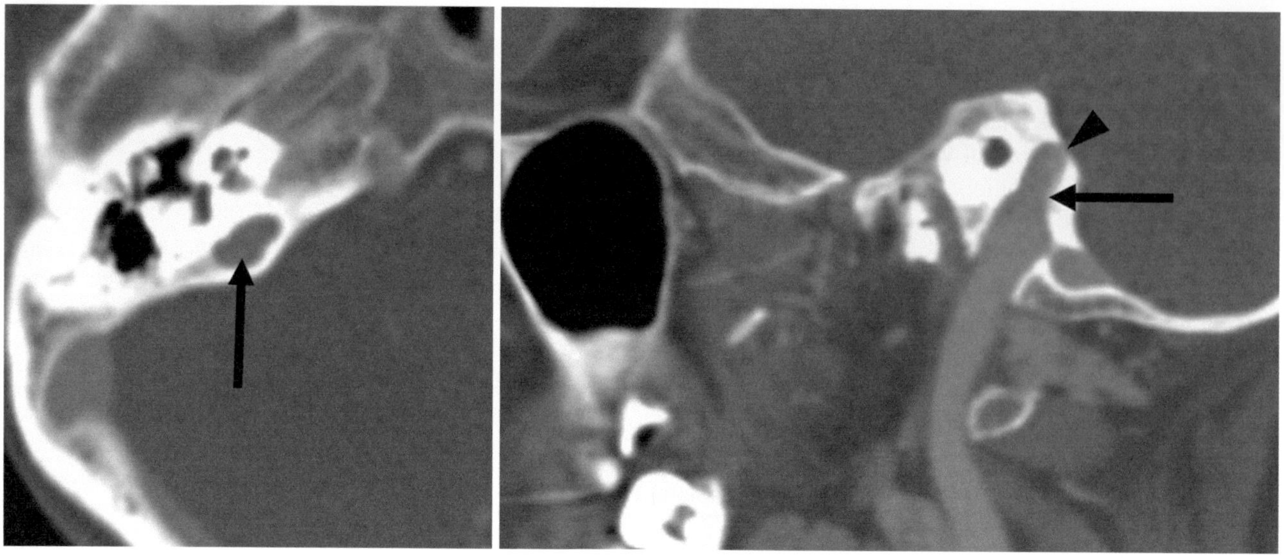

Fig. 5.36 On a neck CECT, a 23-year-old female with stridor had an otherwise negative examination. Axial (*left*) and sagittal (*right*) reconstructions demonstrate a diverticulum of the right internal jugular vein (*arrows*) high into the temporal bone (a so-called "high-riding jugular," which is focally dehiscent along the posterosuperior margin (*arrowhead, right*). Such diverticula are more commonly asymptomatic and as such are "don't touch lesions," although they are sometimes associated with symptoms

5.8 Petrous Apex Fatty Marrow and Pneumatized/Aerated Petrous Apices

Fatty marrow signal within the petrous apex on MRI, particularly on non-FS SET1WI and even on non-FS turbo-SET2WI or fluid-attenuated inversion recovery imaging (FLAIR), may have the appearance of a bright signal that can mimic lesions such as blood/hemorrhage signal within cholesterol granulomas or hemorrhage (such as from trauma) within the petrous apices. This may also lead to "T1 shine-through" of the T1-bright signal (due to the short T1 time of fat) onto other sequences such as time-of-flight MR angiography (MRA), which may simulate an aneurysm. Such a fatty marrow signal is present within most patients to varying degrees but can be problematic if prominent. This occasionally may occur in tandem with arrested pneumatization-aeration of the sphenoid sinus, another normal variant characterized by lack of aeration with fat within the expected location of the sphenoid sinus. The use of FS to saturate (darken) the T1-bright signal of fat can aid in differentiating this normal tissue from true pathology. Alternatively, NECT can be utilized to identify low density within the petrous apices that is typical of normal fatty marrow as well as the lack of bony expansion that may be seen with cholesterol granuloma, mucocele, or other masses of the petrous apex (or, alternatively, masses that are extra-axial and adjacent to the petrous apex, such as meningioma or schwannoma).

Pneumatization-aeration of the petrous apices has been reported in the range of 20–30% of normal patients as an incidental finding; it is only pathologic if there is a complication by obstruction with infection or inflammation (petrous apicitis) by fluid or debris. While this variant is entirely normal, it can cause susceptibility artifact (usually dark signal but occasionally appears bright) that mimics an aneurysm (such as on TOF-MRA) or cerebral hemorrhage (on SWI or GET2*WI. The concomitant use of spin-echo imaging, particularly SET2WI (which is much less susceptible to artifact from air/gas) and even NECT, can mitigate this artifact and confirm the source of the artifactual signal from air-CSF or air-bone interfaces (Figs. 5.37, 5.38, 5.39, 5.40, 5.41, and 5.42).

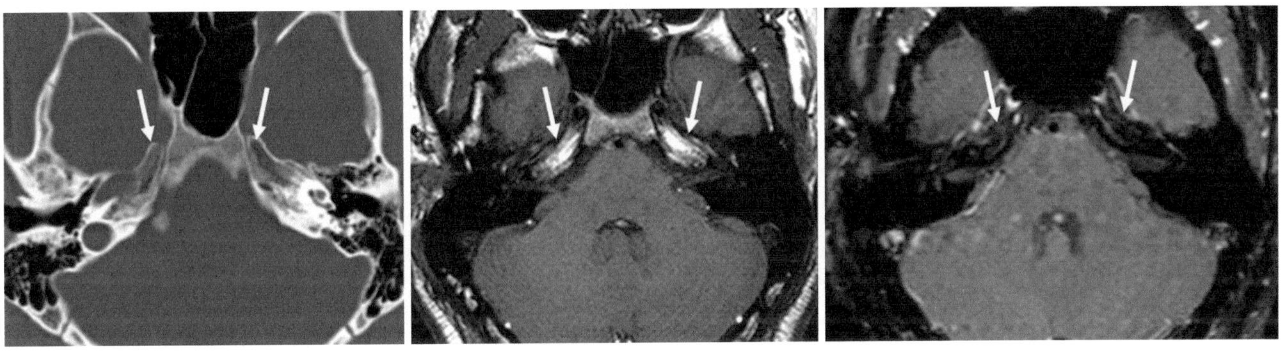

Fig. 5.37 In a 19-year-old male with headaches, incidental fatty marrow is present within both petrous apices (*arrows*) with characteristic hypoattenuation on axial NECT (*left*), 1.5 T MRI axial noncontrast SET1WI (*middle*), and on axial postcontrast FS-SET1WI (*right*). As these areas are not bright on FS-postcontrast SET1WI (they darken-saturate after FS), this normal variant does not represent tumor or cholesterol granuloma

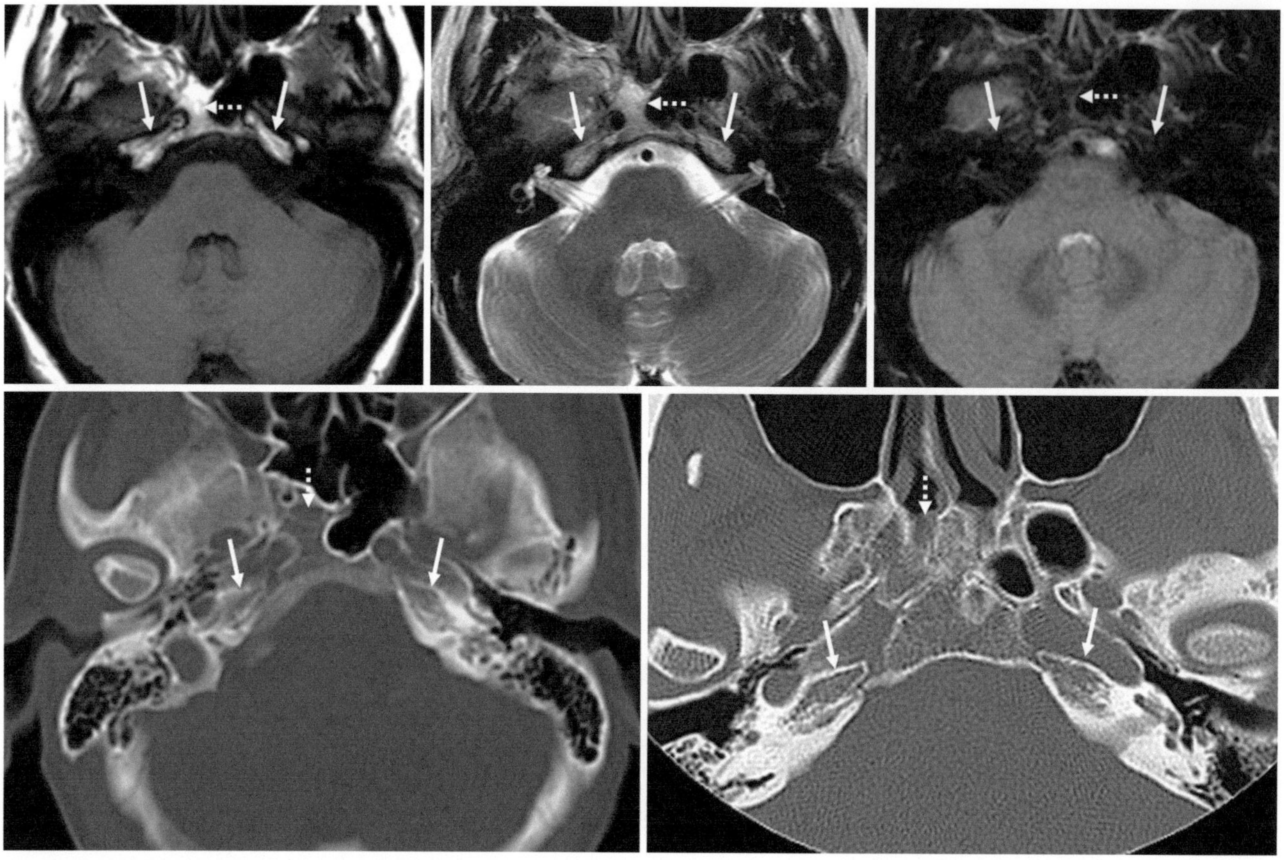

Fig. 5.38 A 16-year-old underwent orbit MRI (which was normal). **Top row:** 1.5T MRI demonstrated normal fatty marrow of the petrous apices bilaterally (*arrows*) on axial SET1WI (*left*), SET2WI (*middle*), and FS-FLAIR (*right*), with incidental adjacent arrested pneumatization of the sphenoid sinus on the right side as well (*dotted arrows*, another normal variant). **Bottom row:** Axial NECT (*left*) and thinner magnified axial NECT reformats (*right*) confirmed the typical low attenuation of fat both within the petrous apices (*arrows*) as well as of the right side of the sphenoid (*dotted arrows*), where fat density is also typical of sphenoid sinus arrested pneumatization. These two normal variants are sometimes found together

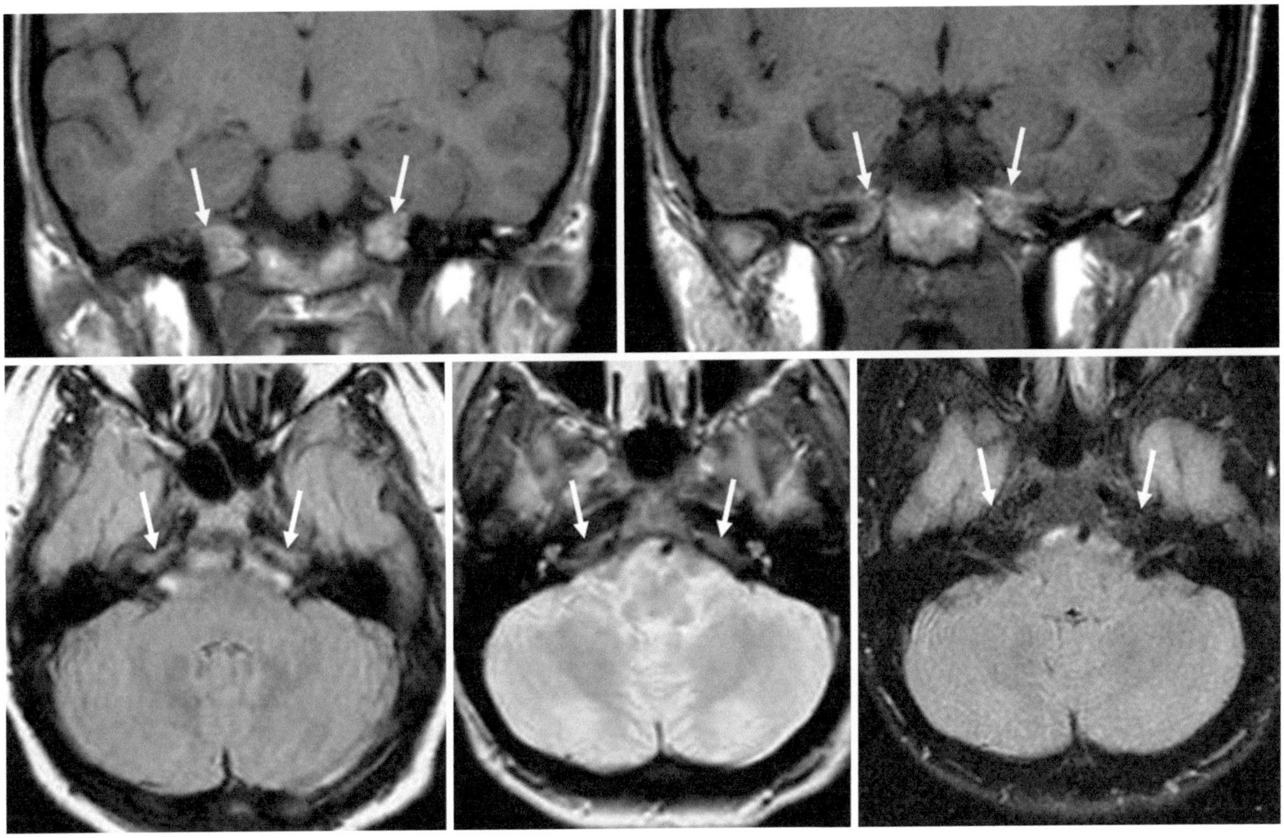

Fig. 5.39 A 15-year-old male with growth hormone deficiency (negative pituitary on MRI) underwent a 1.5T MRI, in which coronal SET1WI (*top row*) demonstrated prominent T1-bright signal (*arrows*), also bright on non-FS FLAIR (*bottom left*). It was of intermediate signal on PDWI (proton density weighted image, *bottom middle*) but darkened on FS-FLAIR (*bottom right*), typical of normal petrous apex fatty marrow

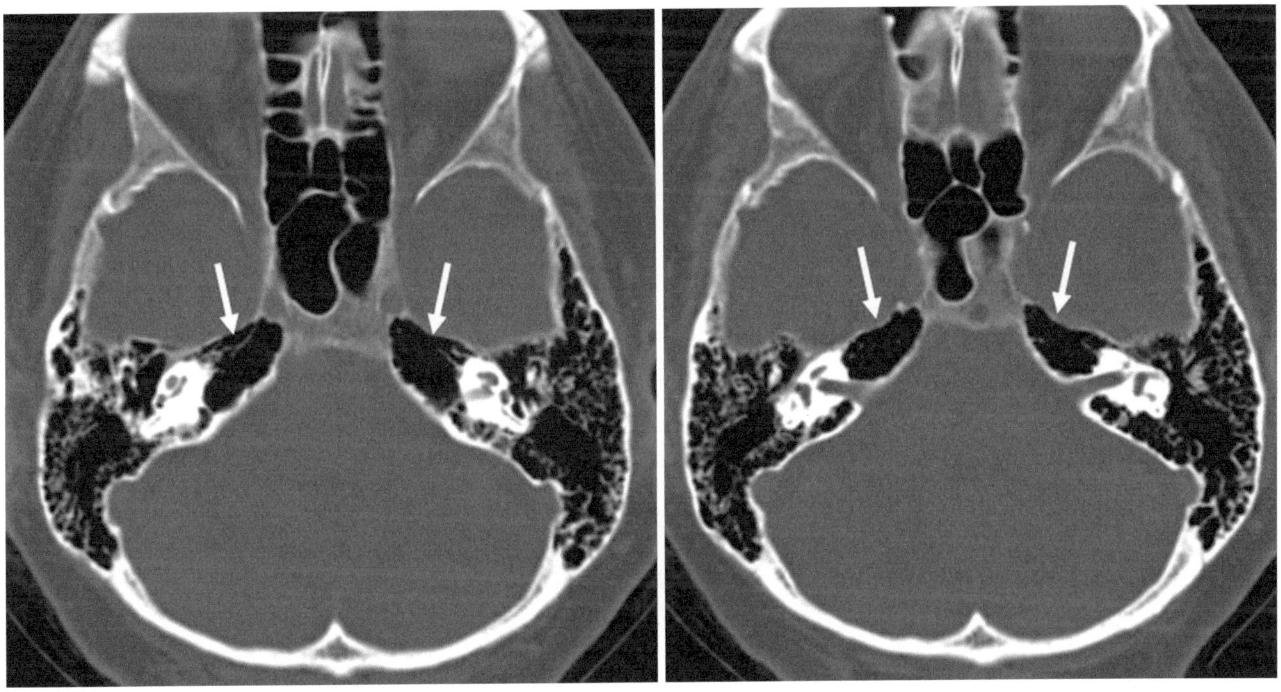

Fig. 5.40 In a 58-year-old female, normal pneumatized-aerated petrous apices are noted bilaterally (*arrows*) on axial NECT reformats

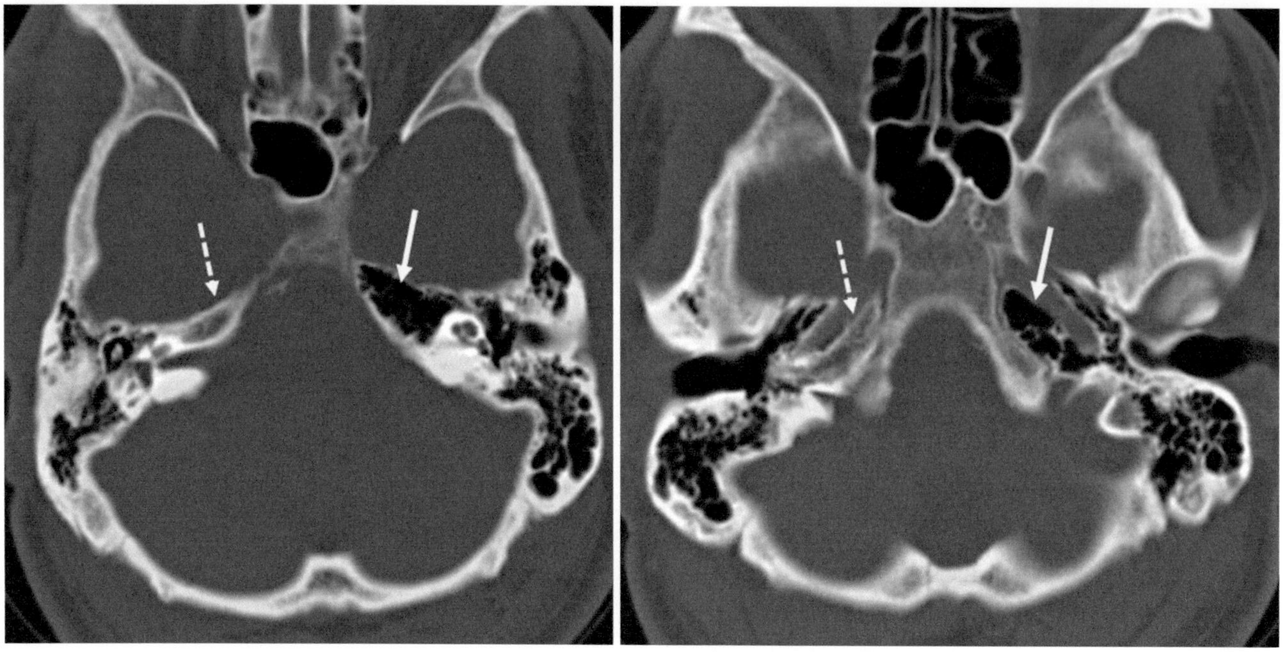

Fig. 5.41 In a 42-year-old male, a unilateral, normal pneumatized petrous apex is noted on the left side *(arrows)* as compared to the right (*dashed arrows*) on axial NECT images. This demonstrates that this common normal variant can occur unilaterally or bilaterally

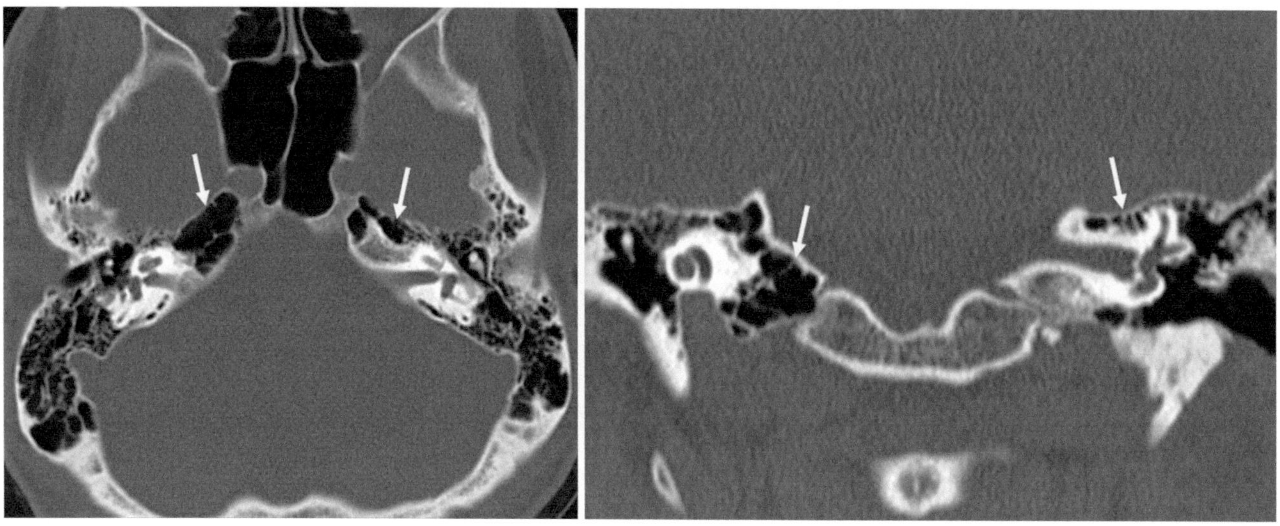

Fig. 5.42 In a 32-year-old male, normal bilateral petrous apex pneumatization (*arrows*) is more extensive on the right side as compared to the left side on axial (*left*) and coronal (*right*) NECT reformats. This demonstrates that the degree of pneumatization can vary between sides

5.9 Petrous and Petrous Apex Exostoses

Exostoses of the petrous apex are uncommon, but their incidence has not been well described, and there is rarely histologic evidence to support their diagnosis because they are overwhelmingly benign. Hence, their terminology varies, and they are often referred to as exostoses, osteomas, or even hyperostosis given the lack of histopathologic confirmation. It is suggested that the term exostosis or osteoma be utilized when they are focal (given the few histologic documented cases of confirmation), while the normal variation hyperostosis would be more appropriate for the situation of diffuse calvarial thickening from hyperostosis frontalis interna or hyperostosis calvaria diffusa. Typically, such "don't touch lesions" are completely ossified, although they may very slowly progressively enlarge in rare cases and do not have a soft-tissue, nonossified component; in such rare cases they may cause symptoms over many years related to adjacent cranial nerve or vascular compression, even though the vast majority are asymptomatic even when the lesions are large. Extremely rare at the petrous apex is the benign calvarial osteochondroma (which also may appear nearly entirely ossified), which may cause confusion in terminology because it is represented by the term "exostosis" in the musculoskeletal radiology literature. Such cases on postcontrast T1WI MRI exhibit contrast enhancement of a cartilaginous cap; they are suspicious for malignant degeneration if the cap is larger than 1.5 cm in thickness. Such exostoses can be multiple throughout the body and rarely involve the cranium in syndromes of hereditary exostosis. Also rare are chondrosarcomas that may involve the petrous apex and protrude, but this low-grade malignancy should be distinguishable from a benign exostosis/hyperostosis/osteoma, since chondrosarcomas typically are composed of mostly cartilaginous elements that enhance on postcontrast imaging.

The difficulty that arises from very dense or T2WI and T1WI dark signal from such petrous apex exostoses/osteomas is that the low signal may mimic a vascular lesion such as an aneurysm, simulate a benign neoplasm such as a meningioma, or may obscure adjacent structures and even cause susceptibility artifact from the bone-air or bone-fat interfaces. FS-SET1WI, FS-SET2WI (rather than GET2WI, which is susceptible to such artifact), or NECT may help identify these "don't touch" lesions. Notably, they also may contain fatty marrow centrally if they are quite large, which can be confirmed by FS-SET1WI and should not be confused with an aneurysm or meningioma simply because they contain a centrally bright signal on T1WI (Figs. 5.43, 5.44, and 5.45).

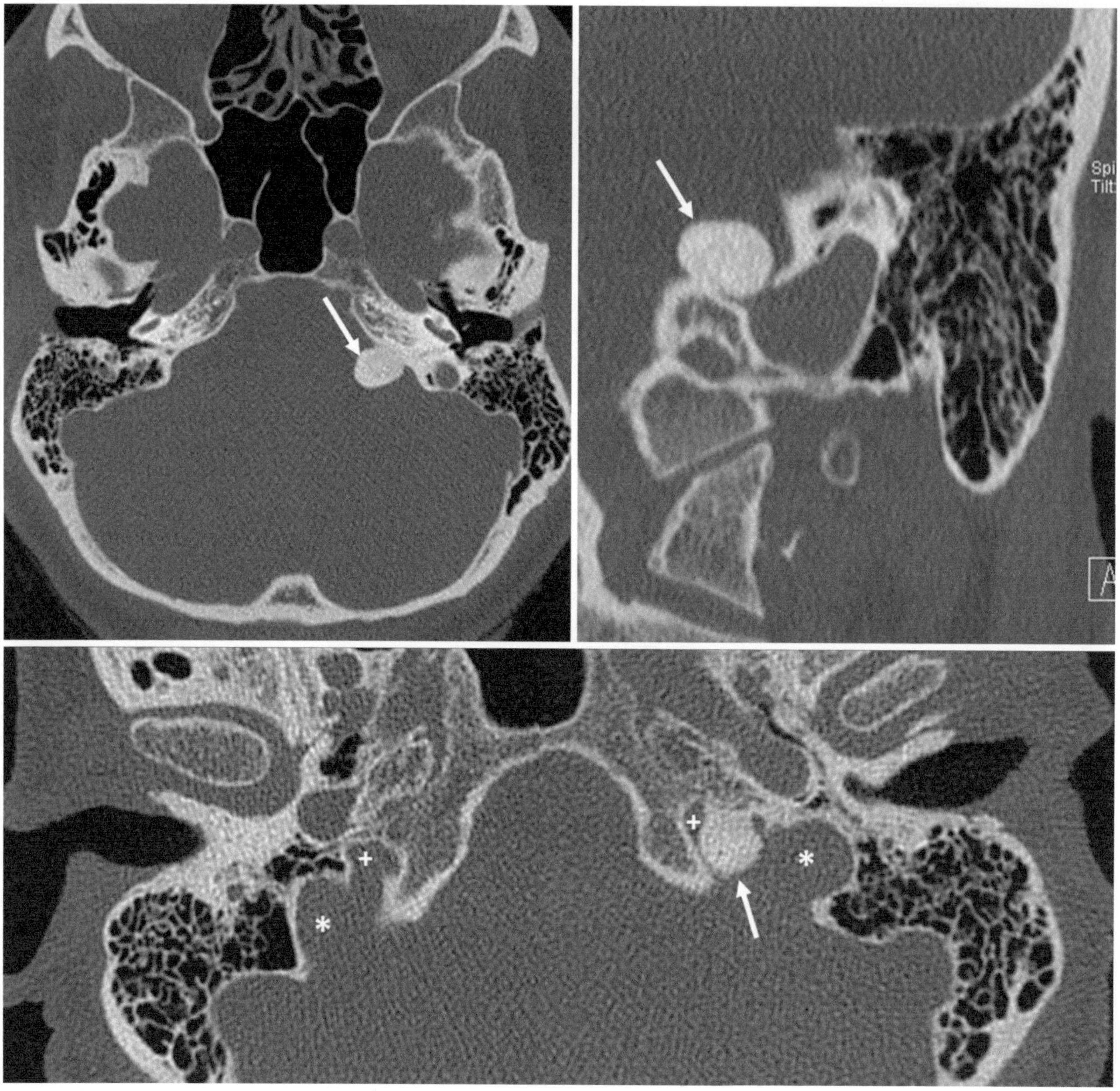

Fig. 5.43 In a 36-year-old female evaluated for sensorineural hearing loss on an otherwise negative NECT, a 1.2-cm sized exostosis (*arrows*) protrudes medially from the left petrous apex on a 0.6-mm thickness HRCT axial image (*top left*), a coronal image of the left side (*top right*), and magnified axial images of the right (*bottom left*) and left (*bottom right*) sides. Note that the exostosis protrudes inferiorly as well as fills a portion of the left jugular foramen, particularly within the pars nervosa portion, which is the anterior portion of the foramen (*plus sign, bottom right*). For comparison, note the normal right side on the *bottom left image*, with the pars nervosa anteriorly (*plus sign*) and pars vascularis posteriorly (*asterisks on both sides*)

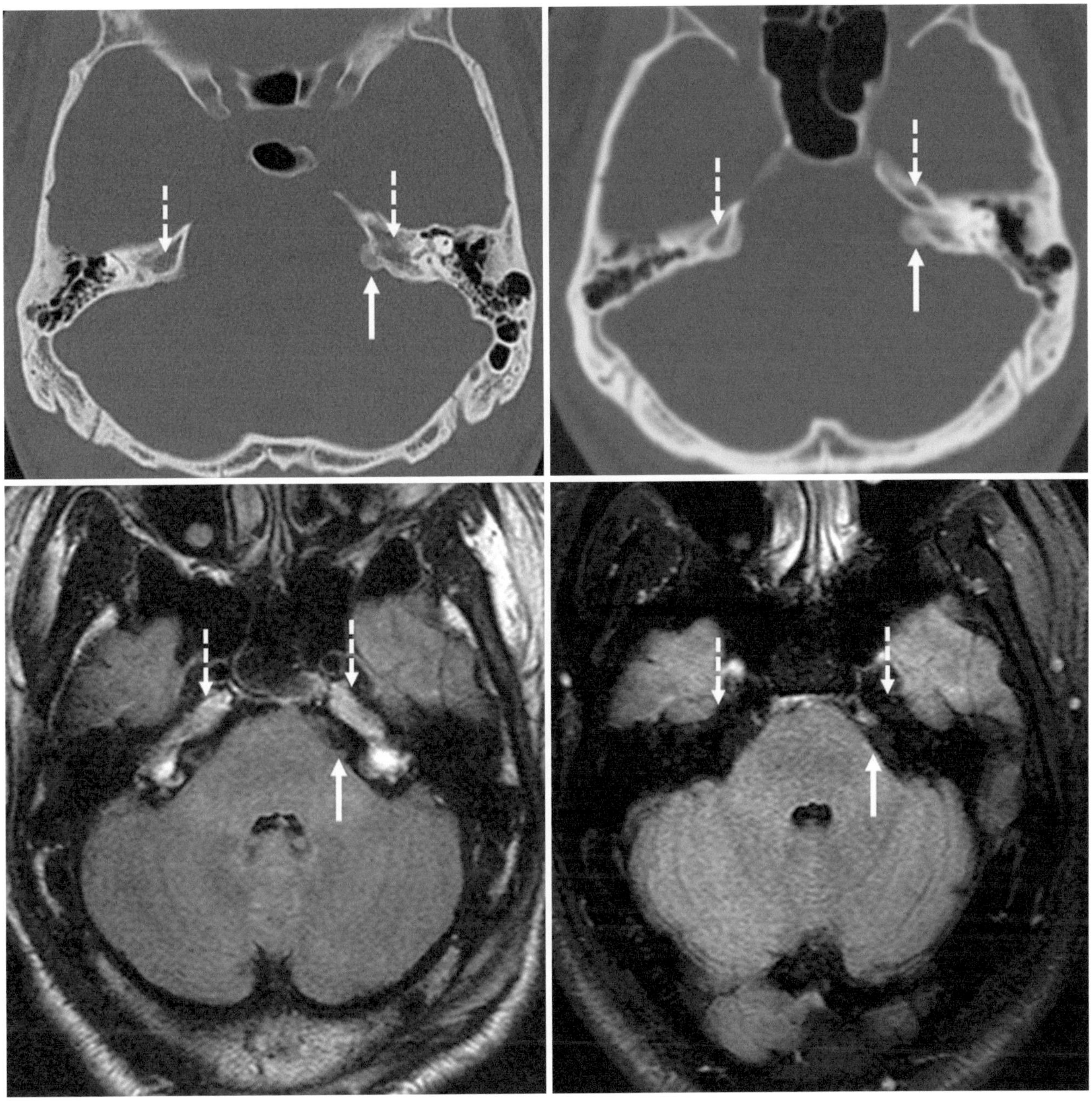

Fig. 5.44 In a 32-year-old male who underwent an otherwise negative temporal bone NECT, an exostosis was noted of the left petrous apex (*arrows*) on axial HRCT images (*top left*); this was unchanged 3 years later on a routine NECT of the head (*top right*). A 1.5T brain MRI soon after, performed for unrelated reasons, demonstrated that the left petrous exostosis (*arrows*) was hardly visible on noncontrast FLAIR without (*bottom left*) and with (*bottom right*) fat suppression (FS). Also note the fatty marrow of the petrous apices bilaterally (*dotted arrows*), a normal variation. Notably, some exostoses contain fatty marrow if large enough, but most do not, as in this example

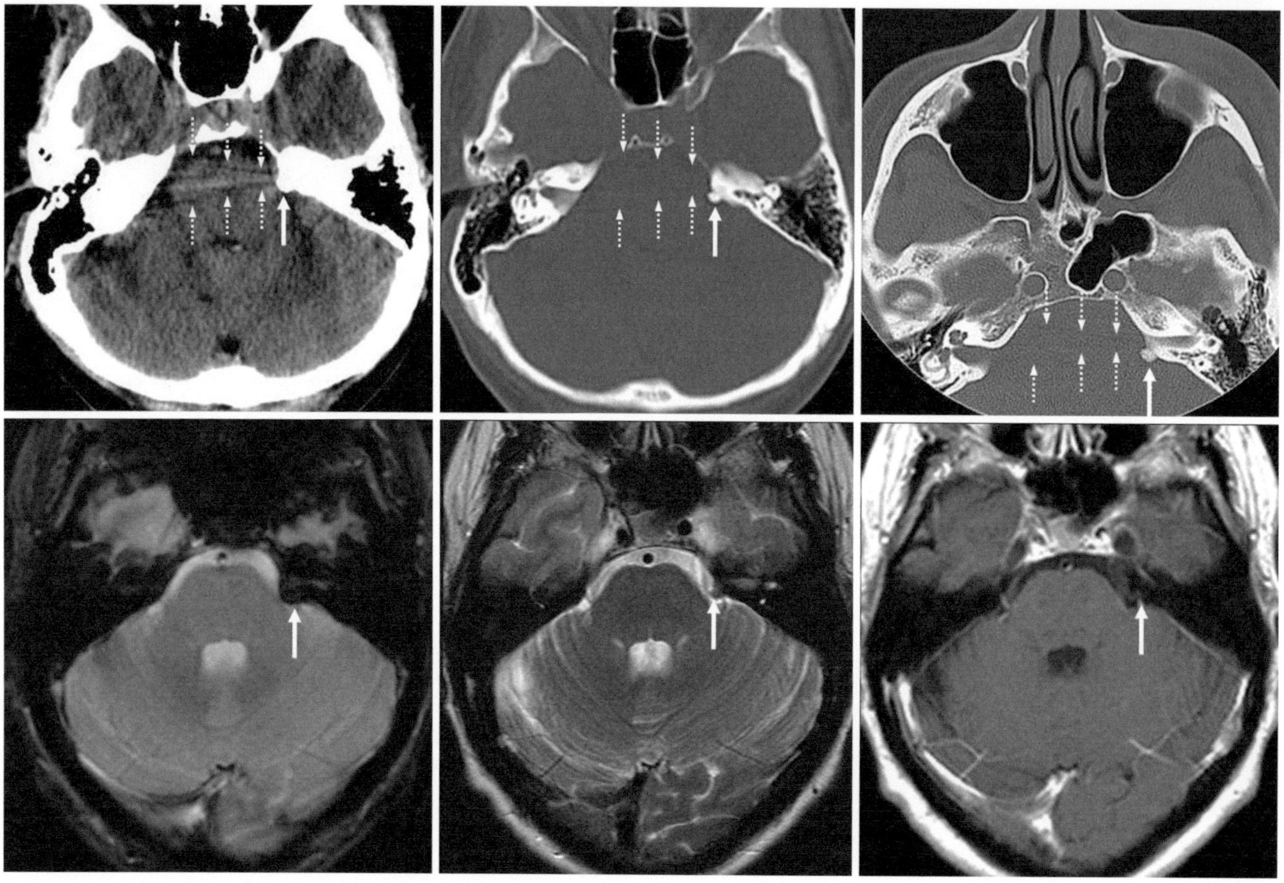

Fig. 5.45 A 53-year-old female with headaches underwent an otherwise negative NECT of the head. **Top row:** A small left petrous exostosis (*arrows*) causing beam hardening streak artifact that obscures the brainstem, with linear streaks (*small dotted arrows*) arising from the exostosis, as shown on axial soft tissue window (*left*) and bone window (*middle*) head CT images. There is also a magnified axial bone window image (*right*) from a facial bone CT the same day. **Bottom row:** On MRI with axial GET2*WI (*left*) there is a blooming susceptibility artifact from the dense bony exostosis (*arrows*), while the exostosis appears smaller on SET2WI (*middle*), since that sequence is less susceptible to artifact. The exostosis does not enhance on postcontrast SET1WI (*right*), distinguishing it from a calcified meningioma. This case demonstrates that although a petrous apex exostosis/osteoma is a "don't touch" lesion, it may obscure adjacent structures, particularly on NECT

5.10 Foramen Tympanicum (Foramen of Huschke)

The foramen tympanicum is an incidental normal variant and is nearly always asymptomatic. It is composed of a small communication/defect in the anteroinferior bony wall of the external auditory canal and the temporomandibular joint (TMJ). This defect perhaps results from a defect in normal development and ossification in the young child. The incidence of this is thought to be in 5–20% of patients who are either normal or have unrelated symptoms and can be either bilateral or unilateral. This variable incidence is likely dependent on the population mix, the modality used to identify it, or on cadaver and anthropologic studies. This variant is readily visible on NECT of the head or neck or HRCT of the temporal bone. It typically is of no consequence, although rare cases of herniation of structures from the temporomandibular fossa or fistulization from the salivary gland have been described. There are also theoretical surgical implications of not being familiar with this normal variant during skull base surgery. Also, this normal variant could potentially simulate a petrous temporal bone fracture (which often extends anteriorly and inferiorly) (Fig. 5.46).

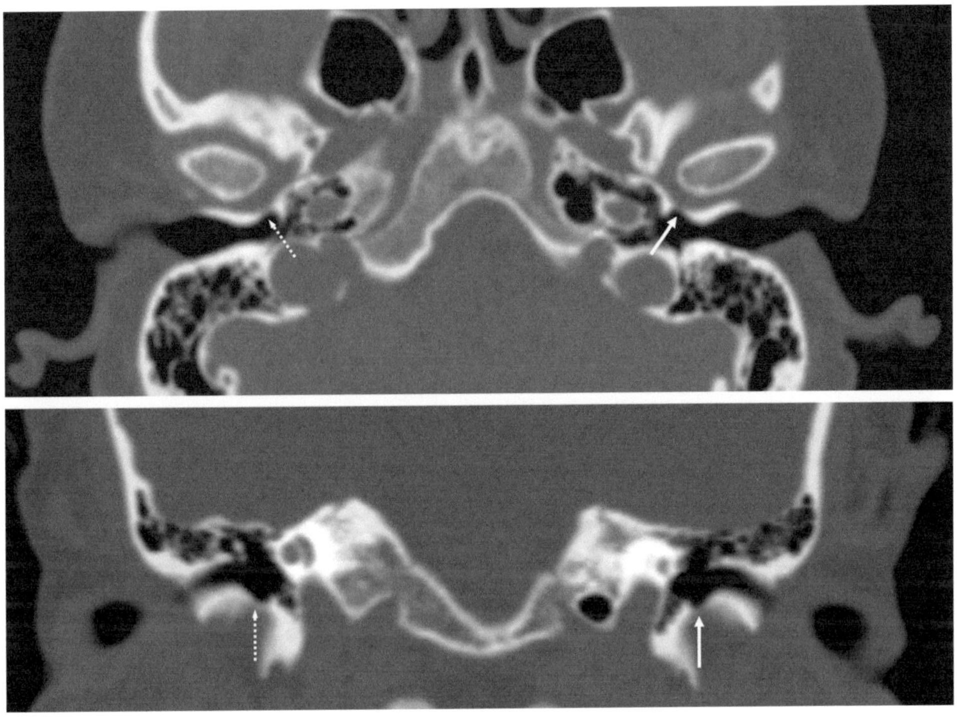

Fig. 5.46 In a 39-year-old female followed for prior episodes of sinusitis (an otherwise negative examination), 1-mm thickness NECT axial (*top*) and coronal (*bottom*) reconstructions demonstrate a normal variant, patent left foramen tympanicum (aka "foramen of Huschke," *arrows*), represented by a bony defect of the anteroinferior bony wall of the external auditory canal. On the right side, a borderline foramen tympanicum (*dotted arrows*) may also be present, while there could be a very thin rim of bone covering the defect that is hard to discern at this imaging resolution

5.11 Calcified Auricular Cartilage ("Petrified Ear")

Calcified (or ossified) auricular cartilage (aka, "petrified ear") is a rare phenomenon with fewer than 50 cases described, although it probably occurs more commonly because the vast majority are asymptomatic, and the occurrence is incidental and hence usually not reported. The bilateral form occurs nearly exclusively in males, and although it is typically asymptomatic, the patient may present with a complaint of rigid or inflexible ears. While it is not a normal variation, it is certainly usually a "don't touch" lesion with a characteristic appearance. Potential causes of such bilateral dystrophic calcification affecting the ears are many, including adrenal insufficiency (adrenocorticotropin insufficiency, or Addison disease), hypopituitarism, parathyroid or thyroid hormone abnormalities, acromegaly, or patients receiving hemodialysis or taking extensive calcium supplements, to name a few. Unilateral causes are less common and may occur in females but include local trauma, frostbite, repeated injury (or exercise such as acrobatics), or focal inflammation. Such data are based mostly on multiple reports or case series in the literature without many large studies; therefore the exact pathophysiologic cause has remained elusive. However, it appears to involve the release of excessive calcium into the extracellular space and is often due to a long-term deficiency in cortisol as well. Hormone replacement therapy can improve other symptoms but does not improve the calcified cartilage or ear stiffness. This can easily be diagnosed on plain films, NECT, or three-dimensional reconstructions of NECT by the appearance of auricular cartilage in the configuration of the ear that is nearly as radiodense/hyperdense as bone (Fig. 5.47).

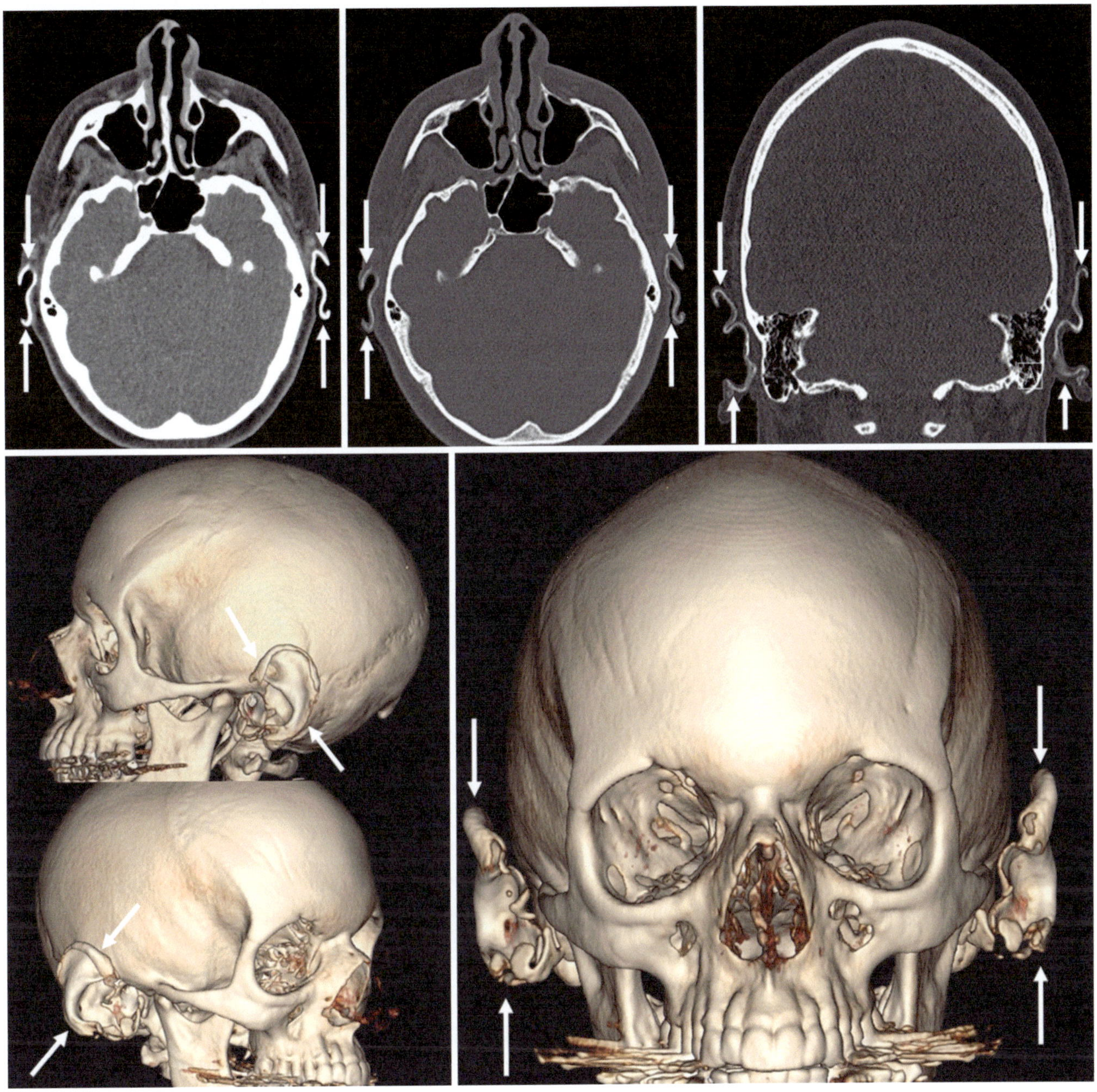

Fig. 5.47 A 40-year-old male with adrenal insufficiency and "petrified ears" who underwent NECT to evaluate the nasal septum. **Top row:** On NECT reformats, axial soft tissue window (*left*), axial bone window (*middle*), and coronal bone window (*right*), there is calcification of the auricular cartilage bilaterally and involving nearly the entire auricular cartilage on both sides, which occurs almost exclusively in males. **Bottom row:** On three-dimensional volume-rendered reconstructions, lateral views of the left side (*left, top image*), right side (*left, bottom image*), and an anteroposterior view (*right*) illustrate how the cartilage is nearly ossified and as dense as the calvarium and facial bones; this leads to the appearance of "petrified ear." This "don't touch" lesion is typically asymptomatic, but further questioning of this patient did reveal that his ears were inflexible

Suggested Reading

Baik FM, Nguyen L, Doherty JK, Harris JP, Mafee MF, Nguyen QT. Comparative case series of exostoses and osteomas of the internal auditory canal. Ann Otol Rhinol Laryngol. 2011;120:255–60.

Barkan A, Glantz I. Calcification of auricular cartilages in patients with hypopituitarism. J Clin Endocrinol Metab. 1982;55:354–7.

Beck DW, Dyste GN. Intracranial osteochondroma: MR and CT appearance. Am J Neuroradiol. 1989;10:7–8.

Brackmann DE, Doherty JK. Facial palsy and fallopian canal expansion associated with idiopathic intracranial hypertension. Otol Neurotol. 2007;28:715–8.

Brant WE, Helms CA. Fundamentals of diagnostic radiology. Philadelphia: Lippincott Williams & Wilkins; 2007.

Brook CD, Buch K, Kaufmann M, Sakai O, Devaiah AK, et al. The prevalence of high-riding jugular bulb in patients with suspected endolymphatic hydrops. J Neurol Surg B Skull Base. 2015;76:471–4.

Burford CM, Mason MJ. Early development of the malleus and incus in humans. J Anat. 2016;229:857–70.

Chadwell JB, Halsted MJ, Choo DI, Greinwald JH, Benton C. The cochlear cleft. Am J Neuroradiol. 2004;25:21–4.

Clarke JT, Clarke LE, Miller JJ. Petrified ears: calcification of the auricular cartilage. J Am Acad Dermatol. 2004;51:799–800.

Clerico DM, Jahn AF, Fontanella S. Osteoma of the internal auditory canal. Case report and literature review. Ann Otol Rhinol Laryngol. 1994;103:619–23.

Cooper MH, Archer CR, Kveton JF. Correlation of high resolution computed tomography and gross anatomic sections of the temporal bone. Part III. Cochlear and vestibular aqueducts. Am J Otol. 1989;10:272–6.

Cox P, Jeffery N. Semicircular canals and agility: the influence of size and shape measures. J Anat. 2010;216:37–47.

Daocai W, Qing W, Ximing W, Cheng L, Xiangxing M. Size of the semicircular canals measured by multidetector computed tomography in different age groups. J Comput Assist Tomogr. 2014;38:196–9.

Deniz Y, Geduk G, Zengin AZ. Examination of foramen tympanicum: cone-beam computed tomography anatomical study. Folia Morphol. 2018;77(2):335–39.

Dolan KD, Babin RW, Jacoby CG. Asymmetry of the internal auditory canals without acoustic neuroma. Ann Otol Rhinol Laryngol. 1978;87:815–20.

Erkoç MF, Imamoglu H, Okur A, Gümüş C, Dogan M. Normative size evaluation of internal auditory canal with magnetic resonance imaging: review of 3786 patients. Folia Morphol. 2012;71:217–20.

Fatterpekar GM, Doshi AH, Dugar M, Delman BN, Naidich TP, Som PM. Role of 3D CT in the evaluation of the temporal bone. Radiographics. 2006;26:S117–32.

Flood LM, Brammer RE, Graham MD, Kemink JL. Pitfalls in the diagnosis of acoustic neuroma. Clin Otolaryngol Allied Sci. 1984;9:165–70.

Friedmann DR, Eubig J, Winata LS, Pramanik BK, Merchant SN, Lalwani AK. Prevalence of jugular bulb abnormalities and resultant inner ear dehiscence: a histopathologic and radiologic study. Otolaryngol Head Neck Surg. 2012;147:750–6.

Gacek RR. Anatomy and significance of the subarachnoid space in the fallopian canal. Am J Otol. 1998;19:358–65.

Glastonbury CM, Harnsberger HR, Hudgins PA, Salzman KL. Lateralized petrous internal carotid artery: imaging features and distinction from the aberrant internal carotid artery. Neuroradiology. 2012;54:1007–13.

Glassman SB, Delbeke D. Nuclear medicine case of the day. Hereditary multiple exostoses. Am J Roentgenol. 1992;158:1384.

Goswami S, Chakraborty PP, Ray S, Ghosh S, Chowdhury S. "Petrified ears" in secondary adrenal insufficiency. J Clin Diagn Res. 2016;10:OD23–4.

Grammatica A, Alicandri-Ciufelli M, Molteni G, Marchioni D, Presutti L. Subarcuate canal and artery: a case report. Surg Radiol Anat. 2010;32:171–4.

Hilding DA. Petrous apex and subarcuate fossa maturation. Laryngoscope. 1987;97:1129–35.

Hongo H, Oya S, Atsushi A, Matsui T. Solitary osteochondroma of the skull base: a case report and literature review. J Neurol Surg Rep. 2015;76:e13–7.

Hourani R, Carey J, Yousem DM. Dehiscence of the jugular bulb and vestibular aqueduct: findings on 200 consecutive temporal bone computed tomography scans. J Comput Assist Tomogr. 2005;29:657–62.

Jackler RK, Hwang PH. Enlargement of the cochlear aqueduct: fact or fiction? Otolaryngol Head Neck Surg. 1993;109:14–25.

Jackler RK, Parker DA. Radiographic differential diagnosis of petrous apex lesions. Am J Otol. 1992;13:561–74.

James HA, Wermers RA. "Petrified ears:" auricular ossification in adrenal insufficiency. Mayo Clin Proc. 2016;91:1487–8.

Juliano AF, Ginat DT, Moonis G. Imaging review of the temporal bone: part I. Anatomy and inflammatory and neoplastic processes. Radiology. 2013;269(1):17–33.

Khangure SR, Wood B. Ossicular fixation—a pictorial review of CT temporal bone findings. Educational Exhibit Poster No. R-0079. The Royal Australian and New Zealand College of Radiologists. Available at: www.ranzcr.edu.au. Accessed 1 Apr 2018.

Lacout A, Marsot-Dupuch K, Smoker WR, Lasjaunias P. Foramen tympanicum, or foramen of Huschke: pathologic cases and anatomic CT study. Am J Neuroradiol. 2005;26:1317–23.

Lasjaunias P, Berenstein A, Ter Brugge KG. Surgical neuroangiography, clinical vascular anatomy and variations. 2nd ed. New York: Springer-Verlag; 2001.

Lee JY, Shin KJ, Kim JN, Yoo JY, Song WC, Koh KS, et al. A morphometric study of the semicircular canals using micro-CT images in three-dimensional reconstruction. Anat Rec (Hoboken). 2013;296:834–9.

Lee TC, Aviv RI, Chen JM, Nedzelski JM, Fox AJ, Symons SP. CT grading of otosclerosis. Am J Neuroradiol. 2009;30:1435–9.

Lemmerling MM, Stambuk HE, Mancuso AA, Antonelli PJ, Kubilis PS. CT of the normal suspensory ligaments of the ossicles in the middle ear. Am J Neuroradiol. 1997;18:471–7.

Leung JY, Ishak GE. Prominent subarcuate canal in children: a normal variant. Pediatr Radiol. 2010;40(Suppl 1):S161.

Li S, Shen N, Cheng Y, Sha Y, Wang Z. The effect of jugular bulb-vestibular aqueduct dehiscence on hearing and balance. Acta Otolaryngol. 2015;135:1103–7.

Lin SR, Lee KF, Stein GN, Lee I. Asymmetrical internal auditory canals. A normal variant. Arch Otolaryngol. 1973;98:164–9.

Lo WW, Solti-Bohman LG, McElveen JT Jr. Aberrant carotid artery: radiologic diagnosis with emphasis on high-resolution computed tomography. Radiographics. 1985;5:985–93.

Manzari L, Scagnelli P. Large bilateral internal auditory meatus associated with bilateral superior semicircular canal dehiscence. Ear Nose Throat J. 2013;92:25–33.

Mastromonaco P, Stöckli S. Hyperostosis of the internal auditory canal: an incidental finding? HNO. 2015;63:516–9.

Masutani H, Takahashi H, Sando I, Sato H. Vestibular aqueduct in Ménière's disease and non-Ménière's disease with endolymphatic hydrops: a computer aided volumetric study. Auris Nasus Larynx. 1991;18:351–7.

Matsushima K, Ribas ES, Kiyosue H, Komune N, Miki K, Rhoton AL. Absence of the superior petrosal veins and sinus: surgical considerations. Surg Neurol Int. 2015;6:34.

Miyashita T, Toyama Y, Inamoto R, Mori N. Evaluation of the vestibular aqueduct in Ménière's disease using multiplanar reconstruction images of CT. Auris Nasus Larynx. 2012;39:567–71.

McKinney AM. Normal variations in calvarial contour, irregular ossification/aeration, and inward/outward projections/protuberances. In: McKinney AM, editor. Atlas of normal imaging variations of the brain, skull, and craniocervical vasculature. Cham: Springer; 2017a. p. 899–907, 911–4.

McKinney AM. Skull base foramina: normal variations and developmental defects. In: McKinney AM, editor. Atlas of normal imaging variations of the brain, skull, and craniocervical vasculature. Cham: Springer; 2017b. p. 805–6, 810.

McKinney AM. Tortuous cervical and intracranial arteries and basilar-carotid dolichoectasia. In: Mc Kinney AM, editor. Atlas of normal imaging variations of the brain, skull, and craniocervical vasculature. Cham, Switzerland: Springer; 2017c. p. 1021–2.

Migirov L, Kronenberg J. Radiology of the petromastoid canal. Otol Neurotol. 2006;27:410–3.

Moore KR, Harnsberger HR, Shelton C, Davidson HC. 'Leave me alone' lesions of the petrous apex. Am J Neuroradiol. 1998;19:733–8.

Moreno RC, Chilvarquer I, Hayek JE, Seraidarian PI. Anatomic and radiograph study of the persistence of foramen of Huschke. Braz J Otorhinolaryngol. 2005;71:676–9.

Moser T, Veillon F, Sick H, Riehm S. The hypodense focus in the petrous apex: a potential pitfall on multidetector CT imaging of the temporal bone. Am J Neuroradiol. 2008;29:35–9.

Nakasato T, Nakayama T, Nakayama M, Ehara S, Ohtsuka H, Sato H. Minor ossicular anomalies in the middle ear: role of submillimeter multislice computed tomography. J Comput Assist Tomogr. 2014;38:655–61.

Noussios G, Chouridis P, Kostretzis L, Natsis K. Morphological and morphometrical study of the human ossicular chain: a review of the literature and a meta-analysis of experience over 50 years. J Clin Med Res. 2016;8:76–83.

Okudera T, Huang YP, Ohta T, Yokota A, Nakamura Y, Maehara F, et al. Development of posterior fossa dural sinuses, emissary veins, and jugular bulb: morphological and radiologic study. Am J Neuroradiol. 1994;15:1871–83.

Park K, Choung YH. Isolated congenital ossicular anomalies. Acta Otolaryngol. 2009;129:419–22.

Patil AR, Bhalla A, Gupta P, Goyal D, Vishnubhatla S, Ramavat A, et al. HRCT evaluation of microtia: A retrospective study. Indian J Radiol Imaging. 2012;22:188–94.

Petrus LV, Lo WW. Spontaneous CSF otorrhea caused by abnormal development of the facial nerve canal. Am J Neuroradiol. 1999;20:275–7.

Prowse SJ, Kelly G, Agada F. Temporomandibular joint herniation and the foramen of Huschke: an unusual external auditory canal mass. J Laryngol Otol. 2011;125:1279–81.

Reardon W, Bellman S, Phelps P, Pembrey M, Luxon LM. Neuro-otological function in X-linked hearing loss: a multipedigree assessment and correlation with other clinical parameters. Acta Otolaryngol. 1993;113:706–14.

Reinshagen KL, Curtin HD, Quesnel AM, Juliano AF. Measurement for detection of incomplete partition type II anomalies on MR imaging. Am J Neuroradiol. 2017;38:2003–7.

Richard C, Courbon G, Laroche N, Prades JM, Vico L, Malaval L, et al. Inner ear ossification and mineralization kinetics in human embryonic development—microtomographic and histomorphological study. Sci Rep. 2017;7:4825.

Roll JD, Urban MA, Larson TC, et al. Bilateral aberrant internal carotid arteries with bilateral persistent stapedial arteries and bilateral duplicated internal carotid arteries. Am J Neuroradiol. 2003;24:762–5.

Saha R, Srimani P, Mazumdar A, Mazumdar S. Morphological variations of middle ear ossicles and its clinical implications. J Clin Diagn Res. 2017;11:AC01–4.

Sato H, Sando I, Takahashi H. Computer-aided three-dimensional measurement of the human vestibular apparatus. Otolaryngol Head Neck Surg. 1992;107:405–9.

Schutt CA, Guo JN, Bagwell KA, Bulsara KR, Malhotra A, Michaelides E. Bilateral osteomas and exostoses of the internal auditory canal. Am J Otolaryngol. 2015;36:583–6.

Shimada R, Kiyosue H, Tanoue S, Mori H, Abe T. Superior petrosal sinus: hemodynamic features in normal and cavernous sinus dural arteriovenous fistulas. Am J Neuroradiol. 2013;34:609–15.

Song JJ, Hong SK, Lee SY, Park SJ, Kang SI, An YH, et al. Vestibular manifestations in subjects with enlarged vestibular aqueduct. Otol Neurotol. 2018; https://doi.org/10.1097/MAO.0000000000001817. [Epub ahead of print].

Stark TA, McKinney AM, Palmer CS, Maisel RH, Truwit CL, et al. Dilation of the subarachnoid spaces surrounding the cranial nerves with petrous apex cephaloceles in Usher syndrome. Am J Neuroradiol. 2009;30:434–6.

Swartz JD, Wolfson RJ, Marlowe FI, Popky GL. Postinflammatory ossicular fixation: CT analysis with surgical correlation. Radiology. 1985;154(3):697–700.

Taguchi T, Yoshida M, Terada Y. Petrified ear auricles with isolated adrenocorticotropic hormone deficiency. Intern Med. 2017;56:3263–4.

Tahir E, Bajin MD, Atay G, Mocan BÖ, Sennaroğlu L, et al. Bony cochlear nerve canal and internal auditory canal measures predict cochlear nerve status. J Laryngol Otol. 2017;131:676–83.

Tanioka H, Kaga H, Zusho H, Araki T, Sasaki Y, et al. MR of the endolymphatic duct and sac: findings in Ménière disease. Am J Neuroradiol. 1997;18:45–51.

Tekdemir I, Aslan A, Elhan A. The subarcuate canaliculus and its artery—a radioanatomical study. Ann Anat. 1999;181:207–11.

Teufert KB, Slattery WH. Cerebrospinal fluid leak of the fallopian canal. Ear Nose Throat J. 2013;92:E20–3.

Thomsen J, Lester J, Zilstorff K. Cerebellopontine pantopaque cisternography and tomography of the internal acoustic meatus in the diagnosis of angle tumors. Arch Otorhinolaryngol. 1976;214:157–65.

Tomura N, Sashi R, Kobayashi M, Hirano H, Hashimoto M, Watarai J. Normal variations of the temporal bone on high-resolution CT: their incidence and clinical significance. Clin Radiol. 1995;50:144–8.

Tozoğlu U, Caglayan F, Harorli A. Foramen tympanicum or foramen of Huschke: anatomical cone beam CT study. Dentomaxillofac Radiol. 2012;41:294–7.

Uthoff H, Wiesli P. Images in clinical medicine. Auricular cartilage calcification and adrenal insufficiency. N Engl J Med. 2011;364:157.

Valvassori GE, Clemis JD. The large vestibular aqueduct syndrome. Laryngoscope. 1978;88:723–8.

Wang RG, Bingham B, Hawke M, Kwok P, Li JR. Persistence of the foramen of Huschke in the adult: an osteological study. J Otolaryngol. 1991;20:251–3.

Weinberg PE, Kim KS, Gore RM. Unilateral enlargement of the internal auditory canal: a developmental variant. Surg Neurol. 1981;15:39–42.

Yan F, Li J, Xian J, Wang Z, Mo L. The cochlear nerve canal and internal auditory canal in children with normal cochlea but cochlear nerve deficiency. Acta Radiol. 2013;54:292–8.

6 Cervical and Thoracic Spine: Normal Variants and Artifacts

6.1 Introduction

Imaging of the cervical spine is a routine part of a radiology practice. Familiarity with the appearance of the cervical and thoracic spinal vertebrae is critical to providing accurate imaging interpretation. In particular, the complex development of the spine, particularly the cervical spine, merits attention to aid in recognition of spinal normal anatomic variants.

CT and MRI are imaging modalities that continue to grow in use for evaluation of the cervical spine, often supplementing or replacing plain radiographs. MRI and CT myelography offer superior evaluation of the spinal cord. Awareness of artifacts frequently observed when imaging the cervical and thoracic spine, particularly with MRI, will aid in avoiding potential pitfalls involved with routine image interpretation.

6.2 Cervical Spine Anatomy and Development

6.2.1 Numbering

The cervical, thoracic, and lumbar vertebrae usually number seven, twelve, and five, respectively. However, it is not uncommon to encounter normal variation in the number of segments, such as eleven to thirteen thoracic vertebrae and four to six lumbar vertebrae. Many authors have advocated that the only true way to number/count cervical, thoracic, and subsequently the lumbar vertebrae is via a craniocaudal approach, beginning from the top of the odontoid-C2 (based on sagittal imaging). Counting can otherwise vary immensely based on the presence of variants such as cervical ribs, supernumerary ribs (i.e., "13th rib" or "lumbar rib"), incompletely fused transverse processes (simulating supernumerary ribs), and transitional lumbosacral vertebrae (further covered in "Lumbar Spine Variants," Chap. 7). Thus, a craniocaudal approach to counting down from the skull base is perhaps the optimal method (i.e., counting down from C2). Awareness of such variants is critical to ensure accurate numbering, which is of particular import to the surgeon or interventionalist for the purpose of performing spinal therapy at the correct level.

A number of techniques have arisen over the years in an attempt to ensure reproducible spinal numbering in the presence of such variants; they have had varying success. However, the use of sagittal "scout" imaging for counting purposes has recently become more facile, since quick sagittal MR imaging with nondiagnostic scout images can now be obtained in under 1 min using various parallel imaging, multiband/multicoil, and phased array techniques. Notably, the technique, acquisition time, and cost of such sequences often vary among MRI vendors.

A. McKinney et al., *Atlas of Head/Neck and Spine Normal Imaging Variants*, https://doi.org/10.1007/978-3-319-95441-7_6

6.2.2 Cervical Ribs

Although *cervical ribs* are most commonly associated with the C7 vertebra, they may also occur very rarely at C4, C5, or C6. They are usually symmetric when bilateral but may be unilateral. When present, cervical ribs often fuse with adjacent structures such as the transverse process or first rib. The reported prevalence of cervical ribs ranges from 0.2% to 8.6%; however, the more recent studies suggest that the prevalence is closer to about 2% of the population. Although most commonly it is an asymptomatic (and thus "don't touch") congenital variant, approximately 10% of patients with cervical ribs also have *thoracic outlet syndrome*. This is typically secondary to a congenital anomalous fibromuscular band that is situated near the brachial plexus and subclavian artery, with resultant compression of these structures. Because of the apparent predisposition of these patients for thoracic outlet syndrome, cervical ribs should be reported but are often overlooked (Fig. 6.1).

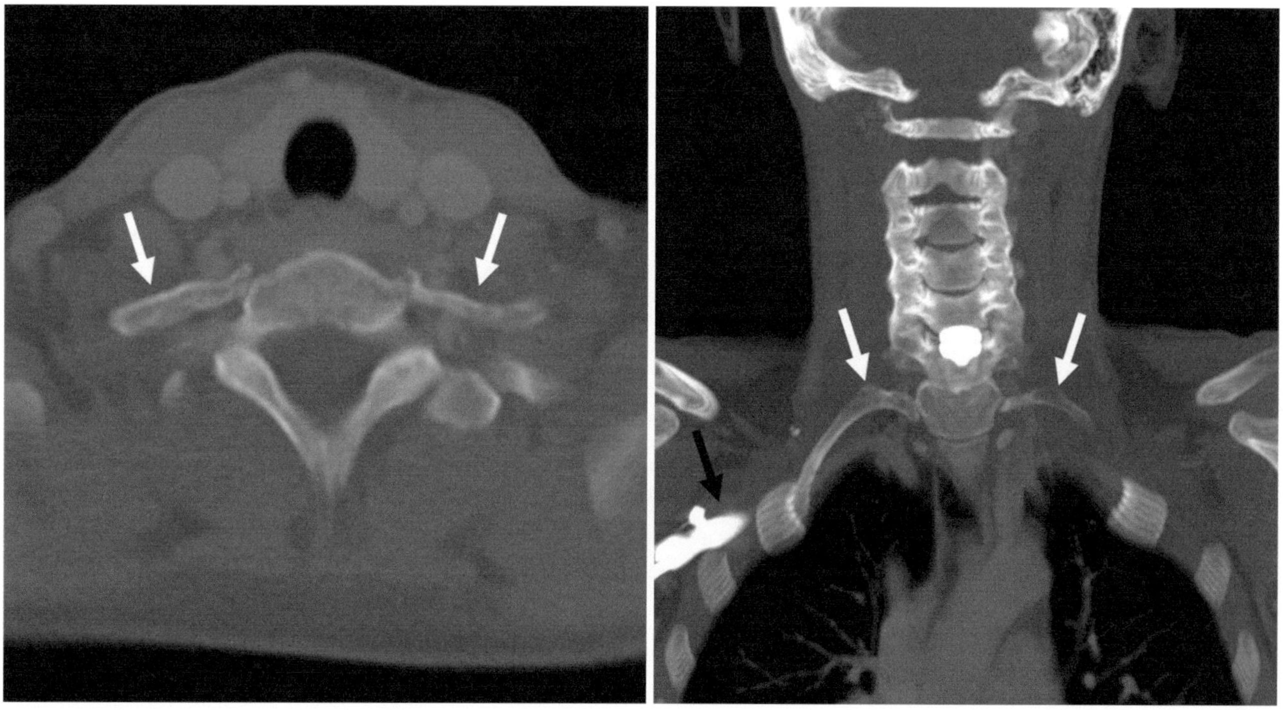

Fig. 6.1 A 35-year-old female underwent CECT imaging of the neck to evaluate the cause of dysphonia. There are normal variant bilateral cervical ribs at C7 (*white arrows*) on axial (*left*) and coronal (*right*) reconstructed images. These paired ribs are mildly asymmetric in this patient, since the right cervical rib is larger than the left. Note the cervical disc arthroplasty changes at C5 to C6 as well. At the time of acquisition of the CECT, there is also persistent dense contrast within the right subclavian vein (*black arrow*) from a right upper extremity contrast injection

6.2.3 Thoracic Rib Variation and Supernumerary ("Lumbar") Ribs

A thoracic vertebra should have a separate costal element along with facets to articulate with the adjacent ribs. The costal elements, or ribs, may be diminutive. Although more than 80% of individuals have twelve paired ribs, some patients may have as few as eleven or as many as thirteen; hence, the presence of a *supernumerary rib* at the thoracolumbar junction is not uncommon (Fig. 6.2). Variability in size of the lower thoracic ribs and the vertebral transverse processes can further complicate the process of segmental classification and numbering. In addition, transitional lumbosacral segments can lead to inconsistent numbering. Correlation with previous imaging examinations, particularly chest radiographs, as well as survey images of the entire spine can help ensure consistent vertebral numbering. Inconsistent or inaccurate numbering can lead to iatrogenic injury or unnecessary incorrect level spine surgery.

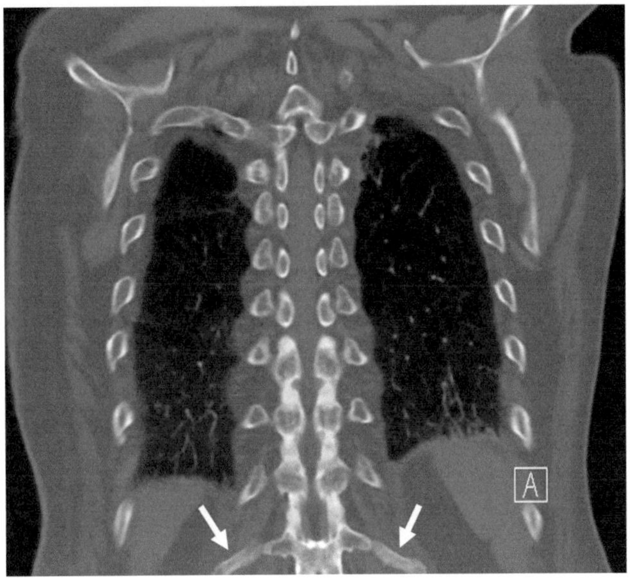

Fig. 6.2 A 66-year-old man underwent CT imaging of the chest for shortness of breath in the setting of non–small cell lung cancer. This reconstructed coronal image shows normal variant paired 13th ribs (*white arrows*). As is commonly associated with such variability in the number of ribs, this patient also had transitional lumbosacral vertebral anatomy (*not shown*)

6.3 Vertebral Embryology Overview and Normal Synchondroses

Embryologically, the vertebrae develop from the mesodermal cells of the *sclerotome*. At each level, these mesodermal cells migrate and condense into one centrum, a paired vertebral arch and paired costal processes. The centrum forms the vertebral body, and the vertebral arch forms the posterior elements. The posterior elements consist of the pedicles, articular processes, transverse processes, laminae, and spinous process. The costal processes form the ribs.

The vertebral body develops from two ossification centers, one ventral and one dorsal, which ultimately fuse. During childhood, from roughly 3–5 years of age, the paired vertebral arches fuse together and also fuse with the centrum. The cartilaginous plate that separates the developing vertebral body from the posterior elements is termed the *neurocentral synchondrosis*. This synchondrosis is commonly observed on pediatric spine imaging. This plate eventually ossifies as the body and posterior elements fuse. This normal synchondrosis can simulate a developmental anomaly or fracture on MRI or CT; however, there will be a lack of associated edema surrounding the synchondrosis on T2-weighted imaging (T2WI) or short tau inversion recovery imaging (STIR) MR sequences, and on CT there will be no fragmentation or prevertebral edema. Also, these are typically present at multiple levels but may not be present at all levels as the vertebrae fuse (Figs. 6.3, 6.4, 6.5 and 6.6).

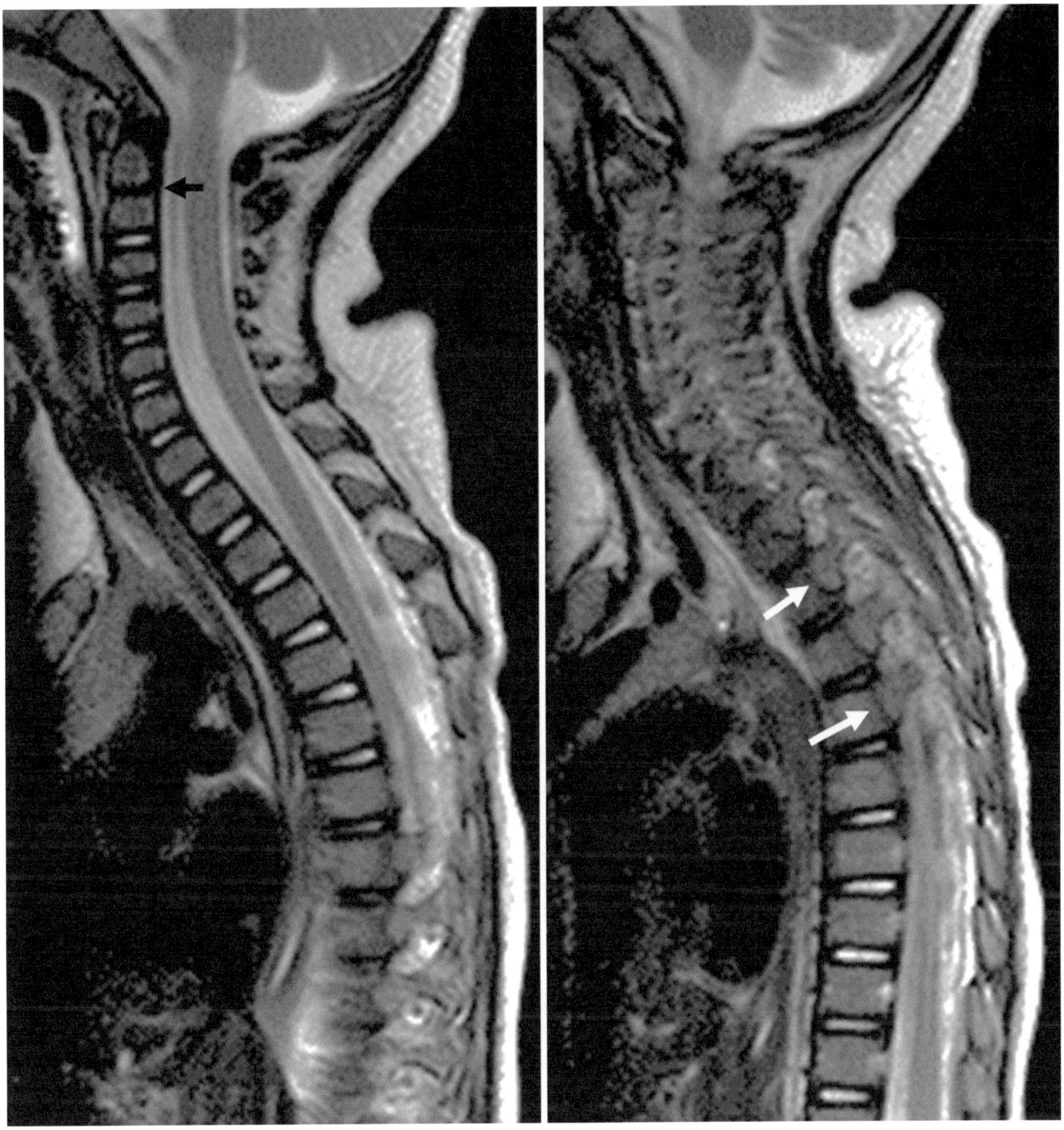

Fig. 6.3 Note the normal, linear hypointense neurocentral synchondroses in the developing thoracic spine of a 4-month-old child (*white arrows, right*) on sagittal SET2WIs. These normal structures should not be confused with fractures. Also note the normal synchondrosis of the developing C2 vertebra, where the base of the dens joins with the remainder of the vertebral body (*black arrow, left*)

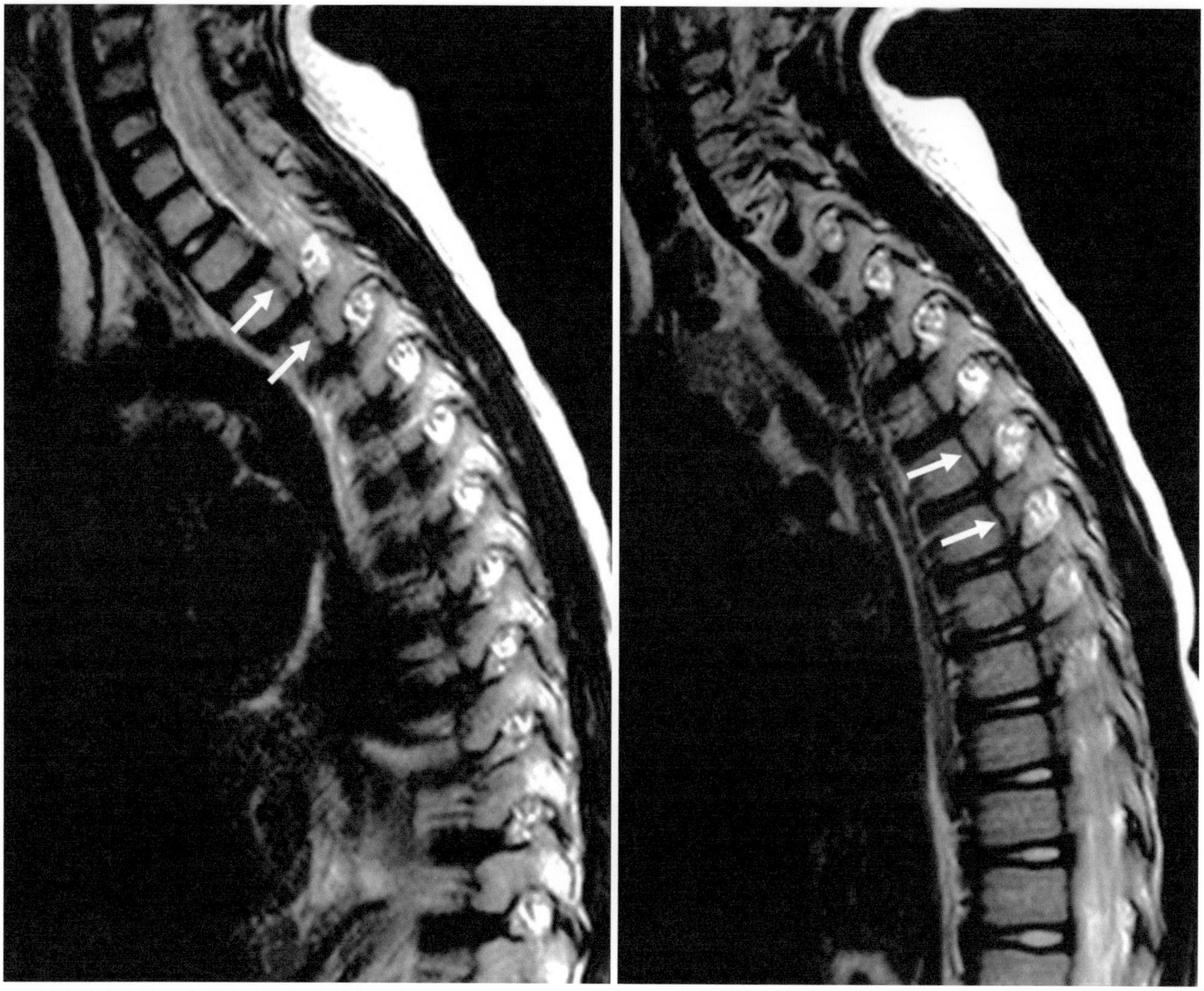

Fig. 6.4 Normal linear hypointense neurocentral synchondroses (*arrows*) in the developing cervical and thoracic spine of a 3-year-old child on sagittal SET2WI

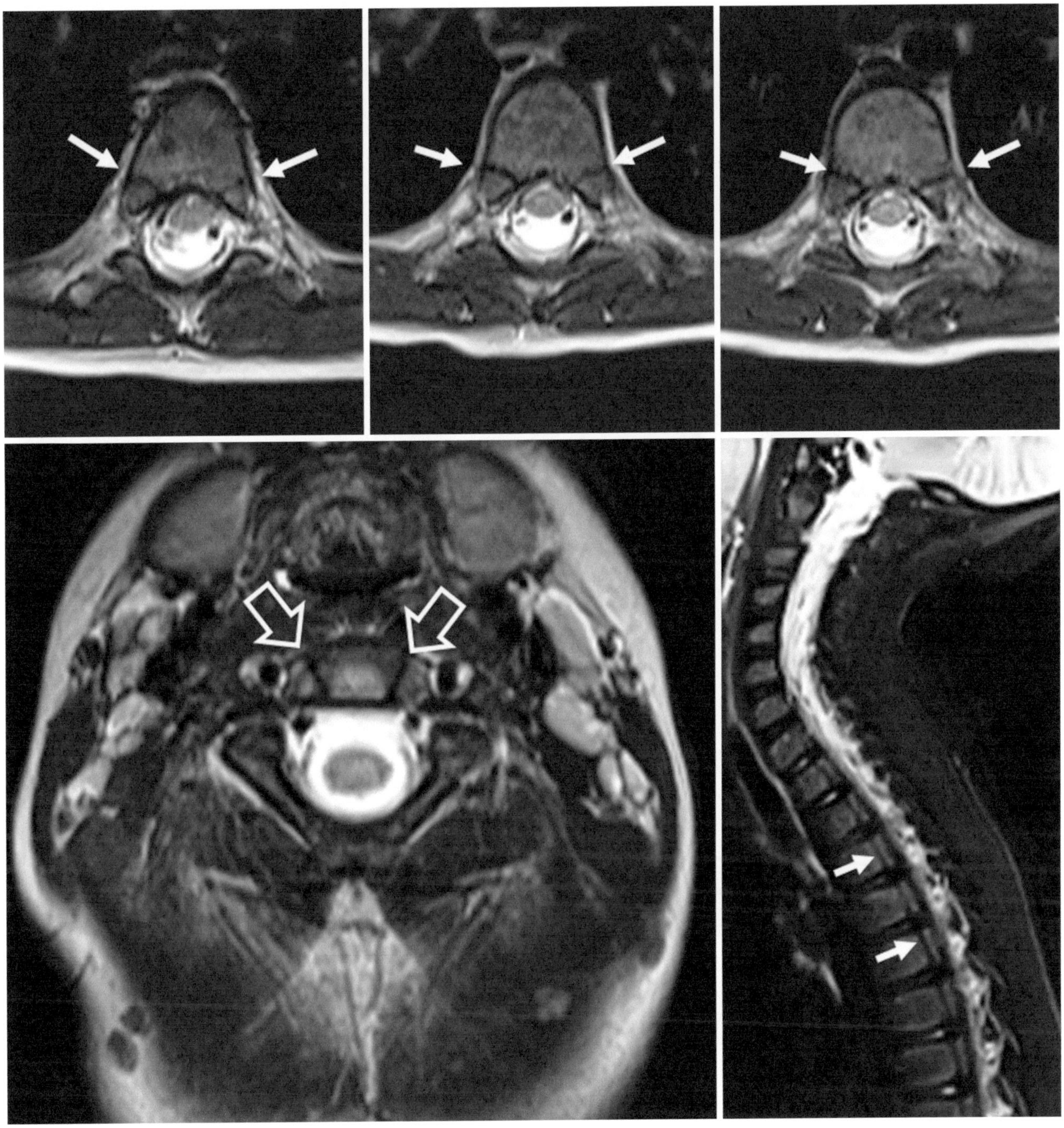

Fig. 6.5 A 4-year-old female undergoing imaging for a potential cranial anomaly (*not shown*) underwent MR imaging that demonstrated normal development of the cervical spine and upper thoracic spine. **Top row:** On axial SET2WIs, normal neurocentral synchondroses (*white arrows*) of the developing pediatric spine are visualized as hypointense lines. As the vertebral bodies continue to fuse with the posterior elements, these eventually disappear. **Bottom row:** On axial SET2WI (*left*), the developing body and posterior arch of the axis (C2) are depicted, with normal bilateral T2 hypointense *cervical* synchondroses (*open white arrows*); on sagittal SET2WI (*right*), note further examples of normal neurocentral *thoracic* synchondroses (*white arrows*)

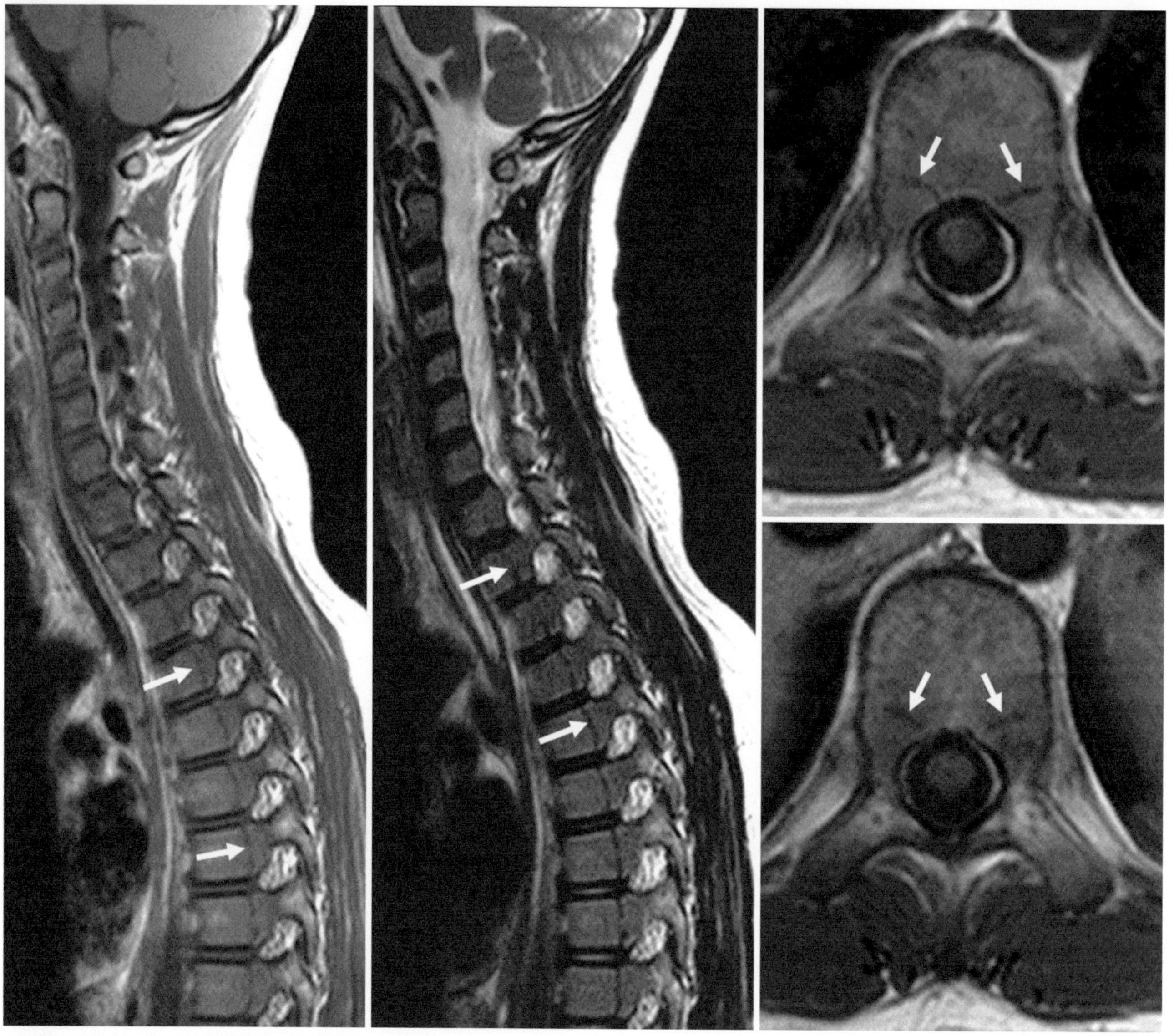

Fig. 6.6 Note normal, linear hypointense neurocentral synchondroses in the developing cervical and thoracic spine of an 11-year-old child (*white arrows*) on sagittal SET1WI MRI (*left*) and SET2WI (*middle*). On axial T1WI (*top right, bottom right*), note the typical orientation of a neurocentral synchondrosis as the developing vertebral body fuses with the posterior elements. When fusion has completed, the synchondrosis becomes normally ossified

6.4 Vertebral Body Development

Variations in development lead to congenital vertebral anomalies. In the most severe form of vertebral body maldevelopment, called *asomia* (or agenesis), a vertebral body entirely fails to form despite the development of its posterior elements. Developmental anomalies range in severity from agenesis to "don't touch" variants on the other end of the congenital spectrum. The more severe anomalies may require surgery, usually because of the resultant scoliosis.

In *hemivertebra*, only half of a vertebral body forms. This developmental anomaly can occur ventrally, dorsally, or ipsilaterally. Often a hemivertebra occurs when either the right or left half of the vertebral body fails to form; the resultant wedge-shaped vertebral body is oriented to the right or to the left and is usually associated with scoliosis. Occasionally, both the right and left portions of the vertebral body form but fail to fuse at the midline, where they are separated by persistent notochordal tissue. This results in a *butterfly (sagittal cleft) vertebral body*. In this situation, as a result of the lack of midline fusion, the vertebral body is widened. The adjacent vertebral endplates above and below the butterfly vertebra tend to have convex margins, thus accommodating the congenital variant. On standard plain films in the setting of trauma, a butterfly vertebra may mimic an acute traumatic fracture, and evaluation of the adjacent endplates may be useful to exclude a fracture. When both halves of the vertebral body form and fuse normally but a small amount of notochord persists, this may manifest as an incidental small central notochordal lucency within the middle of the vertebral body.

If the ventral half of a vertebral body fails to form, this results in a *dorsal hemivertebra*, which is associated with exaggerated kyphosis. Failure of the dorsal half of a vertebral body is extremely rare and is typically associated with exaggerated lordosis. Failure of the ventral and dorsal halves of the vertebral body to fuse can result in a *coronal vertebral body cleft*.

6.4.1 Block (Fused) Vertebrae

Block (fused) vertebrae occur when one or more vertebral bodies fail to develop individually. The appearance is often referred to as congenital vertebral fusion and is often dictated as such in a radiology report, although it may be better described as incomplete segmentation. The resultant block vertebra should be of a height equal to the heights of the involved vertebral bodies as well as the height of the involved intervening intervertebral discs. The block vertebra often has a "waist" at the level of the intervertebral disc, a finding not typically noted with acquired fusion, whether it is postsurgical or traumatic in nature. The degree of fusion may be complete or incomplete, with variable involvement of the vertebral bodies and the posterior elements.

Classically, cervical segmentation anomalies are referred to as Klippel-Feil anomalies (perhaps too general of a term) and are frequently asymptomatic (Figs. 6.7, 6.8 and 6.9). However, cervical segmentation anomalies may be observed along with the classic clinical triad of restricted cervical motion, short neck, and low posterior hairline, known as Klippel-Feil syndrome. As isolated or solitary fusion/block vertebrae are typically asymptomatic, these are considered "don't touch lesions." However, they can occasionally contribute to scoliosis, and there is debate within the literature as to whether and how much congenital block vertebrae contribute to accelerated degenerative disease of the cervical spine and intervertebral discs. Such segmentation anomalies, while common in the cervical spine, may also manifest in the thoracic spine (Fig. 6.10). Additionally, the presence of such block vertebrae is important to note in order to prevent "wrong level surgery," as occasionally inaccurate counting of cervical, thoracic, or lumbar vertebrae can mistakenly occur.

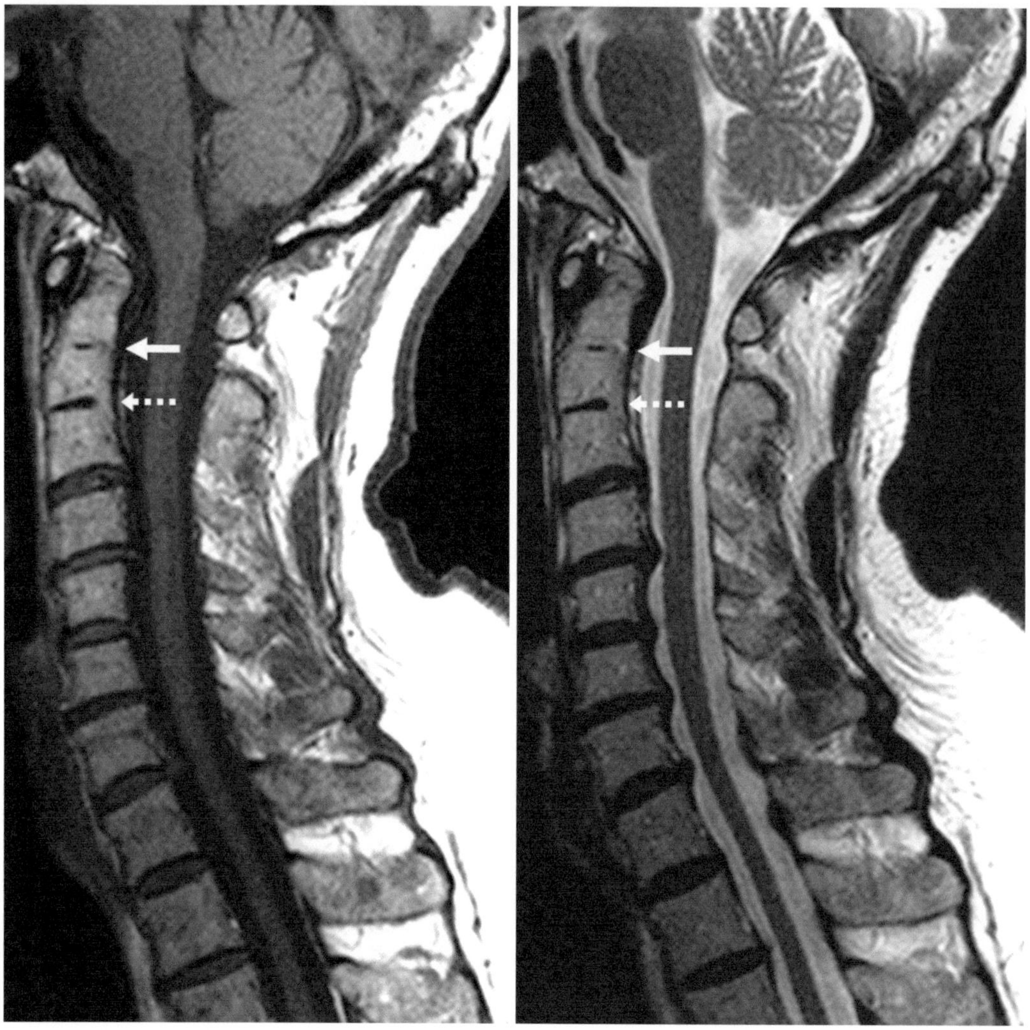

Fig. 6.7 A 67-year-old man underwent MRI of the spine to evaluate for metastases. Sagittal SET1WI (*left*) and SET2WI (*right*) depict congenital fusion/non-segmentation of C2 to C3 (*dotted arrows*), also often referred to as the Klippel-Feil anomaly. However, the patient did not have any clinical features of Klippel-Feil syndrome. Note also the normal hypointense synchondrosis (*white arrows*) where the dens meets the base of the C2 vertebral body. The presence of a concomitant normal cervical synchondrosis with fusion of cervical vertebrae can occasionally lead to inaccurate numbering or counting of vertebrae

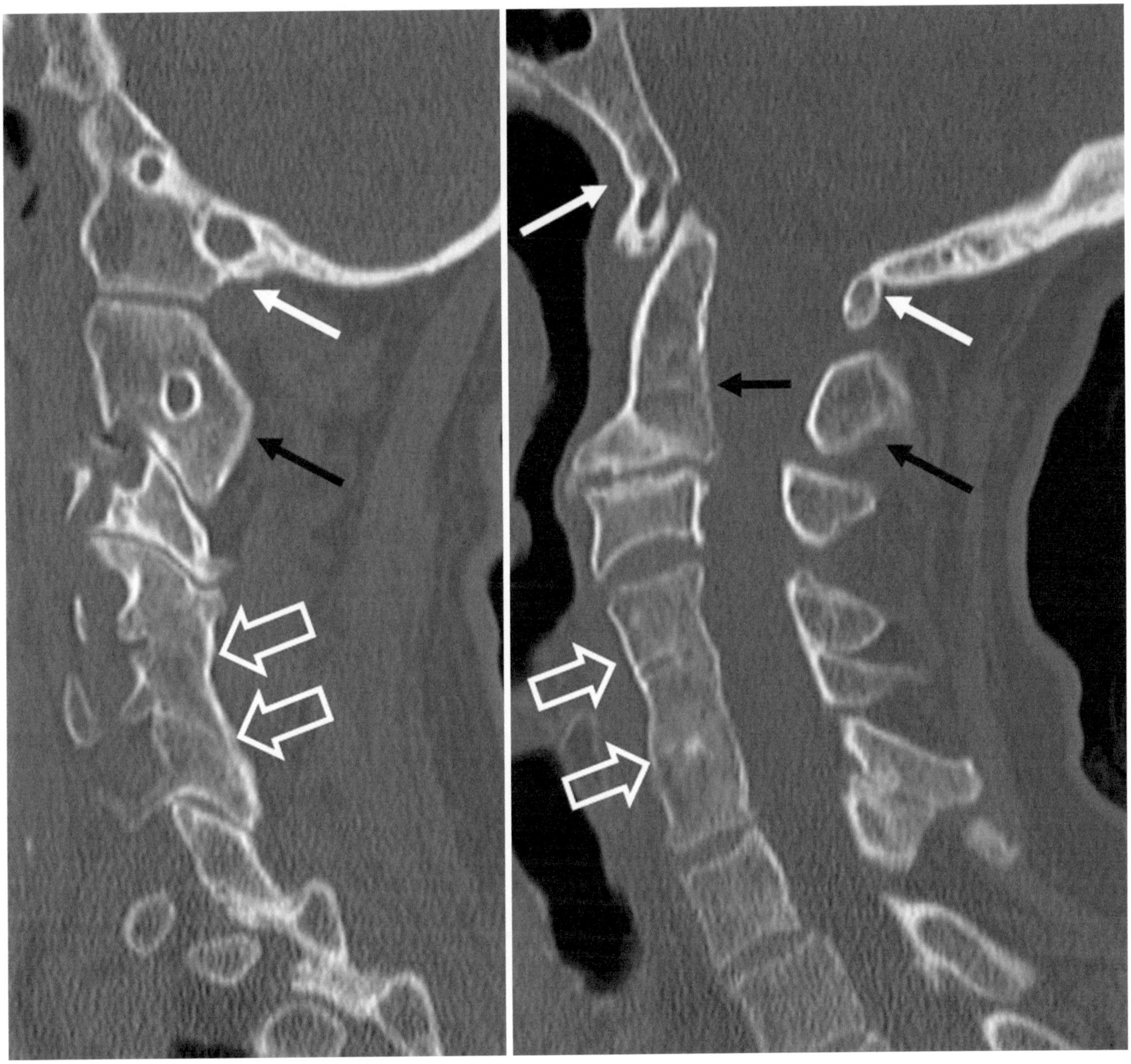

Fig. 6.8 In an 81-year-old female undergoing CT imaging for pain, sagittal NECT images of the cervical spine showed multiple congenital fusion anomalies, including fusion of the occiput with the atlas/C1 (*white arrows*), fusion of the bodies and posterior elements of C3 (*black arrows*), and fusion of the bodies and posterior elements of C5 to C7 (*open white arrows*)

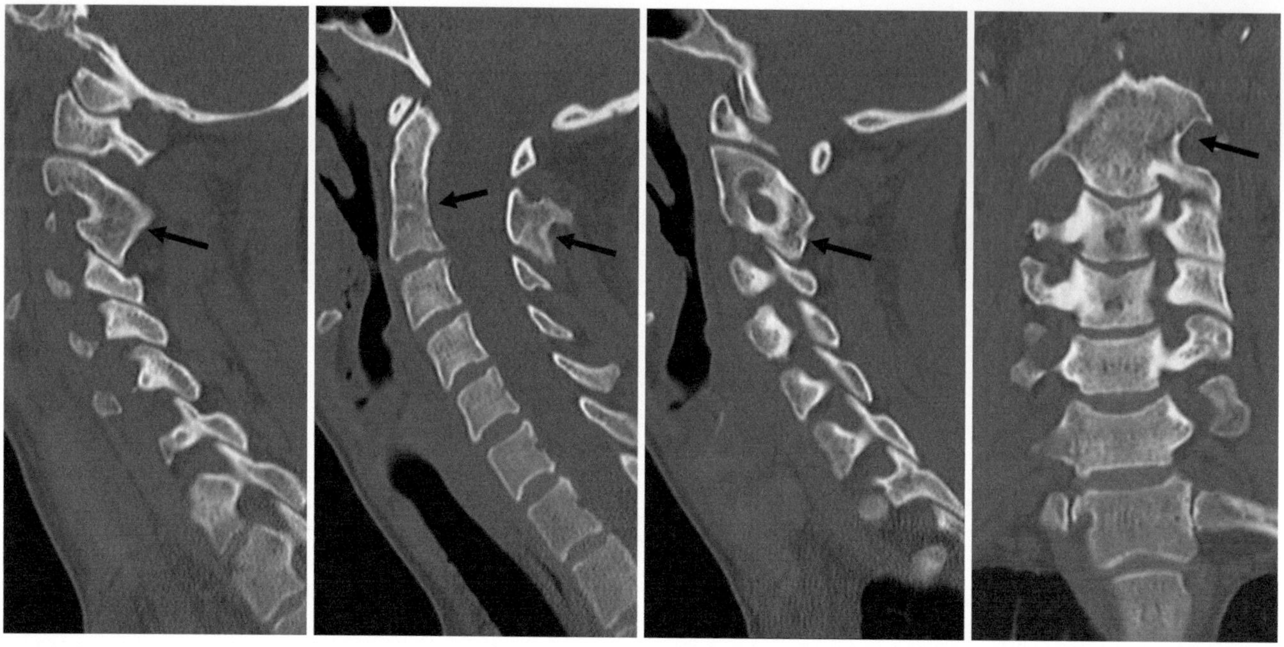

Fig. 6.9 A 27-year-old female underwent CT imaging for trauma. Sagittal (*left three images*) and coronal (*right*) NECT images show normal variant congenital fusion (also described as nonsegmentation), of the bodies and bilateral posterior elements of the C2 and C3 vertebrae (*black arrows*), with normal segmentation of the remainder of the cervical vertebrae. There was no fracture present

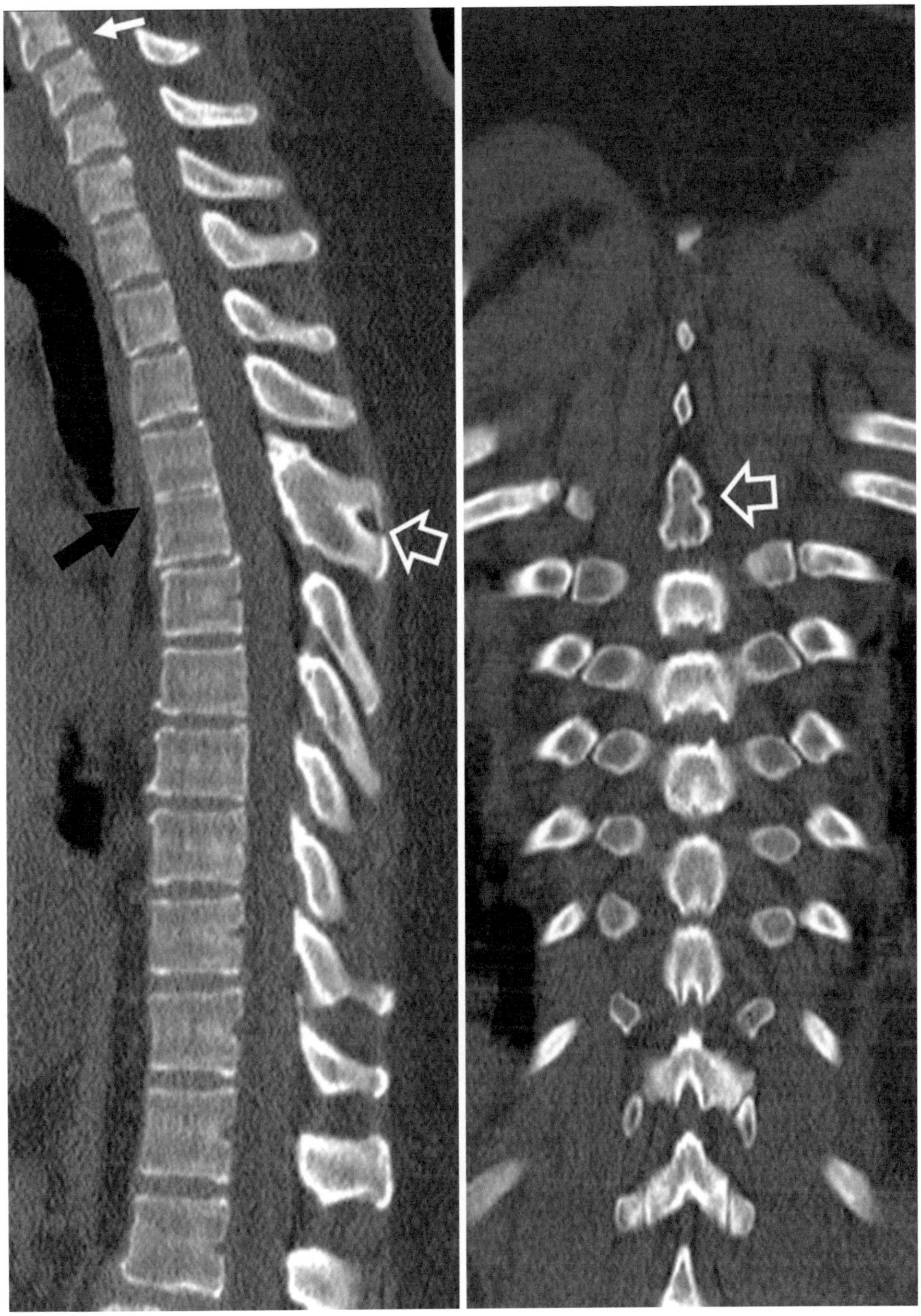

Fig. 6.10 A 49-year-old female undergoing CT imaging for acute trauma. These sagittal (*left*) and coronal (*right*) NECT images show partial fusion (or nonsegmentation) of the T2 and T3 vertebral bodies, with more solid fusion of the posterior elements (*open white arrows*) relative to the anterior segment (*black arrow, left*). Also note normal variant pseudosubluxation of C2 on C3 at the top of the view of the sagittal image (*white arrow, left*)

6.4.2 Vertebral Clefts

Vertebral clefts may be oriented in the sagittal or coronal planes, may be complete or incomplete, and predominantly involve the thoracic and lumbar vertebrae. This normal variant with its typical configuration and well-defined sclerotic margins should not be confused with a fracture.

During fetal vertebral development, mesodermal cells surround the notochord, forming the centrum. The centrum then develops into the vertebral bodies. Other mesodermal cells form the vertebral arch, which develops into the vertebral posterior elements. The components of the centrum and posterior elements fuse from 3–5 years of age. The *sagittal cleft*, or *butterfly vertebra*, is one of several anomalous vertebral configurations that may result from variability in fusion; this variant is typically asymptomatic. In this type of cleft, a persistent notochordal cartilaginous plate separates the two lateral components of the vertebral body. This often results in both a widening of the vertebral body as well as a compensatory convexity in the endplates of the adjacent apposing vertebral bodies. The cleft is often incomplete, as in the provided example (Fig. 6.11), which can also lead to a wedge deformity. This wedge deformity can simulate a compression fracture; however, besides the characteristic midline appearance, a sagittal cleft (butterfly vertebra) can be differentiated from a fracture by the lack of prevertebral edema, the lack of cortical/endplate irregularity, and the symmetry on coronal images.

Coronal clefts are another type of anomaly that results from incomplete fusion. The anterior and posterior ossification centers remain separated by a vertically oriented cartilaginous plate. The radiolucent plate is in the mid-vertebral body or situated slightly posterior to the midportion, involving single or multiple vertebral bodies. These clefts are normally visualized during fetal development and usually resolve by 16 weeks of gestation. When persistent after birth, they are typically transient, are associated with prematurity and delayed vertebral maturation, and disappear by 6 months of life. However, these clefts have also been associated with chromosomal abnormalities and skeletal dysplasias.

Other congenital vertebral body anomalies that may be symptomatic, typically due to scoliosis, include lateral hemivertebra, dorsal hemivertebra, hypoplasia, and agenesis (asomia).

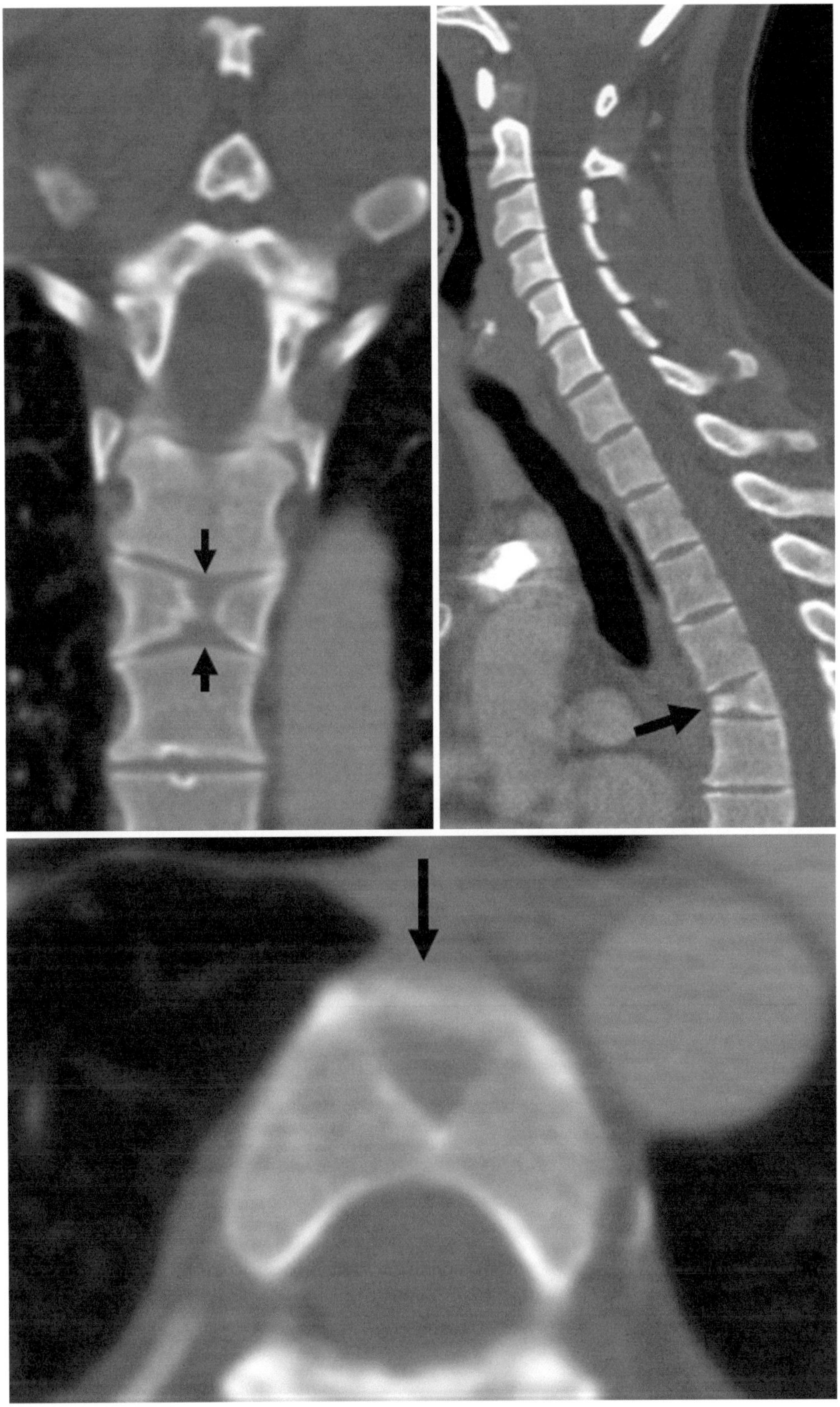

Fig. 6.11 A 34-year-old female underwent a CECT of the neck to evaluate for possible lymphadenopathy (negative). These coronal (*top left*), sagittal (*top right*), and axial (*bottom*) reconstructed images demonstrate a normal variant asymptomatic cleft T4 vertebra (*black arrows*). This sagittal cleft results in a butterfly appearance of the vertebra on coronal imaging, since the two lateral components of the vertebral body failed to fuse. There is associated loss of vertebral body height, most pronounced anteriorly, resulting in an anterior wedge deformity. Using solely sagittal reformats (*top right*), this could mimic an age-indeterminate compression fracture

6.5 Posterior Element Development

Variable genesis of the posterior vertebral elements may result in a wide variety of congenital anomalies, as the vertebral arch forms the pedicles, the transverse processes, the pars interarticularis (or articular pillar), the articular processes, the laminae, and the spinous processes.

Regarding the pedicles, although congenital abnormalities of the pedicles are more commonly encountered in the lumbar spine, they may also occur in the cervical or thoracic spine. The pedicles may simply fail to develop entirely, which can occur unilaterally or bilaterally. If present, an absent cervical pedicle is usually associated with other anomalies of the posterior elements, which range from displacement of the remaining posterior elements to dysplasia. Another variant is that the pedicles can also appear hypoplastic and thin, although this is most common in the lumbar region. They may also be short, elongated, or thickened. The phenomenon of *shortened pedicles* (so-called "short pedicle syndrome") can lead to congenital spinal canal narrowing, exacerbating the narrowing caused by degenerative disease. Clefts in the pedicles, termed *retrosomatic clefts* or *pediculolysis*, are thought to occur as a result of a prior fracture. Unilateral defects may be of no significance, while bilateral defects may lead to instability.

Regarding the transverse processes, there is variability in size, which may be associated with the presence or absence of variable rib development, particularly at transitional levels. For instance, in the setting of normal variant *11 paired ribs*, the transverse processes of T12 may be robust. These processes may be partially fused or incomplete and unilateral or bilateral. From T1 to T9, the thoracic vertebrae usually have a costal facet, while at levels below T10 the costal facet is variable. Note that the foramen transversarium is only present in the cervical vertebrae.

The articular pillar of the cervical spine may be traversed by a cleft that is analogous to the cleft of the pars interarticularis of the lumbar spine, although such defects are rare in the cervical vertebrae (Fig. 6.12). Both are referred to as *spondylolysis*, which is often a bilateral phenomenon.

Regarding the articular processes, these vary normally in morphology along the spinal column, transitioning most dramatically in the cervicothoracic and thoracolumbar regions. The differing orientations of the articular processes and their shape coincide with the variability of vertebral function at different levels. Aside from such regional variations, articular processes may be absent, hypoplastic, or fused. Fusion of the articular processes across adjacent levels is commonly observed in association with fusion of other posterior vertebral elements and the vertebral bodies.

Regarding the laminae, a lamina may also be absent, hypoplastic, or fused. Unilateral congenital anomalies of the laminae are often associated with other posterior element anomalies, such as *facet dysplasia* and *deviation of the spinous process*.

The spinous processes are usually midline in orientation, although mild variability from the midline is not uncommon. More dramatic deviation from the midline is more commonly observed in association with other congenital anomalies of the posterior elements. When the neural arch fails to fuse completely, this results in various forms of *spinal dysraphism*. Spinal dysraphism can be classified into open and closed forms, with a wide spectrum of severity and clinical significance. One of the closed forms, *spina bifida occulta* (SBO*)*, is the most frequently occurring and mildest form of spinal dysraphism, which is typically noted as an incidental finding; the vast majority are considered asymptomatic and "don't touch lesions." In this condition, the spinous processes and/or laminae are incompletely fused. As such, the defect in the posterior arch may be in the midline or off the midline. Although it is usually an incidental finding, SBO has been rarely reported as having an association with skin abnormalities, a tethered cord, or bowel or bladder symptoms. SBO commonly involves the transitional regions of the spine, usually the lumbosacral region, particularly L5 and S1. It can also involve the cervicothoracic region or other vertebral levels. In this mild failure of fusion of the neural arch, the result is an absent, incomplete, or unfused spinous process (Fig. 6.13). Other variants of the spinous processes include *hypoplasia* or a *persistent ossification center*. Such fusion anomalies should be readily identified by their well-defined margins and peripheral sclerosis, which distinguish these variants from fractures and other pathology.

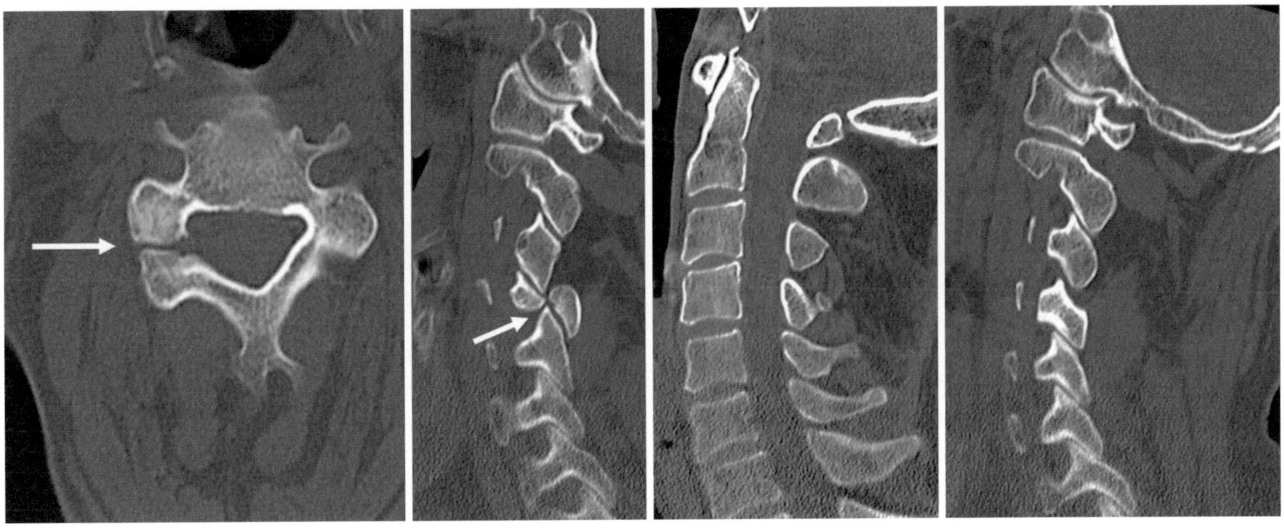

Fig. 6.12 A 51-year-old male underwent imaging of the cervical spine for acute trauma. Axial (*left*) and sagittal (*right three images*) NECT images of the cervical spine demonstrate a rare normal variant pars defect (*arrows*) of the cervical spine. In this patient, the aforementioned lucency (*arrows*) through the right articular pillar of C4 divides the superior and inferior articular processes. Note this variant's well-defined margins, which differentiate this normal variant from an acute fracture. Also, normal cervical spine alignment on the midline sagittal NECT image is seen with essentially normal alignment of the facets on the left side

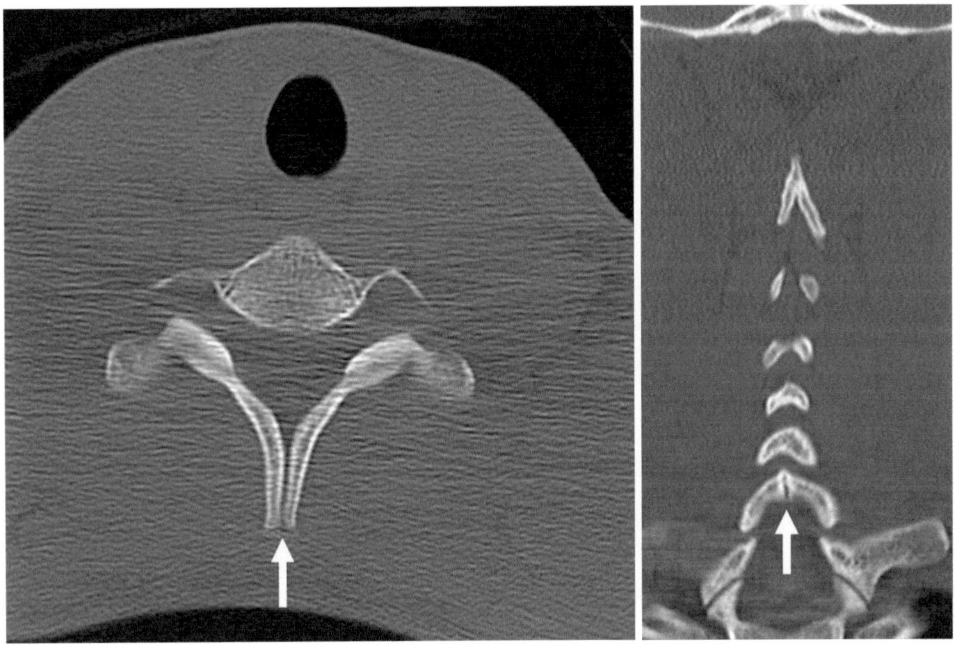

Fig. 6.13 A 17-year-old female underwent NECT imaging of the cervical spine in the setting of acute trauma. Axial (*left*) and coronal (*right*) reconstructed images show nonfusion of the posterior elements of C7 (*arrows*), also referred to as "spina bifida occulta" (SBO), which is more frequently observed within the lumbosacral region. The well-defined sclerotic cortical margins differentiate this normal variant from a fracture deformity

6.6 Atlantooccipital Assimilation and the Paracondylar Process

6.6.1 Atlantooccipital Assimilation

During development of the craniocervical junction, rarely there is a failure of segmentation between the fourth occipital and first cervical sclerotomes, resulting in a fused occiput and atlas. Although it is often described as occipitalization of the atlas, this condition is also referred to as *atlanto-occipital assimilation* (AOA), *nonsegmentation*, or fusion between the clivus, atlas (C1), or odontoid (C2). Although a relatively rare anomaly (described in several studies to be present in just under 1% of the population), AOA is the most common congenital malformation of the craniocervical junction. The degree of fusion is variable, potentially being unilateral or bilateral as well as either partial or complete. The condition is frequently associated with other congenital anomalies, including hypoplasia of the clivus and odontoid process, incomplete posterior arch of C1, fused cervical vertebrae, Chiari malformation, platybasia, and basilar invagination (Fig. 6.14).

While patients with AOA are often asymptomatic on initial presentation, they may present with neck stiffness, headache, or other more pronounced symptoms. In fact, when associated with additional fused cervical vertebrae, particularly C2 to C3 fusion, patients may be at increased risk of developing a myelopathy owing to atlantoaxial instability and compensatory motion at C1 to C2. Hence, while the presence of AOA is most commonly a "don't touch lesion" and most often is noted incidentally, it is important to make the neurologist or neurosurgeon aware of the craniovertebral junction fusion anomaly because the patient occasionally has associated symptoms when unstable, particularly after trauma. Hence, there is also the possibility of an increased risk for vertebral injury (fracture), subluxation, or spinal cord injury. This is particularly important to note if the patient has other congenital anomalies or associated subluxation.

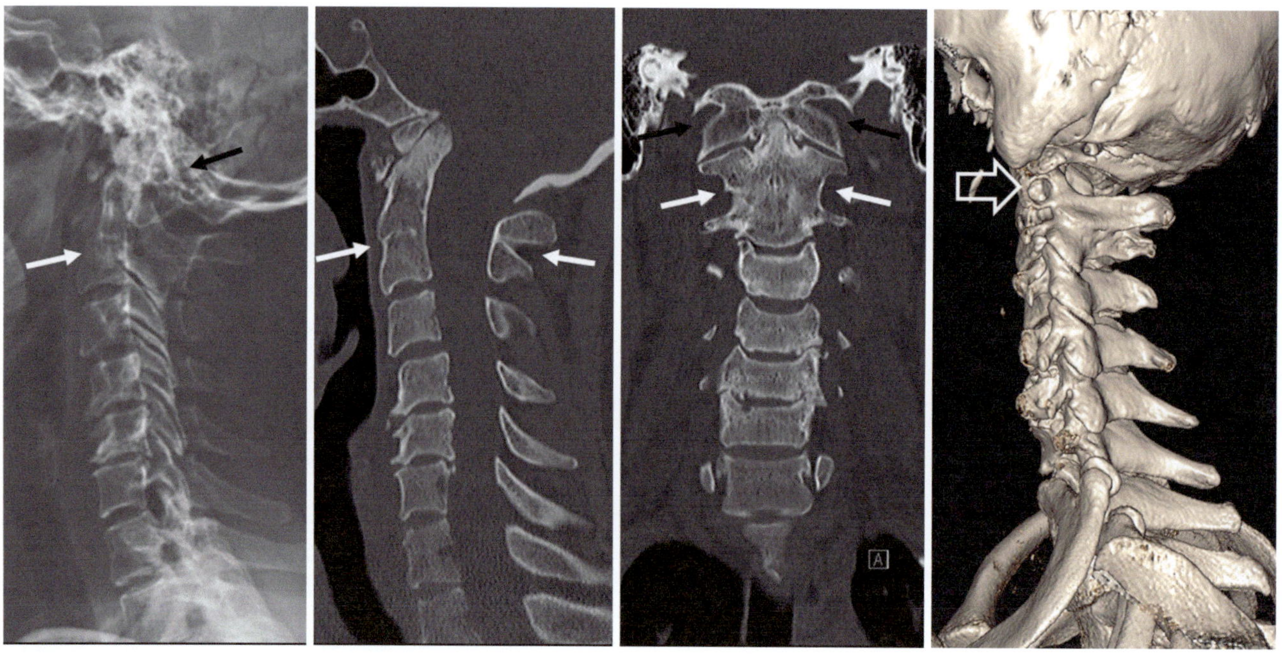

Fig. 6.14 A 43-year-old man with neck pain underwent imaging for a preoperative evaluation. This patient demonstrates multiple congenital fusion anomalies. Specifically, a lateral cervical spinal radiograph (*left*) and NECT images reconstructed in the sagittal (*left middle*) and coronal (*right middle*) planes demonstrate complete atlanto-occipital fusion (*black arrows*) as well as C2 and C3 fusion (*white arrows*). On the lateral radiograph, it is difficult to delineate the margins of the occipital condyles and the C1 vertebra, since they are fused. In this case of C2 and C3 fusion, the vertebral bodies and the posterior elements are fused bilaterally. Careful attention to such fusion anomalies also ensures accurate cervical vertebral numbering. Three-dimensional reconstructions (*right*) from the NECT data also nicely depict the fusion across multiple levels. The three-dimensional reconstructions also show that this patient has a normal variant arcuate foramen (*open white arrow, right*)

6.6.2 Paracondylar Process

The *paracondylar process* is another variant of craniocervical development, having a prevalence of less than 1%. Being along the spectrum of atlanto-occipital assimilation, this variant is derived from the fourth occipital or first cervical sclerotome. Since it may be variable in size, the paracondylar process may be an isolated bone fragment. Alternatively, the accessory process may fuse with the transverse process of the atlas (C1). When large enough, it may form an accessory joint with the occiput (Fig. 6.15). Larger processes are rarer than their smaller counterparts and tend to be unilateral. In contrast, smaller tubercles are more likely to be bilateral.

Despite being usually asymptomatic, this typically normal variant has been occasionally associated with headaches, neck pain, and restricted craniocervical rotation. The larger processes tend to be more frequently associated with symptoms. While it is usually treated conservatively, curative surgical resection has been reported to be necessary in rare cases.

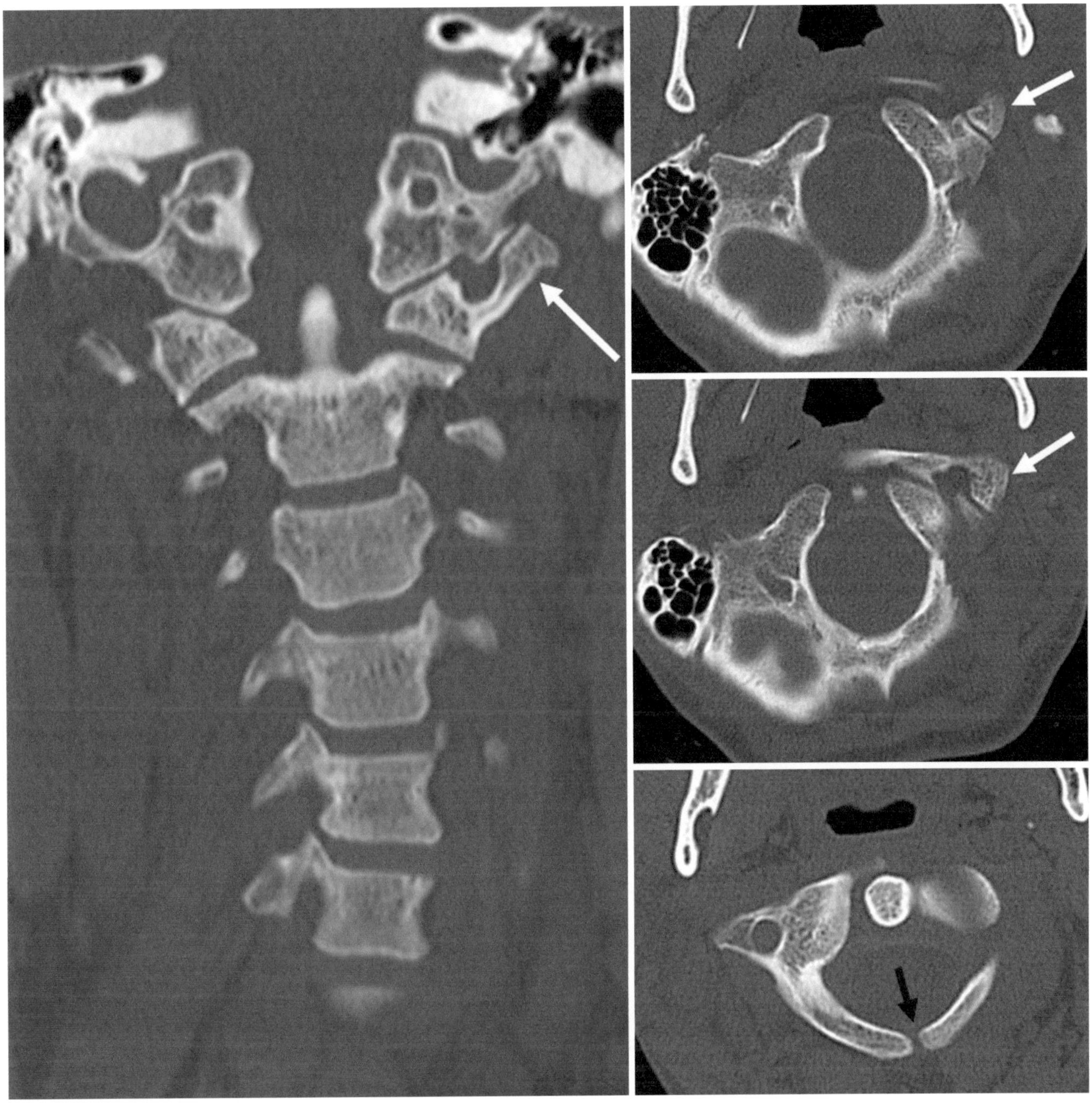

Fig. 6.15 In this 35-year-old male who underwent imaging for acute trauma, coronal (*left*) and axial (*right side: top, middle, and bottom*) NECT images illustrate a unilateral paracondylar process (*white arrows*) on the left side, which is fused with the transverse process of the atlas and articulating with the occiput. Also note normal variant incomplete fusion of the posterior arch of C1 (*black arrow, right bottom*). There was no fracture present

6.6.3 Development of the Atlas (C1)

Knowledge of the development of the atlas is important to avoid confusing normal variant or "don't touch" findings with fractures. The development of the atlas is complex, with thirteen different types and subtypes of ossification patterns described in the literature. Brief descriptions of the normal ossification of the axis and atlas are given below.

Typically, the atlas (C1) forms from three primary ossification centers, one forming the anterior arch and two forming the lateral masses and posterior arch. However, occasionally the anterior arch is formed from two ossification centers. Also, rarely, an additional ossification center may contribute to forming the posterior tubercle.

Ossification of the atlas begins in the lateral masses and progresses posteriorly during the second month of gestation, usually remaining incomplete at birth. The remainder of the posterior arch normally ossifies by 4 years of age.

Ossification of the anterior arch generally follows a more protracted course, typically occurring between 5 and 8 years of age and completing by the age of 10 years (Fig. 6.16). Although anterior arch anomalies are less common than posterior arch anomalies, in some patients the anterior arch never completely fuses. Notably, the process of ossification is also not always symmetric.

Congenital anomalies of the posterior arch of C1 range from clefts to complete agenesis (Figs. 6.17, 6.18 and 6.19). The posterior arch of C1 may be hypoplastic or short and can result in cervical spinal canal stenosis (Fig. 6.20). One theory explaining posterior arch hypoplasia describes premature posterior fusion resulting from failure of dorsal expansion of the two lateral primary ossification centers of C1. Although it is most commonly asymptomatic and akin to the phenomenon of congenital spinal canal stenosis at other levels, *congenital C1 spinal canal stenosis* may predispose the spinal cord to compression secondary to spondylosis or trauma. This may ultimately lead to cervical myelopathy. When atraumatic, this may be treated by posterior decompression, even including removal of the posterior arch of C1.

The location and well-defined sclerotic margins of such congenital defects and awareness of the process of C1 ossification should aid in avoiding mistaking such congenital variants for traumatic injury, as the vast majority of these variants in anterior or posterior C1 arch fusion are asymptomatic and considered "don't touch lesions." Additional helpful findings include a lack of associated soft-tissue swelling and a lack of displacement. Such congenital defects are sometimes referred to as pseudofractures. In the uncommon case of congenital stenosis caused by C1 arch hypoplasia/shortening, the lack of spinal cord compression suggests that the hypoplasia is an incidental finding.

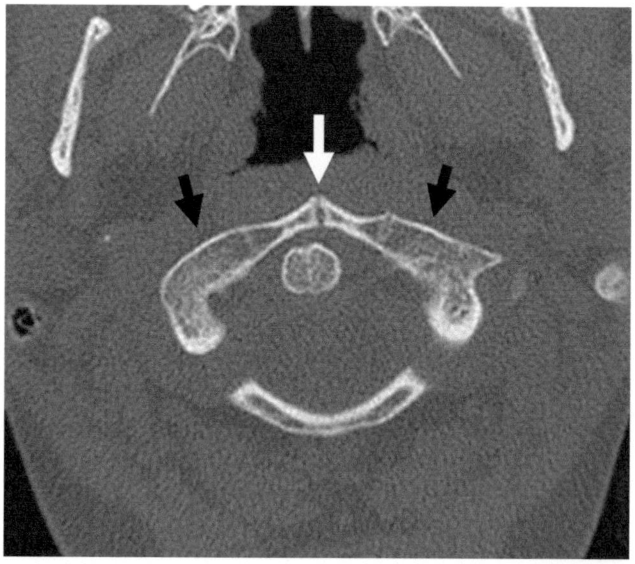

Fig. 6.16 An axial NECT image shows normal variant developing ossification of the anterior arch of C1 in this 5-year-old boy. In this case, the two ossification centers that originated within the anterior arch have not yet completely fused at the midline (*white arrow*), nor have they entirely fused with the ossification sites extending from the lateral masses (*black arrows*). There is also normal variant slight asymmetry of C1 relative to C2 secondary to craniocervical rotation

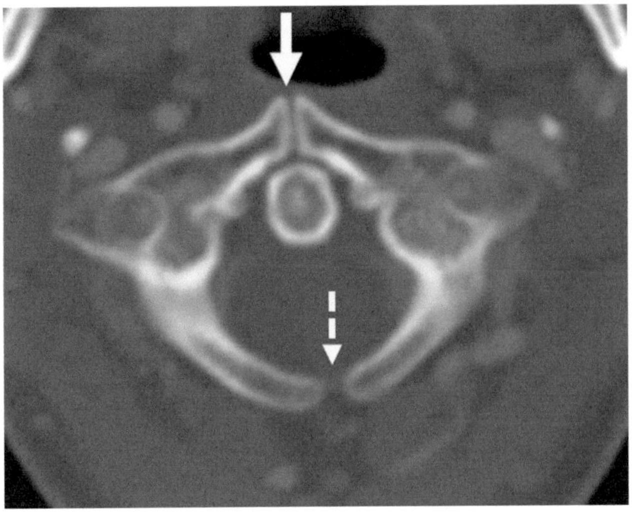

Fig. 6.17 A 51-year-old female underwent CECT imaging of the neck for evaluation of the salivary glands. An axial image shows incidental, normal variant nonfusion of the anterior arch of C1 (*white arrow*) as well as normal variant nonfusion of the posterior arches (*dashed arrow*). The well-defined and sclerotic cortex along the margins of the opposing nonfused components differentiate these normal variants from true fracture deformities

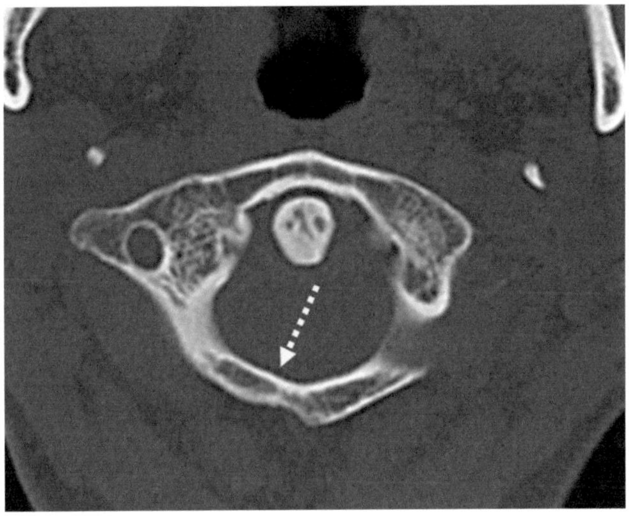

Fig. 6.18 A 48-year-old female who underwent NECT imaging of the cervical spine for upper extremity paresthesias. An axial image shows a mildly hypoplastic posterior arch of C1, which is thinner on the right side (*dotted arrow*)

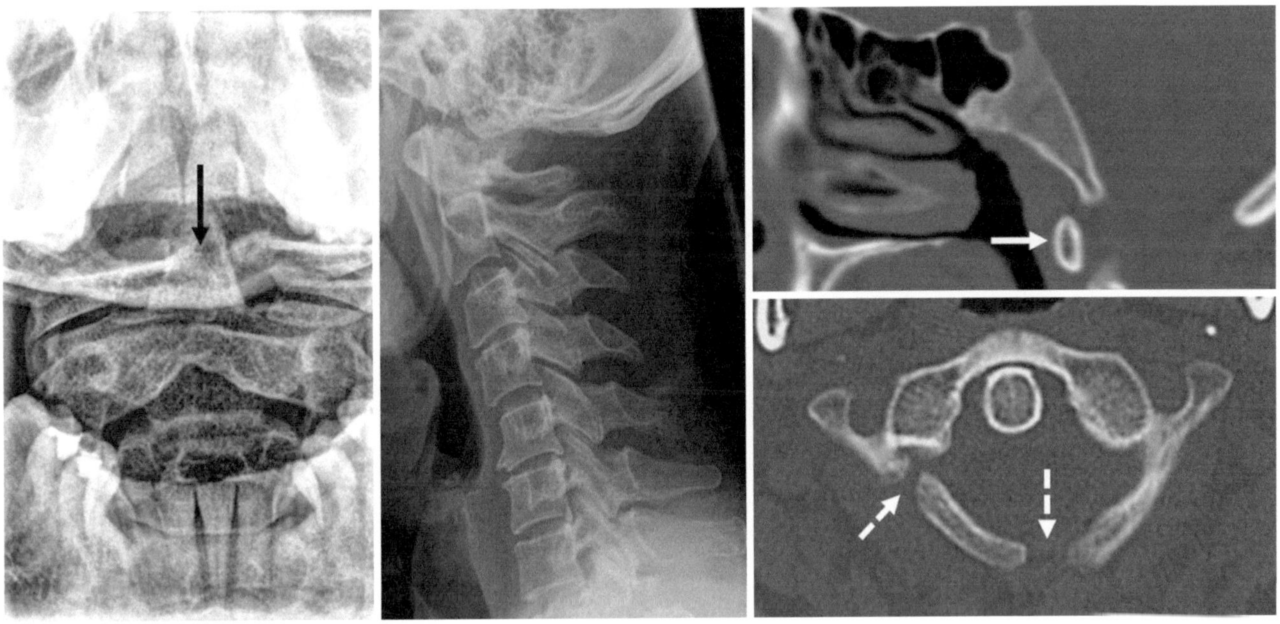

Fig. 6.19 A 49-year-old female with a normal variant incomplete posterior arch of the atlas (C1). On the odontoid view radiograph *(left)*, there is a lucent defect in the midline of the atlas (*black arrow*). The well-defined margins of the defect as well as the normal orientation of C1 on C2 are consistent with an incomplete arch. The incomplete arch is rather subtle on the lateral radiograph *(middle)*. A parasagittal NECT image (*right, top*) depicts the anterior arch of C1 (*white arrow*), but no posterior elements of C1 are present in this imaging plane. The axial NECT image (*right, bottom*) shows the incompletely ossified posterior arch at two different sites posteriorly (*dotted arrows*), further clarifying that this is a normal variant that should not be misinterpreted as a fracture

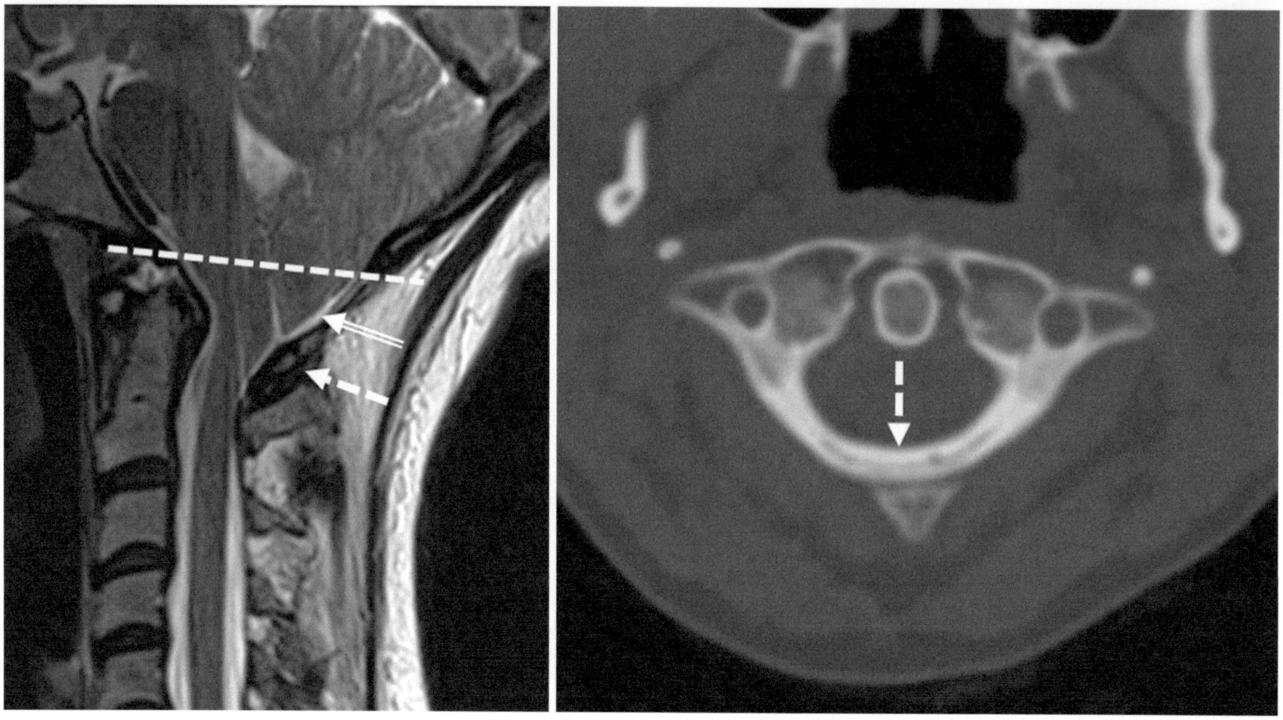

Fig. 6.20 A 31-year-old male with worsening headaches and a short posterior arch of C1 (*dashed arrows* in both images). A sagittal SET2WI MRI of the cervical spine demonstrates what would typically be normal variant mild narrowing of the cervical spinal canal at C1. However, in addition to the variant (typically "don't touch") short posterior arch of C1, this patient also exhibits features of a Chiari 1 malformation, including a small posterior fossa and cerebellar tonsillar ectopia. The cerebellar tonsils (*beveled arrow, left*) are displaced inferiorly through the foramen magnum, being situated about 1.3 cm below the basion-opisthion line (as delineated by the *dashed white line, left*). There is associated crowding of the craniocervical junction. An axial NECT image (*right*) shows the narrow spinal canal at the level of C1. Thus, in the setting of the patient's worsening headaches and the presence of a Chiari 1 malformation, this patient would likely undergo a suboccipital craniectomy (and potentially a C1 posterior arch laminectomy) to decompress the posterior fossa malformation

6.6.4 Development of the Axis (C2)

The axis (C2) normally develops from a total of six separate ossification centers and four synchondroses. It arguably possesses the most complex development of the vertebrae. Before birth, the odontoid forms from two separate ossification centers. At birth, the axis (C2) has four ossification centers: one for the odontoid process, one for the body, and two (one on each side) for the neural arch. Usually between 3 and 6 years of age, the body of the odontoid fuses with the odontoid process; when this ossification center fails to fuse and remains independent, it is referred to as an *os odontoideum*. The os odontoideum variant is usually well-defined, variable in size, and more commonly asymptomatic, but it can predispose to injury. With this normal variant there is often subluxation of the os odontoideum relative to the body of C2. There is also often associated compensatory thickening of the anterior arch of C1, especially with increasing age; this helps to delineate a chronic congenital os odontoideum from a type II dens fracture. Although this variant is most commonly asymptomatic and thus a "don't touch lesion," the failure of complete fusion of the os odontoideum and an associated risk of subluxation in acute trauma increase the likelihood of cord injury with this variant.

At about the same time as the body of the odontoid fuses with the odontoid process, a secondary ossification center termed the *os terminale* develops at the apex of the odontoid process. This secondary ossification center usually fuses with the odontoid process by 12 years of age. When it fails to fuse, it is called a *persistent ossiculum terminale* (or Bergmann ossicle). Awareness of this variant is critical, since it can be mistaken for a type I dens fracture. Hence the location, appearance, and patient age distinguish this normal variant from a true fracture of C2 (odontoid tip).

It is also important to note that the neural arches of the axis normally fuse with one another by about 2–3 years of age. The neural arches then fuse with the vertebral body by about 3–6 years of age. As with the atlas (C1), normal variant incomplete fusion of the posterior neural arches of C2 can also mimic a fracture (Figs. 6.21, 6.22, 6.23 and 6.24).

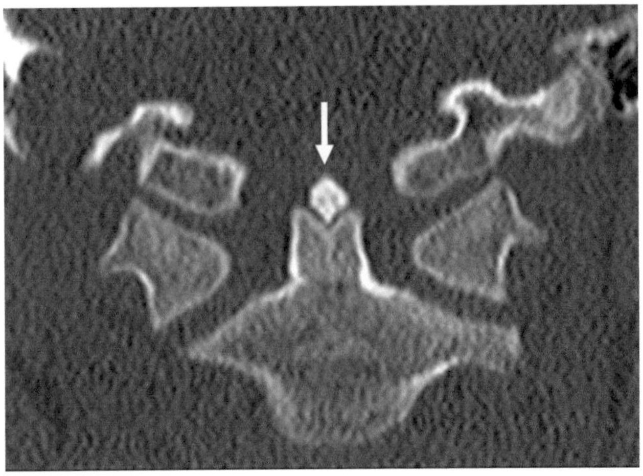

Fig. 6.21 A 6-year-old boy undergoing imaging of the paranasal sinuses for possible sinusitis. A coronal reconstruction from a NECT examination in a plane through the anterior craniocervical junction shows incidental normal ossification of the tip of the odontoid. The odontoid has fused normally with the body of C2, usually occurring between 3 and 6 years of age. At the same time, the secondary ossification center for the tip of the odontoid, the *os terminale* (*arrow*), forms. The os terminale usually fuses with the dens by approximately 12 years of age. If it persists into adulthood, it is termed a *persistent ossiculum terminale*

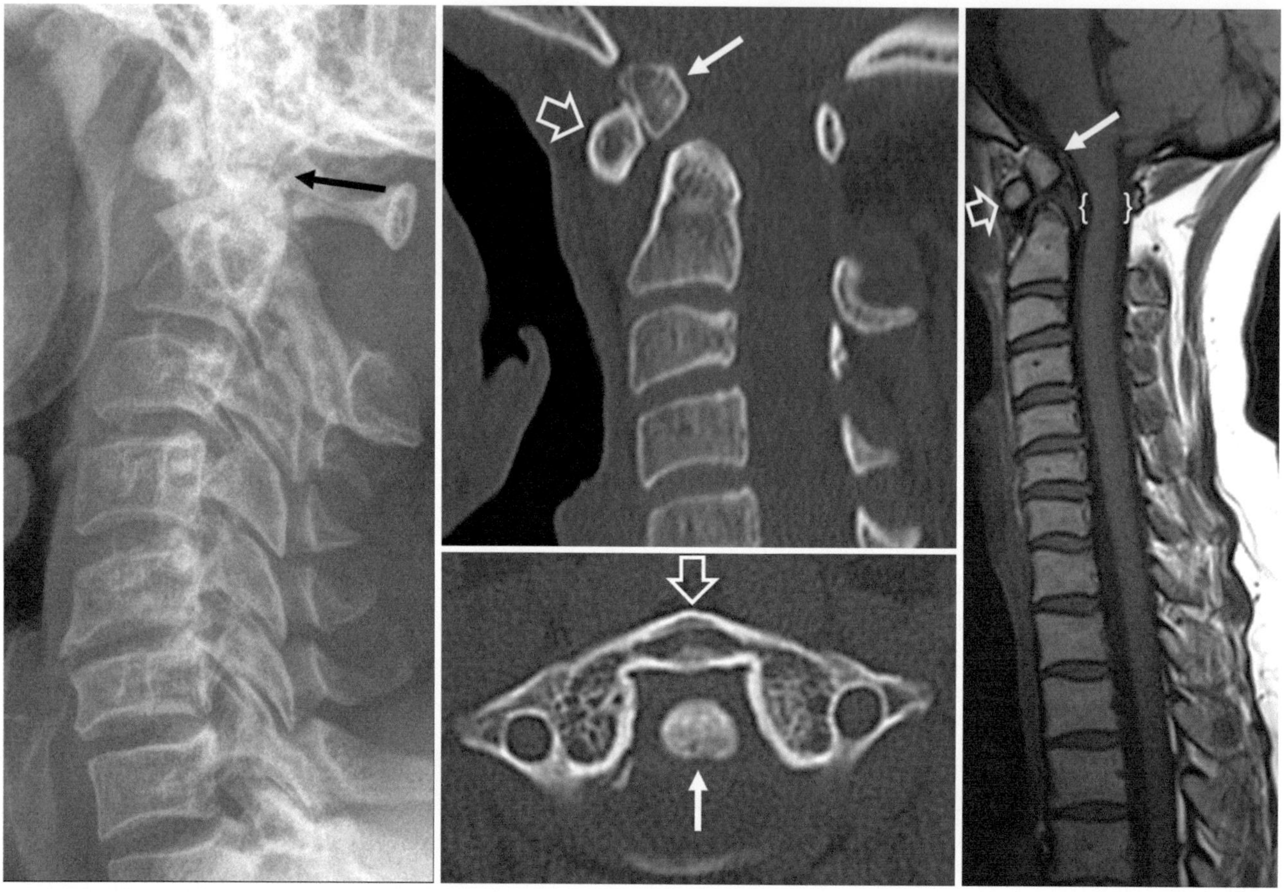

Fig. 6.22 A 45-year-old female underwent imaging of the spine following a motor vehicle collision. The lateral cervical spine radiograph (*left*) shows a subtle lucency (*black arrow*) at the base of the odontoid. On NECT sagittal (*middle, top image*) and axial (*middle, bottom image*) reconstructions, the well-defined margins and bulky (or thickened) anterior arch of C1 (*open white arrows*) together suggest an os odontoideum variant (*white arrows*) rather than a true fracture; the well-defined cortical margins of the os and the upper body of C2 are also identifying characteristics. These NECT images also show the compensatory hypertrophy of the anterior arch of C1 (*open white arrows*) in better detail. On MRI, a sagittal SET1WI (*right*) of the cervical spine depicts these same features. Note the narrowing of the upper cervical spinal canal (between *brackets, right*) secondary to the altered morphology of the upper cervical spine with anterior subluxation of the os odontoideum (*white arrow, right*). This patient also had focal myelomalacia of the upper cervical spinal cord, best demonstrated on SET2WI (*not shown*). This case demonstrates that although an os odontoideum is more commonly a "don't touch lesion," it can be associated with instability and occasionally predispose to cord injury in the setting of trauma

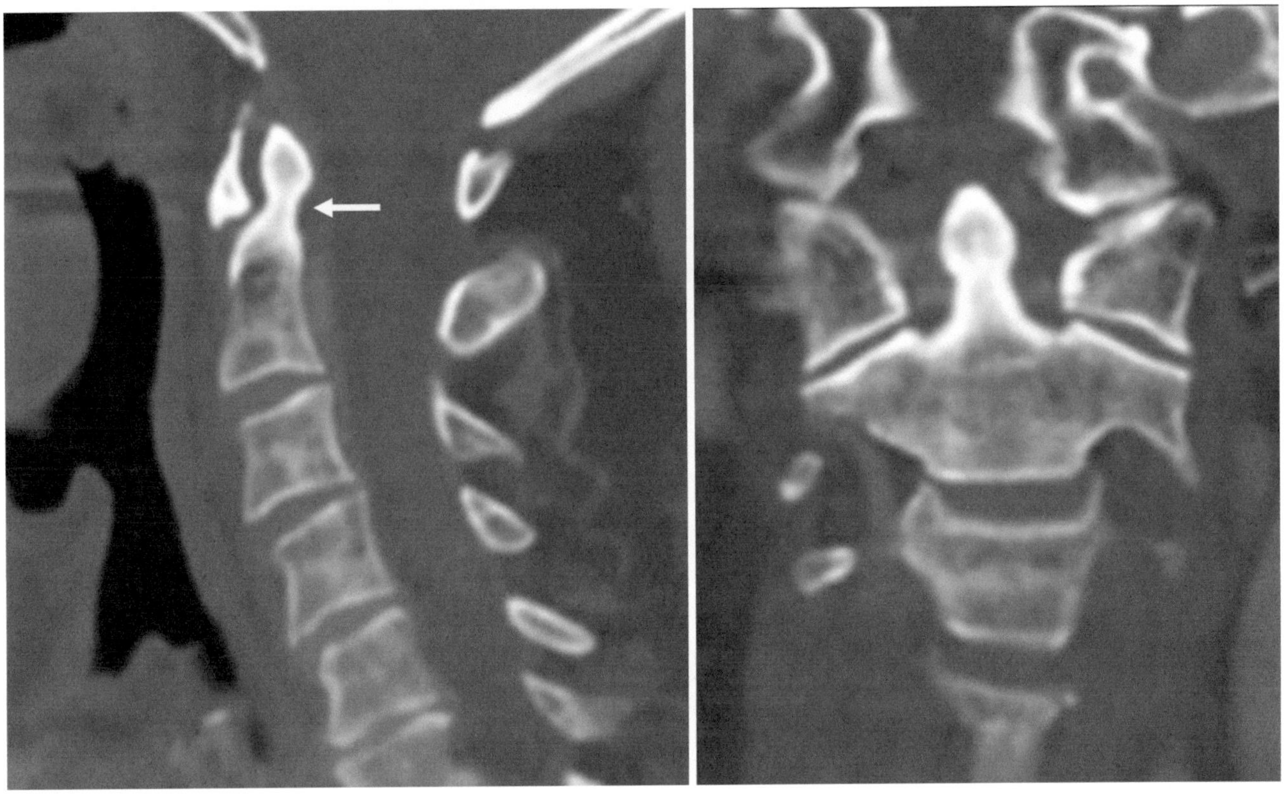

Fig. 6.23 A 50-year old male undergoing imaging of the neck for follow-up of head and neck cancer. Sagittal (*left*) and coronal (*right*) CECT images through the upper cervical spine show normal variant congenital hypoplasia (mild) of the odontoid process. A normally formed odontoid process would not show the "waist" (*arrow, left*) of the base of the dens seen here

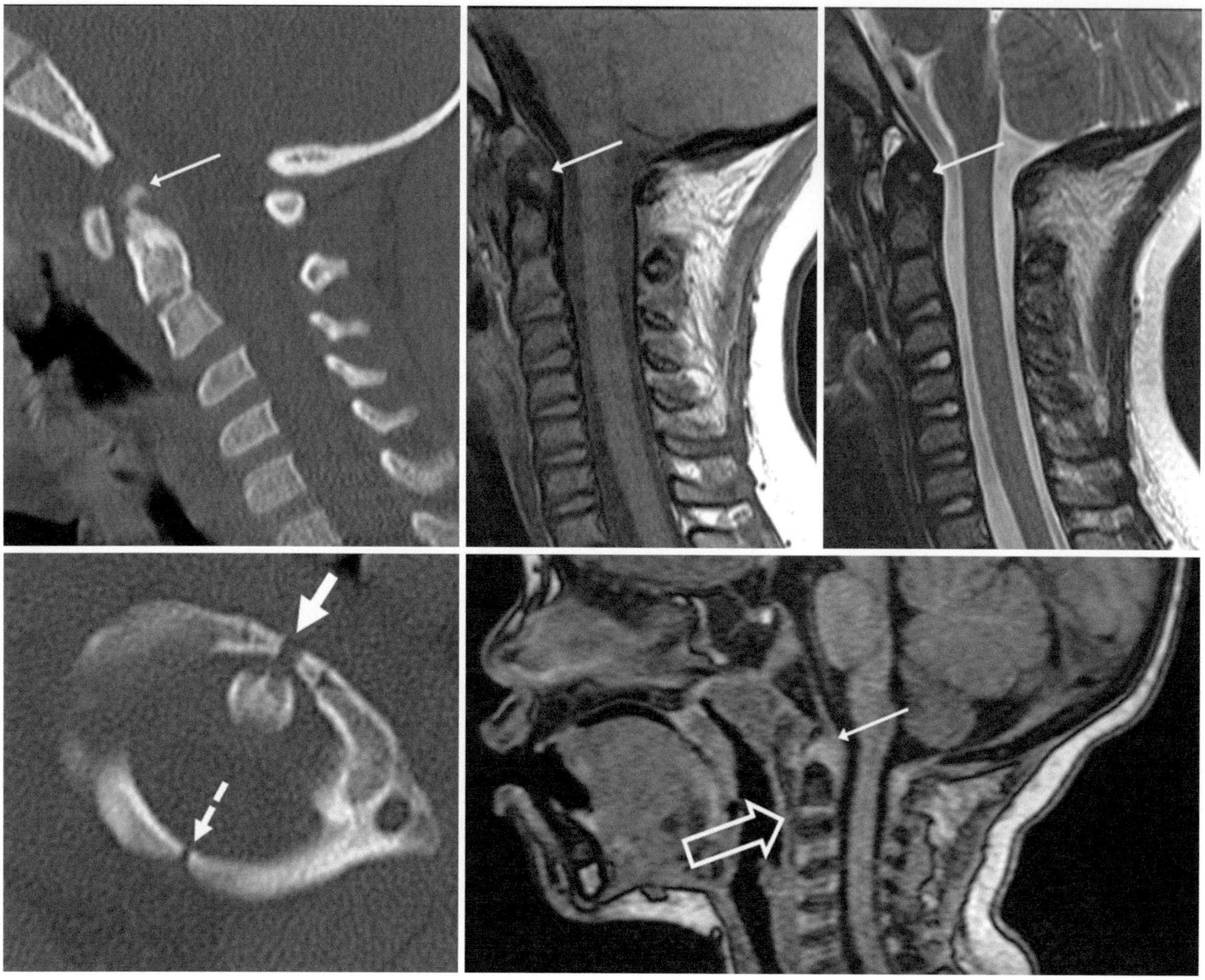

Fig. 6.24 Normal synchondroses and os terminale were found in a young male who underwent imaging of his head and cervical spine on separate occasions. On sagittal (*top left*) and axial NECT (*bottom left*) images of the cervical spine, there is normal cervical spine development where both the anterior arch (*thick white arrow*) and posterior arch (*dashed arrow*) are not yet fused at 4.5 years of age. Similarly, the base of the dens has not yet fused with the body of C2, which is normal at this age; hence, the os terminale (*thin arrow*, *top left*) has only recently formed and is expected to completely fuse with the odontoid by the age of 12 years. An MRI with sagittal SET1WI (*top middle*) and T2WI (*top right*) of the cervical spine, also performed at 4.5 years of age, further depicts normal development; note only very little central marrow signal within the os terminale on both sequences (*thin white arrows*). Notably, a prior sagittal T1WI MR image through the craniocervical junction performed earlier at 2.5 years of age (*bottom right*) shows normal absence of the os terminale (*thin arrow*), or it is quite tiny and hardly visible; the dens is also not yet fused with the C2 vertebral body, as depicted by the normal synchondrosis (*open white arrow*)

6.6.5 Vertebral Artery Dominance and Foraminal Variation

Regarding the vertebral arteries (VAs), the left VA (LVA) is dominant in 50% of patients, while the right VA (RVA) is dominant in 25%; the VAs are codominant (i.e., nearly equal in size) in the remaining 25% of patients. The V1 segment of the vertebral artery extends from its origin to the point where it enters the cervical transverse foramina, beginning its V2 segment. After the VA exits the transverse foramen at the level of the C2 vertebra, it courses superiorly as the V3 segment, usually also crossing the transverse foramen of C1; it becomes the V4 segment as it extends intracranially once it crosses the atlanto-occipital membrane.

As the VA courses superiorly from its origin, its V2 segment usually courses through the transverse foramina of the cervical vertebrae from the levels of C6 up through C2. However, there is notable variation, as the VA may also enter the transverse foramina at a level other than C6 in less than 15% of cases (so-called anomalous vertebral artery entry). For instance, the VA may enter the transverse foramen at C7, C5, or even above the level of C5; the frequency progressively decreases the higher the cervical level. Of note, the presence of a transverse foramen at a particular level, for instance at C7, does not imply that the VA traverses or travels within that particular foramen; this also holds true for the vertebral veins (VVs). In fact, the VA may bypass multiple transverse foramina before beginning its V2 segment. Another important anatomic consideration is that the perivertebral venous plexus and the sympathetic nerve plexus also course within the transverse foramina.

There is considerable variability in the size of the transverse foramina that can vary between sides regardless of the size of the VA. In one study, the mean anteroposterior and transverse dimensions of the transverse foramina measured 5.7 x 5.2 mm on the right and 5.9 x 5.1 mm on the left. The transverse foramina also tend to be smaller more superiorly (i.e., more cephalad). A correlation between the size of the transverse foramen and the corresponding VA has been described, although there is not always a direct or clear correlation. It is also important to consider that a tortuous or dolichoectatic loop of the VA in association with a larger transverse foramen may result in thinning of the adjacent bony pedicle, although such a tortuous loop is typically a normal variant that may progress with age. There is debate as to whether such loops, when extending into an adjacent neural foramen, predispose to development of a cervical radiculopathy. These can simulate lytic neoplasms. Less common (and pathologic) causes of transverse foraminal enlargement include nerve sheath tumors, meningiomas, lytic metastases, arteriovenous malformations, and aortic coarctation.

Regarding the presence of accessory transverse foramina, it is important to mention certain other anatomic considerations. The transverse foramen (or foramen transversarium) is the foramen situated in the transverse process of the cervical vertebrae, formed as the costal bar fuses with the vertebral body and transverse process. This foramen plays an important role, usually transmitting the VA, VVs, or plexi and sympathetic nerves, which often are divided from each other by a fibrous band; however, vasculature does not necessarily have to be located within these foramina.

Occasionally, a normal variant *accessory transverse foramen* may be identified. When present, it is smaller and typically situated posterior to the primary foramen and is usually more lateral. Although this variant is most commonly located at the level of C6, accessory foramina may be in adjacent vertebrae, may be incomplete, and may be unilateral or bilateral. The incidence of structures coursing through the accessory transverse foramina has not yet been comprehensively studied. Nevertheless, it is important to consider the possibility of an accessory or fenestrated VA coursing through the accessory transverse foramen, particularly in the setting of surgery or intervention. In this regard, the VA develops from the intersegmental arteries. While the seventh intersegmental arteries contribute to the formation of the VA, a series of anastomoses connecting the second to sixth cervical intersegmental arteries fuse to develop the majority of the VAs. Hence, incomplete intersegmental artery occlusion is postulated as the source of persistent VA duplication-fenestration (Figs. 6.25, 6.26, 6.27 and 6.28).

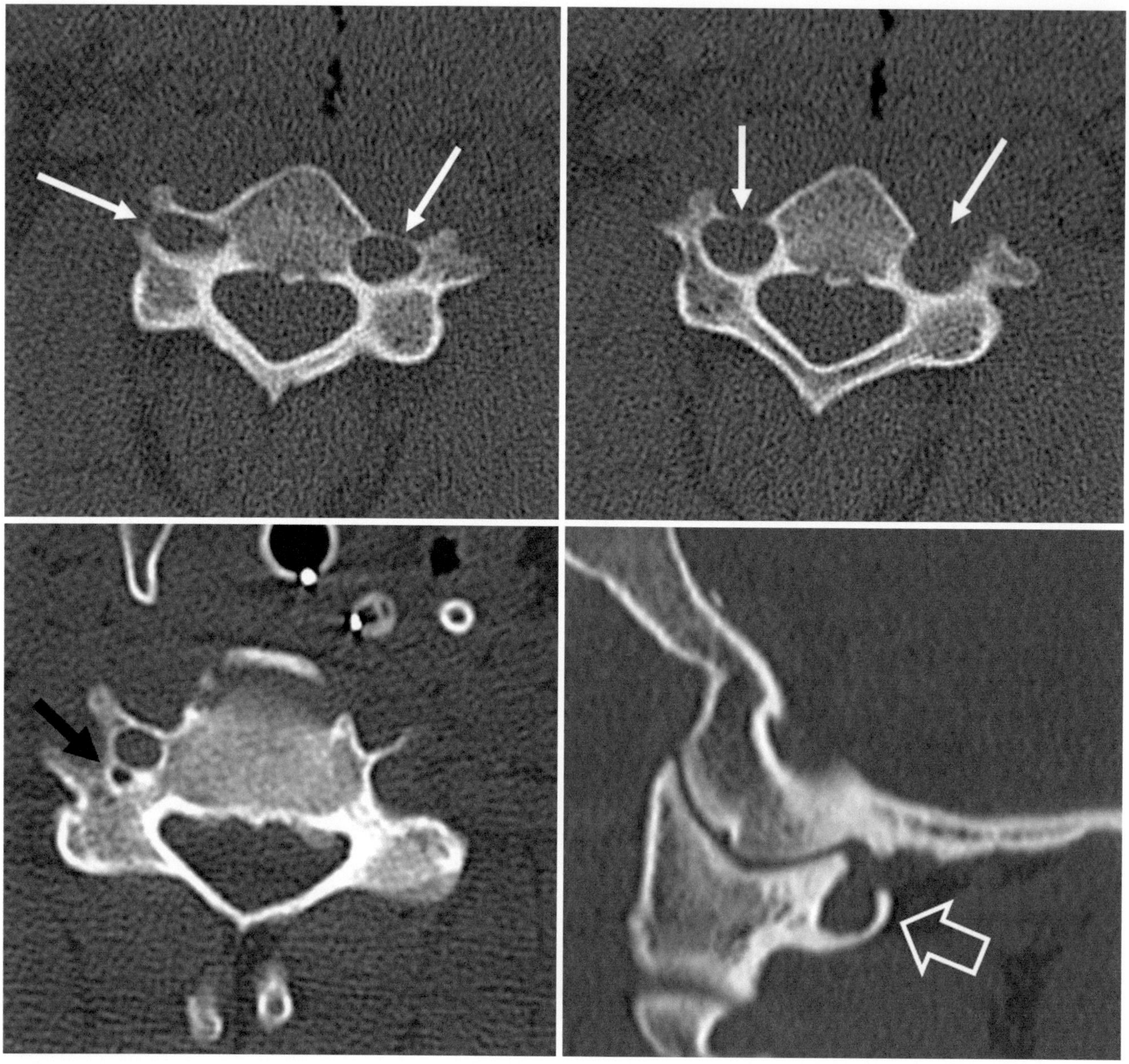

Fig. 6.25 A 38-year-old male underwent a NECT of the cervical spine in the setting of trauma. Three contiguous axial images (*top row and bottom left*) show normal variant enlargement of the transverse foramina of C3 bilaterally (*white arrows*). There is also a normal variant accessory transverse foramen on the right at C5 (*black arrow, bottom left*). Additionally, note that on the sagittal reconstructed image (*bottom right*), selected through the right side of C1, there is normal variant partial ossification of the atlanto-occipital ligament that results in an incomplete ponticulus posticus with a partially formed arcuate foramen (*open arrow*)

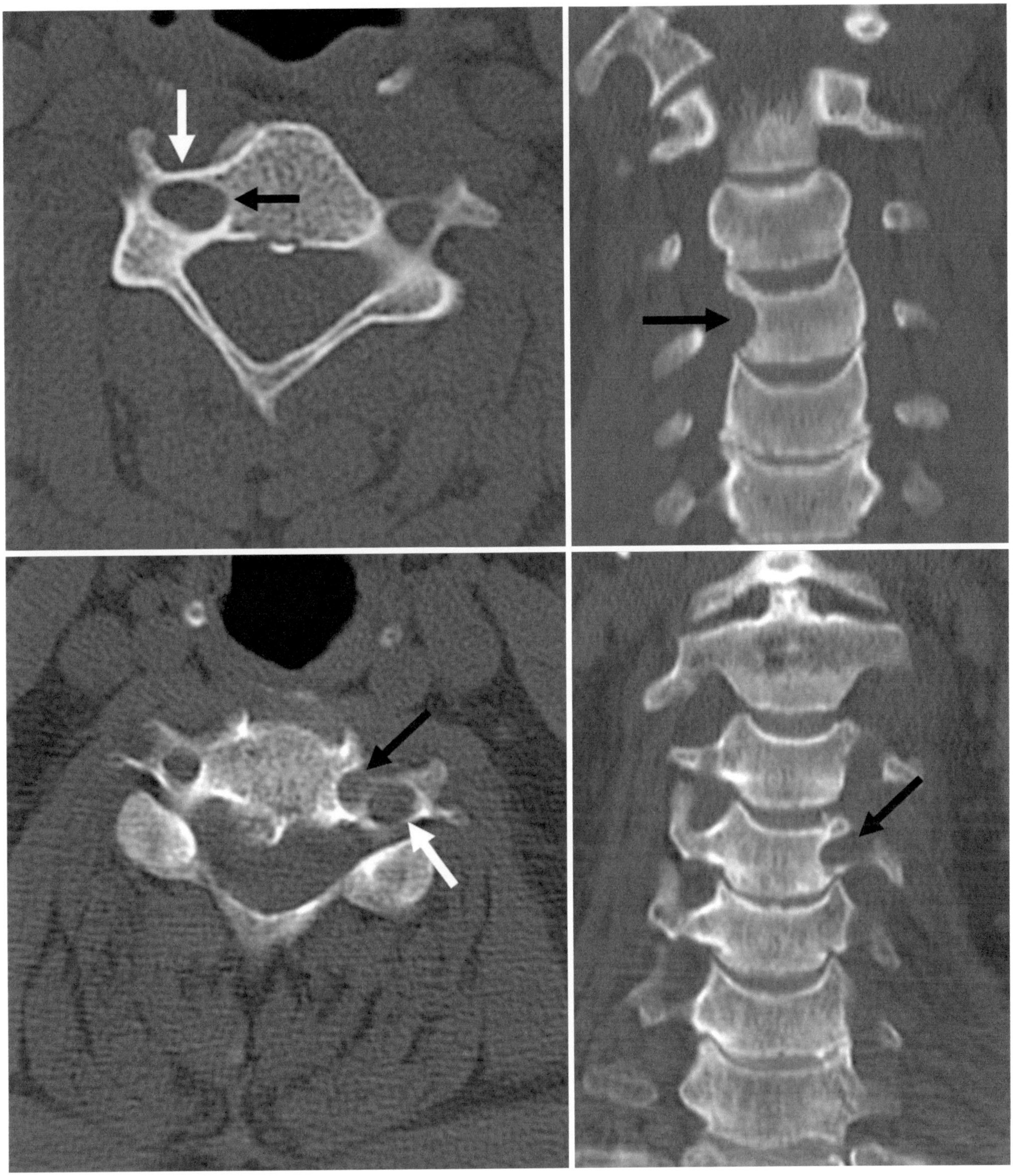

Fig. 6.26 Two different patients with tortuous vertebral arteries (VAs) that loop into the vertebral body. **Top row:** A 47-year-old male who underwent NECT imaging of the cervical spine in the setting of trauma. On axial (*left*) and sagittal (*right*) reconstructions, note the normal asymmetric enlargement of the right transverse foramen of C4 (*white arrow*, *left*) accommodating a focally tortuous right VA. This normal variant enlarged transverse foramen also results in normal variant scalloping of the right lateral C4 vertebral body (*black arrows*). **Bottom row:** In a 68-year-old male evaluated for trauma, a NECT was negative for fracture but axial (*left*) and coronal (*right*) reformats depicted a loop of the left VA scalloping and looping into the left side of the C4 vertebral body (*black arrows*); this simulated a lytic lesion on axial images because the loop initially appeared to be separate from the transverse foramen (*white arrow, left*) on axial images. This shows how a tortuous VA can occasionally simulate a lytic lesion

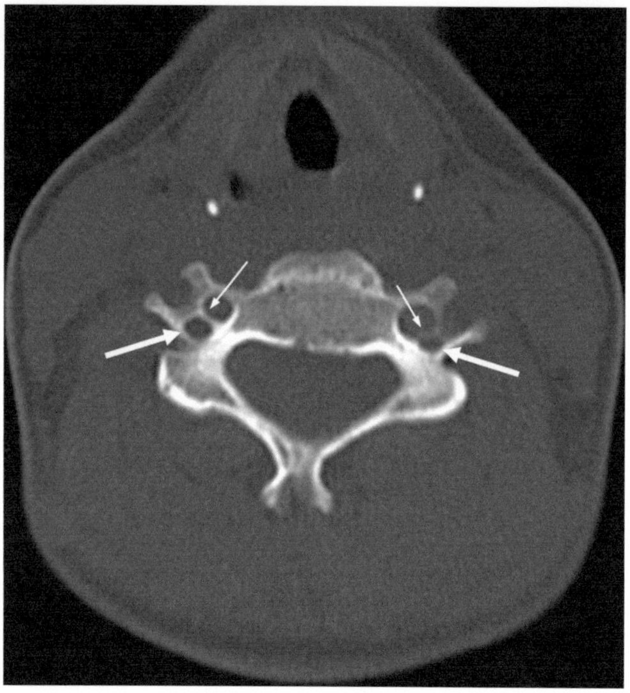

Fig. 6.27 A 21-year-old female who underwent NECT imaging of the cervical spine in the setting of trauma. An axial CT image shows normal variant accessory transverse foramina of C5 bilaterally (*white arrows*). Note the thin osseous septations (*thin arrows*) separating the primary transverse foramina (located more anteriorly) from the adjacent accessory foramina (more posterior)

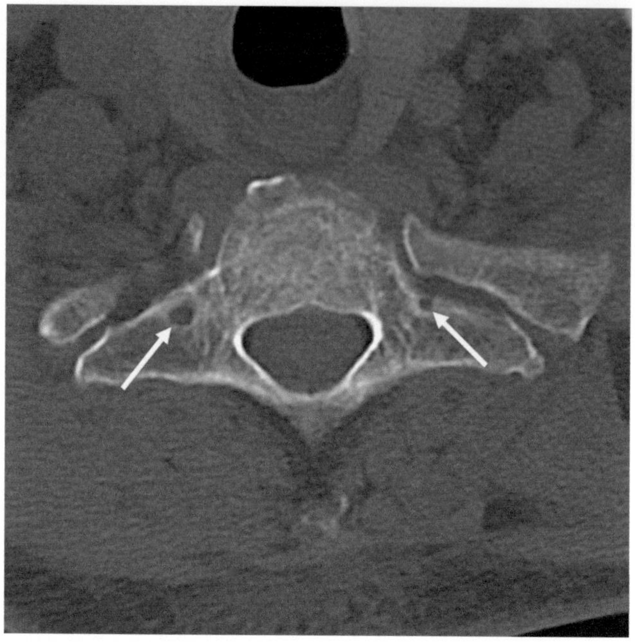

Fig. 6.28 A 72-year-old male underwent NECT imaging of the cervical spine in the setting of trauma. There are bilateral normal variant hypoplastic transverse foramina of T1 (*arrows*); typically, the T1 vertebra does not have transverse foramina. In this patient, the vertebral arteries do not course through these foramina. Also, note the osteoporotic appearance of the T1 vertebra and adjacent ribs

6.6.6 Arcuate Foramen (Foramen of C1)

Normally, the V3 segment of the VA courses along a groove located on the superolateral surface of the posterior arch of the atlas (*C1*). Superior to the VA, as it courses along this groove, the oblique atlanto-occipital ligament forms a bridge over the artery. Ossification of this atlanto-occipital ligament results in the formation of the *ponticulus posticus*, which is Latin for "little posterior bridge." This normal variant arch may be partial or complete; when complete, it creates a horizontally oriented foramen of C1 (Fig. 6.29). The foramen is sometimes called the Kimmerle anomaly, atlantal posterior foramen, foramen sagittale, foramen arcuale atlantis, or the preferred term, *arcuate foramen*. There is wide variability of its reported incidence. It occurs in roughly 5% to 35% of individuals, in whom it is more readily identified on CT than on plain radiographs; this variable incidence also depends on whether the foramen is considered "partial" or "complete" (i.e., fully and circumferentially formed). Notably, the degree of ossification of the ponticulus posticus may vary from side to side, leading to the possibility of a partially formed ipsilateral arcuate foramen with a fully formed contralateral arcuate foramen. When the arcuate foramen is incomplete with a partially ossified ponticulus posticus, this normal variant may simulate a fracture; such pseudofractures can be confusing, particularly when there is normal segmentation of the incompletely formed ponticulus posticus (Figs. 6.30 and 6.31).

While this is typically an asymptomatic normal variant, it is important to avoid injury to the VA trapped in the foramen in the setting of surgical planning, particularly for atlantoaxial instrumentation. In addition to careful review of preprocedural imaging, adequate lateral dissection and surgical exposure by the surgeon might help avoid mistaking the presence of this variant for a broad posterior arch of the atlas. In addition to the possible surgical implications, the presence of an arcuate foramen has also been reported in association with cervicogenic headache and as a possible cause of traumatic VA dissection, particularly in children.

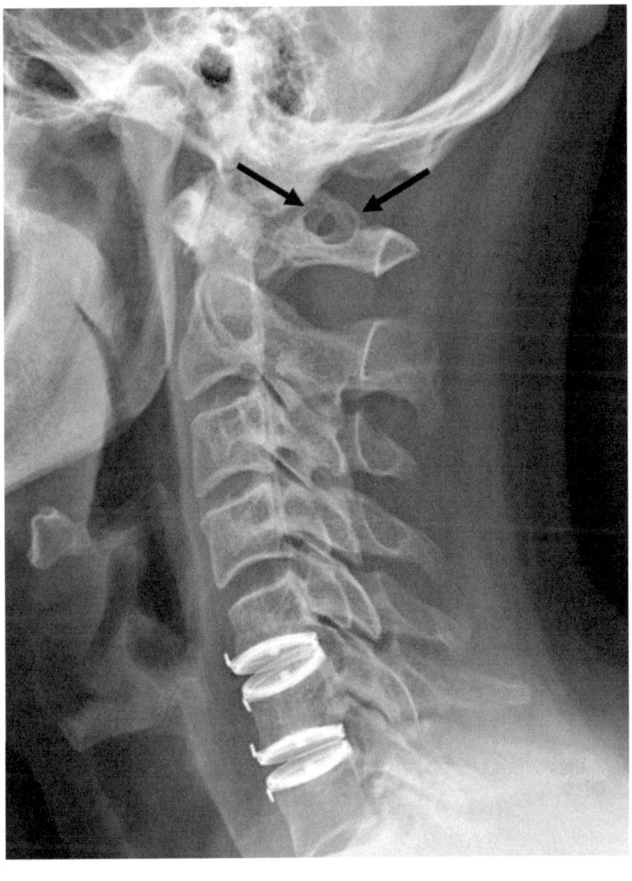

Fig. 6.29 A 51-year-old male with neck pain and prior arthrodesis. A lateral-sagittal radiograph of the cervical spine shows a normal variant arcuate foramen (*black arrows*). A complete bony arch over the groove for the VA completes the foramen. This normal variant is bilateral in this case. Disc prostheses are noted at C5-C6 and C6-C7

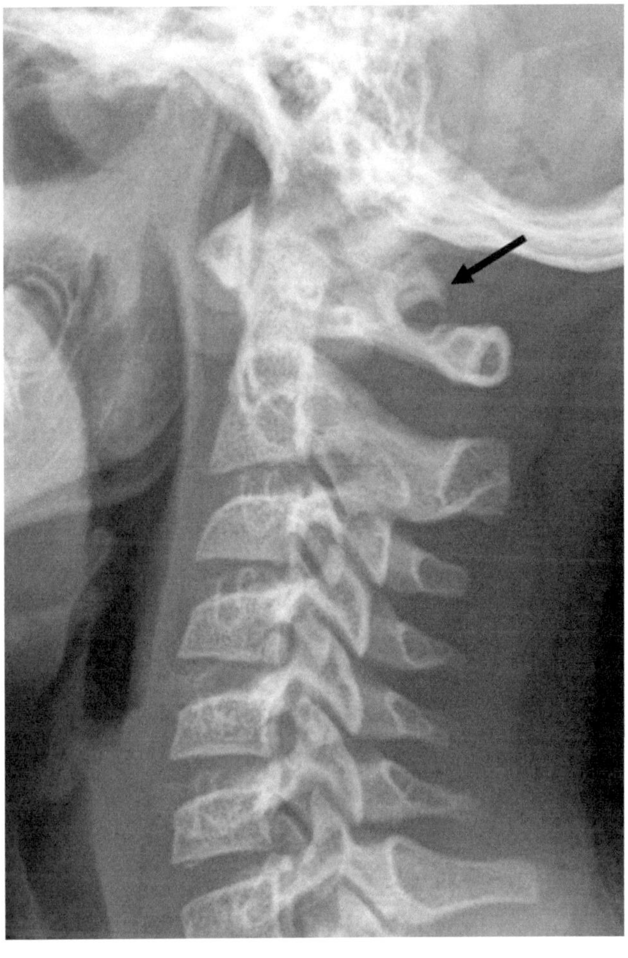

Fig. 6.30 A 19-year-old male with an incomplete ponticulus posticus (the bony contour of the arcuate foramen). This lateral radiograph of the cervical spine reveals an incomplete bony arch (*black arrow*) over the expected course of the VA

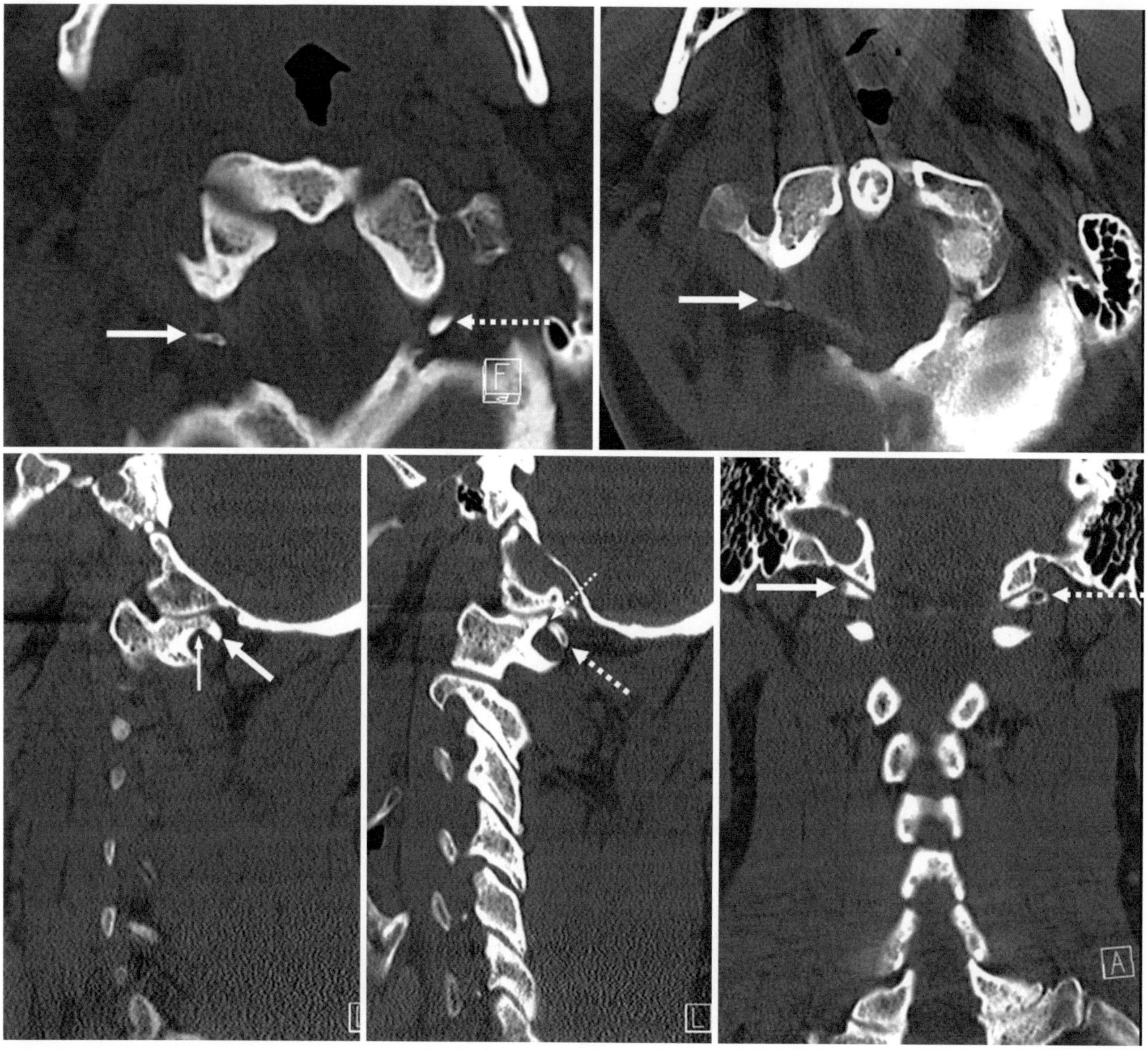

Fig. 6.31 A 55-year-old male, post–motor vehicle accident trauma, underwent a NECT examination to evaluate for fracture (negative). **Top row:** On serial axial reconstructions, note an incomplete ponticulus posticus on both the right (*arrows*) and left (*dotted arrows*) sides. **Bottom row:** On sagittal reformats of the left (*left*) and right (*middle*) sides as well as on a coronal reconstruction (*right*), the incomplete right arcuate foramen with a partial ponticulus posticus (*arrow, left and right images*) has a small defect (*tiny arrow, left*) that simulates a fracture because of its normal incomplete formation. Meanwhile, on the left side the incomplete ponticulus posticus (*dotted arrow, middle and right*) might also simulate a fracture (*thin dotted arrow, middle*). However, no soft-tissue swelling, subluxation, or other injuries are noted. This case demonstrates both how a normal variant arcuate foramen can be partial and how the presence of a partial/incomplete ponticulus posticus can mimic traumatic fractures

6.6.7 Vascular Channels

Intrinsic channels, specifically *vascular channels* traversing the vertebrae, may mimic a fracture or a pathologic lesion at first glance, especially if they are viewed in a single plane. These vascular channels may transmit small veins or arteries. When transmitting an artery, the channel may also be termed a *nutrient foramen*. When large enough, these channels may be observed on plain radiographs. On CT, when large enough, the typical mild hyperdensity of blood may be observed within the vascular structure transmitted by the channel (Figs. 6.32 and 6.33). With careful evaluation, aided by review of multiplanar imaging, the typical well-defined sclerotic margin surrounding a tubular vascular channel is readily identified.

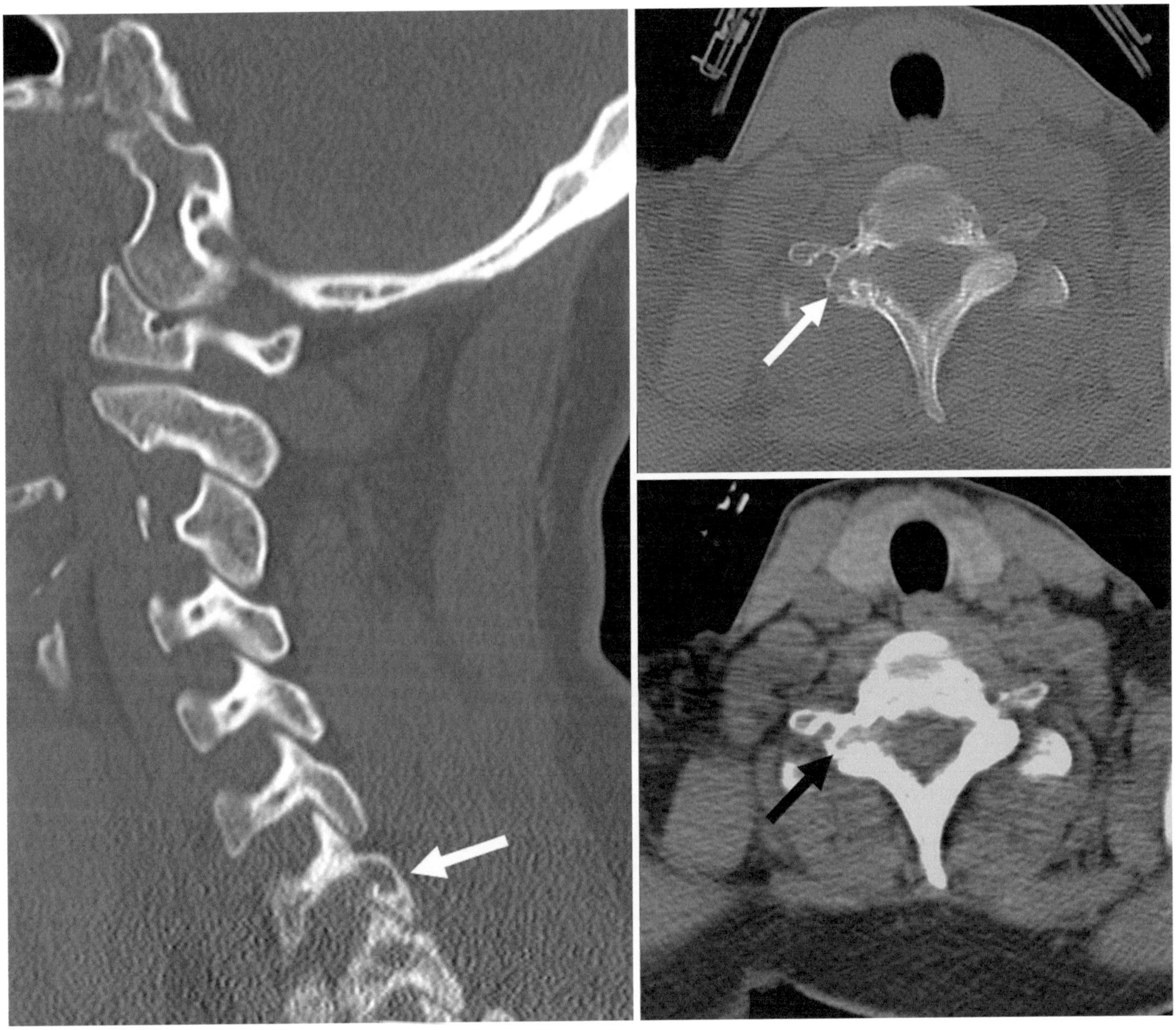

Fig. 6.32 A 31-year-old woman underwent NECT imaging of the cervical spine in the setting of trauma. Sagittal (*left*) and axial (*top right: bone windows, bottom right: soft-tissue windows*) reconstructions demonstrate a prominent vein traversing the epidural space and a portion of the inferior articular process of C7 (*white arrows*). There is well-defined sclerosis surrounding the margins of the vein in the posterior elements of the vertebra. On the axial NECT image with a soft-tissue reconstruction algorithm (*bottom right*), note the normal venous density (*black arrow*) of the blood coursing through this vein, appreciable in this patient given the vessel's size

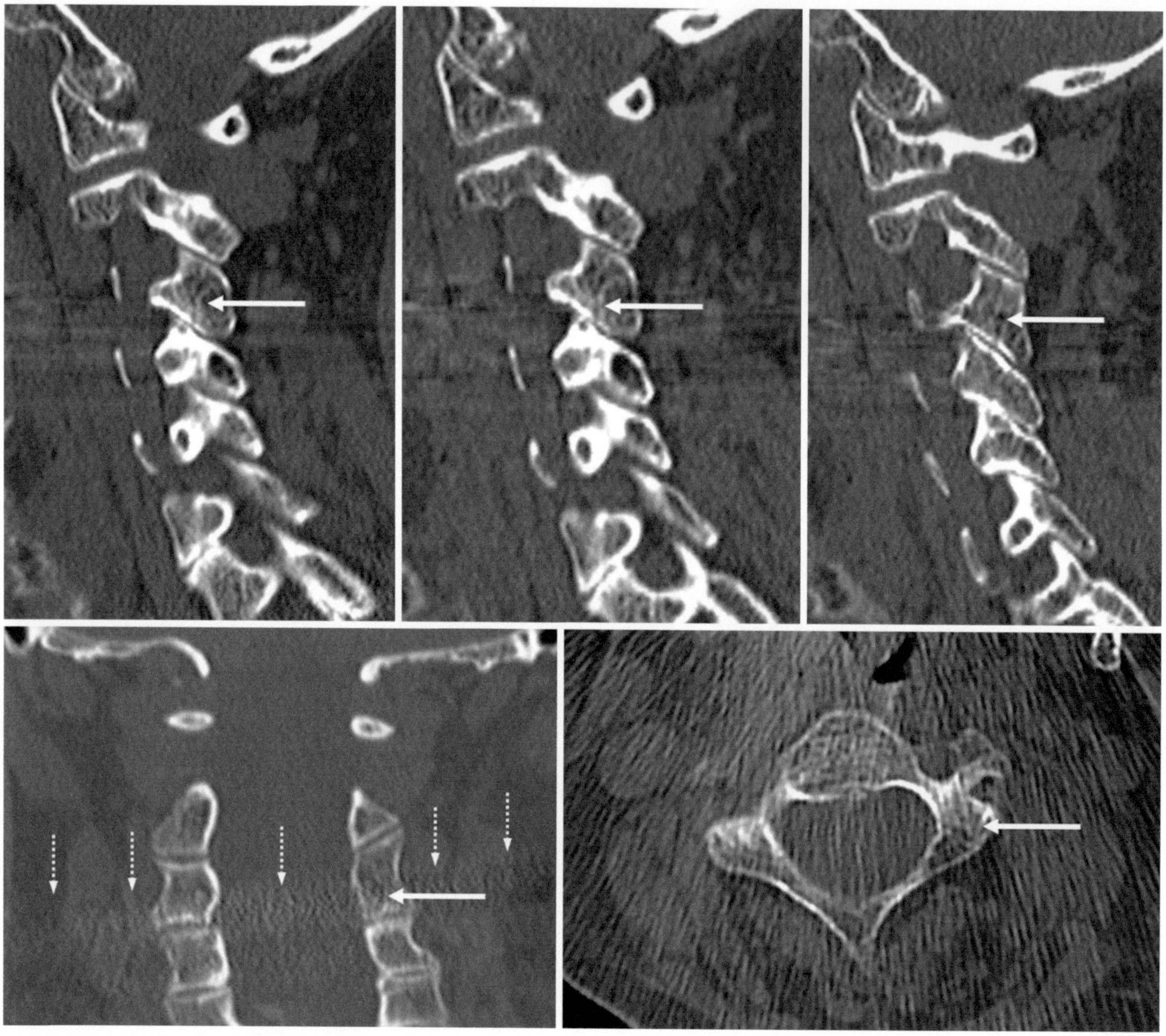

Fig. 6.33 This patient is a 71-year-old post-trauma with a small nutrient channel initially simulating a fracture. **Top row:** A sagittal 2-mm thickness reconstruction (*left*) from a cervical spine NECT was initially questioned as having a thin hairline fracture by a resident physician on call because of the presence of an apparent linear defect along the posterior edge of the left C3 pedicle (*arrows*); however, thinner 1-mm reformats (*middle, right*) showed that this defect did not traverse the cortical margin, and the margin was partially sclerotic, typical of a normal tiny vascular channel. **Bottom row:** On a 2-mm thickness coronal reconstruction (*left*), the channel is noted (*arrow*), the evaluation of which is exacerbated by beam hardening artifact (*thin dotted arrows*) arising from dental amalgam. An axial 2-mm reformatted image (*right*) depicts the extensive beam hardening artifact with subsequent "photon starvation" that causes the normal variant C3 pedicle vascular channel (*arrow*) to be nearly invisible. This case demonstrates the utility of thinner section imaging in distinguishing true fractures from normal vascular channels as well as how a beam hardening artifact can create or exacerbate "pseudo-fractures"

6.7 Spinal Canal

6.7.1 Congenital Spinal Canal Narrowing

A narrow spinal canal at multiple levels independent of degenerative or pathologic change is typically termed a *congenitally narrow spinal canal*, which can occur to varying degrees. Although commonly asymptomatic, congenital narrowing of the cervical spinal canal may also predispose to myelopathy, particularly in conjunction with degenerative spondylosis or trauma, especially from hyperextension injuries. As such, patients with congenital cervical spinal canal narrowing generally present at an earlier age than patients with degenerative canal narrowing.

Although there is variability in the measurement criteria for the definition of congenital cervical spinal canal narrowing, a cervical spinal canal anteroposterior diameter of less than 14 mm is considered uncommon in normal adults (Fig. 6.34). Other measurements, such as the angles created by the orientation of the posterior elements relative to the vertebral bodies, laminar length, lateral mass length, and posterior canal length, may prove useful in identifying patients with congenital cervical spinal canal narrowing. Other techniques utilizing cervical spine radiographs have been described to help screen for and identify congenital cervical spinal canal stenosis. These include estimating the degree of facet overlap and calculating the Torg ratio (a ratio of the diameter of the cervical canal to the width of the cervical body, in which less than 0.8 on a lateral view is considered abnormal).

Congenital thoracic spinal canal stenosis, similar to congenital cervical spinal canal stenosis, also predisposes patients to myelopathy, particularly in the settings of severe degenerative spondylosis or trauma. However, symptomatic thoracic spinal canal stenosis is rare, with less than 1% of patients with congenital thoracic spinal canal stenosis experiencing related symptoms. In general, the normal upper thoracic spinal canal is slightly tapered, decreasing in cross-sectional area from T1 as it courses inferiorly and then increasing in cross-sectional area further inferiorly/caudally, maintaining its largest diameter at T12. There is variability in the reported narrowest thoracic level, ranging from T2 to T10, depending on the measurement parameter and patient population.

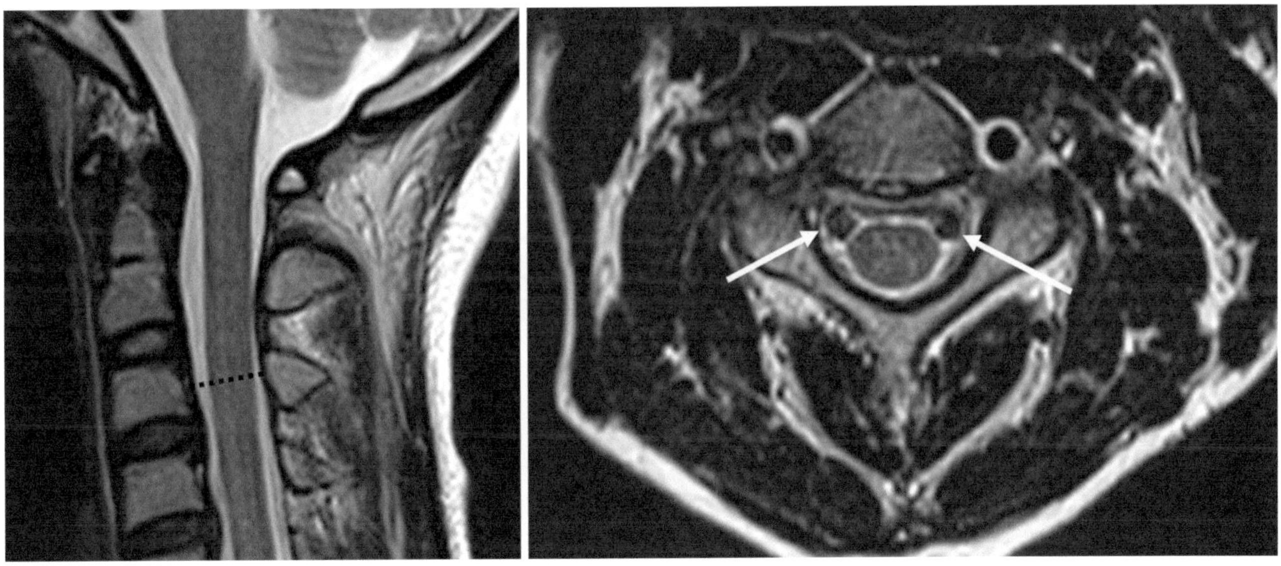

Fig. 6.34 In this 26-year-old female with a cervical spine MRI performed for paresthesias and prior trauma, the narrow cervical spinal canal is readily identified with an anteroposterior diameter of 11 mm at C3 (*dashed black line*), as measured on sagittal SET2WI (*left*). There is no cord signal abnormality on these images, as confirmed on axial SET2WI (*right*). Also note the hypointense signal resulting from CSF flow artifact on the axial T2WI (*white arrows, right*)

6.8 Spinal Cord

6.8.1 Normal Central Grey Matter

The spinal cord is composed of both grey matter and white matter. In contrast to the brain, the grey matter of the cord is generally centrally located and surrounded by peripheral white matter tracts. This central grey matter can at times be more readily delineated from the surrounding white matter on gradient echo T2-weighted imaging (GET2WI) MRI when compared to spin-echo T2-weighted imaging (SET2WI) MRI. On GET2WI, the central grey matter of the cord can be mildly hyperintense relative to the surrounding white matter (Fig. 6.35). This normal hyperintensity can occasionally simulate a myelopathic cord lesion, such as gliosis from prior insult, demyelination, or myelitis. The characteristic location and H-shape of central grey matter, lack of contrast enhancement, and lack of cord swelling all confirm this normal appearance, which can be more pronounced at higher field strengths (such as at 3 Tesla or 7 Tesla), or with higher resolution MR imaging.

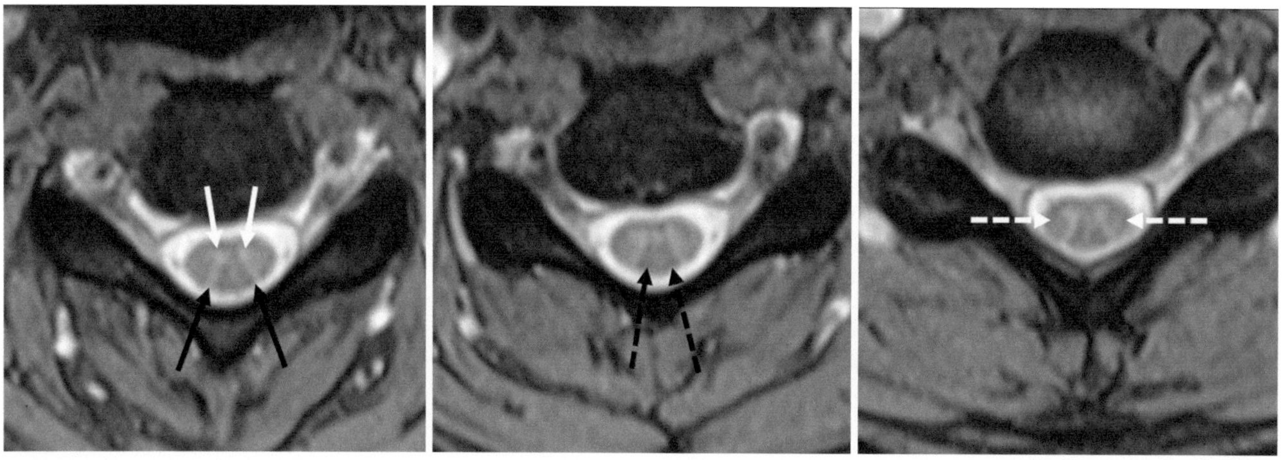

Fig. 6.35 A 27-year-old male underwent an MRI of the cervical spine to evaluate radiculopathy. Axial GET2*WI MR images at different cervical levels showed normal relative hyperintensity of the central grey matter within the spinal cord. Note normal, mildly hyperintense ventral horns (*white arrows*) and dorsal horns (*black arrows*) of the grey matter, together representing an "H-shape" appearance. Also, note the normal relatively hypointense white matter tracts of the lateral columns (*dashed white arrows, right*) and dorsal columns (*dashed black arrows, middle*)

6.8.2 Ventral Median Fissure

The spinal cord is largely divided in the sagittal plane anteriorly by the *ventral* (or anterior) *median fissure* and posteriorly by the *dorsal median fissure*. The ventral median fissure, although not always visible, is wider and much more readily apparent on CT myelography or MRI than its dorsal counterpart (Fig. 6.36). Although not necessary for visualization, spinal cord atrophy may increase the conspicuousness of the ventral median fissure. Notable tracts coursing through the white matter adjacent to the ventral median fissure include the medial longitudinal fasciculus, the anterior corticospinal tract, the medial reticulospinal tract, and the tectospinal tract. Although the normal ventral median fissure might simulate a syrinx (syringmyelia) in the coronal and sagittal planes, review of the axial images easily shows this normal anatomic structure in its typical location (Figs. 6.36 and 6.37).

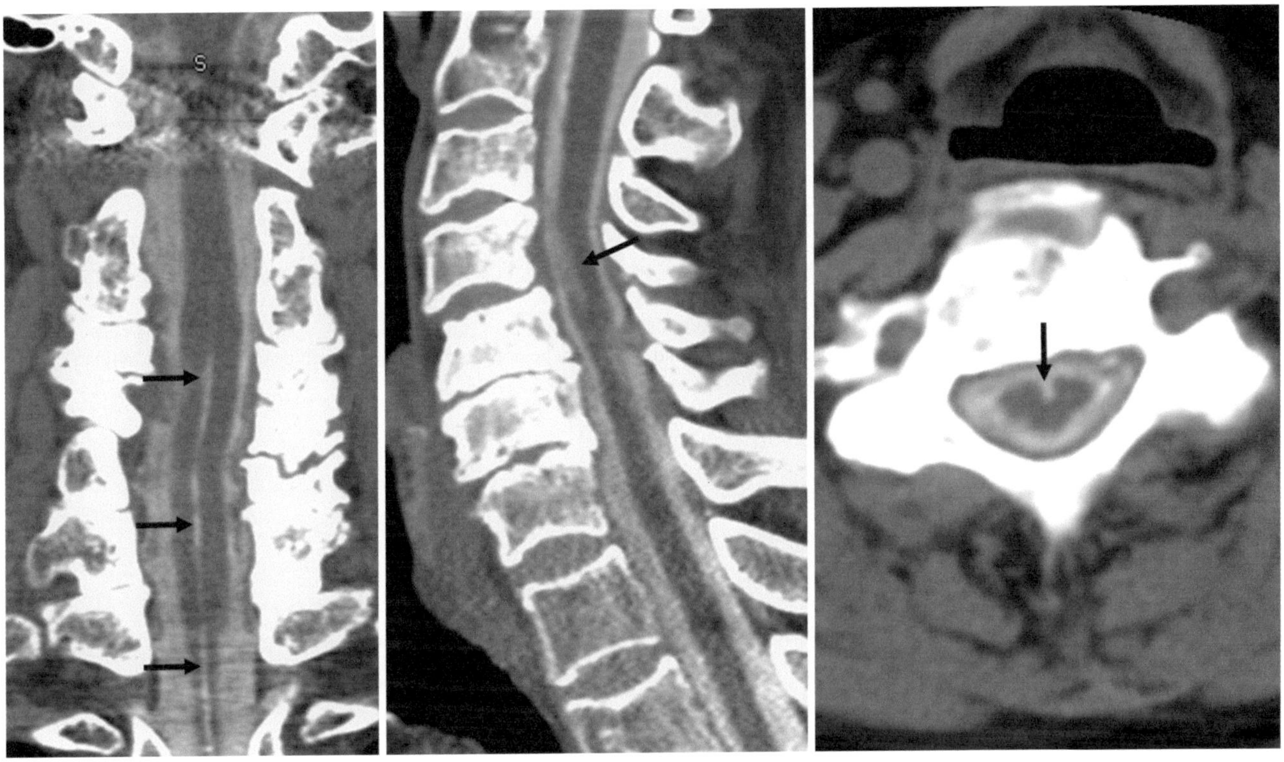

Fig. 6.36 A 71-year-old woman underwent CT myelography of the cervical spine for hyperreflexia. These coronal (*left*) and sagittal (*middle*) reconstructed images show linear increased density (*black arrows*) in the midline of the ventral spinal cord, simulating a syrinx. However, an axial image (*right*) at the level of C6 shows this to be a normal prominent ventral median fissure (*black arrow, right*)

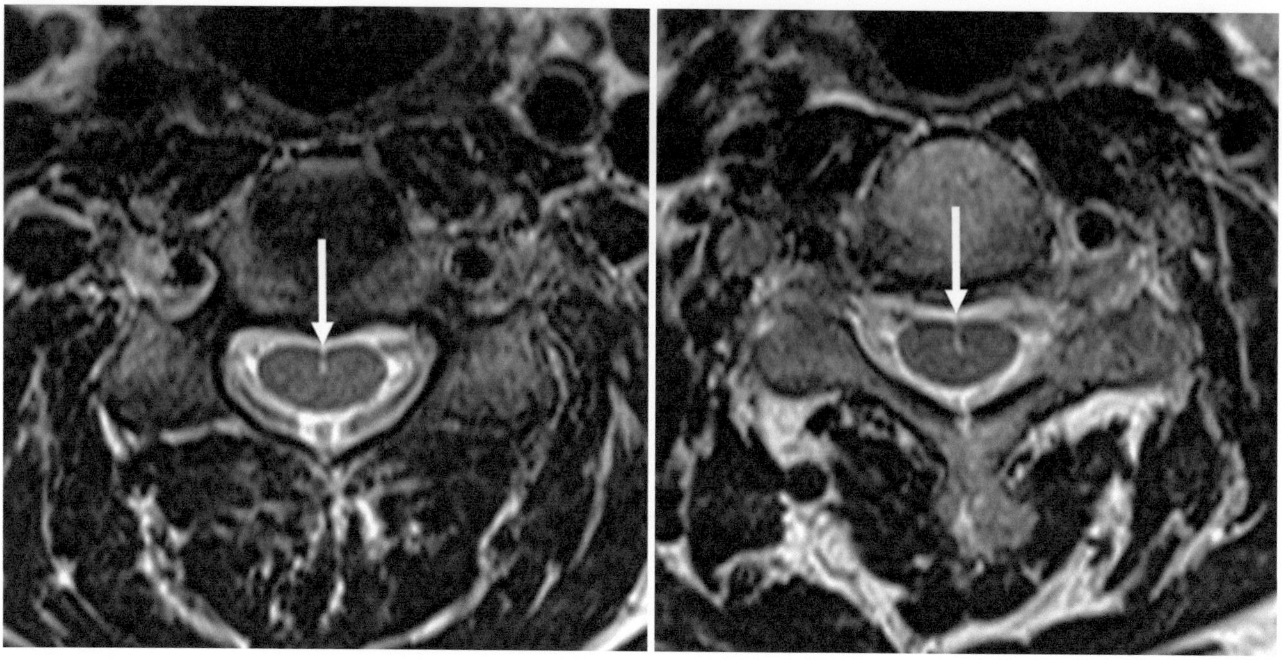

Fig. 6.37 A 51-year-old man underwent an MRI of the cervical spine to evaluate neck pain and radiculopathy. Axial T2WIs show a normal ventral median fissure of the spinal cord (*arrows*). This is a normal finding and should not be confused with myelopathic cord signal or a syrinx

6.8.3 Central Canal Prominence

The *central canal of the spinal cord* develops from the neural groove, courses from the obex (located near the craniocervical junction) down to the conus medullaris (located near the thoracolumbar junction), and it is lined by ependymal cells. It transmits cerebrospinal fluid (CSF) between the spinal region and skull base. It remains present at birth and then usually progressively shrinks until it disappears. Occasionally, it persists into childhood or it may persist even later into adulthood.

On imaging, identification of the central canal is made easier as the spatial resolution of MRIs continues to improve. The MRI is considered the imaging modality of choice to evaluate for syringohydromyelia, followed by CT myelography. In fact, on high resolution heavily weighted SET2WI MRI sequences, the central canal is readily identified in most normal patients if one pays close attention (Fig. 6.38).

There is considerable debate about how to identify and differentiate a normal central canal from a true pathologic syrinx; this involves several considerations, including size, location (centrally within the cord versus ventrally or dorsal), and extent. When present, the normal central canal (and thus normal variant central canal prominence) is typically situated at the junction of the ventral third of the cord with the posterior two thirds of the cord. It is fluid-filled and fusiform in contour, with tapered cephalad and caudal ends. When the central canal of the spinal cord measures less than 3 mm in diameter, it can be considered an incidental normal finding. Thus, most sources consider it unnecessary to recommend follow-up imaging or to call a normal, dilated central canal a syrinx if it measures less than 2 mm in maximum diameter and if it lacks an irregular or extensive appearance. When it is greater than 3 mm in diameter, it is appropriate to image the remainder of the neuraxis to evaluate for evidence of congenital malformation, inflammation, stenosis, trauma, or neoplasm as a cause of the obstruction that led to the syrinx formation. In the absence of any such abnormality, contrast administration is not required.

In the setting of a greater than 3-mm diameter canal that is suspicious for being a syrinx, an initial MRI with gadolinium-based contrast is perhaps prudent for the initial evaluation (usually if no apparent history of trauma or overt severe spinal canal stenosis is present), while contrast is probably not necessary on follow-up MR imaging in the absence of an enhancing mass. Regarding a greater than 3-mm diameter prominence that is suggestive of a normally dilated central canal, follow-up MR imaging is reasonable to ensure at least 12 months of stability. Most of these prominent central canals will remain stable or decrease in size on such annual follow-up imaging. Therefore, only when the fluid-filled cavity in the spinal cord is enlarged, irregular, and related to the presence of a tumor, spinal cord tethering, trauma, or abnormal CSF flow should it be called a syringomyelia or a syrinx.

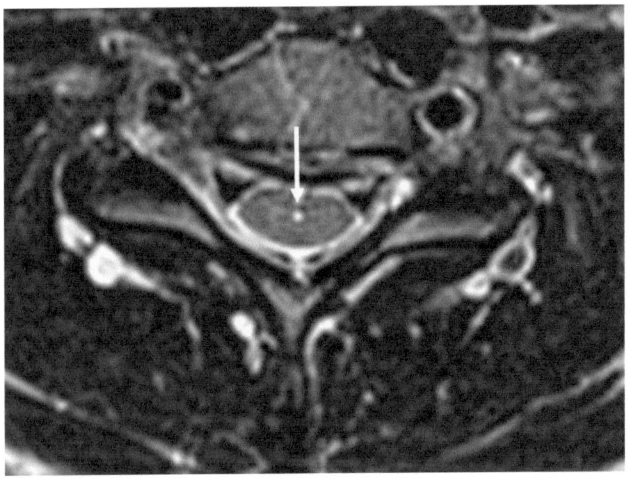

Fig. 6.38 A 26-year-old woman underwent a cervical spine MRI examination for paresthesias and headache. This axial SET2WI shows a normal variant prominent central canal of the spinal cord (*arrow, 1.5 mm diameter*). This could mimic a syrinx, but it measured less than 2 mm in size, was regular, centrally located within the cord, and was not extensive. These characteristics are typical for a normal variant prominent central canal. This was not changed on serial annual follow-up examinations (*not shown*)

6.9 Accessory Ossification and Ligamentous Ossification Simulating Fractures

6.9.1 Craniocervical Accessory Ossicles

Accessory ossicles frequently form along ligaments, perhaps most commonly noted on imaging of the feet. Less commonly, such ossicles occur at the craniocervical junction. These normal variant *craniocervical accessory ossicles* typically exhibit well-defined sclerotic cortical margins, aiding in their differentiation from true fractures. When they are large enough and if the imaging resolution is high enough, they can exhibit central marrow density/signal on CT and on MRI (Fig. 6.39).

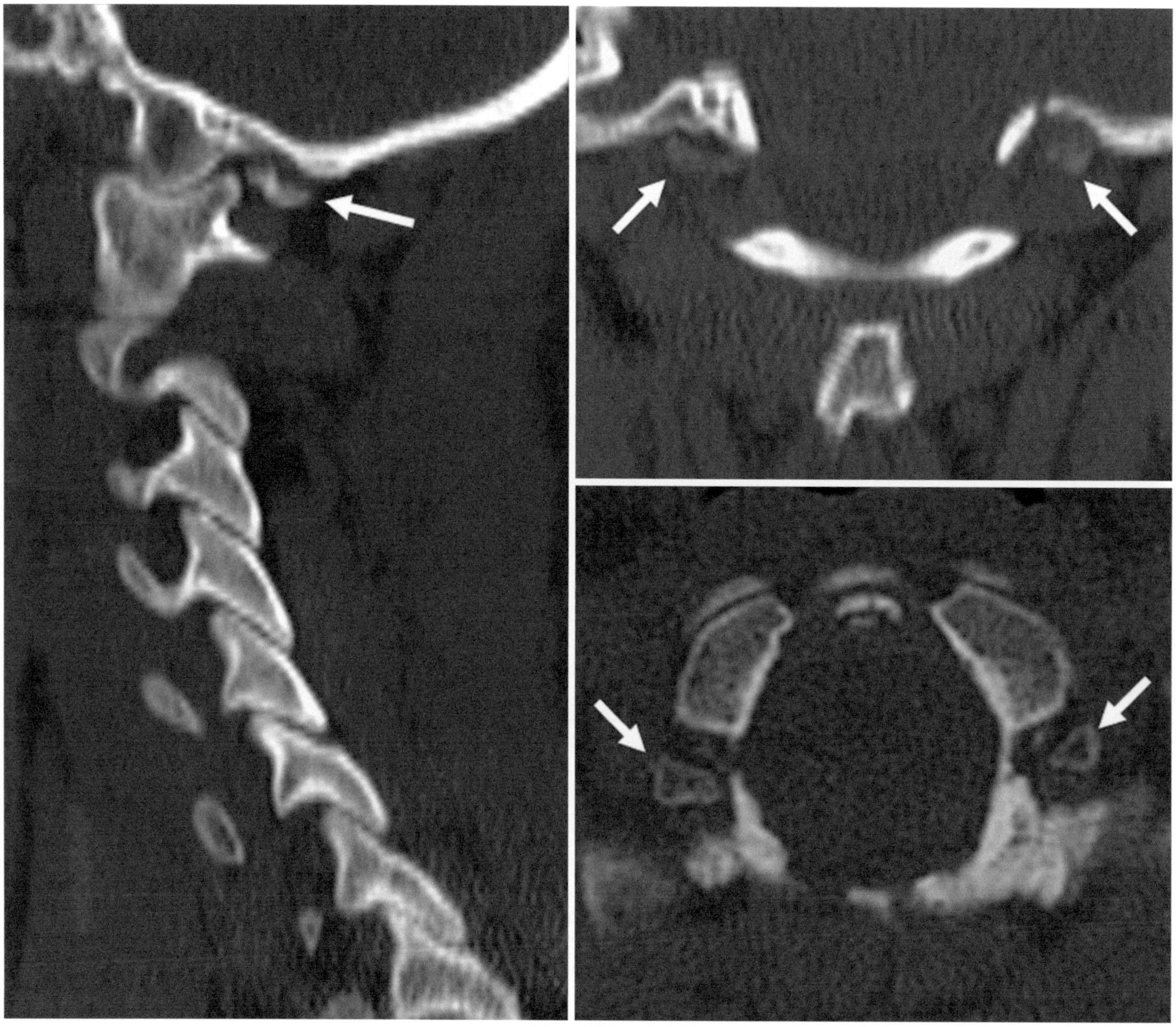

Fig. 6.39 This 41-year-old woman underwent a NECT of the cervical spine in the setting of acute trauma. Note the small, incidental and normal variant symmetric accessory ossicles (*arrows*) located directly posterior to the atlanto-occipital joints bilaterally, as depicted in the sagittal (*left*), coronal (*top right*), and axial (*bottom right*) planes. Note the central hypoattenuation typical of marrow density. There was no acute fracture. While close to the skull base, these ossicles are in a position where they also could in theory represent another example of normal variant partially ossified ponticulus posticus (forming an incomplete arcuate foramen of C1)

6.9.2 Ossification of the Posterior Longitudinal Ligament and Diffuse Idiopathic Skeletal Hyperostosis

Also notable is calcification or *ossification of the posterior longitudinal ligament* (OPLL). This ligament is anteriorly situated relative to the cord and located along the posterior margin of the vertebral bodies and the intervertebral discs. OPLL is not considered a normal variation but can initially be asymptomatic in milder cases; it then can progress and lead to severe spinal canal stenosis and myelopathy. Cervical OPLL (present in about 3% of patients) is more common than thoracic OPLL (in just under 1%), with a difference in prevalence of 0.01–2% in the non-Asian population versus 2–4% in the Asian population. Four subtypes have been noted, ranging from localized to continuous, where more diffuse forms are more likely to cause spinal canal stenosis and myelopathic or radiculopathic symptoms. Interestingly, the rate of progression has been associated with an earlier age of presentation, while presentation in late middle age or in the elderly is less likely to be symptomatic.

Also, OPLL can be associated with *diffuse idiopathic skeletal hyperostosis* (DISH), which in itself is often asymptomatic and an incidental "don't touch" finding. It is present in up to 10–15% of the elderly population and appears as large, "flowing" osteophytes anteriorly between the anterior vertebral segments of the cervical and thoracic vertebrae (Fig. 6.40). Histologically, DISH typically involves calcification or ossification of the anterior longitudinal ligament with fibrosis and perhaps hypervascularity. DISH is usually asymptomatic, although rarely it can result in compression of adjacent structures anteriorly such as the esophagus, causing dysphagia. However, the coexistence of both DISH and OPLL (present in about half of DISH cases) can predispose to myelopathy. Both DISH and OPLL may progressively ossify over time, and both can simulate fractures of degenerative osteophytes when partially/incompletely fused across vertebral segments. Partial or incomplete ossification can be correctly distinguished by the lack of associated edema.

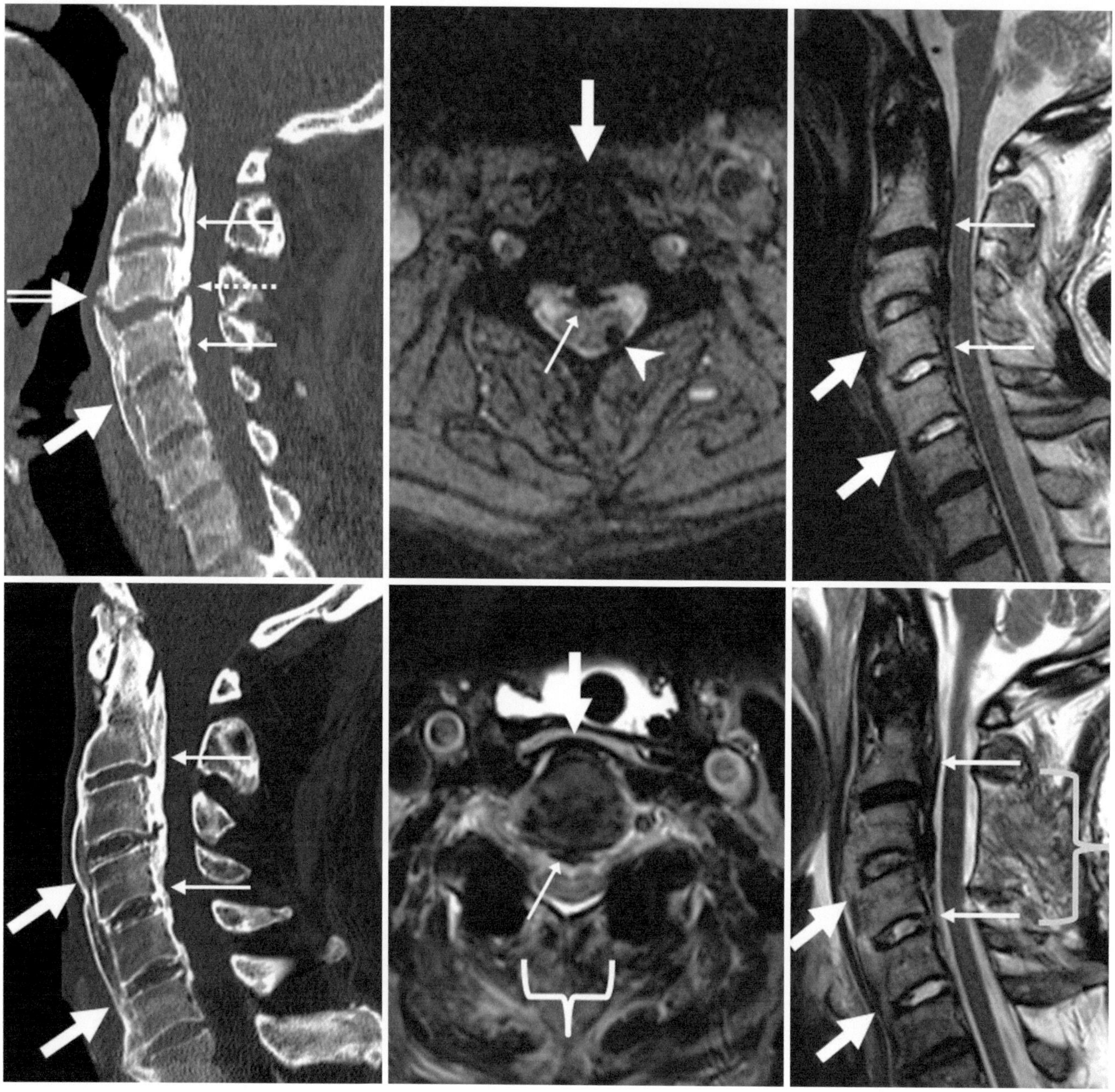

Fig. 6.40 OPLL- and DISH-inducing myelopathy. **Top row:** In a 49-year-old male with myelopathic symptoms, sagittal NECT (*left*) demonstrated both OPLL (*thin arrows*) and DISH (*thick arrow*), with small "gaps" between the "flowing" osteophytes of OPLL (*thin dotted arrow*) and DISH (*thick beveled arrow*). On MRI, axial GET2*WI (*middle*) depicts similar findings, with a focus of hemosiderin (*arrowhead*) within the left side of the cord, attributed to remote hemorrhage from cord injury caused by the OPLL in the setting of prior trauma; sagittal SET2WI (*right*) shows marrow signal within both the OPLL (*thin arrows*) and DISH (*thick arrows*). **Bottom row:** The patient's symptoms worsened over the next 8 years, and both the OPLL (*thin arrows*) and DISH (*thick arrows*) had worsened on sagittal NECT (*left*) with subsequent filling in of the "gaps" between the bony osteophytes. Surgical decompression of the posterior elements was performed. Axial SET2WI (*middle*) and sagittal SET2WI (*right*) confirmed improved patency of the spinal canal after multilevel laminectomy (*surgical defect outlined by brackets*), although both the OPLL (*thin arrows*) and DISH (*thick arrows*) remained

6.9.3 Ossification of the Ligamentum Flavum

Ossification of the ligamentum flavum (OLF) is a rare finding that tends to involve the lower thoracic spine, typically located below the level of the T8 vertebra in more than 70% of cases (Fig. 6.41). It is most commonly reported in Asian countries. It may be asymptomatic but can present with back pain and can predispose to the development of myelopathy. Many patients also have ossification of the adjacent dura mater, or alternatively the ossified ligament is adherent to the dura mater. In that setting, patients are at risk of developing a CSF leak following surgical posterior decompression. Notably, there is a reported case of OLF with associated dural erosion, resulting in a CSF leak and subsequent intracranial hypotension.

Calcification of the ligamentum flavum (CLF) is a similar rare condition that may predispose or progress to myelopathy, although it is often asymptomatic in early cases. CLF, as distinct from from OLF, is a crystal deposition disease. As such, it is often associated with other mineral deposits elsewhere in the body. Although CLF is occasionally difficult to delineate from OLF, the calcification of CLF is usually not in continuity with the laminae and affects the central portion of the ligamentum flavum, sparing the superficial and deep layers (Fig. 6.42).

OLF and CLF have been attributed to disorders resulting in abnormal growth hormone levels and abnormal calcium and phosphorus levels. While these are not considered normal, milder cases may be asymptomatic but can progress and cause spinal canal stenosis and myelopathy. Although they are most frequently associated with hypoparathyroidism, other cited causes include diffuse idiopathic skeletal hyperostosis, hyperthyroidism, hemochromatosis, fluorosis, rickets, Paget disease, diabetes mellitus, and adenocarcinomatous metastasis.

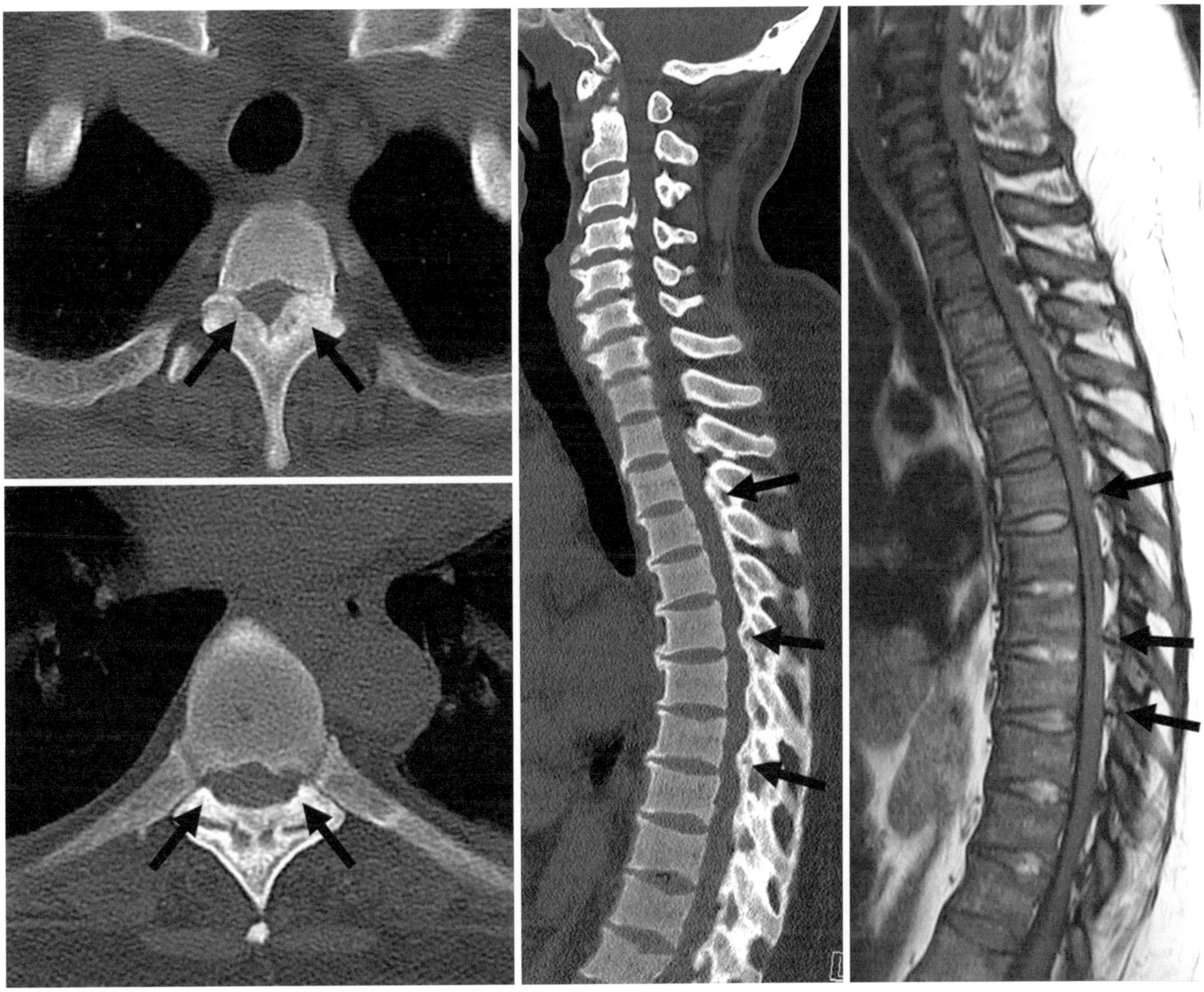

Fig. 6.41 A 47-year-old man underwent imaging of his cervical and thoracic spine to evaluate spondylosis with myelopathy. In this case of ossification of the ligamentum flavum (OLF), the ossified ligamentum flavum (*black arrows*) bridging the thoracic laminae is readily identified on axial (*upper left, bottom left*) and sagittal (*middle*) reconstructions from NECT. A sagittal SET1WI MR image (*right*) of the thoracic spine shows these same changes, illustrating the marrow signal within the ossified ligamentum flavum

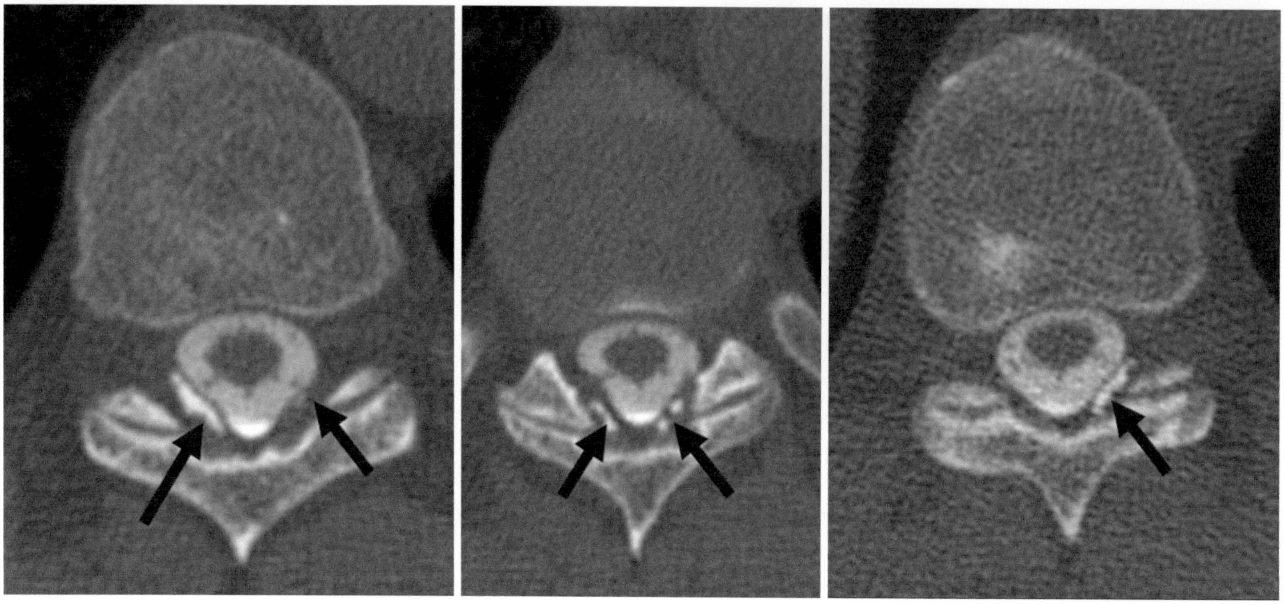

Fig. 6.42 A 60-year-old man with calcification (*arrows*) of the ligamentum flavum, as demonstrated on axial CT myelography images. Ligamentous calcification (*arrows*) lacks the central relative hypoattenuation associated with ossification. This calcification should not be confused with extravasation of contrast media, in which extravasated (extradural) contrast would not be expected within the ligament over multiple levels and would have a different density from bone

6.9.4 Ossification of the Nuchal Ligament

The nuchal ligament extends from the occipital protuberance to the spinous process of C7. This ligament may partially calcify or ossify. A focus of *nuchal ligament ossification* is also sometimes referred to as a sesamoid ossicle of the nuchal ligament. Ossification usually has well-defined cortical margins but may be mildly irregular. Ossification will also exhibit central hypoattenuation on CT and signal isointense to marrow signal on MRI. Calcification of the ligament is often less well-defined and generally hypointense on all MRI sequences.

Ossification (or calcification) of the nuchal ligament is usually asymptomatic, most commonly occurs at C4 to C5 and C5 to C6, and it is considered a "don't touch lesion" or even normal (Figs. 6.43 and 6.44). This can occasionally be mistaken for a chronic fracture of the spinous processes, but the characteristic location and a regular contour (without cortical irregularity) suggest this variant. Although it is often seen in conjunction with ossification of the posterior longitudinal ligament, ossification of the nuchal ligament can also occur in isolation. Interestingly, when spondylosis is present, the level of ossification of the nuchal ligament has been reported to generally correspond to the level of the most pronounced spinal canal stenosis.

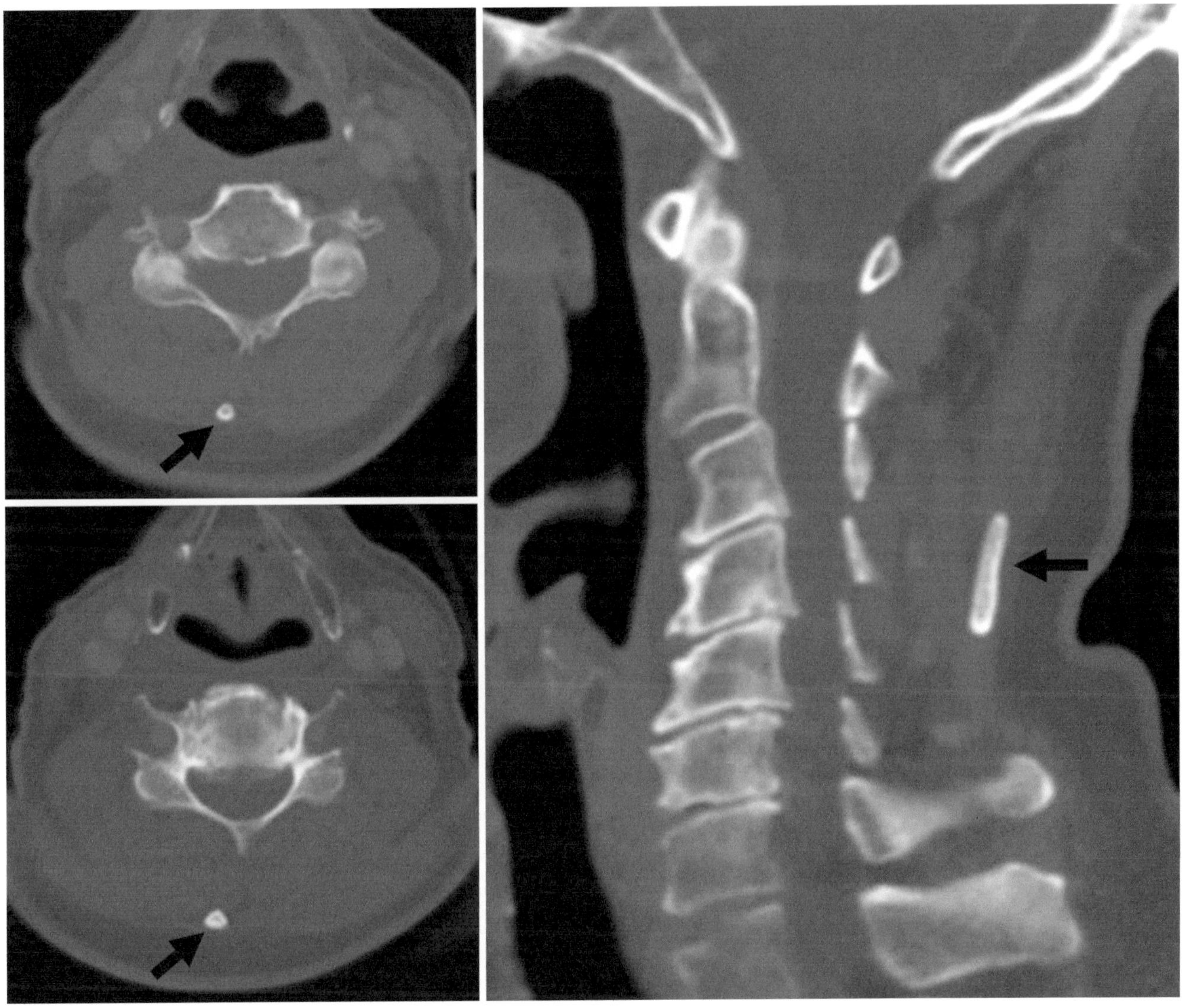

Fig. 6.43 A 63-year-old male undergoing neck imaging for laryngeal carcinoma. There is normal variant ossification (*black arrows*) along a portion of the nuchal ligament at the level of approximately C4 to C5. Note the well-defined sclerotic margins and central density similar to that of the marrow of the adjacent vertebrae on these NECT axial (*top left and bottom left*) and sagittal (*right*) reformatted images. On MRI (*not shown*), the central signal within the area of ossification would be expected to be isointense to marrow (both T1- and T2-hyperintense)

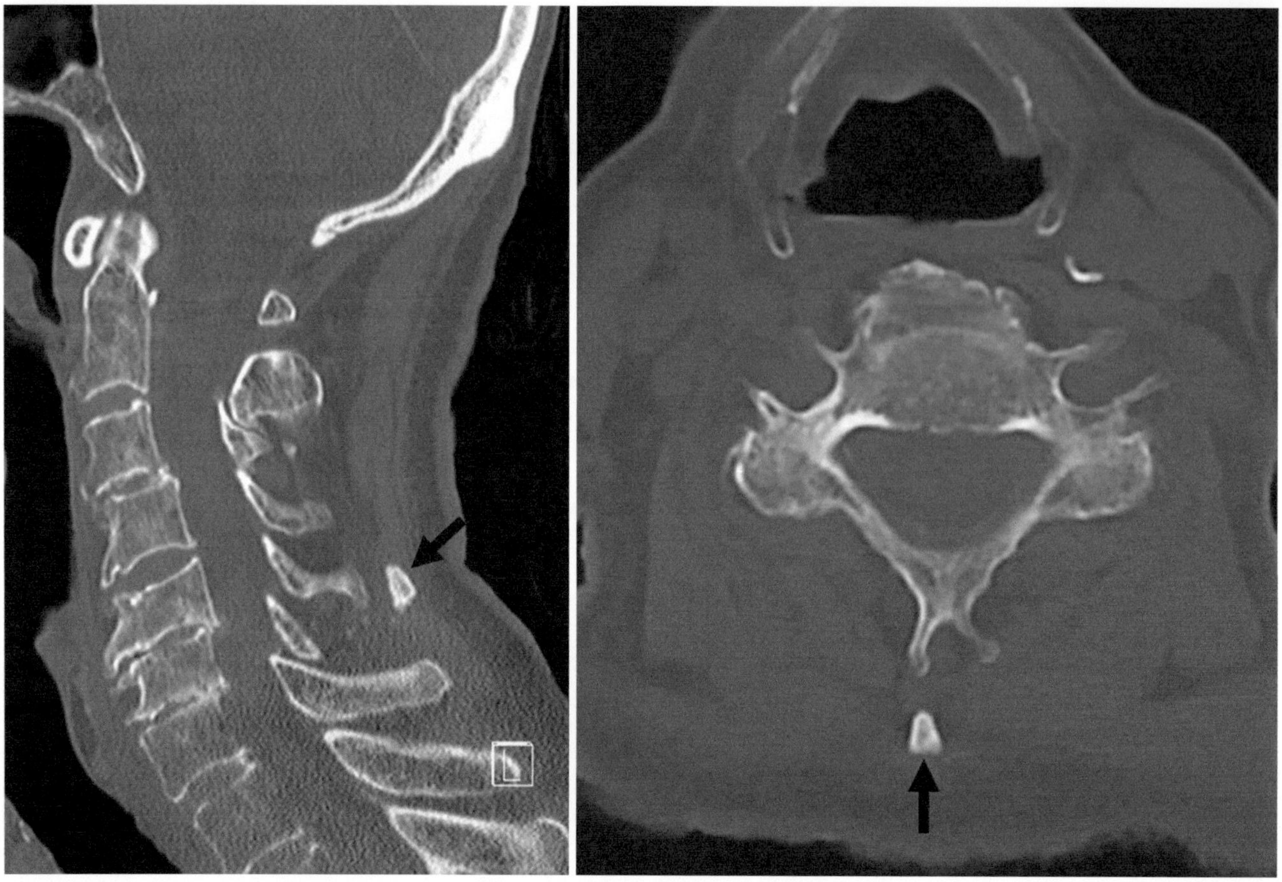

Fig. 6.44 An 89-year-old male undergoing NECT imaging of the cervical spine for trauma. Sagittal (*left*) and axial (*right*) reconstructions show a small focus of normal variant ossification along the lower nuchal ligament (*black arrows*). The well-defined sclerotic cortical margin and the central marrow density are typical of such ligamentous ossification. These characteristics aid in its correct identification as ligamentous ossification as opposed to a fracture. Note the lack of a donor site from the adjacent spinous process, further indicating that this does not represent a fracture

6.9.5 Old Fractures

Although they are not a normal variant, old vertebral fractures may mimic congenital abnormalities, and ligamentous ossification (such as described above) may simulate old fractures. It is also important to differentiate old vertebral fractures (Figs. 6.45 and 6.46) from acute vertebral fractures. Thus, as nuchal ligament calcification/ossification within the interspinous spaces posteriorly can mimic spinous process fractures, some characteristics can be helpful in identifying remote fractures. These include the presence of displacement of bony fragments, well-defined sclerotic margins of the fracture's edges, the presence of ankylosis across the old fracture line(s), and the presence of concomitant remote injuries.

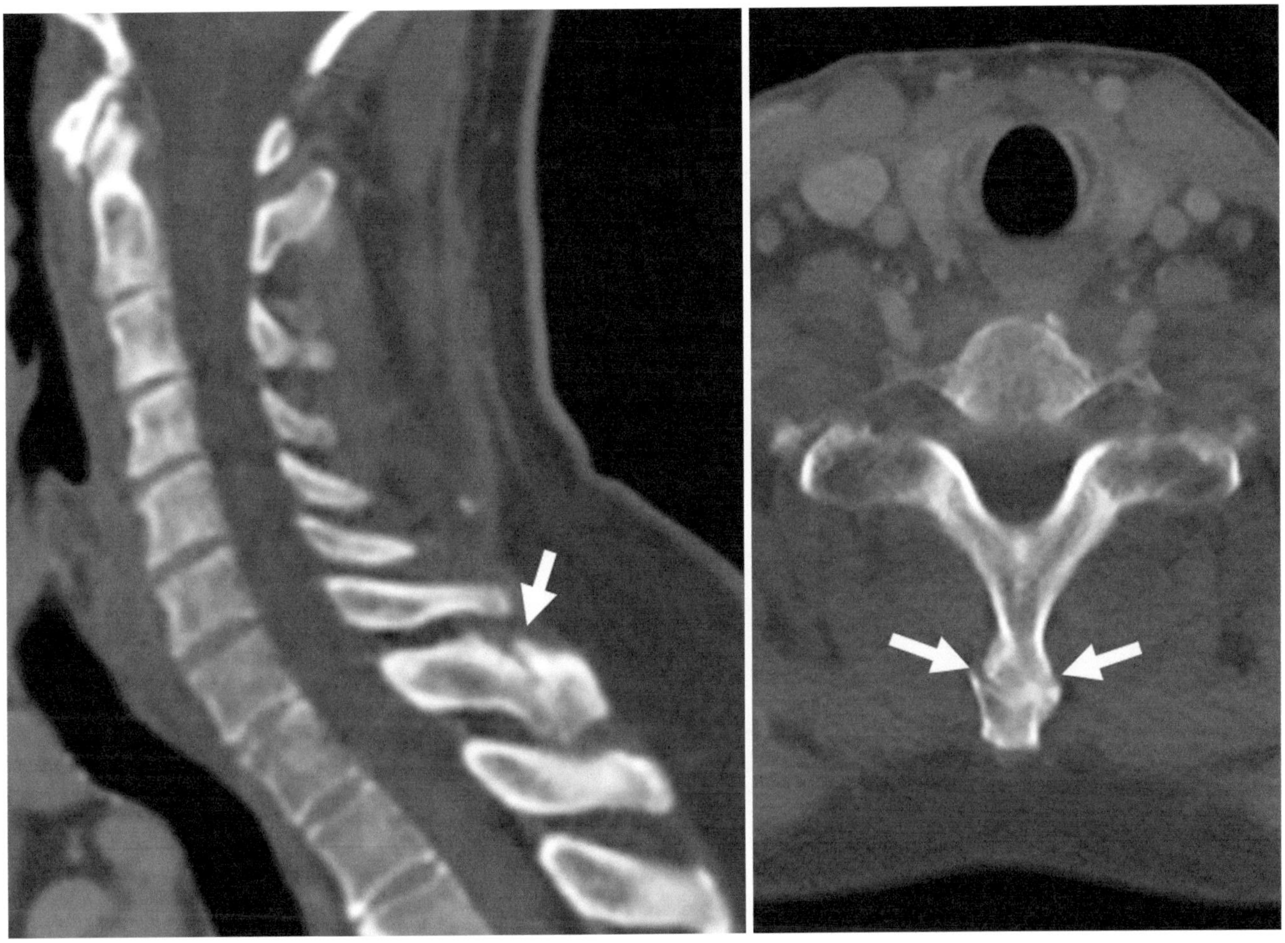

Fig. 6.45 Comparison case of an old spinous process fracture. A 49-year-old male undergoing CECT imaging of the neck for head and neck cancer. Sagittal (*left*) and axial (*right*) images show a well-defined lucency (*arrows*) traversing vertically through the posterior aspect of the T1 spinous process. This old fracture was documented following a prior traumatic injury, although imaging from that traumatic encounter was unavailable. The well-defined margins and lack of soft-tissue edema indicate a chronic process, which corroborates the clinical history. The overall length of the spinous process, perhaps most notable on the sagittal image, is also typical of an old fracture at this location

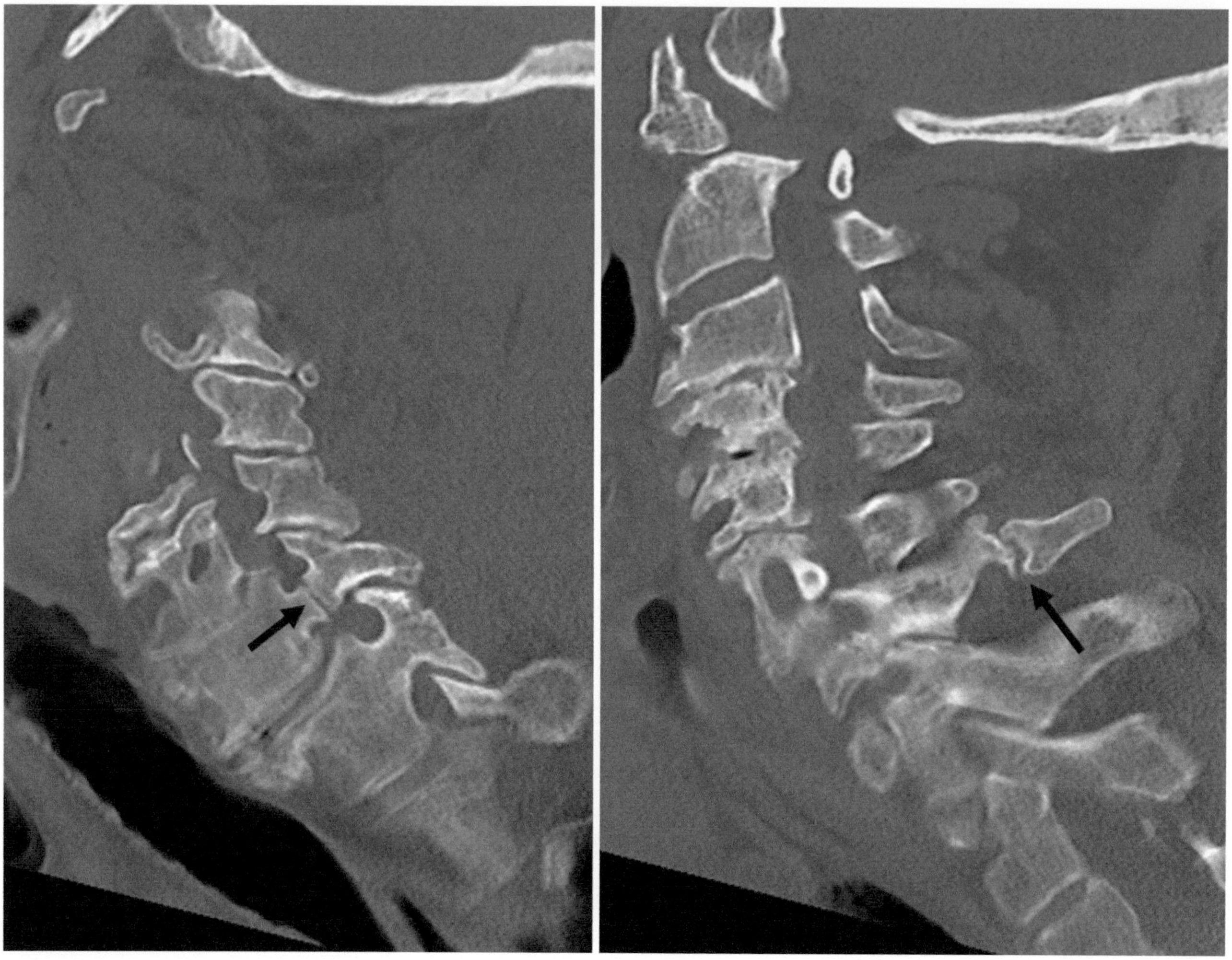

Fig. 6.46 Comparison case of old spinous process fracture. Per the clinical history, a 57-year-old male sustained remote but substantial trauma more than 10 years prior to this NECT examination, but no comparison images were available. On sagittal NECT reconstructed images, in addition to the presence of multilevel degenerative spondylosis, there are old fractures with well-defined sclerotic margins (*black arrows*). Despite the fact that the fractures occurred years ago, there is a lack of bony ankylosis across the old fracture lines, potentially caused by a lack of sufficient immobilization following the injury

6.10 Accessory Findings

6.10.1 Craniocervical Rotation and Asymmetry of the Odontoid Lateral Mass Interval

Craniocervical rotation occurs primarily at C1 to C2. The normal range of rotation of C1 on C2 is 25–53°. Normal physiologic atlantoaxial rotation in the horizontal plane from a neutral rotation accounts for the first approximately 23 degrees of head turn to each side. After 23 degrees of rotation, C1 and C2 both rotate until a head turn of 65 degrees is achieved. Beyond 65 degrees, additional craniocervical rotation occurs at segments below the level of C2.

Asymmetry of the odontoid lateral mass interval (OLMI) can be seen in the normal physiologic state, particularly with craniocervical rotation in the horizontal plane that potentially approaches 3 mm. This can be noted in children or adults, although it can be more prominent in the former. Such asymmetric widening of the OLMI that can be normal occurs most commonly with the head turned toward the side of widening. However, asymmetry may also be an indication of potentially severe ligamentous injury. As such, if no fracture is present on nonenhanced CT (NECT) but a widened OLMI is encountered, it is important to correlate for the presence or absence of predictive clinical findings such as cervical tenderness or torticollis, for imaging findings of trauma (e.g., prevertebral edema), and to note the degree of head turn (Figs. 6.47 and 6.48). Thus, with an atlantoaxial interval of less than 2.6 mm and the head turned toward the side of OLMI widening, such asymmetry is likely to be secondary to positioning. Therefore, in the event of an indeterminate plain film or initial cervical spine NECT caused by asymmetric OLMI with possible head turning, a limited focal scan (to minimize irradiation) can be performed of the clivus down to C3 in the neutral position and with the head turned to confirm that the asymmetry of the OLMI is positional. If the widening of the OLMI persists on the side opposite the direction of head turning, then the findings are suspicious for ligamentous injury with possible atlantoaxial rotational fixation or subluxation; this can be further confirmed by MRI to evaluate for ligamentous or prevertebral edema.

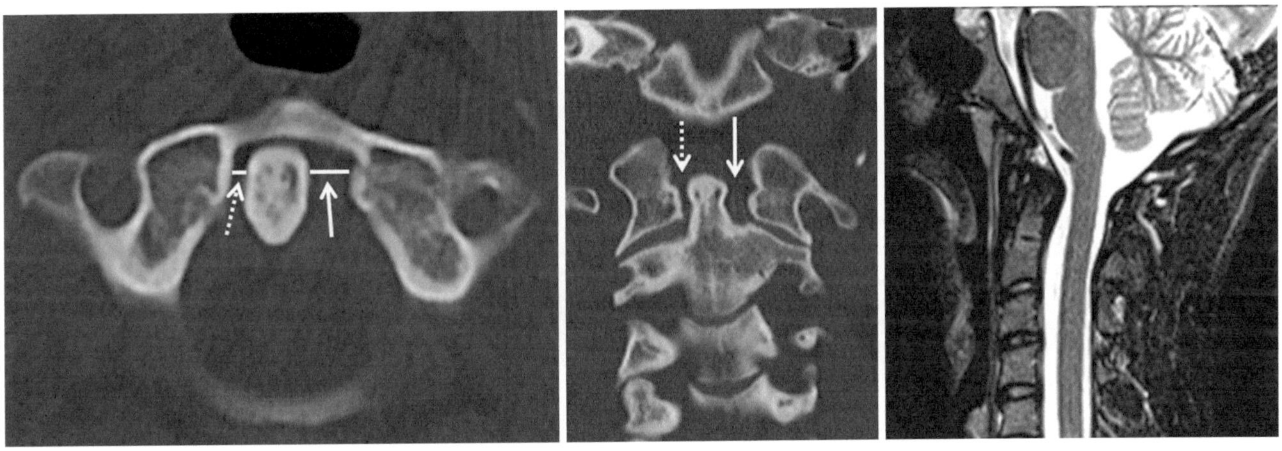

Fig. 6.47 A 22-year-old female who underwent imaging evaluation in the setting of trauma after a motor vehicle accident, lacking torticollis, neck swelling, or prevertebral edema. On NECT, axial (*left*) and coronal (*middle*) reconstructions showed asymmetry of the odontoid lateral mass interval (OLMI) on the left side (*arrows*) that was more than 3 mm (measured 4.7 mm), while the OLMI on the right side was much smaller (*dotted arrows*) and being less than 2 mm; however, it was noted that the patient's head was mildly turned to the left. A follow-up MRI of the cervical spine with sagittal STIR imaging (*right*) was performed the following day for persistent pain, confirming a lack of ligamentous edema and no injury at that location

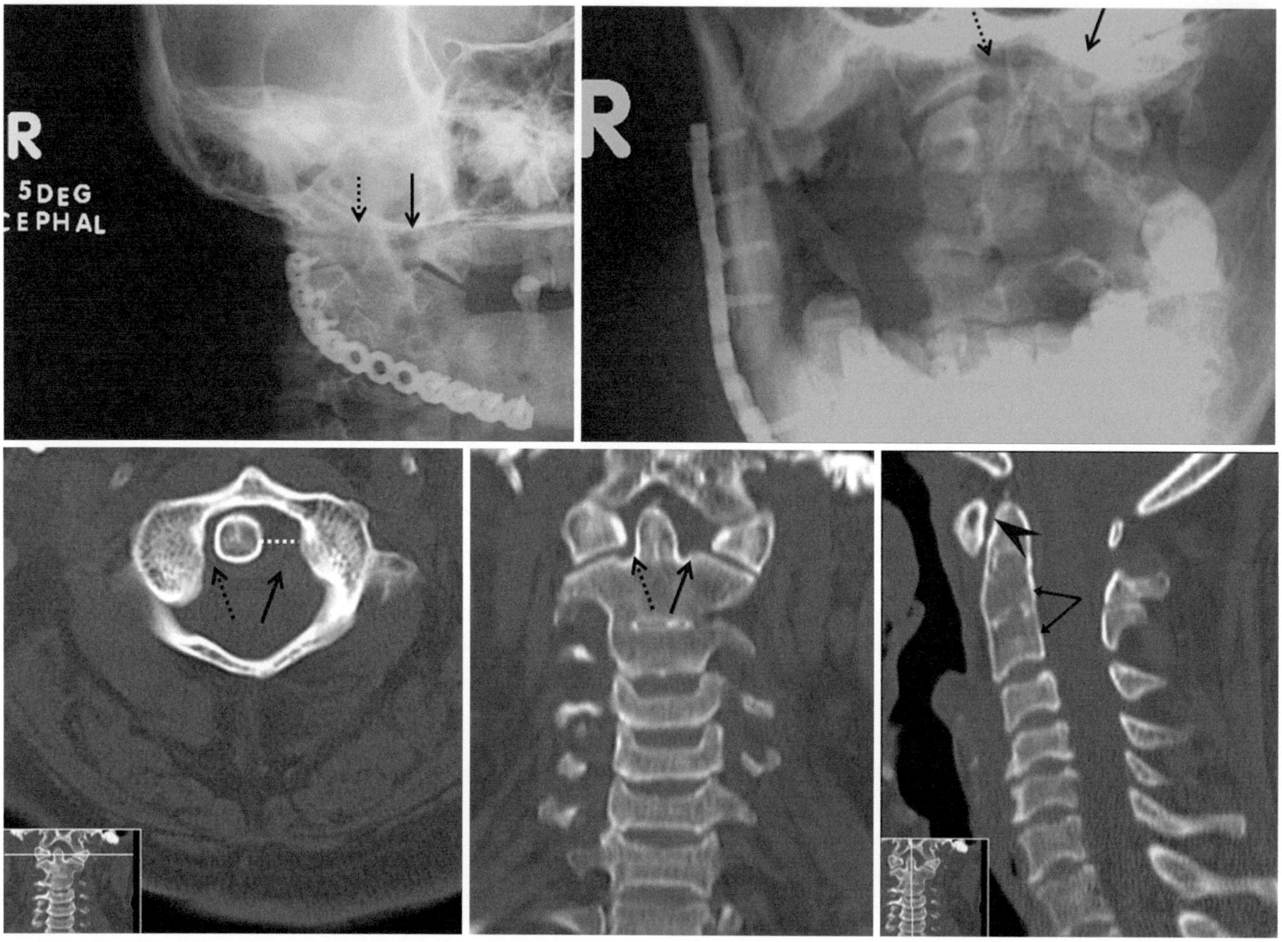

Fig. 6.48 Comparison case of atlantoaxial rotatory fixation-subluxation in trauma. A 44-year-old female presented to the emergency room with cervical pain and torticollis following a motor vehicle accident. **Top row:** On a screening cervical spine anteroposterior plain film (*left*) no fracture was noted, but the patient's head was turned to the left, where a widened left OLMI (*arrows*) was identified, while the right OLMI (*dotted arrows*) was normal; a repeat anteroposterior image with the intention of keeping the head in the neutral position (*right*) was indeterminate because the right OLMI (*dotted arrows*) widened a bit, but the left OLMI (*arrows*) was partially obscured. **Bottom row:** As the patient's pain persisted, a NECT the next day with the head in neutral position showed that the left OLMI (*arrows*) remained widened (just greater than 5 mm, as measured by the *white dotted line, bottom left*), while the right OLMI (*dotted arrows*) was normal, as confirmed on axial (*left*) and coronal (*middle*) reconstructions. Note that on a sagittal reformat (*right*), the cervical vertebral alignment in the sagittal plane and the predental space (*arrowhead*) remained normal, while variant congenital fusion of C2 to C3 was present (*double arrows, right*). Together these findings confirmed ligamentous injury with atlantoaxial rotatory fixation-subluxation in the absence of a cervical spine fracture

6.10.2 Pseudosubluxation of C2 on C3

Imperfect cervical spine alignment is frequently seen in children under 7–10 years of age, most commonly at C2 to C3 with slight anterolisthesis, and is seen less commonly at C3 to C4. This is considered physiologic and is attributed to a combination of ligamentous laxity and the more horizontal orientation of the juvenile facet joints, which become less horizontally oriented in adulthood. This is typically less than 3 mm of listhesis when normal (Fig. 6.49). Such normal variant anterolisthesis or "*pseudosubluxation*" may manifest in the neutral position and in flexion, but it should reduce with extension. When pseudosubluxation is present, the offset along the posterior cervical line, a line extending along the anterior cortex of the posterior arches from C1 to C3, should not exceed 1.5 mm. If it exceeds 1.5 mm, or if the C2 to C3 pseudosubluxation is more than 3 mm, then true subluxation/dislocation should be considered. Also, if the offset from the posterior cervical line is greater than 2 mm, a fracture of the posterior elements (i.e. hangman's fracture) should be considered.

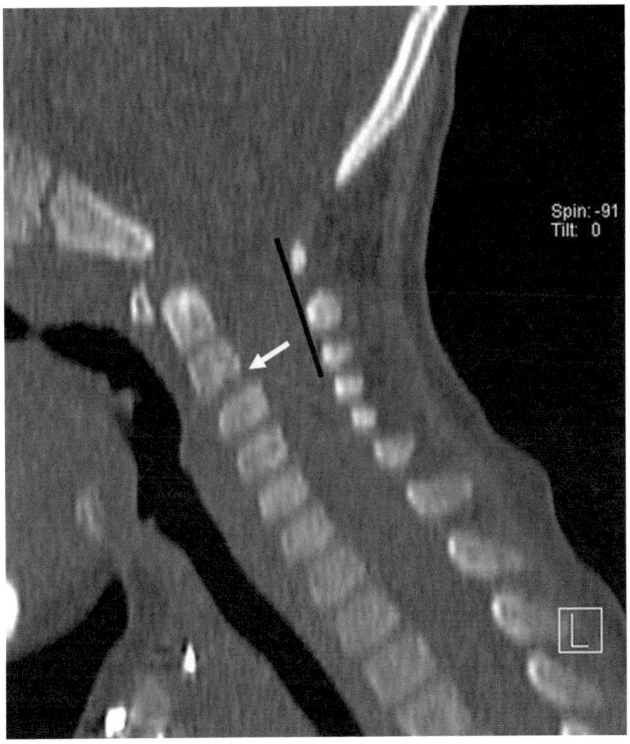

Fig. 6.49 A 2-year, 6-month-old male underwent NECT imaging of the cervical spine after a fall. There is normal variant anterior pseudosubluxation of C2 on C3 (*white arrow*). There is no offset along the posterior cervical line (*solid black line*) that extends along the anterior cortex of the posterior arches from C1 to C3

6.10.3 Loss (or Reversal) of Cervical Lordosis

Although the cervical spine normally exhibits a physiologic lordotic curvature, normal deviation from this may manifest at imaging and is a "don't touch" phenomenon. Straightening, loss, or *reversal of lordosis* is not a definitive sign of injury and may occur secondary to patient positioning. Notably, in the setting of trauma, cervical collar immobilization frequently results in straightening of the cervical spine. Similar normal variant straightening or reversal of lordosis may occur with cervical flexion, which can also cause normal variant pseudosubluxation (i.e., faux anterolisthesis) when the degree of flexion is marked (Fig. 6.50). Other benign causes of altered cervical curvature are fusion instrumentation and muscle spasm. More worrisome causes of loss of cervical lordosis include posterior ligamentous injury and fracture/subluxation. Although variation in patient position is the most likely cause of loss of cervical lordosis, it is important to evaluate for other potential causes. Not surprisingly, more variability in the cervical curvature and less straightening is observed in the absence of cervical collar immobilization. Finally, no reliable correlation has been identified between a loss of cervical lordosis and nonspecific neck pain.

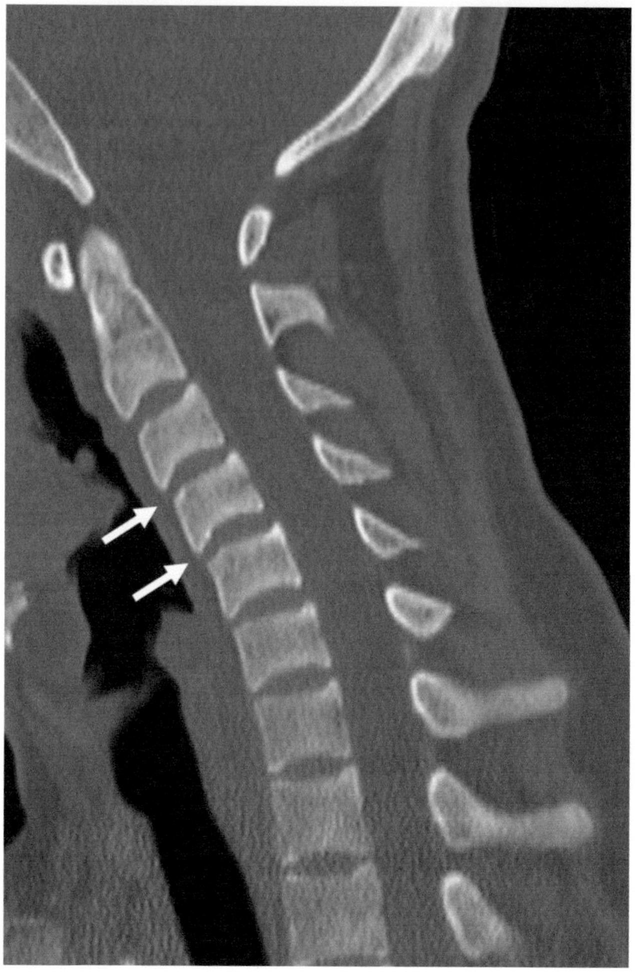

Fig. 6.50 A 22-year-old male underwent cervical NECT to evaluate soft tissue swelling. This sagittal reconstruction shows normal variant reversal of the normal cervical lordosis, most likely a consequence of patient positioning with marked flexion. There is no associated osseous injury or traumatic subluxation. In such cases of marked flexion, the flexion may cause mild pseudosubluxation such as noted here, with minimal normal pseudosubluxation anteriorly of both C3 on C4, and of C4 on C5 (*arrows*)

6.10.4 Epidural Lipomatosis

Epidural lipomatosis is the proliferation of normal adipose tissue in the epidural space. This condition occurs most commonly in the thoracic and lumbar spine. Although it is occasionally idiopathic, exogenous steroid administration and conditions with increased endogenous steroid levels such as Cushing syndrome, diabetes, and obesity are risk factors for the development of epidural lipomatosis.

While epidural lipomatosis is typically a "don't touch lesion," the presence of excess or progressive additional adipose tissue can result in narrowing of the spinal canal (Fig. 6.51). This can occur in the cervical, thoracic (most common), or lumbar region. Depending on the severity of lipomatosis, there can be variable compromise of spinal canal patency, potentially leading to spinal cord and/or nerve root compression with myelopathic symptoms. In the setting of superimposed degenerative change, patients with epidural lipomatosis are at a higher risk of resultant compression. When epidural lipomatosis is symptomatic, correction of the underlying condition, weight loss, analgesics, and in severe cases surgical decompression may be employed in an attempt to alleviate the myelopathy or radiculopathy symptoms.

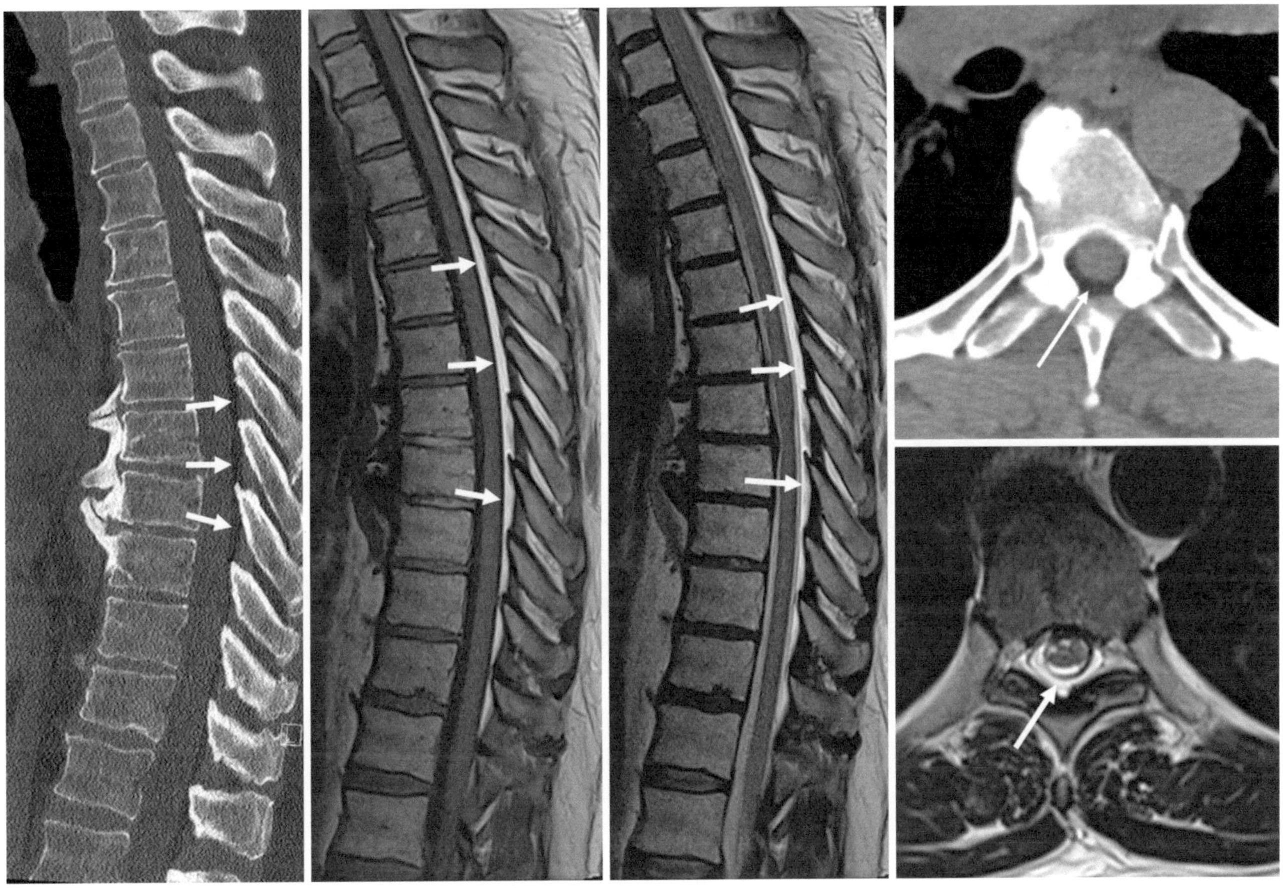

Fig. 6.51 A 63-year-old male underwent imaging of the thoracic spine to evaluate back pain. On sagittal NECT (*left*), sagittal SET1WI (*left middle*), and sagittal SET2WI (*right middle*), there is epidural lipomatosis (*arrows*) along the dorsal epidural space of the thoracic spinal canal. On an axial NECT image (*right, top*) and axial T2WI (*right, bottom*), there is also fat density/signal (*arrows*) representative of epidural lipomatosis. There is also associated narrowing of the thecal sac with a diminished subarachnoid space surrounding the spinal cord

6.10.5 Perineural Cysts

Perineural cysts are found in roughly 5% of patients. As the name implies, these are cysts along the nerve roots, near the dorsal root ganglion, and filled with CSF. Perineural cysts are typically asymptomatic and are only rarely associated with radiculopathy. They can be found through the spinal axis but are most common in the lumbar region. They are round, ovoid, or oblong and well-defined with a thin T2-hypointense rim and central fluid signal/density. They may be solitary or multilevel. In contrast to a peripheral nerve sheath tumor, perineural cysts do not enhance (Fig. 6.52).

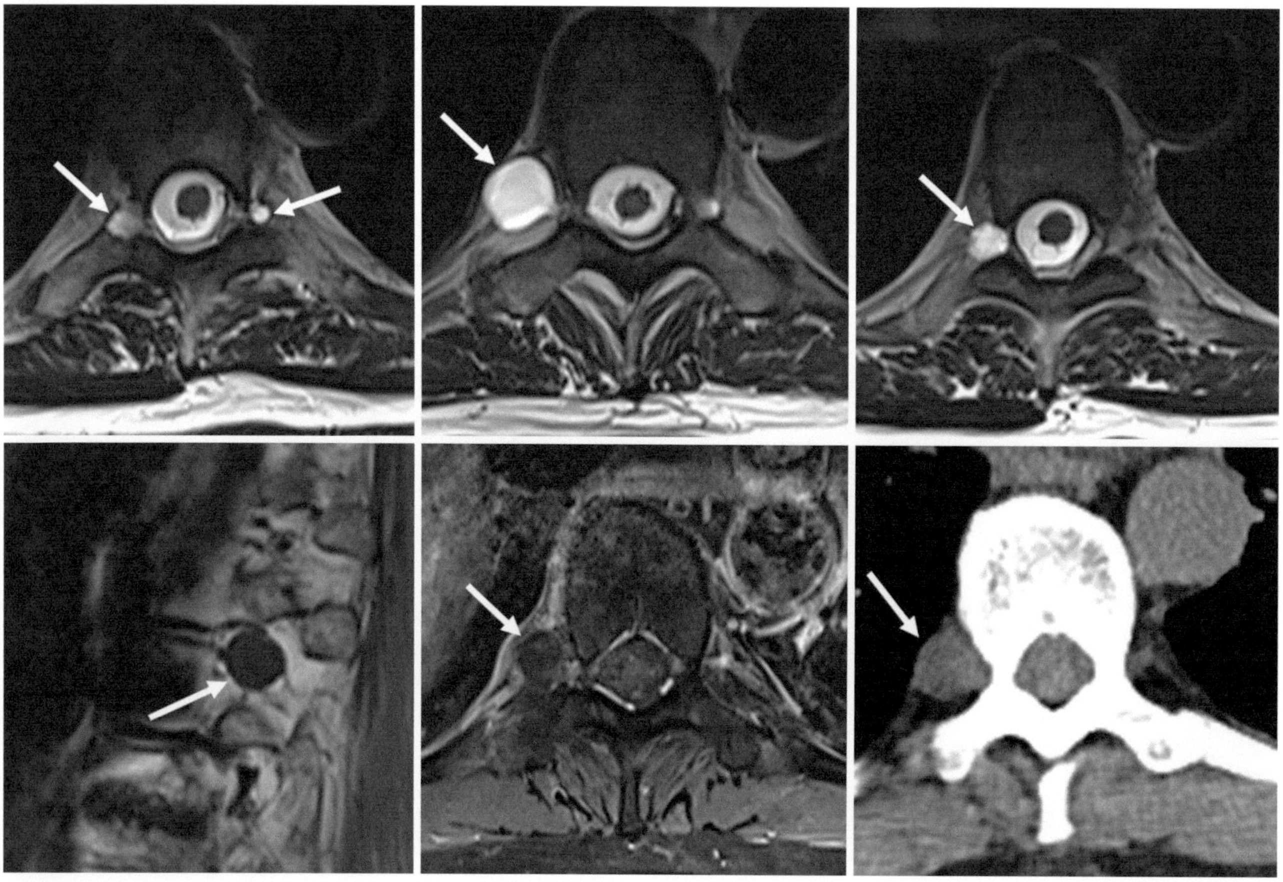

Fig. 6.52 A 74-year-old woman underwent a chest CT to evaluate her known non–small cell lung cancer. Following the chest CT, she underwent an MRI of the thoracic spine. **Top row:** On an MRI with axial SET2WI, there are incidental perineural cysts at multiple thoracic levels (*arrows*), particularly on the right side. The largest of these cysts is on the right at T10-T11 and exhibits the typical features of a perineural cyst. **Bottom row:** The characteristics of the cyst at T10-T11 (*arrows*) that are typical for a perineural cyst (rather than metastatic tumor) include that it is located along the course of the exiting nerve root (T10), it is well defined, it exhibits central T2-hyperintense signal, it does not enhance on sagittal (*left*) or axial (*middle*) postcontrast SET1WI, it is T1 hypointense on sagittal T1WI (*left*), and it is of fluid density on axial NECT (*right*)

6.10.6 Pneumorrhachis

Air can extend throughout much of the human body from another site. For instance, pneumoperitoneum can be seen in association with a gastrointestinal perforation or following intra-abdominal surgery. Similarly, pneumomediastinum can occur following median sternotomy and can track up into the cervical soft tissues. Pneumopericardium can occur following cardiac surgery. Pneumothorax can be found in association with thoracic surgery, following trauma, or even spontaneously. Intravenous air may be associated with peripheral intravenous catheter placement, a contrast injection, or other medication administration. Air in the subcutaneous tissues is called subcutaneous emphysema and can occur following trauma or in the setting of drain or tube placement. It can also occur in the presence of air elsewhere, such as in association with a pneumothorax.

Air may even extend into the spinal canal, typically into the epidural space. This phenomenon is called pneumorrhachis (Fig. 6.53). Potential sources of *pneumorrhachis* include blunt or penetrating skull fracture, spinal trauma, spine therapy, pneumomediastinum, pneumothorax, cranial surgery, or thoracic surgery. As mentioned above, pneumorrhachis can be related to severe trauma or extensive open surgery, but it can also be spontaneous, such as related to spontaneous pneumomediastinum or spontaneous pneumothorax. Pneumorrhachis is not a normal variant, but it is usually a benign (and thus "don't touch") finding unless it causes severe compression of the cord (i.e., tension pneumorrhachis). It can also occur anywhere along the spinal axis. Its presence is important to note, since the search for a potential source of air should be conducted.

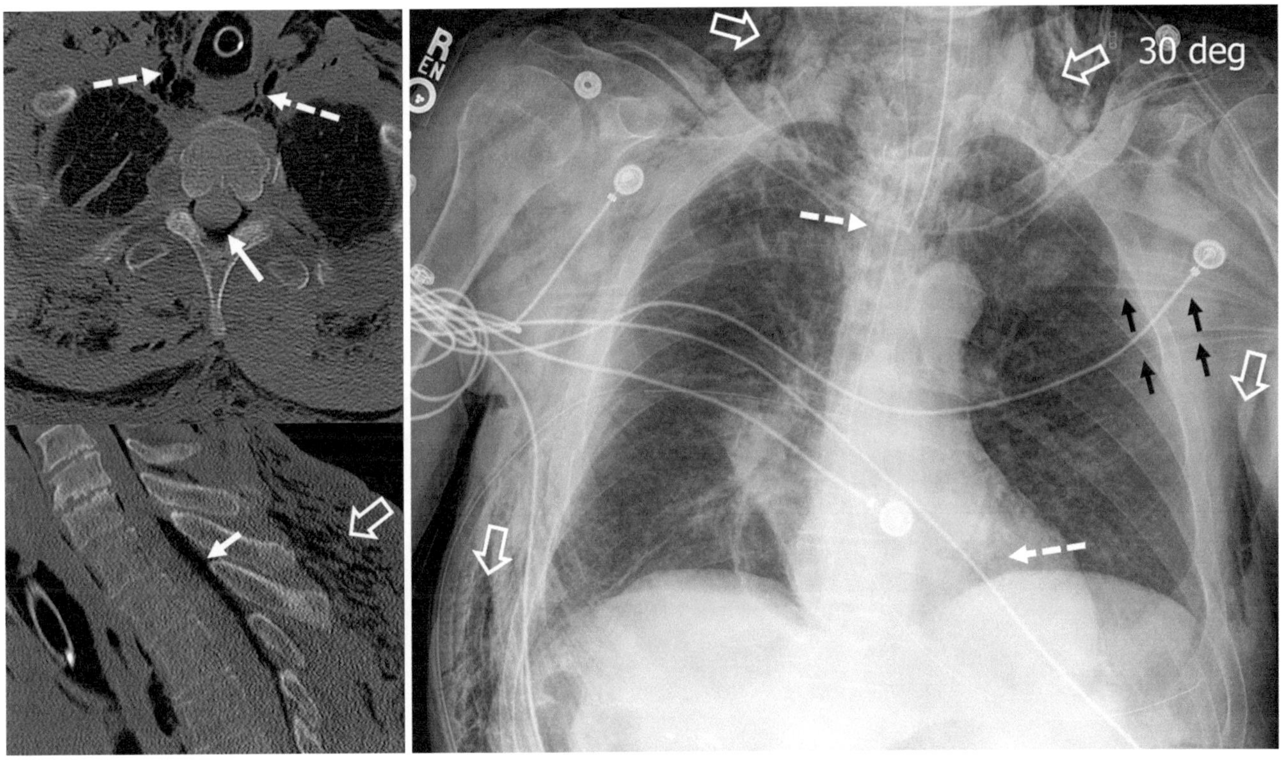

Fig. 6.53 A 65-year-old male in the setting of acute trauma. Axial and sagittal reconstructed NECT images (*top left and bottom left, respectively*) of the cervicothoracic spine show epidural pneumorrhachis (*solid white arrows*), pneumomediastinum (*dashed white arrows*), and subcutaneous emphysema (*open white arrow, right*) accompanying a traumatic pneumothorax. Although the pneumorrhachis is not readily apparent on a portable anteroposterior chest radiograph (*right*) performed on the same day as the NECT, the pneumomediastinum and subcutaneous emphysema are well demonstrated. The striations of the pectoralis muscles are also well delineated as they are outlined by air (*black arrows, right*)

6.10.7 Contrast Reflux into Paraspinous Veins and Plexi

Contrast-enhanced CT (CECT) examinations are common, and more so when imaging the neck compared with dedicated imaging of the spine. With a bolus administration of intravenous iodinated contrast, *reflux of intravenous contrast* commonly occurs. Another commonly observed phenomenon is *venous stasis of contrast* (Fig. 6.54). This occurs when contrast agent persists in a venous structure despite normal venous flow, and it should spontaneously clear, particularly after the imaging examination is completed. Stasis and reflux of contrast are usually benign but may be more pronounced when there is impaired central venous flow, such as with central venous thrombosis, stenosis, or compression. Such contrast reflux, particularly in the setting of stasis, heart failure, or thrombosis, may demonstrate venous plexi in paraspinous locations not normally visible on routine CECT, such as the anterior internal vertebral venous plexus, the posterior internal vertebral venous plexus, the posterior external vertebral venous plexus, vertebral veins (or plexi), or even veins traversing the neural foramina. Thus, while the central venous cause of obstruction or stenosis is not normal, the appearance of such paraspinal veins or plexi that can appear prominent in their normal locations is not pathologic in and of itself. Such vertebral/paravertebral/paraspinous vein or plexus prominence may simulate vascular lesions such as arteriovenous malformation or dural arteriovenous fistula, or it can mimic enhancing neoplastic lesions such as leptomeningeal carcinomatosis (from metastatic disease) or lymphoma.

When present, the persistent venous contrast may be quite dense, often denser than bone, but it may also be of intermediate density if mixing with normal venous blood occurs. The dense contrast could mimic dense embolization material, although the use of embolization material in the cervical and thoracic spines is uncommon and is usually not as widespread as reflux of contrast material. The high density, particularly when concentrated within the subclavian vein, is also prone to streak artifact, which can obscure visualization of structures adjacent to the dense contrast. Adjustments to imaging protocols, including timing of image acquisition relative to the contrast bolus and saline administration as well as recognizing a patient with central venous stasis or thrombosis issues, can often reduce this potential artifact and thus improve image quality.

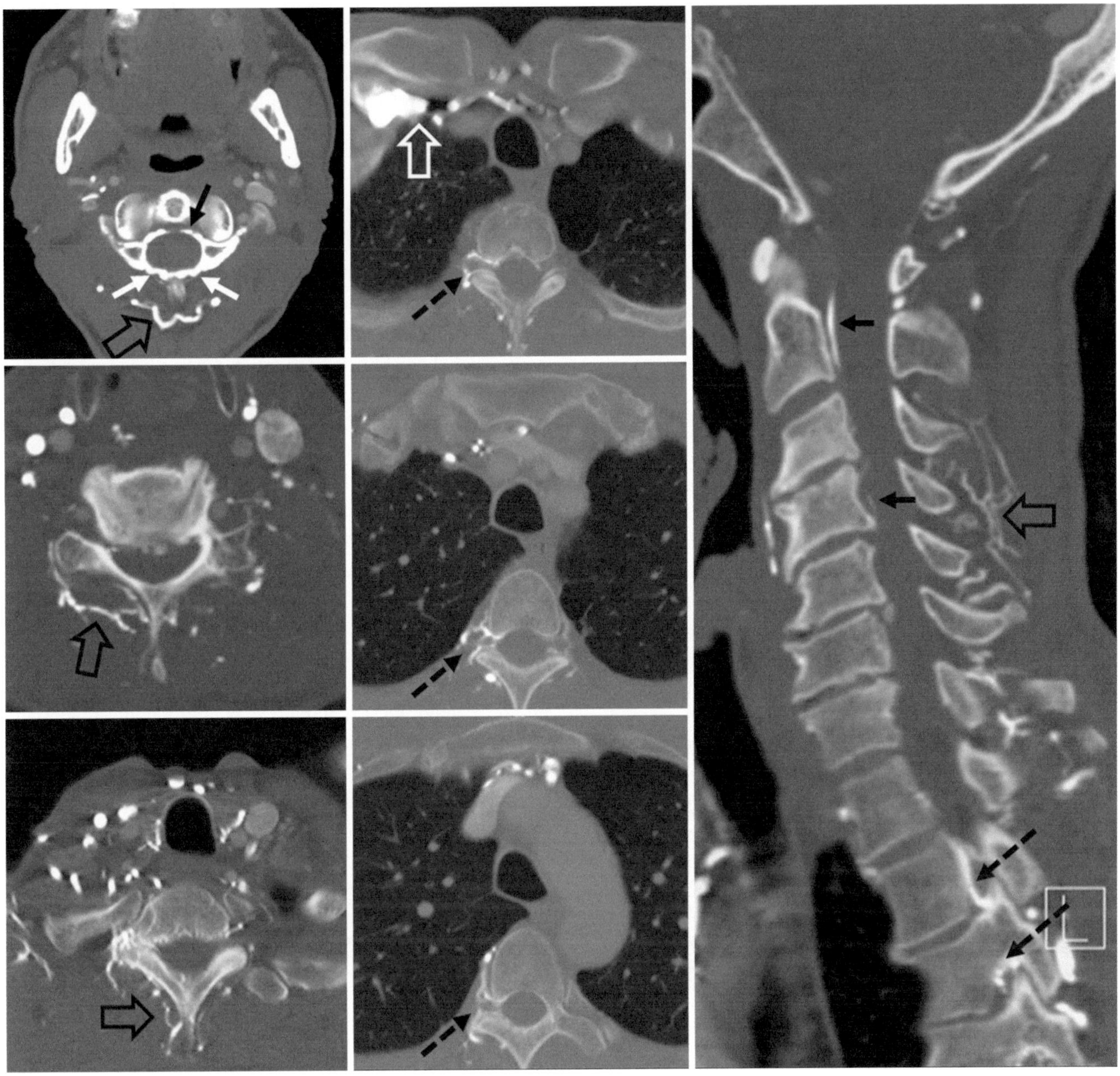

Fig. 6.54 A 64-year-old male underwent contrast-enhanced CT (CECT) of the neck for tonsillar cancer. In this case, there is widespread reflux of contrast, particularly pronounced owing to a chronic central right subclavian vein obstruction (*open white arrow, top middle image*), as demonstrated on axial CECT reformats (*left column and middle column*) and on a sagittal reconstruction (*right*). Aside from reflux into the anterior veins of the neck, there is also reflux of contrast into the interconnected anterior internal vertebral venous plexus (*solid black arrows, top left and right*), the posterior internal vertebral venous plexus (*solid white arrows, top left*), and the posterior external vertebral venous plexus (*open black arrows, left column and right*). Also note the contrast reflux into multiple right neural foramina (*dashed black arrows, middle column and right*)

6.11 Artifacts That Simulate Spinal Lesions

6.11.1 CSF Flow Artifact

Motion during MRI often leads to artifact, and the manifestation of such artifact depends on the source, imaging sequence, and severity. Vascular and CSF flow from pulsation can result in signal voids, particularly on conventional spin-echo or inversion recovery imaging,such as spin-echo T1-weighted (SET1WI), spin-echo T2-weighted (SET2WI), or fluid-attenuated inversion recovery (FLAIR) sequences owing to the changing of positions of protons between the two echoes that prevents the accumulation/registration of signal in a particular location. *CSF flow artifact* phenomena may also manifest due to a combination of time-of-flight (TOF) effect and turbulent flow. This artifact can be reduced or eliminated by using sequences that implement a single radiofrequency (RF) excitation pulse such as echo-planar imaging (EPI), gradient echo imaging (GE), or by other much faster image acquisition sequences such as single shot fast spin echo (SS-FSE), single shot turbo spin echo (SS-TSE), or the half-Fourier-acquired single-shot turbo spin-echo (HASTE) techniques, or even by motion-correction parallel imaging techniques (such as BLADE and PROPELLER). In general, a shorter echo time (TE) used with these techniques results in less phase incoherence and thus less signal loss. The potential pitfall of suspecting pathology caused by hypointensity on conventional SET2WI can be readily accounted for by repeat imaging using GET2WI. As in the examples provided, CSF flow can result in marked signal loss of the subarachnoid space surrounding the spinal cord; this can be multifocal, diffuse, unilateral, or bilateral. Such CSF flow artifacts can mimic an arteriovenous malformation (AVM), dural arteriovenous fistula (DAVF), subarachnoid or subdural hemorrhage, disc hernation, or extramedullary mass. Other benefits of utilizing GET2WI include improved delineation between grey and white matter and the higher sensitivity relative to SET2WI for detecting intraspinal hemorrhage. However, the signal-noise ratio and thus detection of intrinsic cord lesions may be slightly lower than those of SET2WI.

6.11.2 Gibbs Artifact Phenomenon

Gibbs phenomenon (also known as "truncation artifact") occurs when oscillations that result from high-contrast anatomic boundaries lead to abrupt transitions in signal magnitude. This phenomenon is associated with the appearance of alternating bright and dark lines, also described as "ripples" or "ringing" oriented perpendicular to the anatomic boundary. Gibbs artifact is predictable and commonly observed on sagittal SET2WI of the spine as a vertically oriented signal abnormality; this phenomenon can also be noted on STIR imaging. In addition to the typical linear band of T2 hyperintensity within the cord, decreased sharpness along the edges of the cord may be manifest. Gibbs/ringing artifact can be reduced by decreasing pixel size (e.g., increasing the acquisition matrix or decreasing the field-of-view) and by selecting a phase encoding direction perpendicular to the prominent edges of anatomic structures. The phenomenon is potentially problematic when it involves the spinal cord, and awareness of this artifact helps to prevent misconstruing it as myelopathic cord signal or a dilated central canal such as a syrinx. Also, respiratory motion artifact may further degrade visualization of the spinal cord, although this artifact is restricted to the phase-encoding direction. In the event that respiratory motion artifact mimics a lesion, phase swapping (changing the phase-encoding direction) or respiratory gating can help confirm or eliminate the finding (Figs. 6.55, 6.56, 6.57 and 6.58).

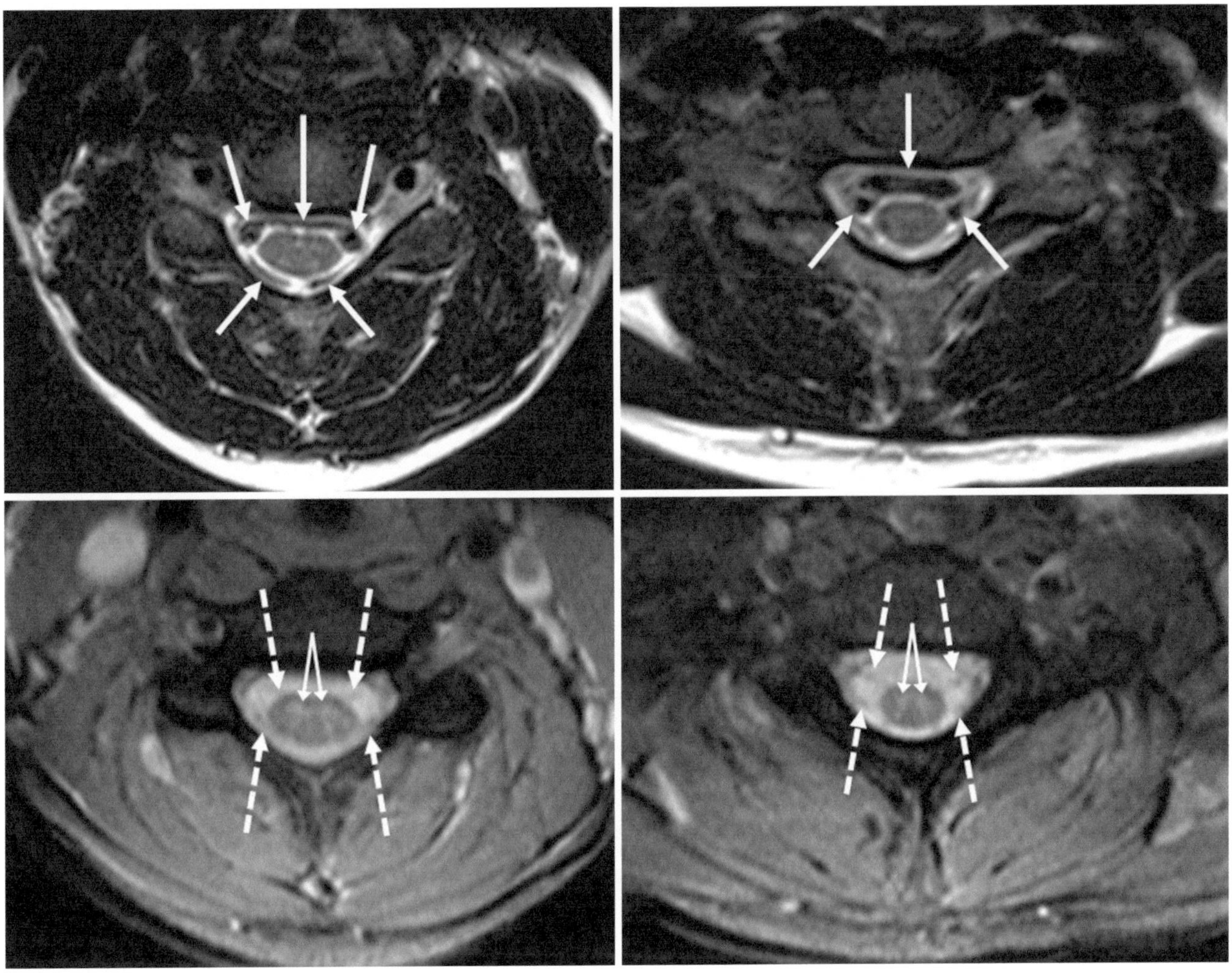

Fig. 6.55 A 2-year-old girl underwent MRI of the cervical spine to evaluate neck pain, where MR imaging revealed a normal cervical spine. **Top row:** There were multifocal regions of hypointense signal on axial SET2WI, as such artifact on this spin-echo sequence; dark artifact surrounding the cord within the spinal canal results from normal dynamic CSF flow during imaging (*arrows*). **Bottom row:** These regions of flow artifact completely resolve on axial GET2WI. On GET2WI, now that the CSF flow voids are no longer visible, note the relatively subtle and normal appearance of the nerve roots traversing the subarachnoid space (*dashed arrows*) as well as the now normally visible and mildly hyperintense central grey matter (*double arrows*)

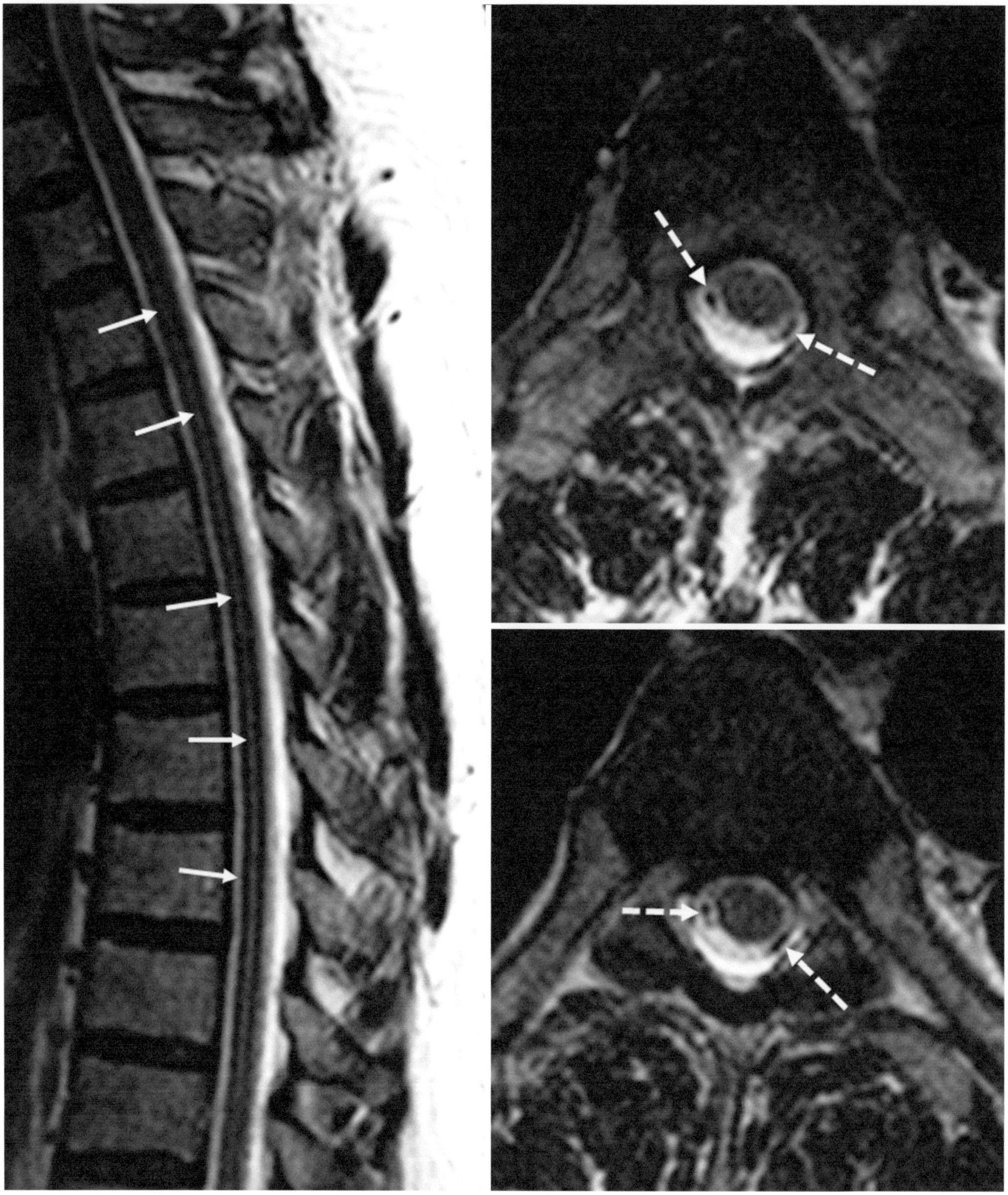

Fig. 6.56 A 56-year-old male with a thoracic spine MRI to evaluate for a possible spinal cord lesion. On sagittal SET2WI of the thoracic spine (*left*), there is central linear hyperintense T2 signal coursing through the middle of the spinal cord (*arrows*) typical of Gibbs phenomenon. Axial SET2WI (*right, top, and bottom images*) shows normal signal within the thoracic spinal cord, verifying that the finding on the sagittal images was related to Gibbs artifact; thus pathology was excluded. Also note small areas of T2 hypointensity on axial SET2WI (*dashed white arrows, right*) that should not be confused for pathology because they represent normal CSF flow voids. Axial GET2WI (not performed in this patient) could be performed to verify that the areas of hypointensity are simply CSF flow voids

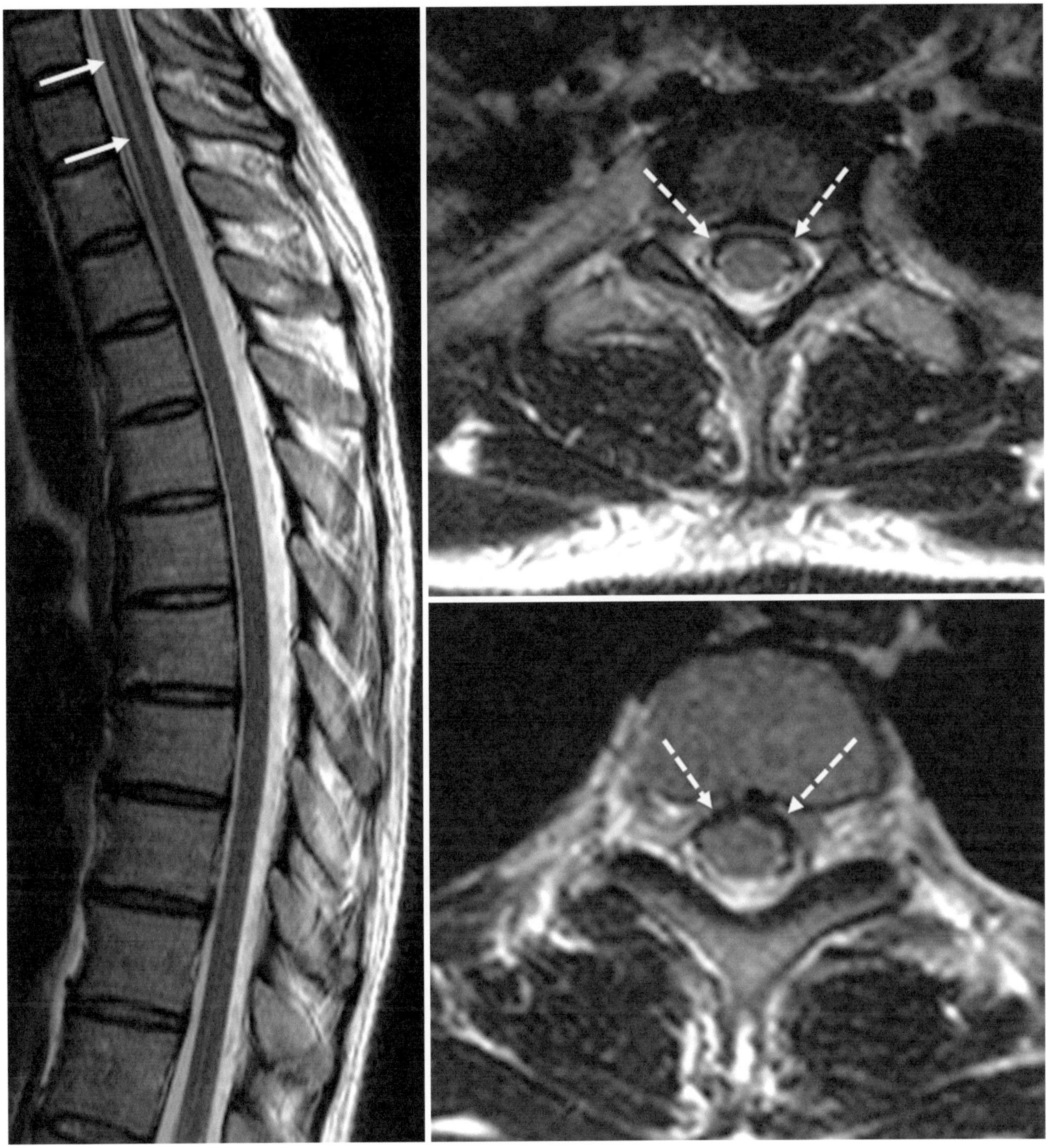

Fig. 6.57 A 32-year-old female underwent MRI of the thoracic spine to further evaluate possible central cord signal abnormality identified on prior MRI imaging. On sagittal SET2WI (*left*), a contiguous central line of increased signal coursing through the middle of the lower cervical and upper thoracic spinal cord is present at the top of the field of view (*arrows, left*). Axial SET2WI (*right, top and bottom images*) shows normal intramedullary signal of the spinal cord at those levels, verifying Gibbs phenomenon. Normal CSF flow void artifactual dark signal is present within the subarachnoid space (*dashed white arrows, right*), surrounding portions of the spinal cord on the axial SET2WI

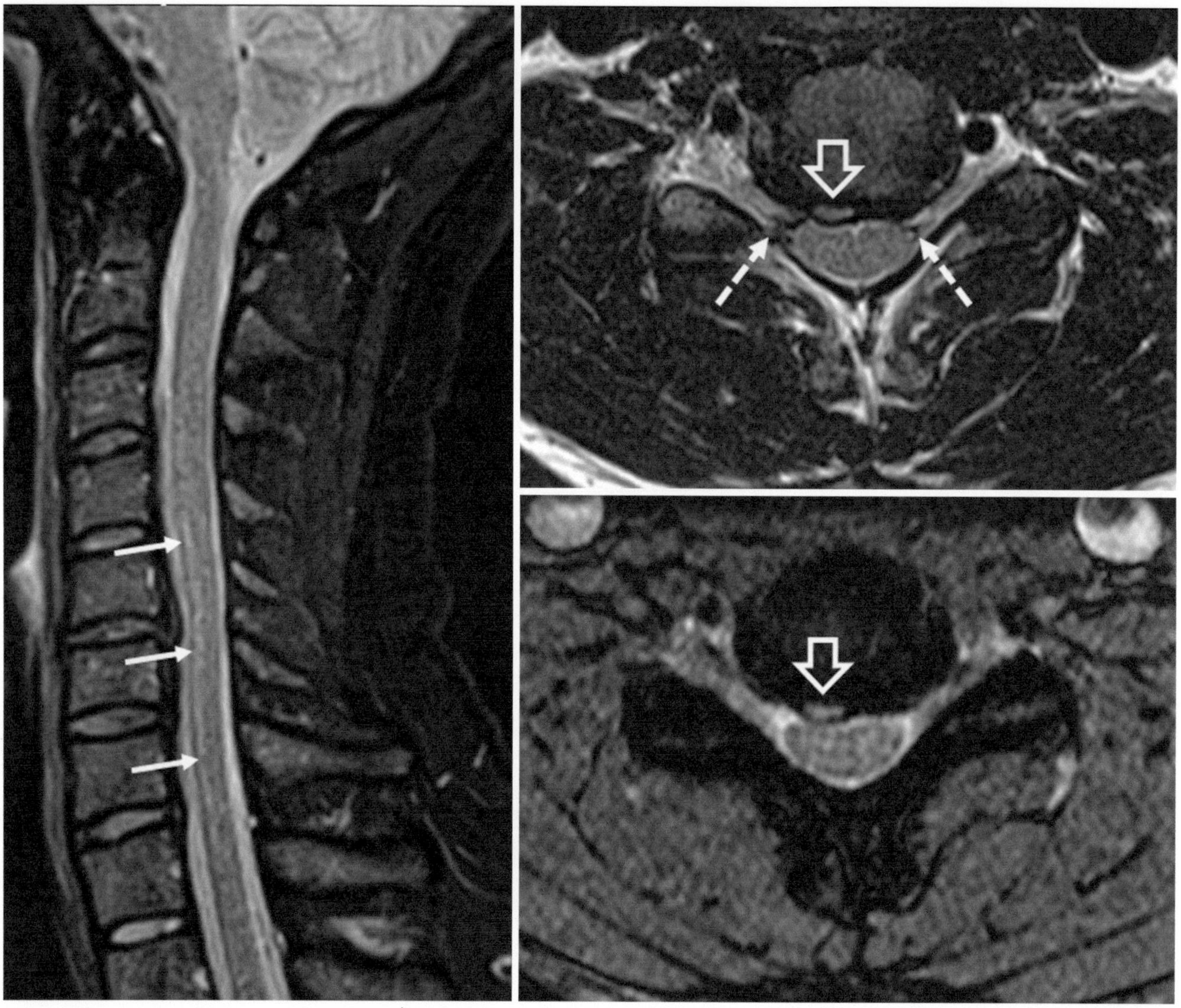

Fig. 6.58 A 31-year-old male with chronic neck pain having both Gibbs artifact and CSF flow void artifact. On the midline sagittal STIR image (*left*) of the cervical spine, there is a central line of increased signal coursing through the lower cervical spinal cord (*arrows*); this is typical of a Gibbs phenomenon–related artifact that mimics myelopathic cord signal. However, on axial SET2WI (*top right*) there is normal signal within the spinal cord, verifying Gibbs artifact; note the right central disc protrusion at C5 and C6 (*open arrows*) that abuts the cord, representing true degenerative pathology and causing spinal canal stenosis. These images also nicely illustrate CSF flow artifact, where there are small areas of T2 hypointensity on SET2WI (*dashed arrows, top right*) ventral to the brain stem and lateral to the cervical spinal cord that represent normal CSF flow voids and should not be confused with pathology. Axial GET2WI of the cervical spinal cord (*bottom right*) confirms resolution of the areas of hypointensity indicative of the CSF flow void-related artifact as well as the true disc protrusion (*open arrows*) resulting in mild spinal canal stenosis

6.11.3 Vacuum Phenomenon

The *vacuum phenomenon* has been postulated to occur as air, previously dissolved in solution, that accumulates within the otherwise negative space within a joint. This process would explain why it is more readily visualized with extension or traction. In the intervertebral disc space, this air is at least 90% nitrogen and is most commonly associated with disc degeneration. The prevalence of this phenomenon has been reported to range from 2% of patients to nearly 21% of asymptomatic elderly patients, which may depend on the ages of the study cohorts. Notably, the air may extend beyond the disc space into the epidural space or alternatively into the adjacent vertebrae (Fig. 6.59). The vacuum phenomenon is usually readily identified on imaging, since this air is hypointense on MRI and hypodense on radiographs and CT.

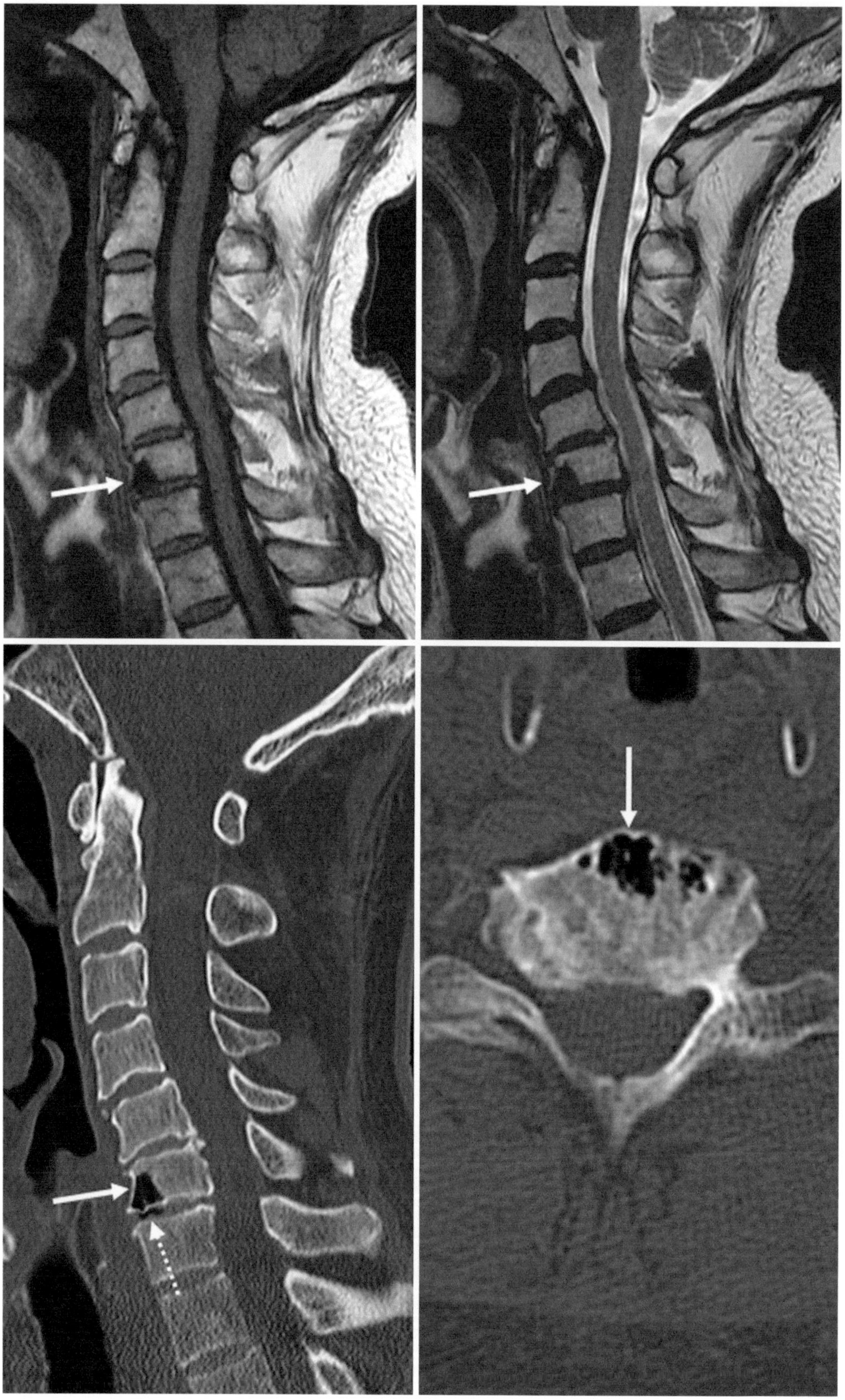

Fig. 6.59 A 56-year-old male underwent a cervical spine MRI for cervical pain. Sagittal SET1WI (*top left*) and sagittal SET2WI (*top right*) demonstrate a focal region of hypointense signal (*arrows*) in the anterior C6 vertebral body. Owing to a suspicion of sclerotic metastasis, this was further evaluated with CT. Sagittal (*bottom left*) and axial (*bottom right*) CT images confirm the presence of hypodense air (*arrows*) within the anterior C6 vertebral body, corresponding to the region of hypointense signal on the prior MRI. There is also air inferiorly in the adjacent C6–C7 disc space (*dotted arrow, bottom left*), demonstrating that this benign finding is commonly associated with disc degeneration

6.11.4 Vertebroplasty Cement

Vertebral augmentation, although somewhat controversial in terms of its effectiveness, is a treatment option for some vertebral compression fractures. Typically, from a transpedicular approach, the proceduralist can inject cement into the collapsed vertebral body. When cement is injected in isolation, this is called vertebroplasty. When a balloon is inflated within the collapsed vertebral body prior to cement injection, this is called kyphoplasty. Vertebroplasty cement is typically rather dense. Its high density is readily appreciated on CT. On MRI, vertebroplasty cement is hypointense (Fig. 6.60). Lucent defects from the procedure, similar to pedicle screw tracts, may also be seen. Knowledge of this intervention is helpful in correctly identifying the cement. Otherwise, on MRI, the presence of cement may be misconstrued as a sclerotic lesion.

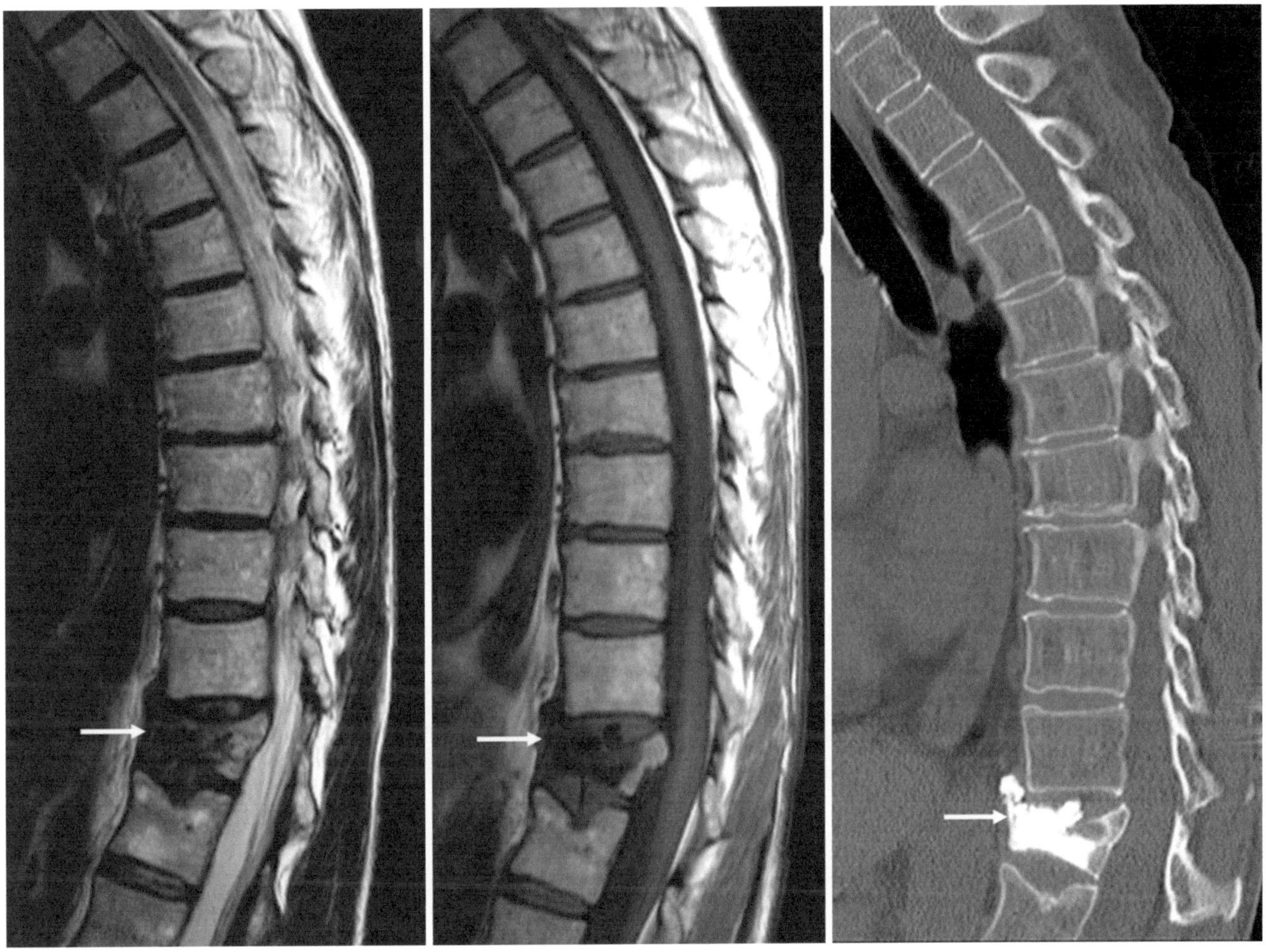

Fig. 6.60 A 49-year-old woman underwent imaging of the thoracic spine to evaluate back pain. These sagittal SET2WI (*left*) and SET1WI (*center*) MR images show a compression fracture of the T12 vertebral body with anterior wedging. There is central hypointense signal within the compressed vertebral body and within the adjacent disc space. At first glance, and in the absence of adequate historical information, this appearance could potentially be misinterpreted as a sclerotic metastasis. A sagittal NECT image (*right*) clearly demonstrates hyperdense vertebroplasty cement, accounting for the hypointense signal on the prior MRI examination. The presence of older imaging or an appropriate clinical history can help prevent this conundrum

Suggested Reading

Abiola R, Rubery P, Mesfin A. Ossification of the posterior longitudinal ligament: etiology, diagnosis, and outcomes of nonoperative and operative management. Global Spine J. 2016;6:195–204.

Adib O, Berthier E, Loisel D, Aubé C. Pediatric cervical spine in emergency: radiographic features of normal anatomy, variants and pitfalls. Skelet Radiol. 2016;45:1607–17.

Akbar JJ, Weiss KL, Saafir MA, Weiss JL. Rapid MRI detection of vertebral numeric variation. Am J Roentgenol. 2010;195:465–6.

Aljuboori Z, Yaseen A, Simpson J, Boakye M. Surgical excision of a symptomatic thoracic nerve root perineural cyst resulting in complete resolution of symptoms: a case report. Cureus. 2017;9:e1343.

Al-Khawaja D, Seex K, Eslick GD. Spinal epidural lipomatosis--a brief review. J Clin Neurosci. 2008;15:1323–6.

Arvin B, Fournier-Gosselin M-P, Fehlings MG. Os odontoideum: etiology and surgical management. Neurosurgery. 2010;66:22–31.

Baeesa SS, Bokhari RF, Bajunaid KM, Al-Sayyad MJ. Prevalence of the foramen arcuale of the atlas in a Saudi population. Neurosciences. 2012;17:345–51.

Bajwa NS, Toy JO, Ahn NU. Establishment of parameters for congenital thoracic stenosis: a study of 700 postmortem specimens. Clin Orthop Relat Res. 2012;470:3195–201.

Barnett GH, Hardy RW Jr, Little JR, Bay JW, Sypert GW. Thoracic spinal canal stenosis. J Neurosurg. 1987;66:338–44.

Bayrakdar IS, Miloglu O, Altun O, Gumussoy I, Durna D, Yilmaz AB. Cone beam computed tomography imaging of ponticulus posticus: prevalence, characteristics, and a review of the literature. Oral Surg Oral Med Oral Pathol Oral Radiol. 2014;118:e210–9.

Billmann F, Bokor-Billmann T, Burnett C, Kiffner E. Occurrence and significance of odontoid lateral mass interspace asymmetry in trauma patients. World J Surg. 2013;37:1988–95.

Brewin J, Hill M, Ellis H. The prevalence of cervical ribs in a London population. Clin Anat. 2009;22:331–6.

Cakmak O, Gurdal E, Ekinci G, Yildiz E, Cavdar S. Arcuate foramen and its clinical significance. Saudi Med J. 2005;26:1409–13.

Carrino A, Campbell PD Jr, Lin DC, Moorison WB, Schweitzer ME, Flanders AE, et al. Effect of spinal segment variants on numbering vertebral levels at lumbar MR imaging. Radiology. 2011;259:196–202.

Chen MY, Elster AD. Simulation of syringomyelia by ventral median fissure. J Comput Assist Tomogr. 1990;14:841–2.

Chen Y, Zhuang Z, Qi W, Yang H, Chen Z, Wang X, Kong K. A three-dimensional study of the atlantodental interval in a normal Chinese population using reformatted computed tomography. Surg Radiol Anat. 2011;33:801–6.

Chiba K, Yamamoto I, Hirabayashi H, Iwasaki M, Goto H, Yonenobu K, et al. Multicenter study investigating the postoperative progression of ossification of the posterior longitudinal ligament in the cervical spine: a new computer-assisted measurement. J Neurosurg Spine. 2005;3:17–23.

Cloud GC, Markus HS. Diagnosis and management of vertebral artery stenosis. QJM. 2003;96:27–54.

Cushing KE, Ramesh V, Gardner-Medwin D, Todd NV, Gholkar A, Baxter P, et al. Tethering of the vertebral artery in the congenital arcuate foramen of the atlas vertebra: a possible cause of vertebral artery dissection in children. Dev Med Child Neurol. 2001;43:491–6.

de Graauw N, Carpay HA, Slooff W-BM. The paracondylar process: an unusual and treatable cause of posttraumatic headache. Spine. 2008;33:E283–6.

Doberentz E, Schumacher R, Gembruch U, Gasser JA, Müller AM. Coronal vertebral clefts: a radiological indicator for chromosomal aberrations. Pediatr Dev Pathol. 2013;16:1–6.

Doberentz E, Madea B, Müller AM. Coronal clefts in infants – rare differential diagnosis of traumatic injuries of vertebral bodies in battered children. Legal Med. 2014;16:333–6.

Dorne HL, Lander PH. CT recognition of anomalies of the posterior arch of the atlas vertebra: differentiation from fracture. Am J Neuroradiol. 1986;7:176–7.

Drevelengas A, Kalaitzoglou I, Petridis A. Pneumorrhachis associated with spontaneous pneumomediastinum. Eur J Radiol. 1994;18:122–3.

Elgafy H, Pompo F, Vela R, Elsamaloty HM. Ipsilateral arcuate foramen and high-riding vertebral artery: implication on C1–C2 instrumentation. Spine J. 2014;14:1351–5.

Emiralioğlu N, Ozcan HN, Oğuz B, Yalçın E, Doğru D, Özçelik U, Kiper N. Pneumomediastinum, pneumorrhachis and subcutaneous emphysema associated with viral infections: report of three cases. Pediatr Int. 2015;57:1038–40.

Epstein BS, Epstein JA, Jones MD. Cervical spinal stenosis. Radiol Clin N Am. 1977;15:215–26.

Eran A, Yousem DM, Izbudak I. Asymmetry of the odontoid lateral mass interval in pediatric trauma CT: do we need to investigate further? Am J Neuroradiol. 2016;37:176–9.

Esakkiammal N, Chauhan R. Clinical significance of presence of accessory foramen transversarium in typical cervical vertebrae. Int J Res Med Sci. 2016;4:5231–6.

Fassett DR, Schmidt MH. Spinal epidural lipomatosis: a review of its causes and recommendations for treatment. Neurosurg Focus. 2004;16:E11.

Ford LT, Gilula LA, Murphy WA, Gado M. Analysis of gas in vacuum lumbar disc. Am J Roentgenol. 1977;128:1056–7.

Ford LT, Goodman FG. X-ray studies of the lumbosacral spine. South Med J. 1966;59:1123–8.

Freilich M, Virapongse C, Kier EL, Sarwar M, Bhimani S. Foramen transversarium enlargement due to tortuosity of the vertebral artery. Computed tomographic appearance. Spine. 1986;11:95–8.

Gay RE. The curve of the cervical spine: variations and significance. J Manip Physiol Ther. 1993;16:591–4.

Gershon-Cohen J, Schraer H, Sklaroff DM, Blumberg N. Dissolution of the intervertebral disk in the aged normal; the phantom nucleus pulposus. Radiology. 1954;62:383–7.

Gholve PA, Hosalkar HS, Ricchetti ET, Pollock AN, Dormans JP, Drummond DS. Occipitalization of the atlas in children. Morphologic classification, associations, and clinical relevance. J Bone Joint Surg Am. 2007;89:571–8.

Goddard AJ, Annesley-Williams D, Guthrie JA, Weston M. Duplication of the vertebral artery: report of two cases and review of the literature. Neuroradiology. 2001;43:477–80.

Goh BK, Yeo AW. Traumatic pneumorrhachis. J Trauma. 2005;58:875–9.

Gohil I, Vilensky JA, Weber EC. Vacuum phenomenon: clinical relevance. Clin Anat. 2014;27:455–62.

Grob D, Frauenfelder H, Mannion AF. The association between cervical spine curvature and neck pain. Eur Spine J. 2007;16:669–78.

Guebert GM, Yochum TR, Rowe LJ. Congenital anomalies and normal skeletal variants. In: Yochum TR, Rowe LI, editors. Essentials of skeletal radiology. Baltimore: Lippincott Williams & Wilkins; 2005. p. 278–87.

Guo Q, Ni B, Yang J, Zhu Z, Yanget J. Simultaneous ossification of the posterior longitudinal ligament and ossification of the ligamentum flavum causing upper thoracic myelopathy in DISH: case report and literature review. Eur Spine J. 2011;20(Suppl 2):S195–201.

Guttentag AR, Salwen JK. Keep your eyes on the ribs: the spectrum of normal variants and diseases that involve the ribs. Radiographics. 1999;19:1125–42.

Hadjigeorgiou GF, Singh R, Stefanopoulos P, Petsanas A, Hadjigeorgiou FG, Fountas K. Traumatic pneumorrachis after isolated closed head injuries: an up-to-date review. J Clin Neurosci. 2016;34:44–6.

Hahn PY, Strobel JJ, Hahn FJ. Verification of lumbosacral segments on MR images: identification of transitional vertebrae. Radiology. 1992;182:580–1.

Hanson EH, Mishra RK, Chang DS, Perkins TG, Bonifield DR, Tandy RD, et al. Sagittal whole-spine magnetic resonance imaging in 750 consecutive outpatients: accurate determination of the number of lumbar vertebral bodies. J Neurosurg Spine. 2010;12:47–55.

Harty JA, Lenehan B, O'Rourke SK. Odontoid lateral mass asymmetry: do we over-investigate? Emerg Med J. 2005;22:625–7.

Helliwell PS, Evans PF, Wright V. The straight cervical spine: does it indicate muscle spasm? J Bone Joint Surg Br. 1994;76:103–6.

Hori T, Kawaguchi Y, Kimura T. How does the ossification area of the posterior longitudinal ligament progress after cervical laminoplasty? Spine. 2006;31:2807–12.

Hori T, Kawaguchi Y, Kimura T. How does the ossification area of the posterior longitudinal ligament thicken following cervical laminoplasty? Spine. 2007;32:E551–6.

Iclal ET, Lomasney LM, Jones NS, Wojewnik B, Aziz A, Alsabban K, Adams W. A practical radiographic visual estimation technique for the prediction of developmental narrowing of cervical spinal canal. Br J Radiol. 2017;90:20170–286.

Ionete C, Omojola MF. MR angiographic demonstration of bilateral duplication of the extracranial vertebral artery: unusual course and review of the literature. Am J Neuroradiol. 2006;27:304–6.

Jenkins TJ, Mai HT, Burgmeier RJ, Savage JW, Patel AA, Hsu WK. The triangle model of congenital cervical stenosis. Spine. 2016;41:E242–7.

Jones BV. Cord cystic cavities: syringomyelia and prominent central canal. Semin Ultrasound CT MR. 2017;38:98–104.

Junewick JJ, Chin MS, Meesa IR, Ghori S, Boynton SJ, Luttenton CR. Ossification patterns of the atlas vertebra. Am J Roentgenol. 2011;197:1229–34.

Kang K-C, Lee C-S, Shin S-K, Park SJ, Chung CH, Chung SS. Ossification of the ligamentum flavum of the thoracic spine in the Korean population. J Neurosurg Spine. 2011;14:513–9.

Karwacki GM, Schneider JF. Normal ossification patterns of atlas and axis: a CT study. Am J Neuroradiol. 2012;33:1882–7.

Kessler JT. Congenital narrowing of the cervical spinal canal. J Neurol Neurosurg Psychiatry. 1975;38:1218–24.

Khalili H, Niakan A, Ghaffarpasand F. Massive pneumocephalus and pneumorrhachis after severe skull base fracture. Bull Emerg Trauma. 2016;4:248–9.

Khamanarong K, Woraputtaporn W, Ratanasuwan S, Namking M, Chaijaroonkhanarak W, Sae-Jung S. Occipitalization of the atlas: its incidence and clinical implications. Acta Med Acad. 2013;42:41–5.

Kim C, Lee S-H, Park SS, Kim BJ, Ryu WS, Yoon B-W, et al. A quantitative comparison of the vertebral artery and transverse foramen using CT angiography. J Clin Neurol. 2012;8:259–64.

Kim MS. Anatomical variant of atlas: arcuate foramen, occipitalization of atlas, and defect of posterior arch of atlas. J Korean Neurosurg Soc. 2015;58:528–33.

Klekamp J. How should syringomyelia be defined and diagnosed? World Neurosurg. 2018;111:e729–45.

Knutsson F. The vacuum phenomenon in the intervertebral discs. Acta Radiol. 1942;23:173–9.

Krupa K, Bekiesińska-Figatowska M. Artifacts in magnetic resonance imaging. Pol J Radiol. 2015;80:93–106.

Kumar R, Guinto FC Jr, Madewell JE, Swischuk LE, David R. The vertebral body: radiographic configurations in various congenital and acquired disorders. Radiographics. 1988;8:455–85.

Larsen DW, Teitelbaum GP, Norman D. Cerebrospinal fluid flow artifact. A possible pitfall on fast-spin-echo MR imaging of the spine simulating intradural pathology. Clin Imaging. 1996;20:140–2.

Lavdas E, Mavroidis P, Kostopoulos S, Ninos C, Strikou A-D, Glotsos D, et al. Reduction of motion, truncation and flow artifacts using BLADE sequences in cervical spine MR imaging. Magn Reson Imaging. 2015;33:194–200.

Lee CK, Weiss AB. Isolated congenital cervical block vertebrae below the axis with neurological symptoms. Spine. 1981;6:118–24.

Leivseth G, Frobin W, Brinckmann P. Congenital cervical block vertebrae are associated with caudally adjacent discs. Clin Biomech. 2005;20:669–74.

Levy LM, Di Chiro G, Brooks RA, Dwyer AJ, Wener L, Frank J. Spinal cord artifacts from truncation errors during MR imaging. Radiology. 1988;166:479–83.

Linsenmaier U, Deak Z, Krtakovska A, Ruschi F, Kammer N, Wirth S, et al. Emergency radiology: straightening of the cervical spine in MDCT after trauma--a sign of injury or normal variant? Br J Radiol. 2016;89:20150996.

Lisanti C, Carlin C, Banks KP, Wang D. Normal MRI appearance and motion-related phenomena of CSF. Am J Roentgenol. 2007;188:716–25.

Lustrin ES, Karakas SP, Ortiz AO, Cinnamon J, Castillo M, Vaheesan K, et al. Pediatric cervical spine: normal anatomy, variants, and trauma. Radiographics. 2003;23:539–60.

McKinney AM. Chapter. 33: Cervical carotid and vertebral arterial variants. In: AM MK, editor. Atlas of normal imaging variations of the brain, skull, and craniocervical vasculature. Cham: Springer; 2017. p. 971–94.

Magge SN, Smyth MD, Governale LS, Goumnerova L, Madsen J, Munro B, et al. Idiopathic syrinx in the pediatric population: a combined center experience. J Neurosurg Pediatr. 2011;7:30–6.

Marr JT. Gas in intervertebral discs. Am J Roentgenol Radium Therapy, Nucl Med. 1953;70:804–9.

Marshall DL, Tuchin PJ. Correlation of cervical lordosis measurement with incidence of motor vehicle accidents. Australas Chiropr Osteopathy. 1996;5:79–85.

Matsunaga S, Sakou T. OPLL: disease entity, incidence, literature search and prognosis. In: Yonenobu K, Nakamura K, Toyama Y, editors. OPLL: ossification of the posterior longitudinal ligament. Tokyo: Springer; 2006. p. 11–7.

Mellado JM, Larrosa R, Martín J, Yanguas N, Solanas S, Cozcolluela R. MDCT of variations and anomalies of the neural arch and its processes: Part 1—Pedicles, pars interarticularis, laminae, and spinous process. Am J Roentgenol. 2011;197:W104–13.

Mellado JM, Larrosa R, Martín J, Yanguas N, Solanas S, Cozcolluela MR. MDCT of variations and anomalies of the neural arch and its processes: Part 2—Articular processes, transverse processes, and high cervical spine. Am J Roentgenol. 2011;197:W114–21.

Merks J, Smets A, Vanrijn R, Kobes J, Caron HN, Maas M, Hennekam RC. Prevalence of rib anomalies in normal caucasian children and childhood cancer patients. Eur J Med Genet. 2005;48:113–29.

Mitra R, Kirpalani D, Wedemeyer M. Conservative management of perineural cysts. Spine. 2008;33:E565–8.

Murlimanju BV, Prabhu LV, Shilpa K, Rai R, Dhananjaya KV, Jiji PJ. Accessory transverse foramina in the cervical spine: incidence, embryological basis, morphology and surgical importance. Turk Neurosurg. 2011;21:384–7.

Murlimanju BV, Chettiar GK, Krishnamurthy A, Pai MM, Saralaya VV, Prabhu LV, Vadgaonkar R. The paracondylar skull base: anatomical variants and their clinical implications. Turk Neurosurg. 2015;25:844–9.

Narayanan R, Shankar B, Paruthikunnan SM, Kulkarni CD. Paracondylar process of the occipital bone of the skull: a rare congenital anatomical variant. BMJ Case Rep. 2014. pii: bcr2014205315: https://doi.org/10.1136/bcr-2014-205315.

Natsis K, Lyrtzis C, Totlis T, Anastasopoulos N, Piagkouet M. A morphometric study of the atlas occipitalization and coexisted congenital anomalies of the vertebrae and posterior cranial fossa with neurological importance. Surg Radiol Anat. 2017;39:39–49.

Newbold RG, Wiener MD, Vogler JB 3rd, Martinez S. Traumatic pneumorrhachis. Am J Roentgenol. 1987;148:615–6.

O'Brien WT Sr, Shen P, Lee P. The dens: normal development, developmental variants and anomalies, and traumatic injuries. J Clin Imaging Sci. 2015;5:38.

Oertel MF, Korinth MC, Reinges MH, Krings T, Terbeck S, Gilsbach JM. Pathogenesis, diagnosis and management of pneumorrhachis. Eur Spine J. 2006;15(Suppl 5):636–43.

Ohtsuka K, Terayama K, Yanagihara M, Wada K, Kasuga K, Machida T, et al. An epidemiological survey on ossification of ligaments in the cervical and thoracic spine in individuals over 50 years of age. Nippon Seikeigeka Gakkai Zasshi. 1986;60:1087–98.

Pang D, Li V. Atlantoaxial rotatory fixation: Part 1—Biomechanics of normal rotation at the atlantoaxial joint in children. Neurosurgery. 2004;55:614–26.

Panjabi MM, Takata K, Goel V, Federico D, Oxland T, Duranceau J, Krag M. Thoracic human vertebrae. Quantitative three-dimensional anatomy. Spine. 1991;16:888–901.

Pavlov H, Torg JS, Robie B, Jahre C. Cervical spinal stenosis: determination with vertebral body ratio method. Radiology. 1987;164:771–5.

Petit-Lacour MC, Lasjaunias P, Iffenecker C, Benoudiba F, Hadj Rabia M, Hurth M, et al. Visibility of the central canal on MRI. Neuroradiology. 2000;42:756–61.

Phan N, Marras C, Midha R, Rowed D. Cervical myelopathy caused by hypoplasia of the atlas: two case reports and review of the literature. Neurosurgery. 1998;43:629–33.

Poustchi-Amin M, Mirowitz SA, Brown JJ, McKinstry RC, Li T. Principles and applications of echo-planar imaging: a review for the general radiologist. Radiographics. 2001;21:767–79.

Rathnakar P, Remya K, Swathi B. Study of accessory foramen transversaria in cervical vertebrae. Nitte Univ J Health Sci (NUJHS). 2013;3:97–9.

Raybaud C. Anatomy and development of the craniovertebral junction. Neurol Sci. 2011;32(Suppl 3):S267–70.

Rea P. Essential clinical anatomy of the nervous system. Cambridge, MA: Academic Press; 2015.

Resnick D, Niwayama G, Guerra J Jr, Vint V, Usselman J. Spinal vacuum phenomena: anatomical study and review. Radiology. 1981;139:341–8.

Rojas CA, Bertozzi JC, Martinez CR, Whitlow J. Reassessment of the craniocervical junction: normal values on CT. Am J Neuroradiol. 2007;28:1819–23.

Roos DB. Congenital anomalies associated with thoracic outlet syndrome. Anatomy, symptoms, diagnosis, and treatment. Am J Surg. 1976;132:771–8.

Sabuncuoglu H, Ozdogan S, Karadag D, Kaynak ET. Congenital hypoplasia of the posterior arch of the atlas: case report and extensive review of the literature. Turk Neurosurg. 2011;21:97–103.

Saleh A, Gruber J, Bakhsh W, Rubery PT, Mesfin A. How common is the ponticulus posticus? A CT based analysis of 2,917 patients. Spine. 2018;43:E436–41.

Saker E, Henry BM, Tomaszewski KA, Loukas M, Iwanaga J, Oskouian RJ, Tubbset RS. The human central canal of the spinal cord: a comprehensive review of its anatomy, embryology, molecular development, variants, and pathology. Cureus. 2016;8:e927.

Sangari SK, Dossous P-M, Heineman T, Mtui EP. Dimensions and anatomical variants of the foramen transversarium of typical cervical vertebrae. Anat Res Int. 2017;35:719–22.

Satti SR, Cerniglia CA, Koenigsberg RA. Cervical vertebral artery variations: an anatomic study. Am J Neuroradiol. 2007;28:976–80.

Shah MJ, Kaminsky J, Vougioukas VI. Surgical removal of a symptomatic paracondylar process: case report. J Neurosurg Spine. 2009;10:474–5.

Sharma V, Chaudhary D, Mitra R. Prevalence of ponticulus posticus in Indian orthodontic patients. Dentomaxillofac Radiol. 2010;39:277–83.

Sharma DK, Sharma D, Sharma V. Atlantooccipital fusion: prevalence and its developmental and clinical correlation. J Clin Diagn Res. 2017;11:AC01–3.

Shilton M, Branney J, de Vries BP, Breen AC. Does cervical lordosis change after spinal manipulation for non-specific neck pain? A prospective cohort study. Chiropr Man Therap. 2015;23:33.

Singh R, Srivastva SK, Prasath CSV, Rohilla RK, Siwach R, Magu NK. Morphometric measurements of cadaveric thoracic spine in Indian population and its clinical applications. Asian Spine J. 2011;5:20–34.

Slouma M, Cheour E, Sahli H, Elleuch M. Congenital butterfly vertebra. Acta Medica Port. 2016;29:491.

Sohail AH, Maan MAA, Khan MS, Masood Q. Isolated ligamentum flavum ossification in primary hypoparathyroidism. Surg Neurol Int. 2018;9:4.

Spadliński Ł, Cecot T, Majos A, Stefańczyk L, Pietruszewska W, Wysiadecki G, et al. The epidemiological, morphological, and clinical aspects of the cervical ribs in humans. Biomed Res Int. 2016;1:8034613.

Spencer HT, Gold ME, Hresko MT. Abnormal rib count in scoliosis surgery: impact on the reporting of spinal fusion levels. J Child Orthop. 2014;8:497–503.

Spiegel D, Shrestha S, Sitoula P, Rendon N, Dormans J. Atlantoaxial rotatory displacement in children. World J Orthop. 2017;8:836–45.

Stathis G, Economopoulos N, Mavraganis D, Kelekis N, Alexopoulou E. Paracondylar process, a rare normal variant: the value of MRI in the diagnosis. Surg Radiol Anat. 2012;34:281–4.

Stevens JM, Chong WK, Barber C, Kendall BE, Crockard HA. A new appraisal of abnormalities of the odontoid process associated with atlanto-axial subluxation and neurological disability. Brain. 1994;117:133–48.

Stubbs D. The arcuate foramen. Variability in distribution related to race and sex. Spine. 1992;17:1502–4.

Swischuk LE. Anterior displacement of C2 in children: physiologic or pathologic. Radiology. 1977;122:759–63.

Swischuk LE. The cervical spine in childhood. Curr Probl Diagn Radiol. 1984;13:1–26.

Szárazová AS, Bartels E, Turčáni P. Vertebral artery hypoplasia and the posterior circulation stroke. Pers Med. 2012;1:198–202.

Szpinda M, Baumgart M, Szpinda A, Woźniak A, Małkowski B, Wiśniewski M, et al. Cross-sectional study of the ossification center of the C1–S5 vertebral bodies. Surg Radiol Anat. 2013;35:395–402.

Taitz C. Bony observations of some morphological variations and anomalies of the craniovertebral region. Clin Anat. 2000;13:354–60.

Takahashi T, Hanakita J, Minami M. Pathophysiology of calcification and ossification of the ligamentum flavum in the cervical spine. Neurosurg Clin N Am. 2018;29:47–54.

Tambawala SS, Karjodkar FR, Sansare K, Motghare D, Mishra I, Gaikwad S, Dora AC. Prevalence of ponticulus posticus on lateral cephalometric radiographs, its association with cervicogenic headache and a review of literature. World Neurosurg. 2017;103:566–75.

Tan SH, Teo EC, Chua HC. Quantitative three-dimensional anatomy of cervical, thoracic and lumbar vertebrae of Chinese Singaporeans. Eur Spine J. 2004;13:137–46.

Tanaka T, Uhthoff HK. Coronal cleft of vertebrae, a variant of normal enchondral ossification. Acta Orthop Scand. 1983;54:389–95.

Tang R, Li F, Chen Q. A case report of atypical long segmental thoracic hypertrophic pachymeningitis with ossification of ligamentum flavum and literature review. Eur Spine J. 2017;26:202–6.

Tatara Y, Shimizu T, Fueki K, Masatake I, Naofumi T, Tanouchi T, Nodoka M. Clinical and anatomical features as well as pathological conditions of surgically treated adult patients with occipitalization of the atlas. Int J Spine Surg. 2016;10:5.

Tins BJ, Balain B. Incidence of numerical variants and transitional lumbosacral vertebrae on whole-spine MRI. Insights Imaging. 2016;7:199–203.

Tokuda K, Miyasaka K, Abe S, Takei H, Sugimoto S, Tsuru M. Angiographic analysis of anomalous vertebral arteries. Neuroradiology. 1985;27(5):410–3.

Travan L, Saccheri P, Sabbadini G, Crivellato E. Bilateral arcuate foramen associated with partial defect of the posterior arch of the atlas in a medieval skeleton: case report and review of the literature. Looking backward to go forward. Surg Radiol Anat. 2011;33:495–500.

Tubbs RS, Muhleman M, Miller J, Shoja MM, Loukas M, Wellons JC, et al. Cervical ribs with neurological sequelae in children: a case series. Childs Nerv Syst. 2012;28:605–8.

Turel MK, Kerolus MG, O'Toole JE. Ossified ligamentum flavum of the thoracic spine presenting as spontaneous intracranial hypotension: case report. J Neurosurg Spine. 2018;28(4):401–5.

Ulusoy OL, Kafadar C, Ozturk E, Mutlu A, Sirvanci M. Idiopathic thoracic epidural lipomatosis presenting with back pain. Spine J. 2016;16:e487–8.

Viertel VG, Intrapiromkul J, Maluf F, Patel NV, Zheng W, Alluwaimi F, et al. Cervical ribs: a common variant overlooked in CT imaging. Am J Neuroradiol. 2012;33:2191–4.

von Lüdinghausen M, Fahr M, Prescher A, Schindler G, Kenn W, Weiglein A, et al. Accessory joints between basiocciput and atlas/axis in the median plane. Clin Anat. 2005;18:558–71.

Walden MJ, Adin ME, Visagan R, Viertel VG, Intrapiromkul J, Maluf F, et al. Cervical ribs: identification on MRI and clinical relevance. Clin Imaging. 2013;37:938–41.

Wang H, Zou F, Jiang J, Lu F, Chen W, Ma X, et al. The correlation between ossification of the nuchal ligament and pathological changes of the cervical spine in patients with cervical spondylosis. Spine. 2014;39:B7–11.

Wang H, Zou F, Jiang J, Lu F, Chen W, Ma X, et al. Analysis of radiography findings of ossification of nuchal ligament of cervical spine in patients with cervical spondylosis. Spine. 2014;39:E7–11.

Weaver AA, Schoell SL, Stitzel JD. Morphometric analysis of variation in the ribs with age and sex. J Anat. 2014;225:246–61.

Weir DC. Roentgenographic signs of cervical injury. Clin Orthop Relat Res. 1975;109:9–17.

Westvik J, Lachman RS. Coronal and sagittal clefts in skeletal dysplasias. Pediatr Radiol. 1998;28:764–70.

Wigh RE. The thoracolumbar and lumbosacral transitional junctions. Spine. 1980;5:215–22.

Young J, Young P, Ackermann M, Anderson PA, Riew KD. The ponticulus posticus: implications for screw insertion into the first cervical lateral mass. J Bone Joint Surg Am. 2005;87:2495–8.

Zong R, Yin Y, Qiao G, Jin Y, Yu X. Quantitative measurements of the skull base and craniovertebral junction in congenital occipitalization of the atlas: a computed tomography-based anatomic study. World Neurosurg. 2017;99:96–103.

Normal Variants of the Lumbar and Sacral Spine

7

7.1 Introduction, Acquisition Techniques, and Basic Anatomy

Normal variants of the lumbar spine are well described but can simulate pathology if not recognized and understood.

MRI is the imaging study of choice for most patients with back pain, but CT can better delineate bony anatomy, evaluate for calcified disc protrusions, or be used for problem solving regarding findings discovered on MRI. CT is also considered front line for most initial trauma evaluations because of better delineation of fractures and subluxations and its ready availability 24/7, since it is often located in close proximity to emergency rooms. MRI should be added if there is concern for ligamentous or soft-tissue injury, in some cases for potential evaluation of epidural or subdural hematoma (especially if suspected on CT), and to better evaluate the integrity of the spinal cord and cauda equina.

Our institution utilizes a typical routine MRI protocol (in patients with no history of surgery) that includes sagittal spin-echo T1-weighted imaging (SET1WI), spin-echo T2-weighted imaging (SET2WI), and short tau inversion recovery imaging (STIR) sequences with axial SET2WI (or sometimes gradient echo T2*-weighted imaging (GET2*WI) sequences, utilizing 4-mm slice thickness for both planes. The goal is to complete such routine *outpatient* examinations in less than 30 min. In order to decrease scan times and improve outpatient throughput, we often replace the sagittal and axial SET2WI sequences with an isotropic T2-SPACE three-dimensional acquisition that is then reformatted into sagittal and axial planes at 1-mm thickness and can be reconstructed in further planes on request. Regarding patients with a history of prior surgery or concerns for infection or malignancy, we obtain sagittal SET1WI, SET2WI, STIR, and diffusion-weighted imaging (DWI), with axial SET2WI and SET1WI without intravenous gadolinium contrast, followed by a weight-based dose of intravenous (macrocyclic) gadolinium-based contrast to obtain fat-suppressed (FS) sagittal and axial SET1WI. Our noncontrast CT (NECT) studies are similar to most standard acquisitions, which typically involve a noncontrast helical acquisition with sagittal, axial, and coronal 3-mm thickness images reconstructed with both bone and soft-tissue kernels. Since some surgeons request myelography, although this is increasingly uncommon with the advent of MRI, the intrathecal contrast is administered by a neuroradiologist with the CT portion obtained in a fashion similar to that described above for NECT. The added caveat is that a radiologist typically checks for the presence of intrathecal contrast before the patient exits the CT scanner.

An in-depth description of normal anatomy is beyond the scope of this text, since numerous references abound (please see the *Suggested Reading* section at the end of this chapter), but an understanding of basic lumbosacral anatomy and embryology assists in recognizing such variants. In the following topics, most of these variants are "don't touch" lesions whether congenital or acquired in nature, although surgery may be necessary in extreme cases such as spinal instability or symptoms from compression/stenosis of the spinal canal, conus medullaris, or roots.

7.2 Epidural Lipomatosis

Epidural lipomatosis is a relatively rare disorder with overgrowth of epidural fat, which is typically seen in patients on chronic corticosteroids and in those with endocrine disorders that produce an elevated cortisol level such as Cushing syndrome. It may also manifest in obese patients or be idiopathic. A small amount of epidural fat and mild prominence

A. McKinney et al., *Atlas of Head/Neck and Spine Normal Imaging Variants*, https://doi.org/10.1007/978-3-319-95441-7_7

can be normal (and actually may assist in epidural pain injections), but compression of the CSF-filled spinal canal and roots is abnormal. A frequent presentation is progressive lower extremity weakness and paresthesias, but back pain and radicular symptoms are fairly common. Decompression is the treatment of choice for progressive symptoms. Conservative therapy includes weaning of corticosteroids and weight loss. Uncommonly, focal epidural lipomatosis can be confused with subacute (T1-bright) epidural hematoma, but these are easily discerned with FS T1-weighted imaging (T1WI) that saturates (darkens) the T1-bright fat in focal lipomatosis (Figs. 7.1 and 7.2).

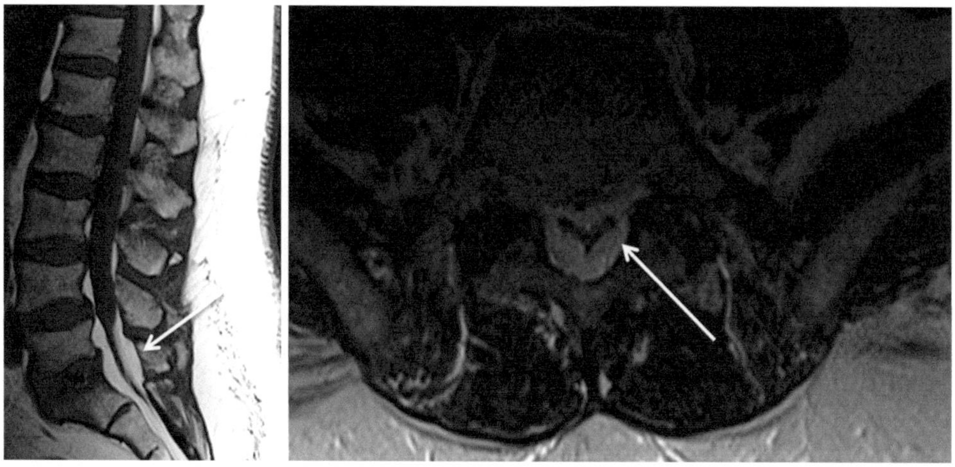

Fig. 7.1 A 60-year-old female with low back and right hip pain and right sciatica. Sagittal (*left*) and axial (*right*) SET1WI demonstrate excessive epidural fat (*arrows*), which can be seen starting at L3 but becomes most notable below the level of L4-L5. While small amounts of epidural fat can be normal, prominent amounts such as in this patient can cause severe narrowing of the thecal sac and occasionally lead to symptomatology

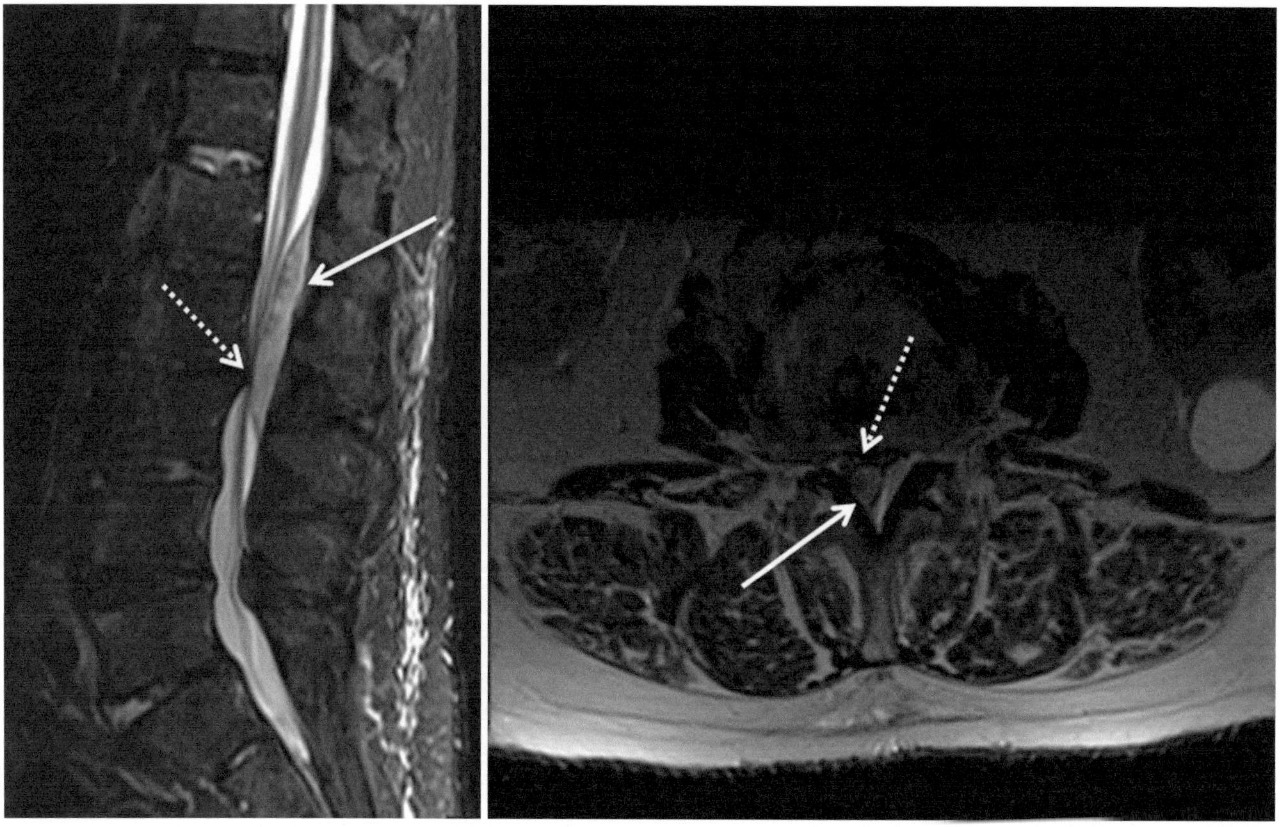

Fig. 7.2 Comparison case of epidural hematoma. A 45-year-old male with sudden onset of lower extremity weakness after a lumbar puncture performed in the clinic; his platelet count was very low, being 12 × 10^9/L. Sagittal STIR (*left*) and axial SET2WI (*right*) images demonstrate a slightly hypointense CSF and a mildly heterogeneous epidural collection (*white arrows*) that displaces the epidural fat and severely compresses the thecal sac (*dotted arrows*). The findings are consistent with an epidural hematoma

7.3 Limbus Vertebra

Limbus vertebra, which is closely related to *Schmorl nodes* (described in the following section), results from interosseous herniation of the nucleus pulposus between the vertebral body and the ring apophysis. In the lumbar spine this is typically situated at the anterosuperior vertebral body corner. The clinical presentation may be an asymptomatic patient with an incidentally noted *limbus vertebra*, or the patient may present with vague back pain, radiculopathy, or rarely inflammatory low back pain. Posteroinferior *limbus vertebra* rarely occurs and may present with nerve compression and radiculopathy. Differentiation from an acute fracture is accomplished by noting the irregular noncorticated fracture fragment border as opposed to the well-corticated margin of a *limbus vertebra*. Also, a limbus vertebra should not be confused with infection, as this would show erosive changes and not a corticated fragment (Figs. 7.3 and 7.4).

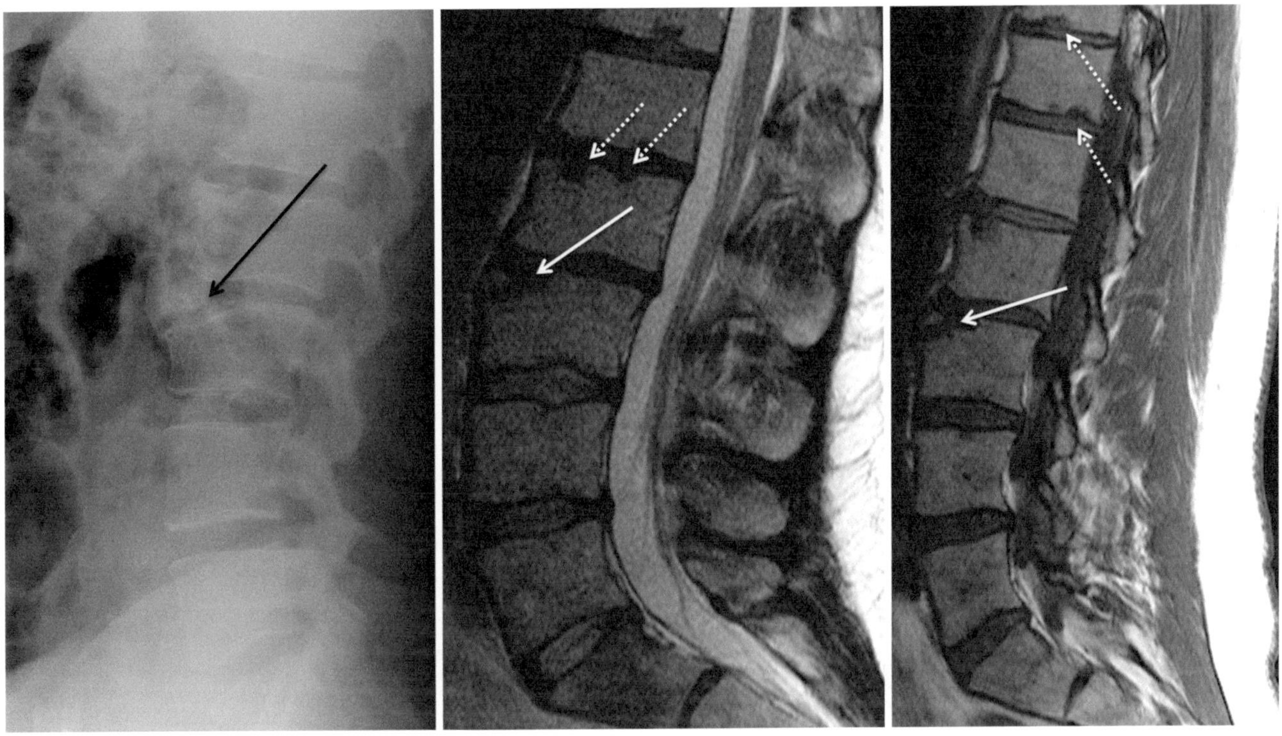

Fig. 7.3 A 31-year-old female with left leg numbness and weakness. A lateral plain film (*left*), sagittal SET2WI (*middle*), and SET1WI (*right*) images are displayed. The plain film (*left*) depicts a corticated fragment of the anterosuperior corner of L3 (*black arrow*), while the MRI images demonstrate separation of the fragment from the vertebral body by material isointense to the intervertebral disc on both T2WI (*middle*) and T1WI (*right*), contiguous with the intervertebral disc (*white arrows*). Superiorly, note the incidental Schmorl nodes as well (*dashed arrows*)

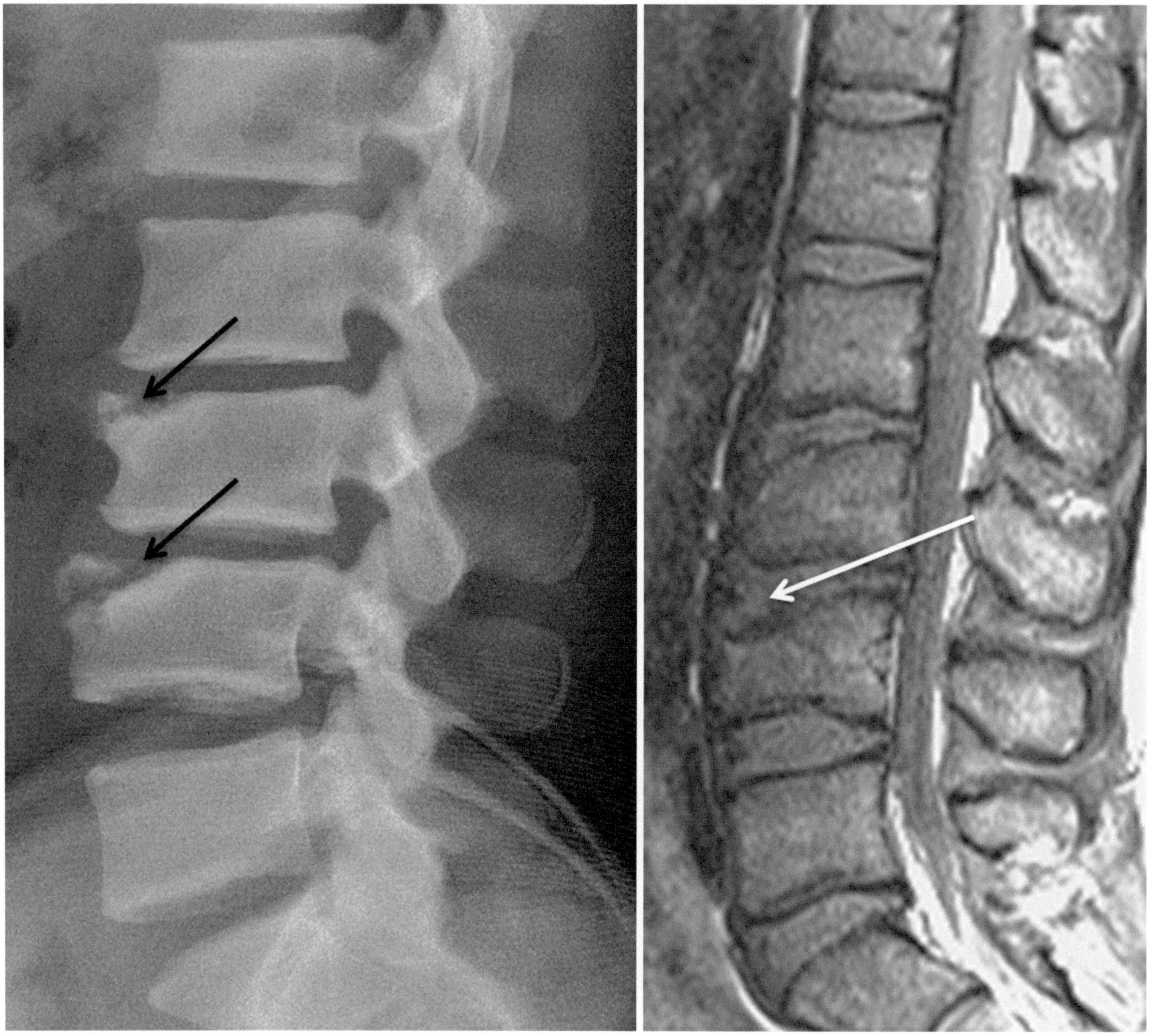

Fig. 7.4 A 17-year-old male with chronic middle to low back pain. A lateral plain film (*left*) demonstrates corticated fragments (*black arrows*) at L3 and L4. A sagittal SET1WI MR image (*right*) demonstrates inter-osseous disc herniations separating the fragment from the vertebral body, which is best seen at L4 (*white arrow*)

7.4 Schmorl Nodes

First described in 1927, *Schmorl nodes* (intrabody disc herniations) are focal herniations of the nucleus pulposus through the bony endplate and into the subjacent vertebral body. Most are incidental and asymptomatic, but they can uncommonly produce back pain, probably caused by the inflammatory reaction from the herniated nucleus pulposus into a well-vascularized vertebral body. Acute Schmorl nodes may peripherally enhance, simulating pathology such as malignancy and discitis-osteomyelitis, while others do not, suggesting that they are quiescent, chronic, and asymptomatic. Additionally, symptomatic nodes usually demonstrate adjacent bone marrow hyperintensity on T2WI and hypointensity on T1WI due to the marrow edema (also seen as bright on STIR images). Established Schmorl nodes typically demonstrate a sclerotic border on NECT imaging. The etiology is unknown, but axial loading injury and degenerative disc disease are both commonly associated with Schmorl nodes. There is no established treatment for symptomatic Schmorl nodes, although fusion surgery and vertebroplasty, among other more esoteric modalities, are reported as potential therapies for symptomatic Schmorl nodes (Figs. 7.5 and 7.6).

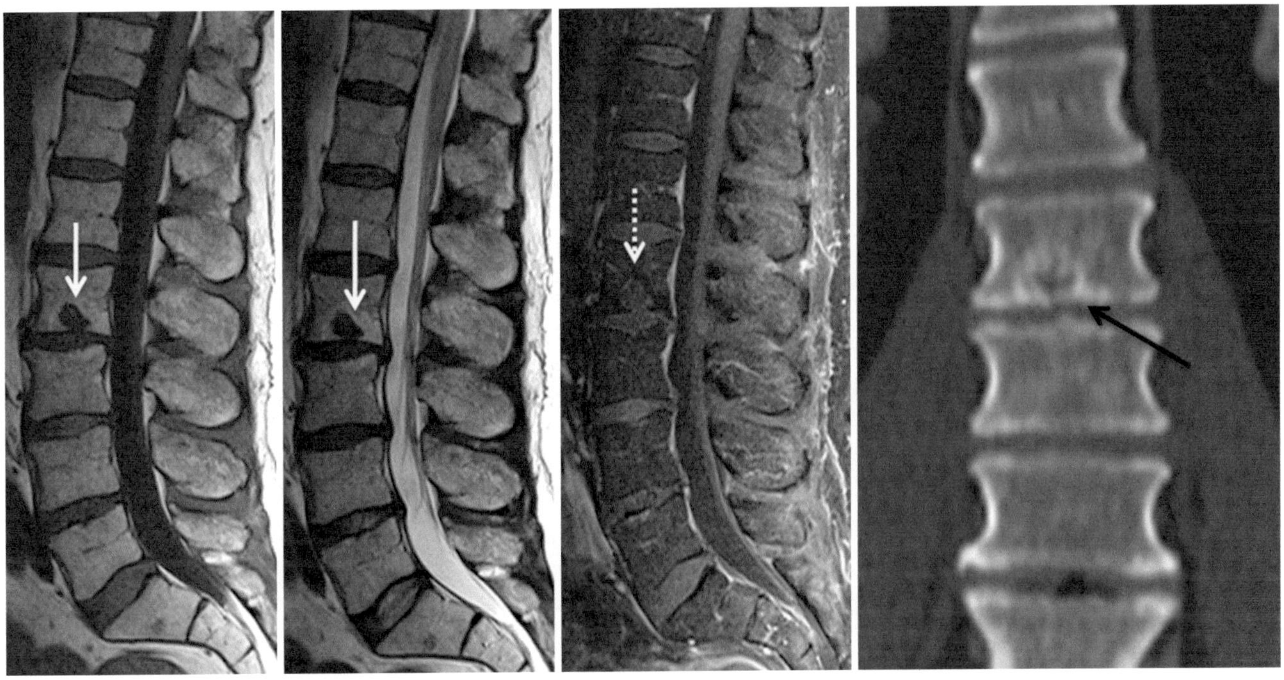

Fig. 7.5 A Schmorl node in a 63-year-old male with a history of renal cell carcinoma, who presented with low back pain. Displayed are sagittal SET1WI (*left*), SET2WI (*left middle*), postcontrast FS SET1WI (*right middle*), and coronal NECT (reconstructed from a positron emission tomography (PET)-CT, *right*). Note the intravertebral disc herniation (*white arrows*) into the inferior endplate of L2, which is isointense to the intervertebral disc on T1WI and T2WI. In this case, there is no significant contrast enhancement associated with the Schmorl node (*dotted arrow, right middle*), but it is common to see enhancement around the periphery of the node, which is presumably secondary to granulation tissue. Note the sclerotic border on the companion NECT (*right*), which is typical of Schmorl nodes (*black arrow*)

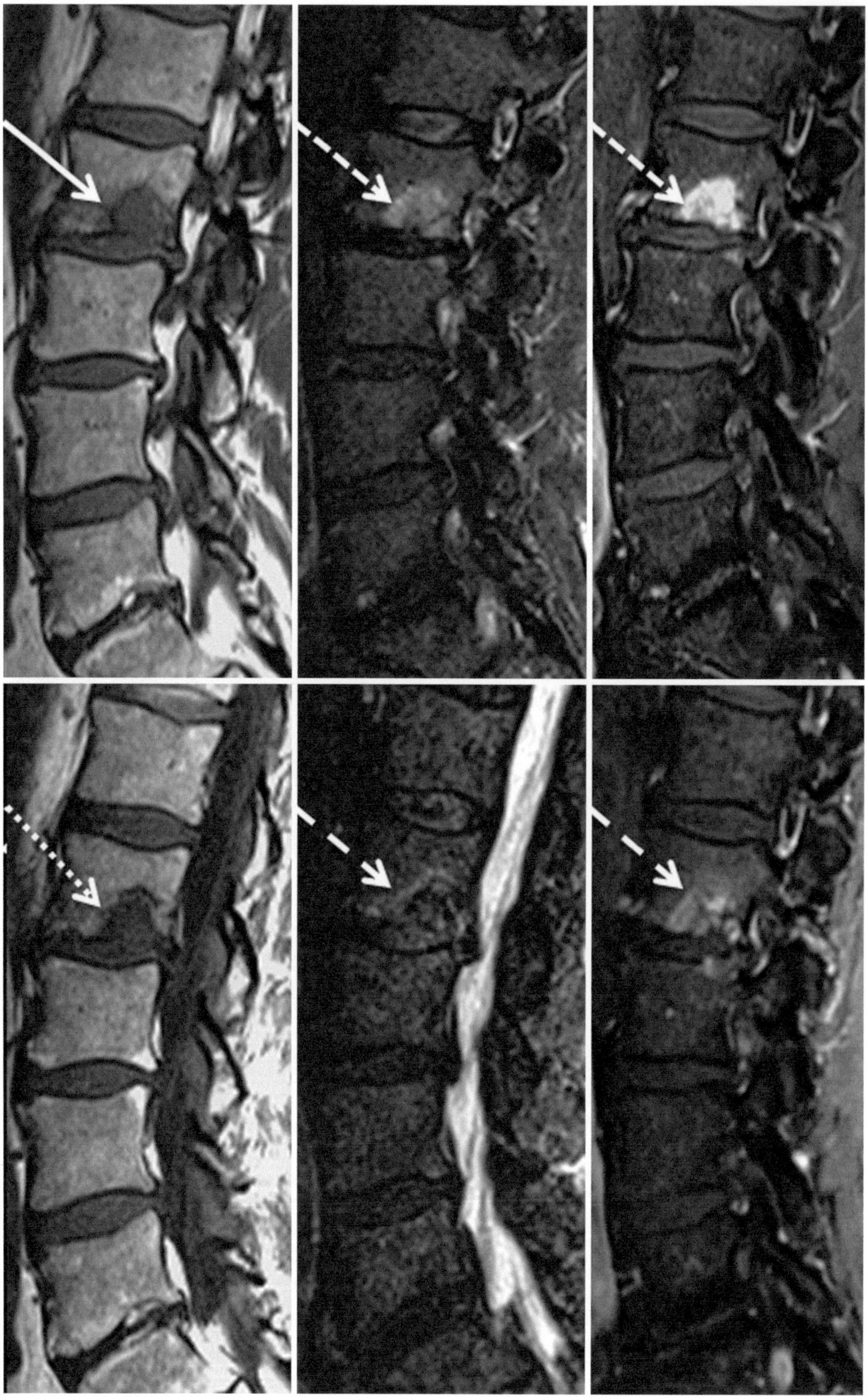

Fig. 7.6 A presumed benign Schmorl node in a 48-year-old female with back pain and no history of malignancy. SET1WI (*left*), STIR (*middle*), and postcontrast FS SET1WI (*right*) are provided on the initial MRI (*top row*) and follow-up MRI at 13 months (*bottom row*). The initial MRI demonstrates hypointensity on T1WI that is isointense to disc material (*white arrow, top left*), This lesion is T2 hyperintense on STIR (*dashed arrows, top middle*) and demonstrates contrast enhancement (*dashed arrows, top right*). With no prior history of malignancy and the appearance of an intravertebral disc herniation (Schmorl node), the lesion was felt to be benign, and a follow-up MRI was recommended. On that MRI 13 months later (*bottom row*), the lesion is again T1-hypointense on SET1WI (*bottom left*), with an intensity similar to that of the disc material (*dotted arrow*). The T2 hyperintensity and contrast enhancement have decreased in intensity on STIR (*bottom middle*) and postcontrast FS SET1WI (*bottom right*), and the lesion is unchanged in size

7.5 Spina Bifida Occulta

Spina bifida occulta is the mildest and most common of the posterior neural arch defects (others are retrosomatic clefts, retroisthmic clefts, and pars defects/spondylolysis), which constitutes a minor form of a neural tube defect. By definition there is skin overlying the bony defect, and there are no abnormalities of the cord or nerve roots. This is a "don't touch" lesion, as there are generally no associated neurologic symptoms, although there is an association with folic acid deficiency. This variant is typically quite apparent, although it can occasionally mimic a fracture of the posterior elements, particularly if it is subtle and obliquely oriented on routine axial image review (Fig. 7.7).

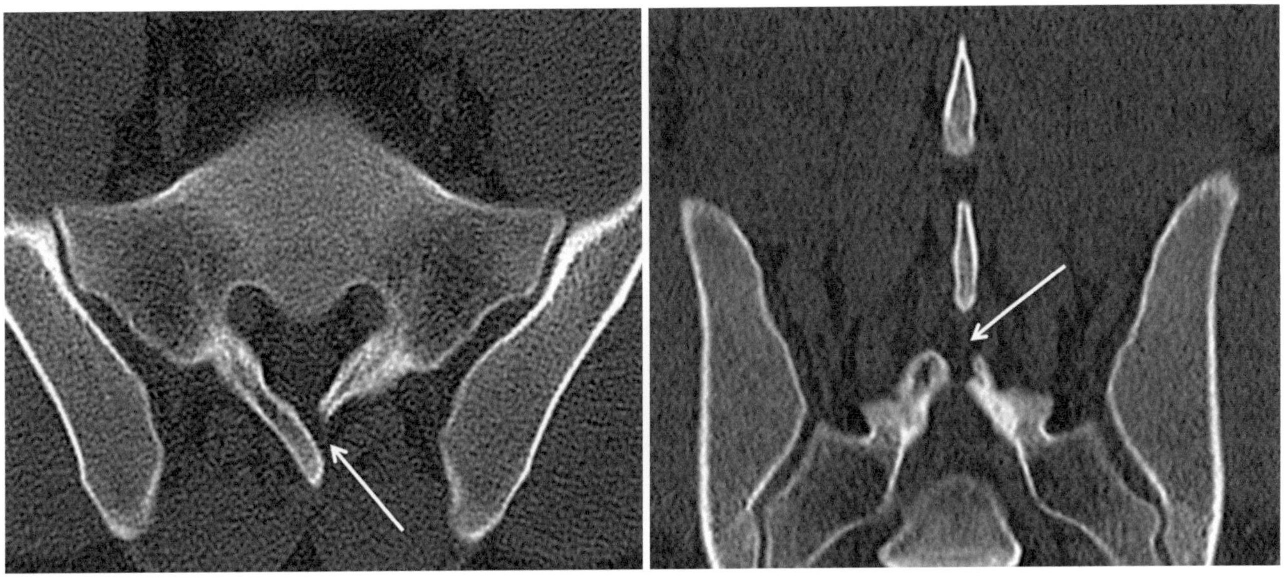

Fig. 7.7 A 30-year-old male with low back pain. Axial (*left*) and coronal (*right*) reformats from a helically acquired CT are provided. Note the sacral spina bifida occulta defect, as indicated by the *white arrows*

7.6 Retrosomatic Cleft

A *retrosomatic cleft* or pediculolysis is a vertical linear defect within the pedicle of the vertebral body. This "don't touch" lesion is controversial as to whether it is derived from prior fractures or whether it is congenital, especially since other congenital anomalies may be present. The clinical consideration is that bilateral clefts can lead to instability of the spine. This may mimic an acute lumbar pedicle fracture (Fig. 7.8).

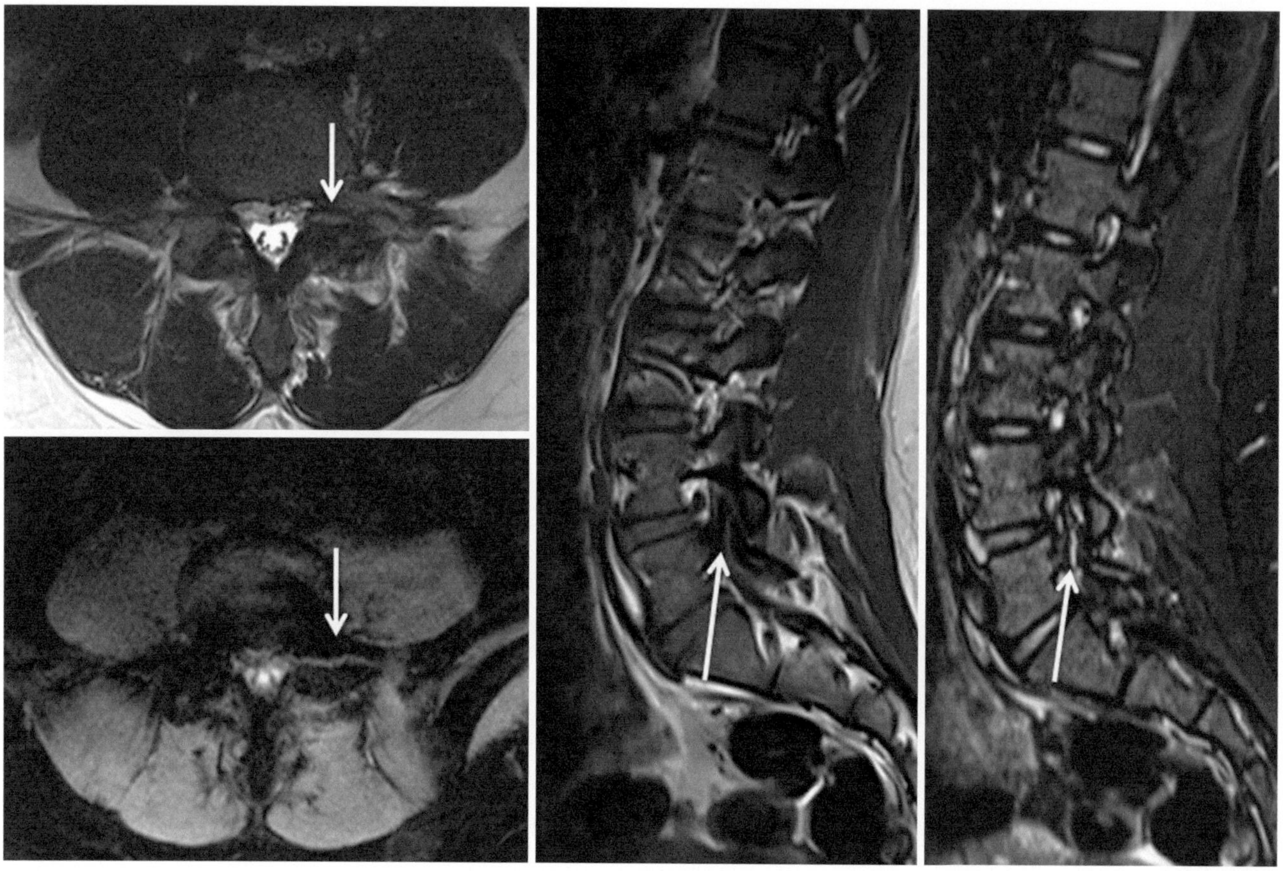

Fig. 7.8 A 29-year-old male with back pain. Axial SET2WI (*upper left*), axial gradient echo T2*-weighted imaging (GET2*WI) (*lower left*), sagittal SET1WI (*middle*), and sagittal SET2WI (*right*) are provided. The MRI demonstrates a retrosomatic cleft (*white arrows*) in each image

7.7 Retroisthmic Cleft

Retroisthmic clefts are rare congenital anomalies of the neural arch that occur within the lamina; they are situated dorsal to the pars interarticularis. They may be the least common of the posterior neural arch defects. Some have suggested that trauma as a cause of this "don't touch" lesion, but as they are associated with other congenital anomalies such as dysplasia of the facet joints or ipsilateral deviation of the spinous process, many feel this is a congenital anomaly (Fig. 7.9).

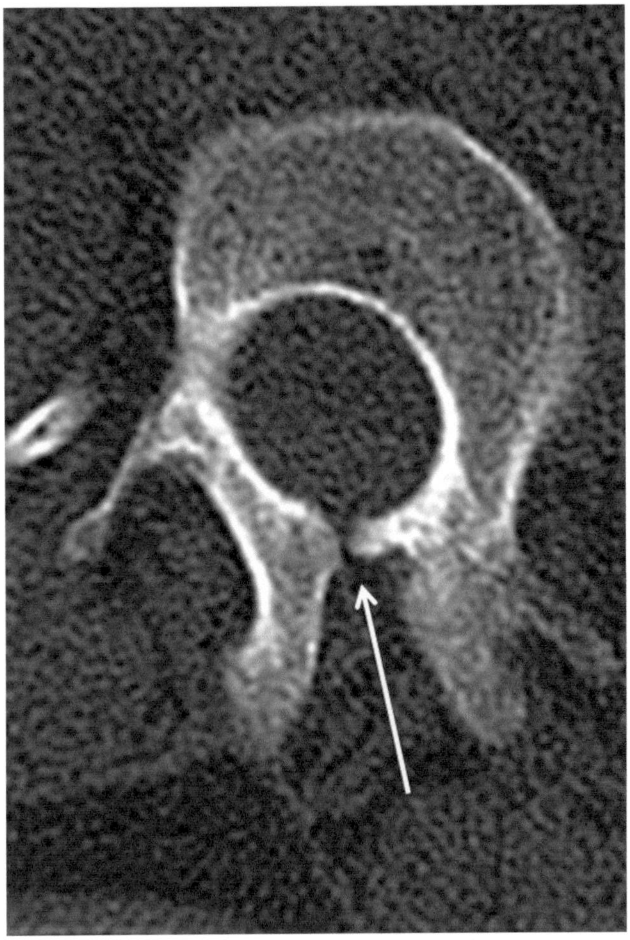

Fig. 7.9 A 40-year-old female with trauma. Axial NECT with a bone reconstruction algorithm demonstrates a well-corticated defect in the left lamina of L1, consistent with a retroisthmic cleft (*white arrow*)

7.8 Pars Interarticularis Defect

The *pars interarticularis,* also known as the "isthmus," is situated between the superior and inferior articular facets, ventral to the lamina and dorsal to the pedicles. Defects of the bridge between the superior and inferior facets of the lumbar spine are referred to as spondylolysis and can cause anterior spondylolisthesis or anterolisthesis of the affected vertebral body, which is the more superior of the two involved vertebral bodies (e.g., spondylolysis of L5 can produce anterolisthesis of L5 on S1). These listheses are typically graded from 1 (25% slippage) to grade 4 (100% full width slippage). Defects can also be unilateral or bilateral and can be either congenital in nature from dysplasia (less common) or acquired from an acute stress fracture (most common). This is most commonly a "don't touch" lesion in which acute spondylolysis secondary to trauma is typically treated by rest, braces, and/or physical therapy, whereas surgery is usually reserved for more severe slippage, instability, and the uncommon onset of neurologic symptoms (Figs. 7.10 and 7.11).

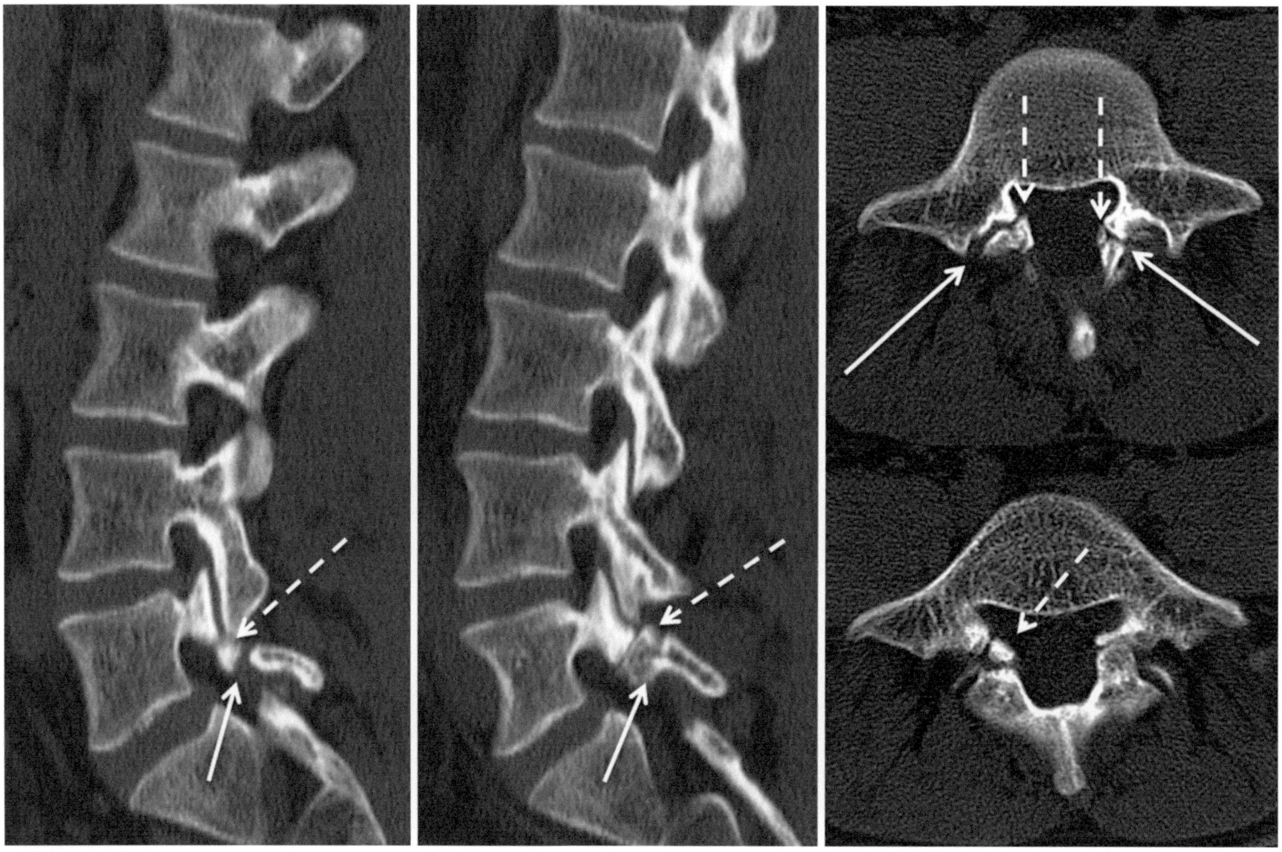

Fig. 7.10 A 25-year-old male with a recent history of motor vehicle trauma. Sagittal (*left, middle*) and axial (*top right, bottom right*) NECT images demonstrate right and left L5 spondylolysis/pars defects (*solid arrows*) with fragmentation (*dashed arrows*). These are at least in part chronic defects given their sclerotic/well-corticated margins

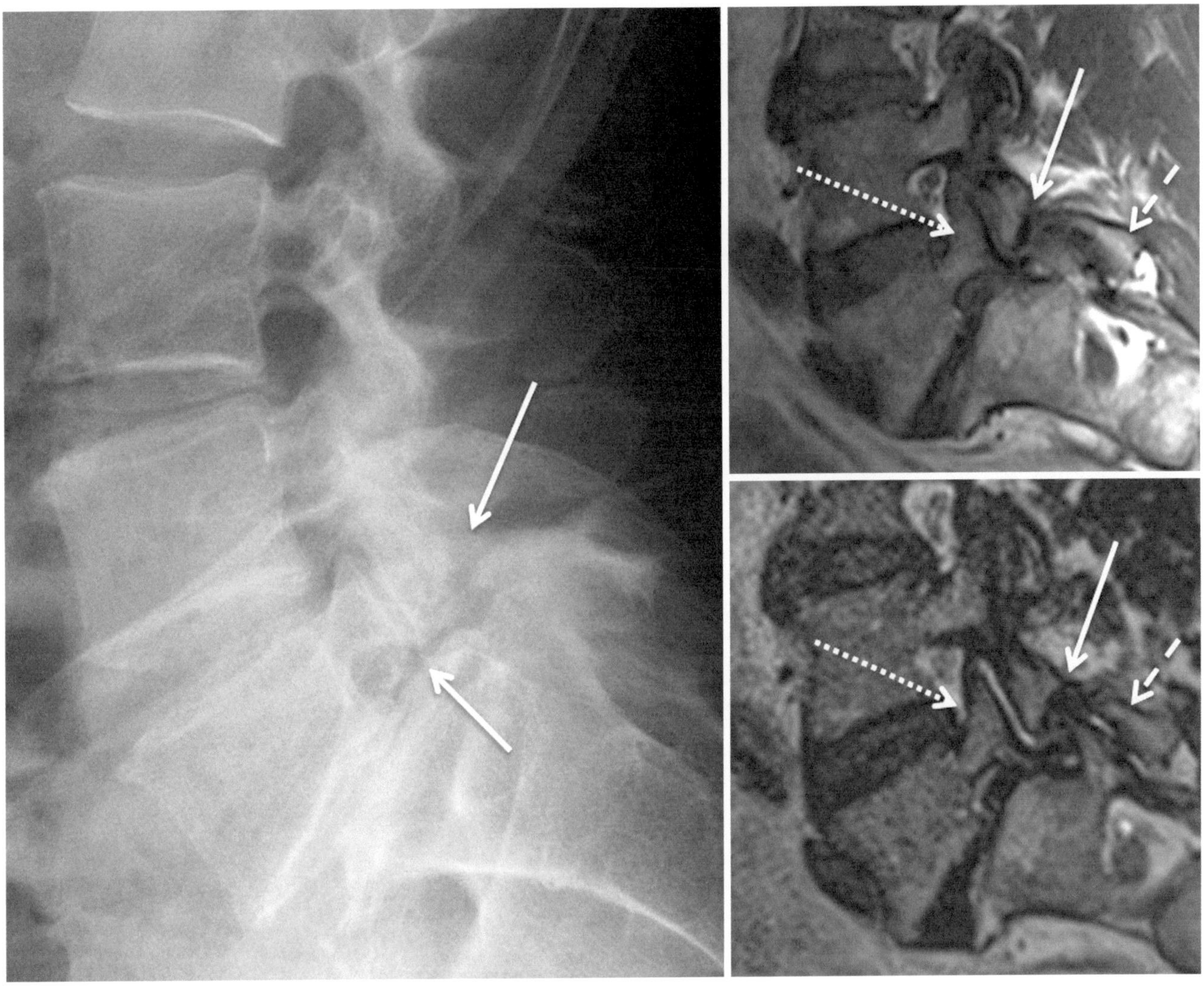

Fig. 7.11 A 21-year-old female with a history of motor vehicle trauma. A lateral plain film (*left*) demonstrates grade 2 anterolisthesis (25–50%) and bilateral spondylolysis at L5-S1 (*white arrows*). Sagittal SET1WI (*upper right*) and SET2WI (*lower right*) images demonstrate the pars defect (*white arrows*) with the L5 superior articular facet (*dotted arrows*) and the L5 inferior articular facet (*dashed arrows*) also depicted, which are widely separated

7.9 Sacral Cleft

Sacral clefts are not well described in the literature. These "don't touch" variants can be considered as a form of anterior spina bifida, with a fibrous band contained within the cleft. Anterior spina bifida (ASB) has been associated with neurenteric cysts, which are secondary to disruption of notochord development from persistence of the embryologic neurenteric canal with resultant prevertebral cyst formation (Fig. 7.12).

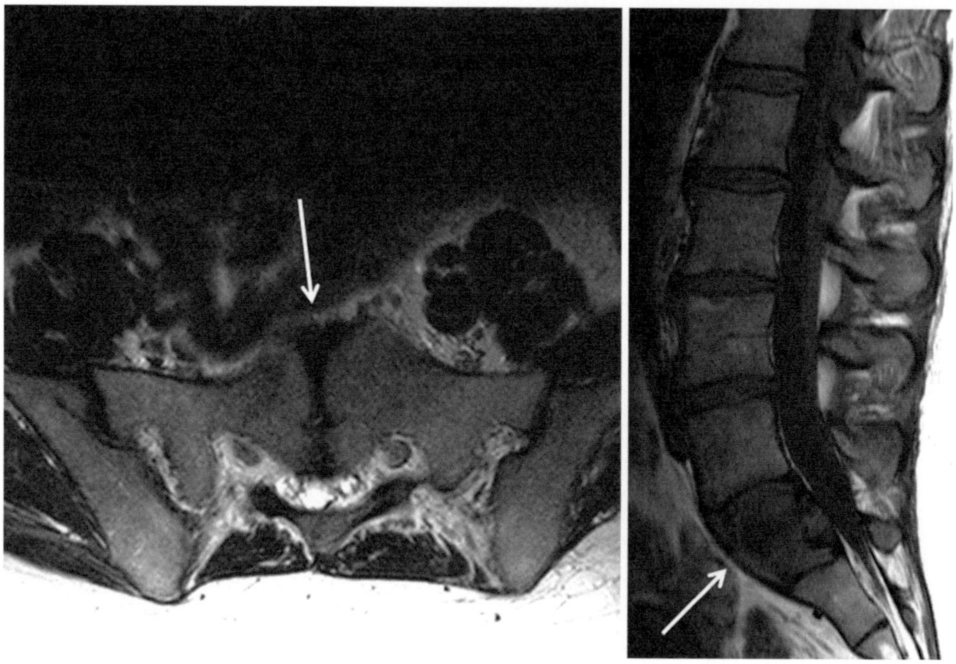

Fig. 7.12 A 50-year-old male with back pain. Axial SET2WI (*left*) and sagittal SET1WI (*right*) demonstrate a sagittally-oriented cleft (anterior spina bifida) containing a fibrous band (*white arrows*), but without a definitely associated presacral neurenteric cyst or myelomeningocele. No definite neurenteric cyst was identified, but it is assumed that the formation of the cleft was caused by a similar embryological disruption. Anterior spina bifida can also be associated with a presacral myelomeningocele, which also was not identified in that patient

7.10 Perineural Cysts (Tarlov Cysts)

Tarlov cysts or *perineural cysts* are CSF-filled nerve root cysts that are located near the dorsal root ganglion and arise between the perineurium and endoneurium. Most frequently, these variants are found involving the sacral nerve roots, but they can be seen at any spinal level. Although technically extradural, they do contain nerve fibers within their walls. They are quite common (an incidence of about 5%) and are found more often in women than in men. The vast majority are asymptomatic and usually incidental on MRI, but a minority can enlarge (particularly after trauma) and become symptomatic, manifesting with lumbosacral pain, sciatica, perineal pain, and even sphincter or sexual dysfunction (Fig. 7.13).

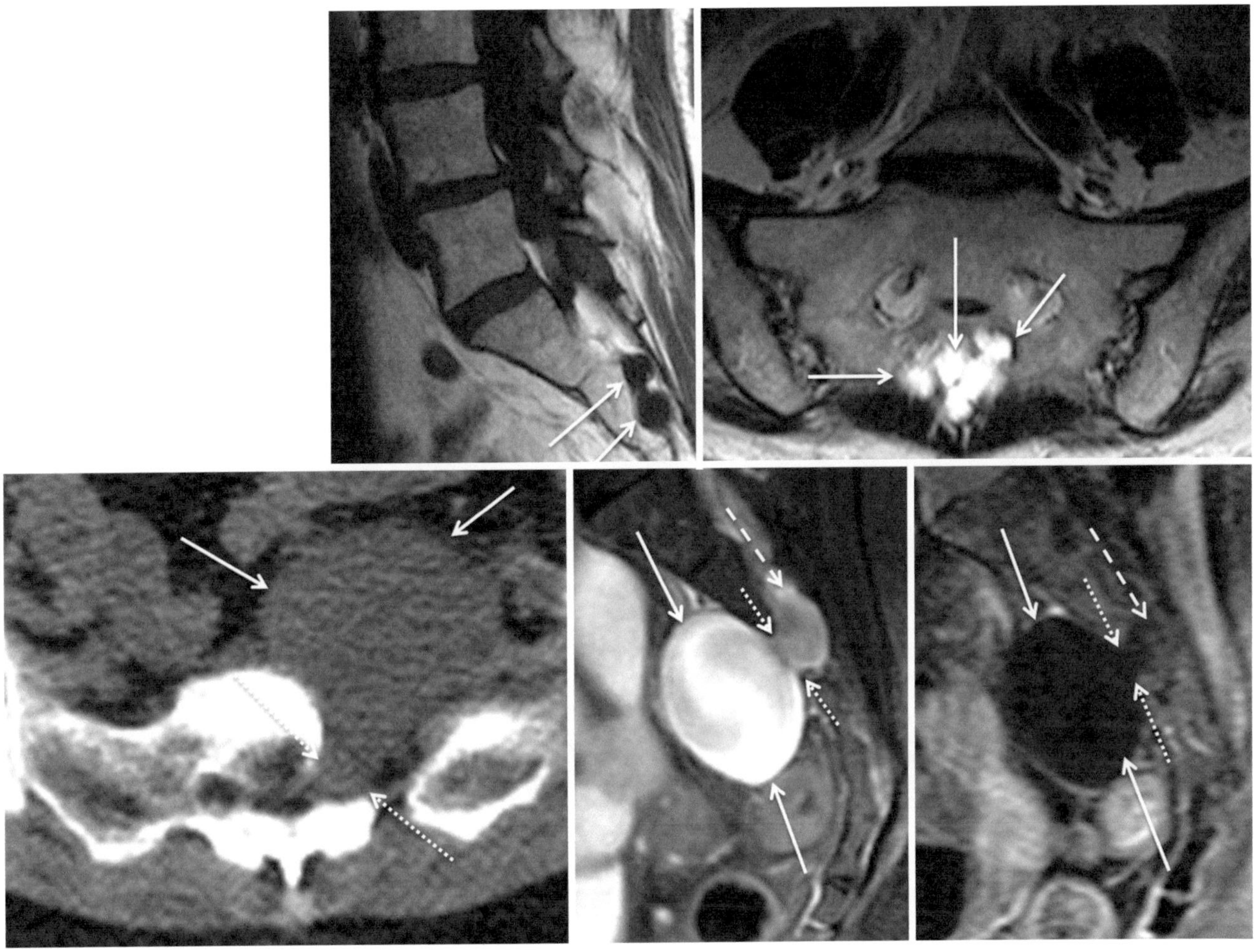

Fig. 7.13 **Top Row:** A 49-year-old woman with right leg pain. Sagittal SET1WI *(left)* and axial SET2WI *(right)* images demonstrate multiple cystic structures in the sacral canal consistent with perineural cysts or Tarlov cysts *(white arrows)*. **Bottom Row:** A 61-year-old female with dysuria. Outside facility axial NECT *(left)* demonstrates a low to intermediate density mass in the posterior left pelvis *(white arrows)* that appears to extend into the left S2-S3 neural foramen *(dotted arrows)*. This was felt to represent a schwannoma and a contrast-enhanced MRI was recommended. Outside facility sagittal STIR *(middle)* and contrast-enhanced sagittal FS SET1WI *(right)* demonstrate a T2 hyperintense mass that does not enhance and that begins in the canal *(dashed arrows)*, widens the left S2-S3 neural foramen *(dotted arrows)*, and extends into the pelvis *(white arrows)*. This is consistent with a giant perineural cyst. In retrospect, when the Hounsfield units (HU) of the mass on the axial NECT image were explored, the CT density was determined to be 7 HU or water density and the MRI was likely not needed to make the diagnosis

7.11 Dermal Sinus Tract

A spinal dermal sinus tract is typically found within the lumbosacral region. A rare spinal dysraphism, it is lined with epithelium and extends variable depths into and can terminate in the spinal canal. These are not "normal variants" since they can present with serious symptoms, including a neurologic deficit, infection (meningitis), or both. These abnormalities are associated with dermal inclusion tumors, tethered cord, and diastematomyelia. Neurologic deficits can increase with age if not addressed in a timely manner. Surgery is the treatment of choice (Fig. 7.14).

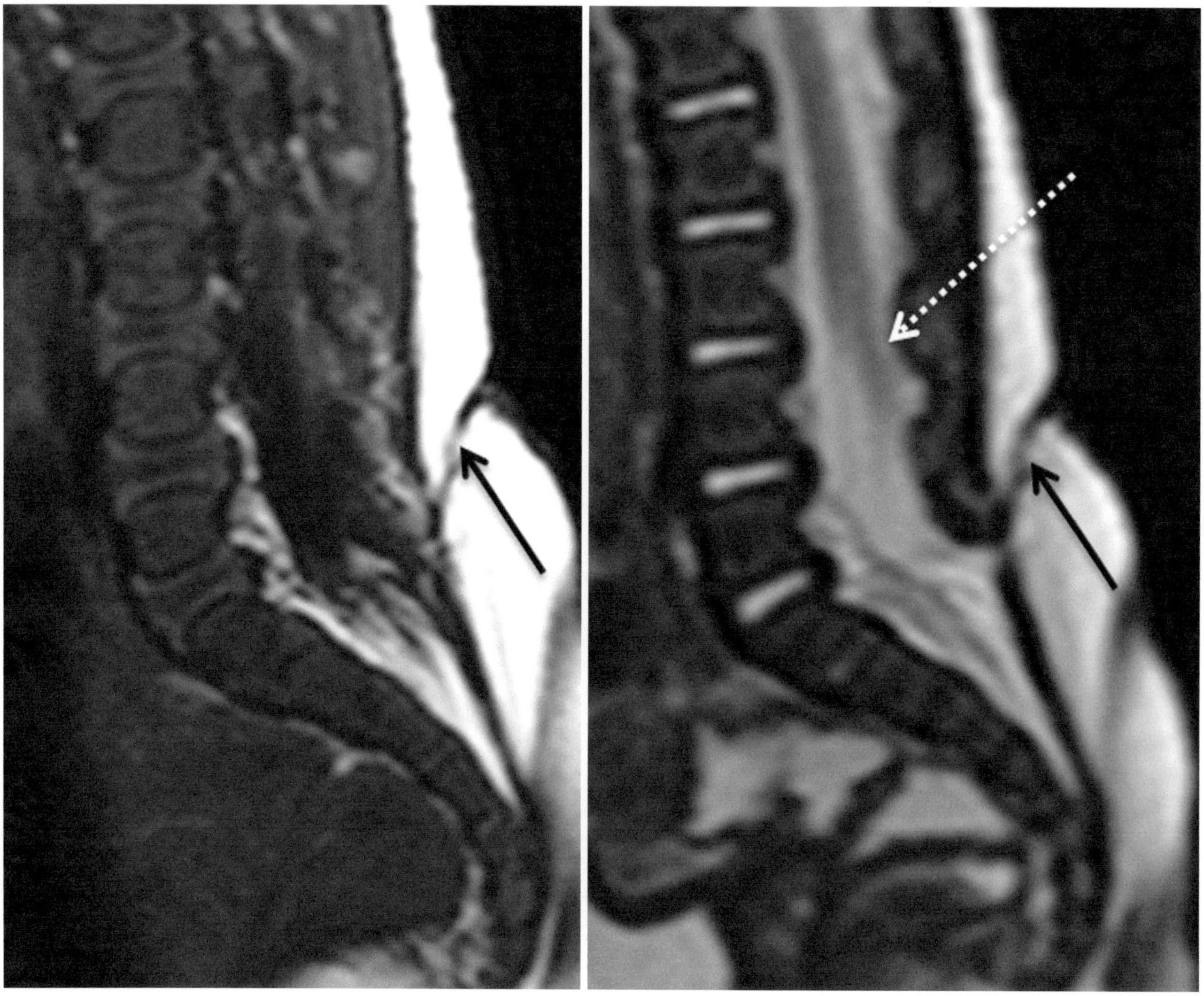

Fig. 7.14 A 2-month-old male with a dimple on his back. Sagittal SET1WI (*left*) and SET2WI (*right*) images demonstrate the dermal sinus tract (*black arrows*) within the lower lumbar subcutaneous tissues, extending under the lamina of L5. There is tethering of the spinal cord with a low-lying conus medullaris (*dotted arrow, right*)

7.12 Sacralization

Lumbosacral *transitional vertebrae* are congenital anomalies that have an intermediate morphologic appearance with characteristic spanning of the lumbar and sacral segments. Their prevalence is fairly common and may be anywhere from 2% to 30% of the population, depending on the source of data. Notably, the only true way to determine the lumbar and sacral levels is to count down from the top of the odontoid process of C2, typically via sagittal plain films or scout MRI images. It is controversial whether these anomalies cause pain or not, and they are usually considered "don't touch lesions" because most individuals are asymptomatic and the transitional vertebra is incidentally found. Sacralization is when the lowest lumbar vertebral body has either one or two enlarged transverse processes that may "pseudoarticulate" or completely fuse to the sacrum (and rarely to the ilium as well). This may be unilateral or bilateral. When this occurs, the L5 to S1 intervertebral disc may be hypoplastic or absent. The most common clinical scenario in which this is of importance is spinal counting on imaging prior to surgery. A clear description of the transitional segment is needed to alert the surgeon, and consistent documentation of the numbering schema is recommended to prevent "wrong level surgery" (Figs. 7.15 and 7.16).

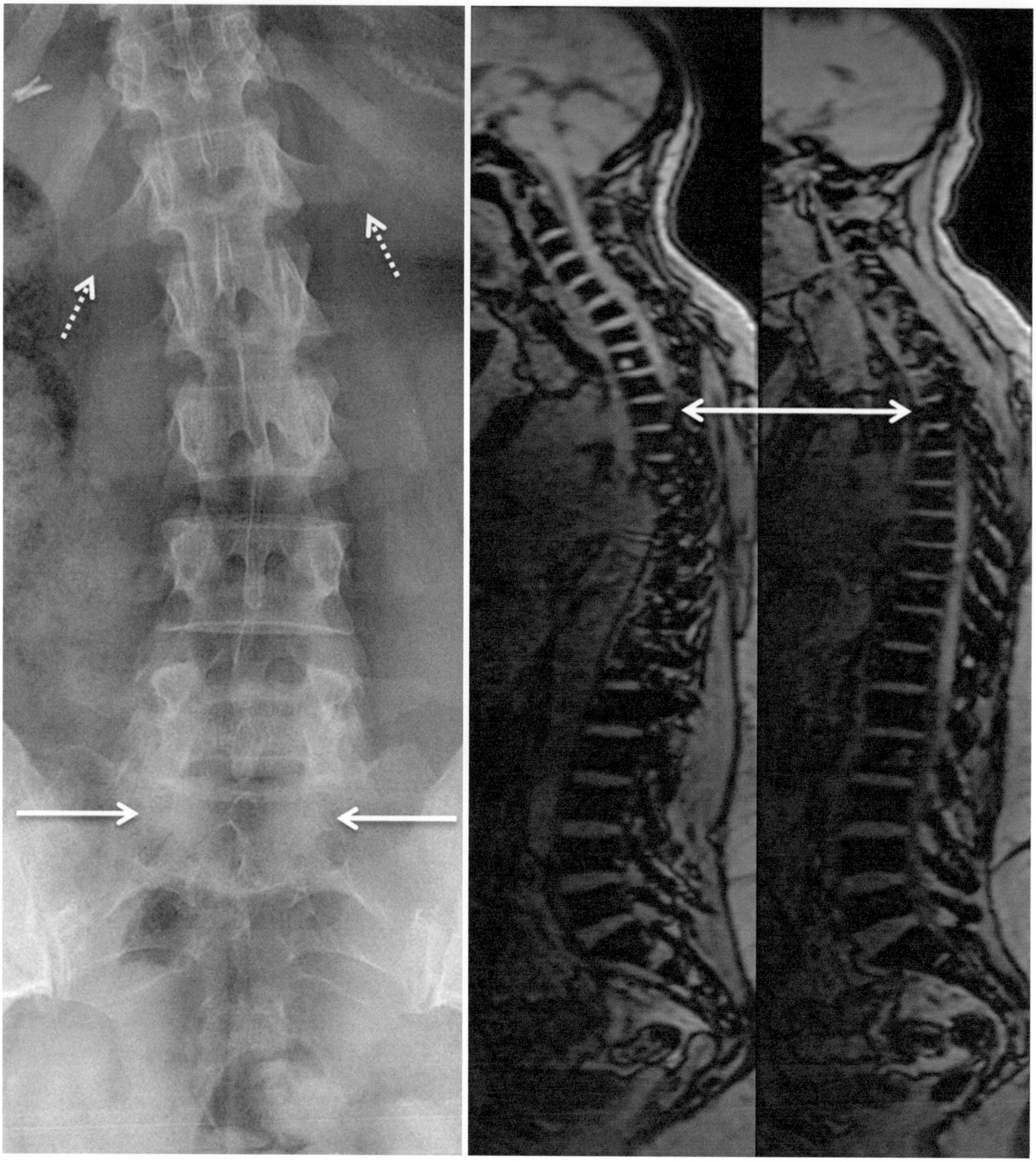

Fig. 7.15 A 40-year-old male with back pain. At first glance, the anteroposterior plain film (*left*) appears to have five lumbar-type vertebral bodies, and the expected numbering would be L1-L5. However, the patient went on to have an MRI of his lumbar spine, and scout images of the entire spine were obtained. He had mild thoracolumbar scoliosis; therefore, the entire spine could not be visualized on a single image. Two sequential GET1WI scout MRI images are presented (*middle and right*); a *double-ended arrow* denotes the superior endplate of T3 on each image. Thus, the inferiormost lumbar-type vertebral body with surrounding fully formed and hydrated discs is actually L4, indicating four "lumbar-type" vertebral bodies. L5 is completely sacralized (*white arrows, left*), while T12 has long transverse processes (*dotted arrows, left*) that can mimic ribs and may cause further discrepancies if only plain films are used for counting/numbering

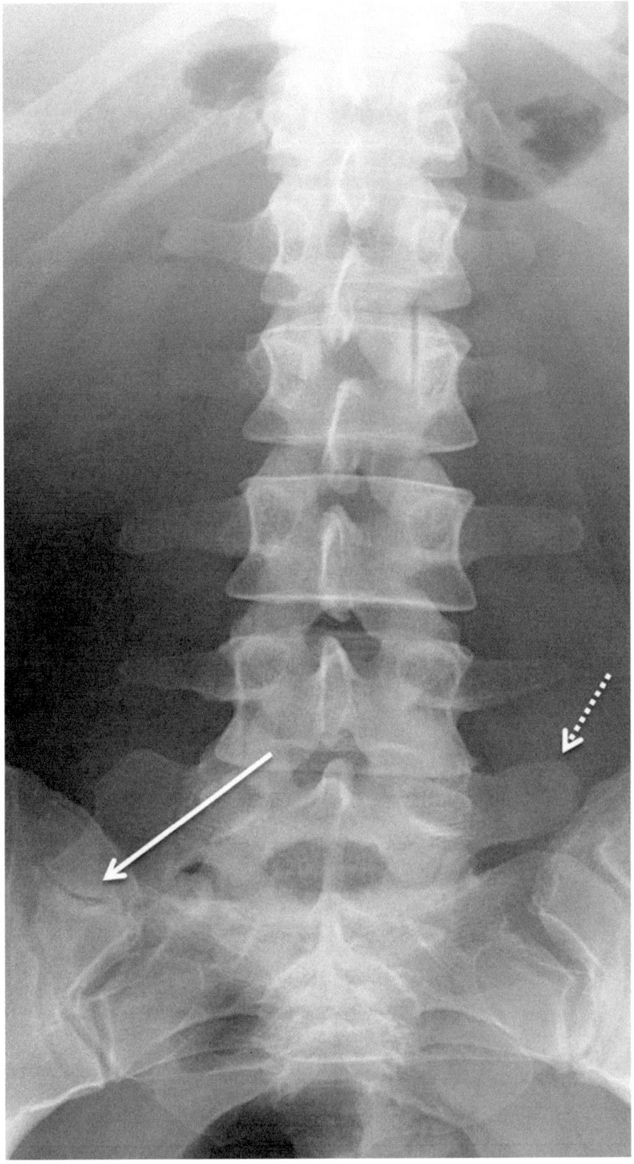

Fig. 7.16 A 25-year-old female with back pain. An anteroposterior plain film demonstrates four lumbar vertebral bodies and a transitional vertebra at L5 with partial sacralization. There is pseudoarticulation of the enlarged right transverse process with the sacrum (*white arrow*). The left transverse process is also enlarged but does not articulate with and is not fused with the sacrum on the left side (*dotted arrow*)

7.13 Lumbarization

Lumbarization is when the S1 and S2 vertebrae fail to fuse, the S1 vertebra appears as a "lumbar-type" vertebral body, and there appear to be six lumbar-type segments, most commonly denoted on sagittal plain films, CT, or MRI. Lumbarization is less common than sacralization. As with sacralization, this phenomenon may be bilateral or unilateral, is usually a "don't touch" lesion, and requires consistent documentation and awareness of the numbering schema in order to prevent "wrong level surgery." This can be best delineated by counting down from the top of the odontoid process of C2, with assistance from the radiologist in ambiguous cases (Figs. 7.17 and 7.18).

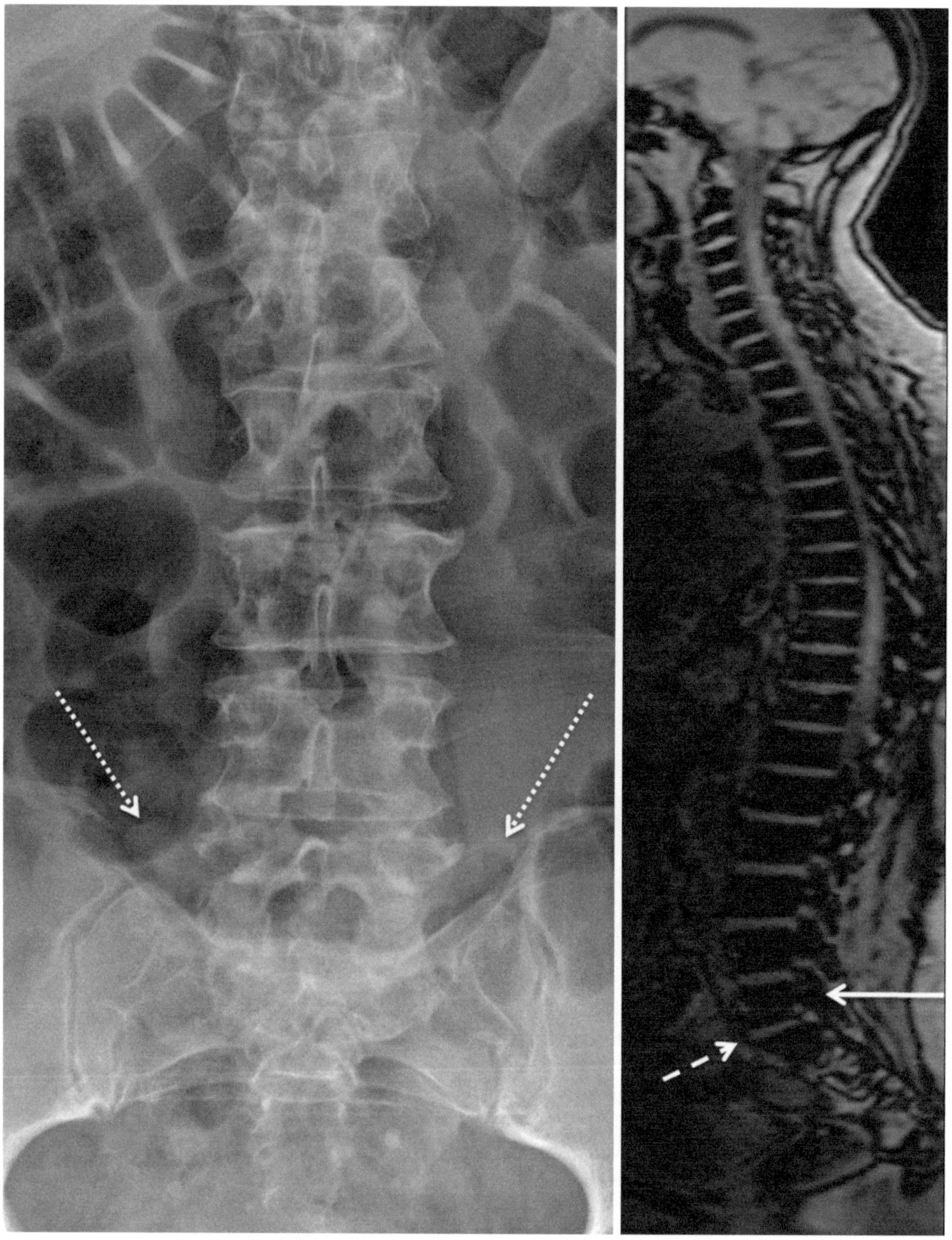

Fig. 7.17 A 65-year-old male with back pain. The anteroposterior plain film (*left*) demonstrates six lumbar-type vertebral bodies. The transverse processes (*dotted arrows, left*) of the lumbarized S1 vertebrae are mildly enlarged but not fused. The sagittal scout GET1WI image (*right*) demonstrates that there is a hydrated S1-S2 intervertebral disc (*dashed arrow, right*) and that S1 is the transitional segment (*white arrow, right*)

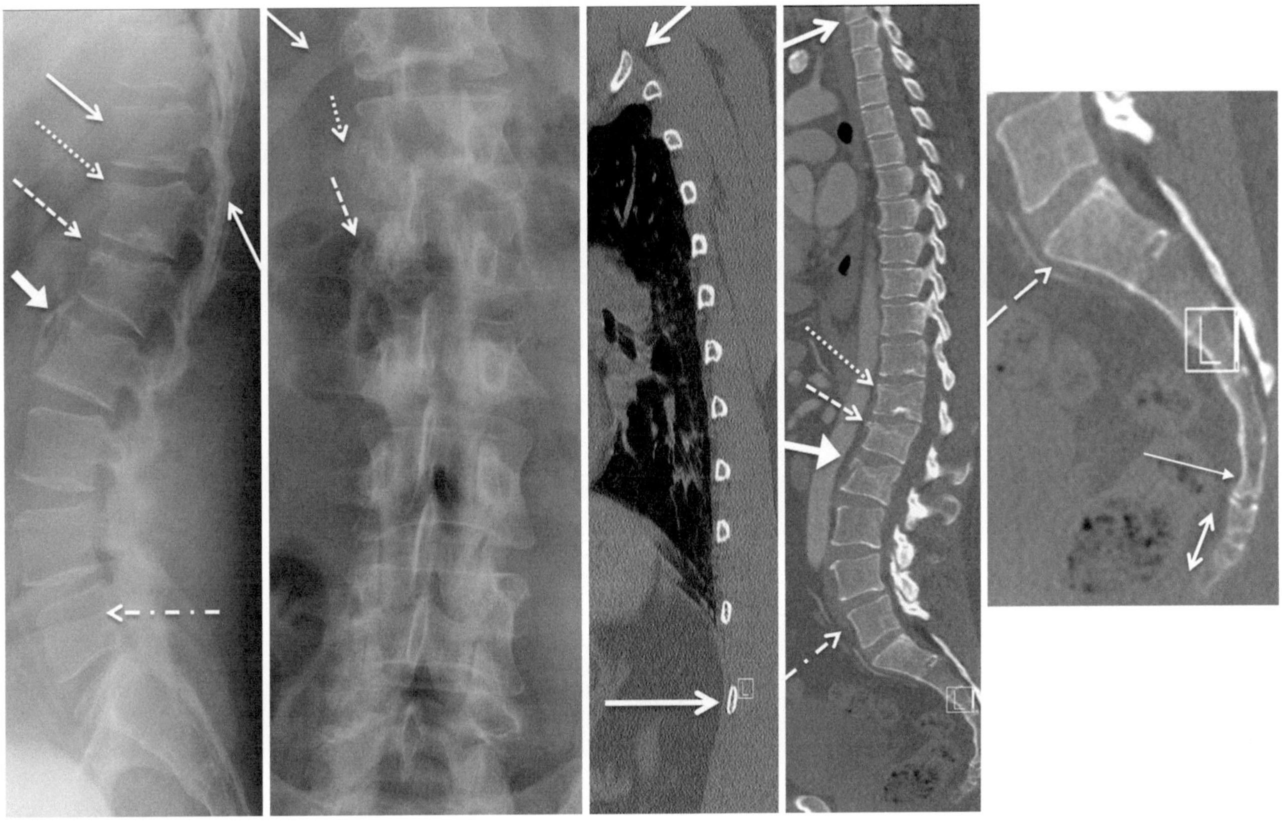

Fig. 7.18 Comparison case of transitional vertebra in traumatic fracture. A 30-year-old male with back pain after a motor vehicle crash. A lateral plain film (*left*) demonstrates superior endplate compression deformities at L1 (*dotted arrow*), L2 (*dashed arrow*), and L3 (*large tip white arrow*). There is fragmentation anteriorly at L2 and L3. There are six lumbar type vertebral bodies with L6 noted (*dash-dot-dash arrow*). The twelfth rib and twelfth vertebral bodies are indicated (*solid white arrows, left*). An anteroposterior plain film (*left middle*) demonstrates no hypoplastic ribs to help explain the appearance of six lumbar type vertebrae, but rather at L1 and L2 there are nonunited hypoplastic transverse processes (*dotted arrow and small dashed arrow, respectively*). The right twelfth rib is indicated (*white arrow, left middle*). A parasagittal CT bone window from the chest, abdomen, and pelvis contrast-enhanced CT (CECT) (*middle image*) demonstrates 12 thoracic ribs with the first rib (*large arrow*) and the twelfth rib (*long white arrow*) indicated. There were seven cervical vertebrae noted on the CT of the cervical spine, and the above number is also based on counting down from the top of C2-odontoid (*not shown*). A sagittal CT bone window (*right middle*) of the thoracic, lumbar, sacral, and coccygeal spine is provided with T1 indicated (*large white arrow*). The compression deformities at L1, L2, and L3 (*dotted, dashed,* and *large tip white arrows, respectively*) and L6 (*dash-dot-dash arrow*) are noted. Further, a coned-down sagittal CT bone window of the sacrum and coccyx (*right*) demonstrates five fused sacral vertebral bodies with S1 (*large dashed arrow*) and S5 (*thin arrow*) indicated. There are three formed coccygeal segments (*double arrow, right*). Thus, there truly are six lumbar vertebrae, and there must be L6 nerve roots which, in theory, would have a neuronal distribution that consists of a mixture of parts of the L5 nerve root and the S1 nerve root distributions

7.14 Hemivertebrae

Discussion of vertebral column embryology and development is beyond the scope of this text, as numerous references exist (please see "*Suggested Reading*" section). Congenital anomalies of the vertebral body include asomia (agenesis), hypoplasia, hemivertebrae (including lateral and dorsal), coronal cleft, butterfly vertebrae, and block vertebrae (congenital fusion). Lateral hemivertebrae will produce scoliosis centered at that level. Dorsal hemivertebrae typically produce kyphosis (Fig. 7.19).

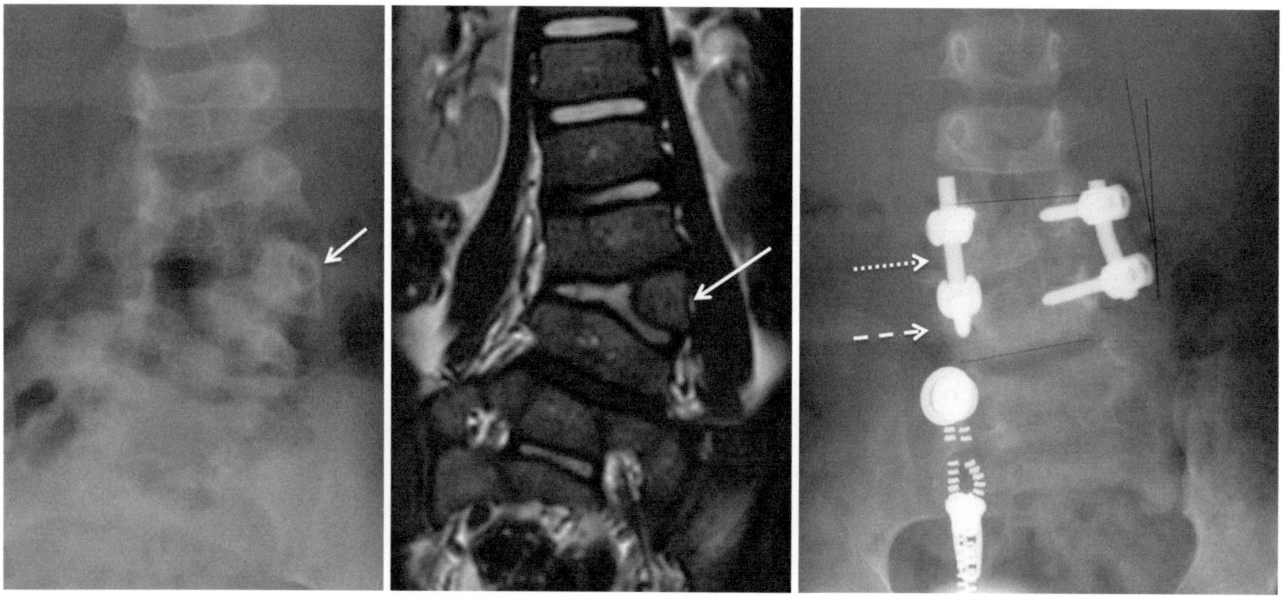

Fig. 7.19 A 6-year-old male with congenital scoliosis. An anteroposterior plain film (*left*) and coronal SET2WI (*right*) demonstrate the left-sided hemivertebra at L4 (*arrows*), with resultant levoconvex scoliosis. After resection and fusion of the hemivertebra, a postoperative anteroposterior plain film (*right*) demonstrates improved alignment. Pedicle screws with dorsal rods are seen in L3 (*dotted arrow, right*) and L5 (*dashed arrow, right*)

7.15 Conus Medullaris at the Level of L3

There is a wide variation regarding the normal level of the conus medullaris. The most common adult position is at L1-L2. In children, the level can vary from the T10-T11 interspace to the superior aspect of the L3 vertebral body; notably, the L3 tip of conus is present in less than 5% of term infants. In adults, the level can range from the middle third of T11 to the middle third of L3 (rare), depending on the study. It is thought that a conus medullaris above the level of the L2-L3 interspace is normal in adolescents and adults, and that one lying at the level of L3 is equivocal, representing either a rare normal variant or being secondary to a tethered cord. A low-lying conus medullaris can also be associated with a fatty filum or thickened filum terminale. A tethered cord is also known as an occult spinal dysraphism sequence (Fig. 7.20).

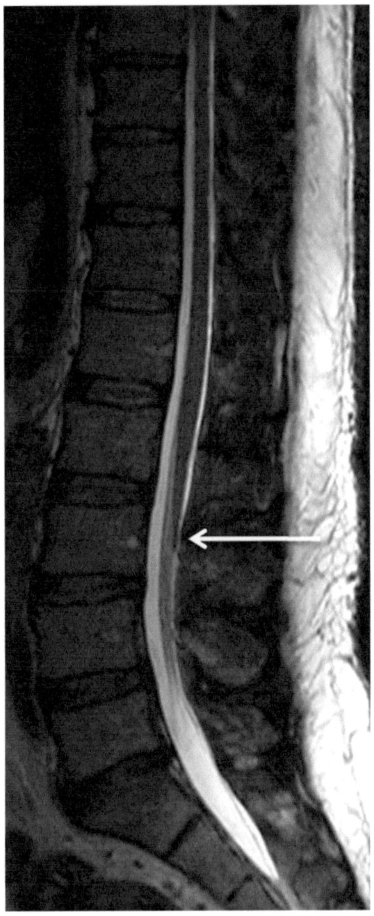

Fig. 7.20 A 46-year-old male with low back pain. Sagittal SET2WI demonstrates the conus at the level of L3 (*arrow*). There was no evidence for a thickened or fatty filum. The patient had been asymptomatic until recently, with nonspecific lower back pain and no symptoms of radiculopathy

7.16 Ventriculus Terminalis

The *ventriculus terminalis* is an ependymal lined space at or near the conus medullaris that represents an anatomic remnant and usually a normal variant when not associated with other findings (such as cord tethering, lipoma, or a longer syrinx). Normally the ventriculus terminalis regresses in infancy and is rarely seen in adults. When seen in an adult, it must be differentiated from a cystic neoplasm of the distal cord or syringohydromyelia (Figs. 7.21, 7.22 and 7.23).

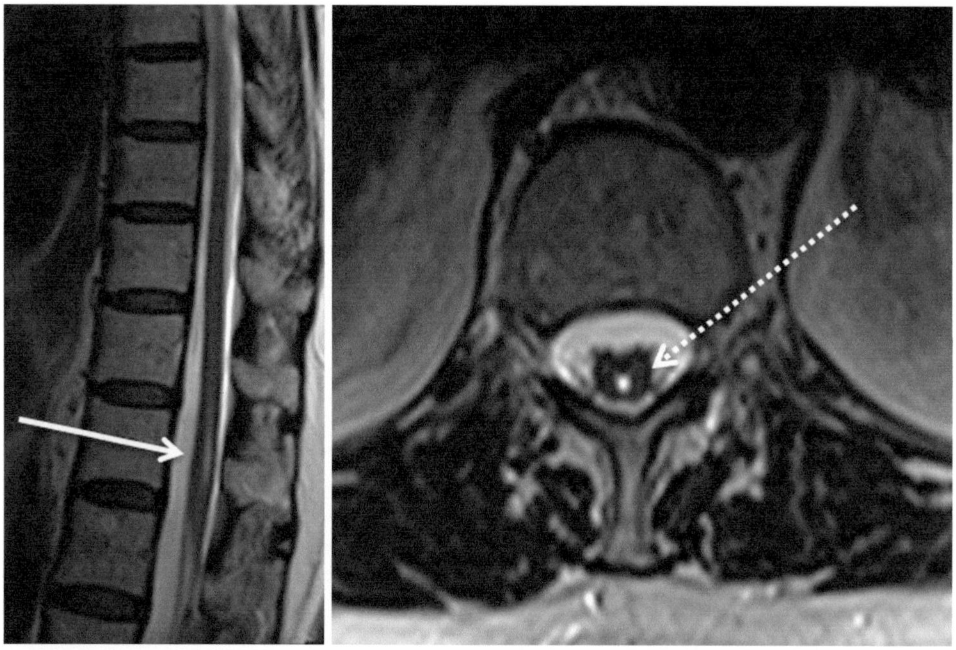

Fig. 7.21 A 76-year-old female with back pain and a questioned signal abnormality in the conus on a previously performed lumbar MRI. However, axial images were not provided through that level on that prior outside examination. On the current examination, a sagittal (*left*) SET2WI demonstrates a linear focus of T2-hyperintensity within the conus medullaris (*white arrow*), which is centrally located on axial SET2WI (*right, dotted arrow*) and consistent with a normal variant ventriculus terminalis

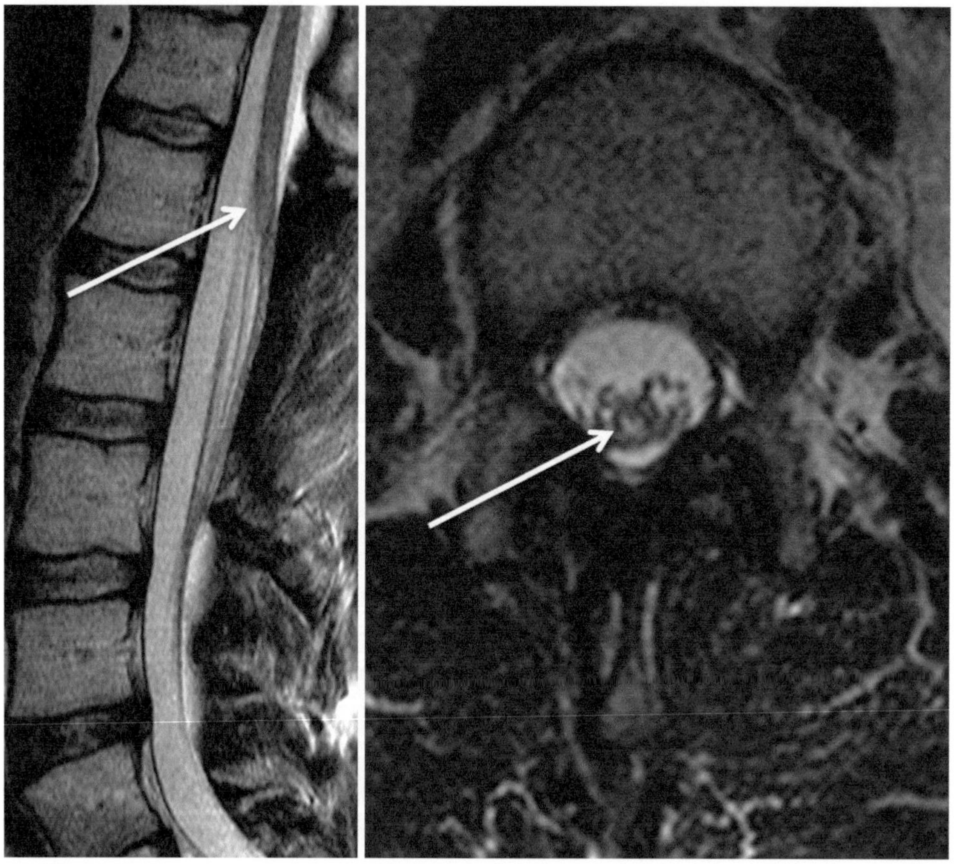

Fig. 7.22 A 35-year-old male status postresection of a known cellular ependymoma, where sagittal (*left*) and axial (*right*) SET2WI demonstrate residual atrophy and myelomalacia within the conus medullaris, simulating a ventriculus terminalis (*white arrows*)

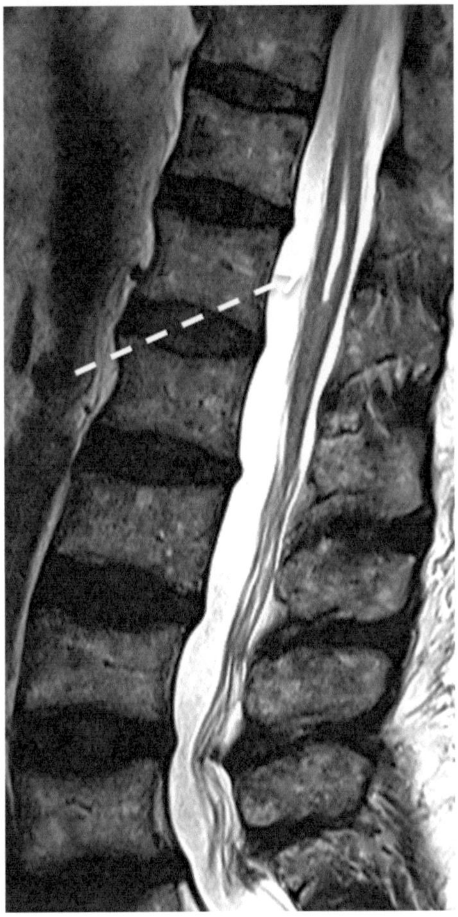

Fig. 7.23 Comparison case of syrinx. A 62-year-old male with low back pain. Sagittal SET2WI (*right*) demonstrates a distal thoracic syrinx (*dashed arrow*), which extends well above the conus medullaris

7.17 Vertebral Bone Island

A *bone island* or enostosis is a dense sclerotic focus of mature, compact bone within cancellous bone. Usually found as an incidental finding on plain film or CT, it can masquerade as a sclerotic metastasis in the clinical context of a patient with a history of primary cancer. This "don't touch" lesion likely represents a hamartoma of bone and is asymptomatic. Differentiation from other sclerotic lesions can usually be accomplished by evaluating clinical symptoms and radiologic features. On plain film and CT, these features are dense foci within cancellous bone that have a feathery brush-like border created by spicules extending outward that blend in with the normal trabeculations. On MRI these are uniformly hypointense on T1WI and T2WI sequences. Although they are usually silent on nuclear medicine scintigraphy, they occasionally show uptake when active, especially the larger lesions (Fig. 7.24).

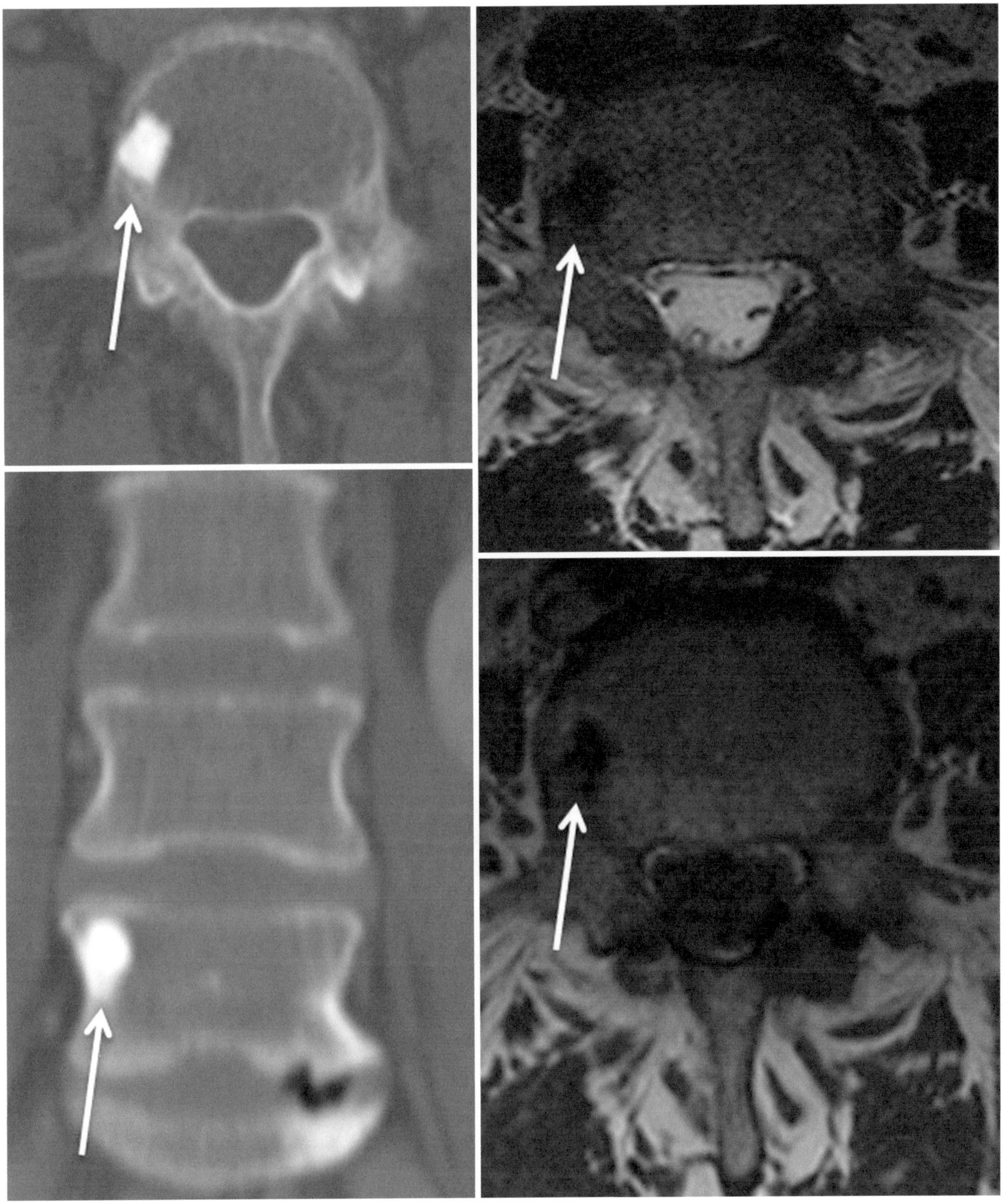

Fig. 7.24 A 51-year-old male with diffuse abdominal pain. Axial and coronal CT bone window images (*top left, bottom left*) that were obtained from an abdomen and pelvic CT (not a dedicated lumbar spine CT) demonstrate a dense sclerotic focus with feathery spicules that align with the normal trabeculations of the bone; this is consistent with a bone island/enostosis (*white arrows*). These are hypointense (*white arrows*) on both T2WI (*top right*) and T1WI (*bottom right*) images

7.18 Osteopoikilosis

Osteopoikilosis ("spotted bones") is a benign, rare, autosomal dominant inherited disorder characterized by innumerable sclerotic foci that are often clustered around the larger joints and around the joints in the pelvis; they are most often seen in the hands and feet. There are usually very few or no clinical manifestations, and the lesions are typically noted as part of an incidental work-up. In general, the axial skeleton is relatively spared. Classified as an osteosclerotic dysplasia, the lesions develop in childhood and do not regress. The lesions are sclerotic foci usually measuring 2–10 mm that align parallel to the trabeculations of the bones and have the same radiographic appearance as bone islands on CT and MRI. Hence, even if there are rarely clinical symptoms from this benign disorder, the innumerable sclerotic foci themselves are typically considered "don't touch" lesions. Although they are typically asymptomatic, there are patients who report mild articular pain. There is an association with osteopathia striata and melorheostosis, which may represent a spectrum of the same condition. It is important to recognize the condition as benign and not confuse it with multifocal sclerotic metastases (Fig. 7.25).

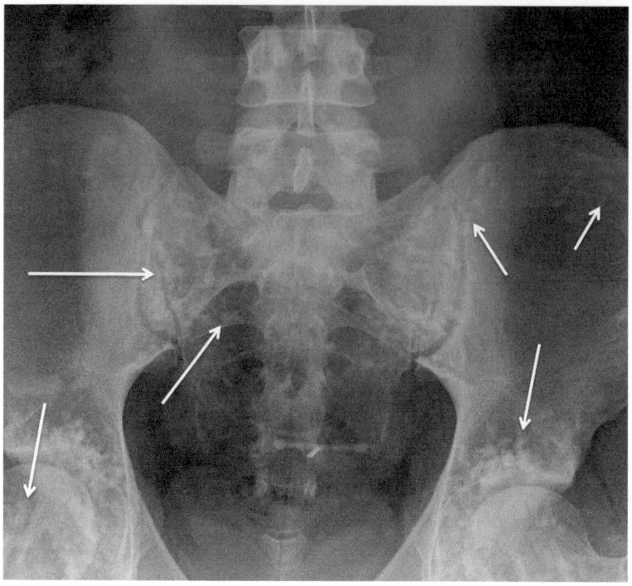

Fig. 7.25 A 25-year-old male with low back pain. An anteroposterior plain film of the lumbar spine/pelvis demonstrates innumerable small sclerotic foci (*white arrows*), that is, bone islands from osteopoikilosis, which are in general clustered about the joints but also involve the entire sacrum and pelvis

7.19 Filum Terminale Lipoma

An incidental and benign lipoma of the filum terminale, which is also known as a *fatty filum* terminale, is created by a developmental error in migration of mesodermal cells. This is a relatively common finding and is present in up to 5% of patients undergoing imaging of the lumbar spine, and it is largely incidental. Although usually asymptomatic, a fatty filum can be associated with cord tethering in a minority of patients, typically if associated with spinal dysraphism/neural tube defects or various neurologic symptoms. In these patients the filum is usually thickened (>2 mm) and associated with a low-lying conus medullaris. This is considered a "don't touch" benign lesion in the setting of a lack of cord tethering (normal conus level at L1-L2 in adults), lack of a spinal dysraphism, and lack of associated neurologic deficits. These can be confirmed by fatty signal on MRI, typically by darkening after FS applied to T1WI or on STIR imaging (Fig. 7.26).

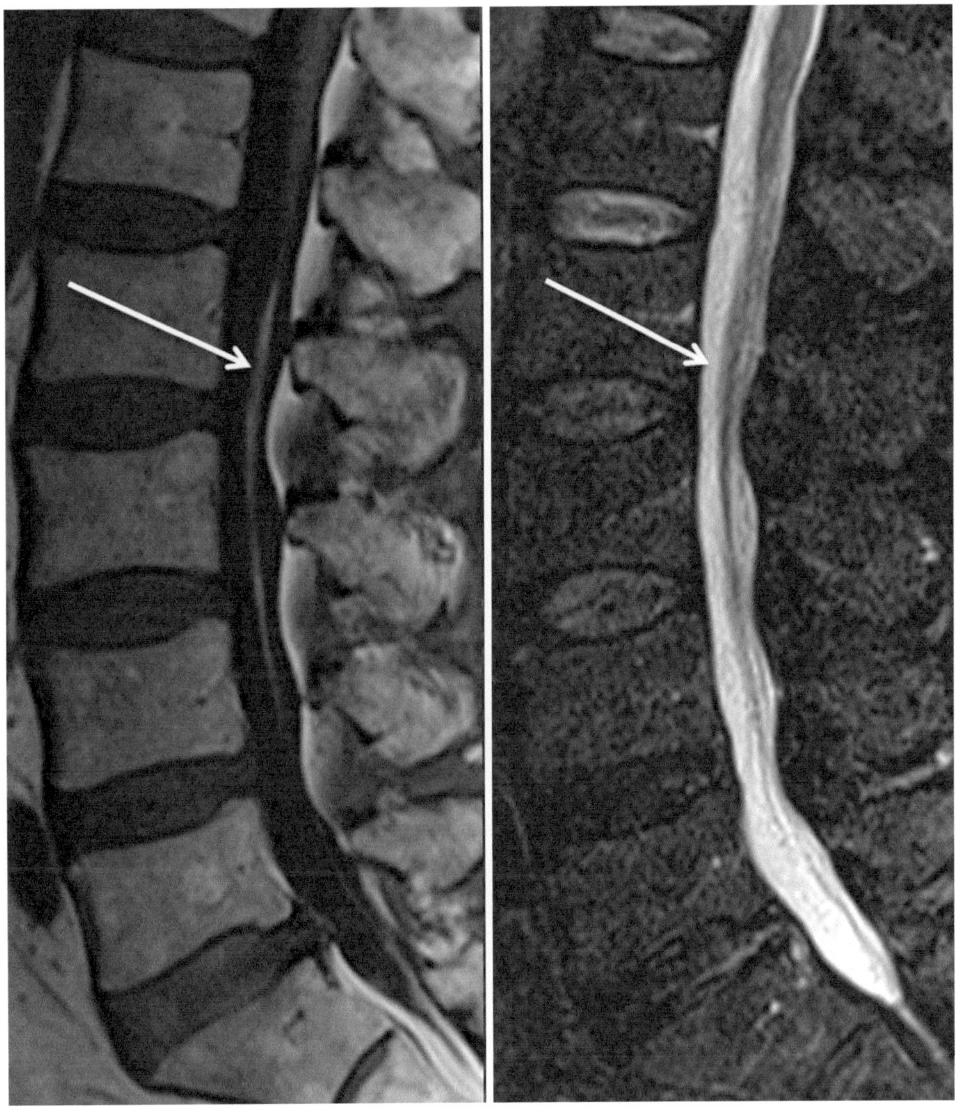

Fig. 7.26 A 35-year-old female with back pain. Sagittal SET1WI (*left*) demonstrates a thickened and T1-hyperintense filum terminale (*white arrows*). This is hypointense on STIR imaging (*right*). The lipoma extends from the upper portion of L2 to the lower portion of L4. Note the lack of cord tethering, as the conus medullaris is in a normal position at L1. The majority of fatty fila are incidental, as in this case

7.20 Supernumerary Ribs

Supernumerary lumbar ribs are not common, but their prevalence varies by studies, perhaps because of the variability in counting technique used throughout the literature. In fact, a true prevalence has not been established, although less than 1% of the population is a rough estimate. Lumbar ribs typically arise from the L1 vertebrae, but they can also arise from the second and third lumbar vertebrae. Supernumerary ribs may also arise from the cervical vertebrae, supernumerary thoracic vertebrae, and the sacrum or coccyx. Their prevalence may also vary, since they may imitate (or overlap with) the appearance of incompletely formed/ossified transverse processes of vertebrae, particularly in the lumbar region. Hence, it is not uncommon for supernumerary ribs to overlap in appearance with incomplete transverse process ossification, even to simulate rib or vertebral fractures in the acute setting, or to cause counting problems of the vertebrae when only a lumbar plain film is present. Thus, again, the only way to be truly certain of such lumbar numbering is counting down from the top of the odontoid process of C2. Generally asymptomatic and considered "don't touch" normal variants, lumbar ribs are occasionally associated with back pain over the kidneys. A discussion of the embryology of the anomaly is beyond the scope of this book, but they have been associated with various gene mutations (Figs. 7.27, 7.28 and 7.29).

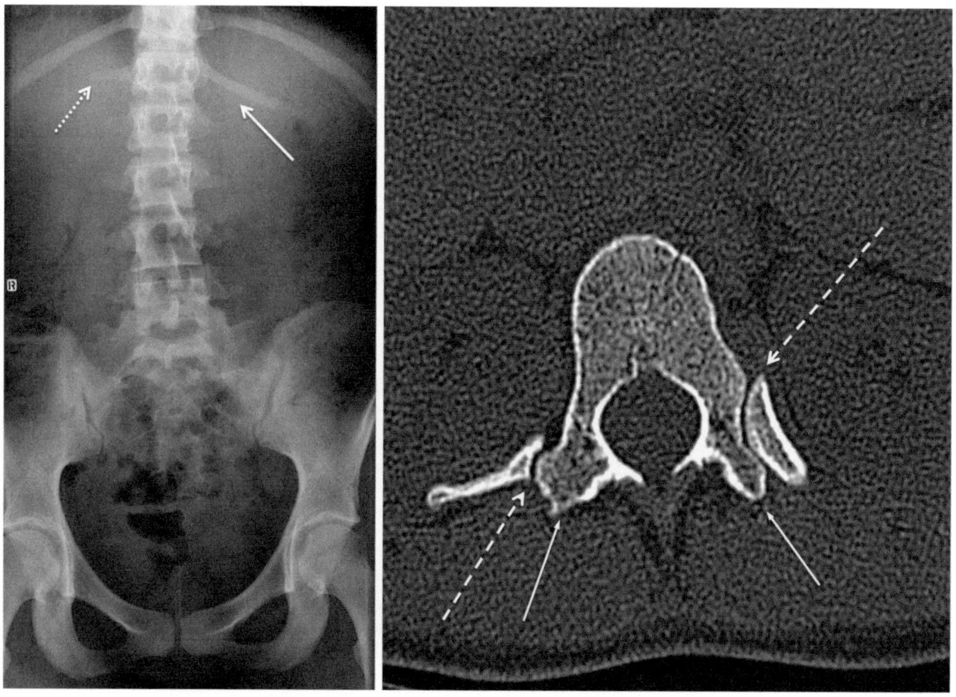

Fig. 7.27 A 23-year-old female with middle and low back pain. An anteroposterior plain film (*left*) demonstrates a fully formed left-sided 13th rib at L1 (*white arrow*). There is a hypoplastic rib on the right, which also could be associated with being an incomplete transverse process (*dotted arrow*). An axial NECT image (*right*) demonstrates the rib articulations with L1 (*dashed arrows*) and the hypoplastic transverse processes (*thin arrows*), which appear analogous to thoracic transverse processes rather than appearing as normal lumbar transverse processes

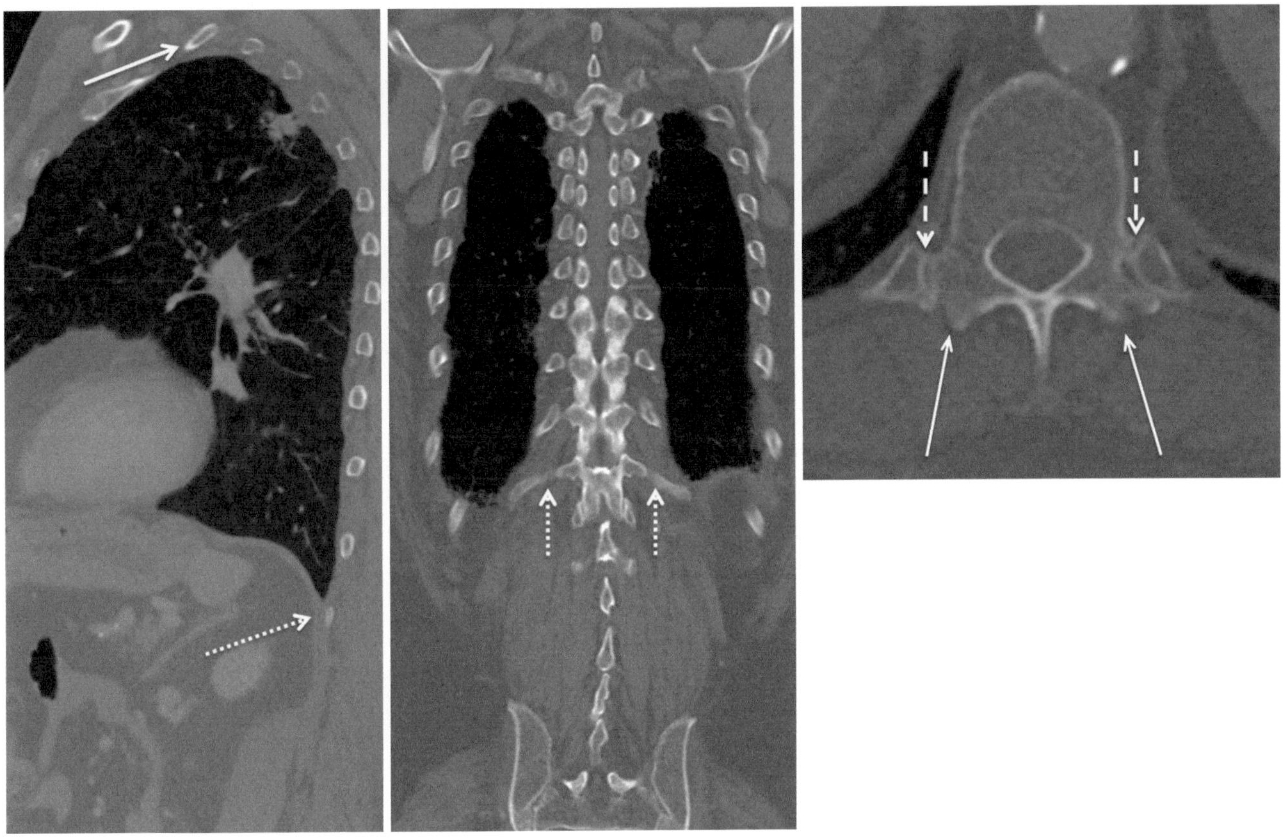

Fig. 7.28 A 67-year-old male with lung cancer and back pain from metastatic disease. A parasagittal reconstruction from a chest/abdomen CECT using bone windowing (*left*) demonstrates 13 ribs; the 1st rib is at T1 (*solid white arrow*), while the 13th rib is at L1 (*dotted arrows*). Notably, on inferiormost imaging (*not shown*), S1 had a transitional appearance and was partially lumbarized. The 13th rib is hypoplastic and bilateral (*dotted arrows*) and is also depicted on coronal reformats from the CECT (*middle*). On axial reconstructions (*right*), the L1 rib articulations are demonstrated (*dashed arrows*), while the transverse processes have an appearance analogous to those seen in the thoracic spine (*thin arrows*)

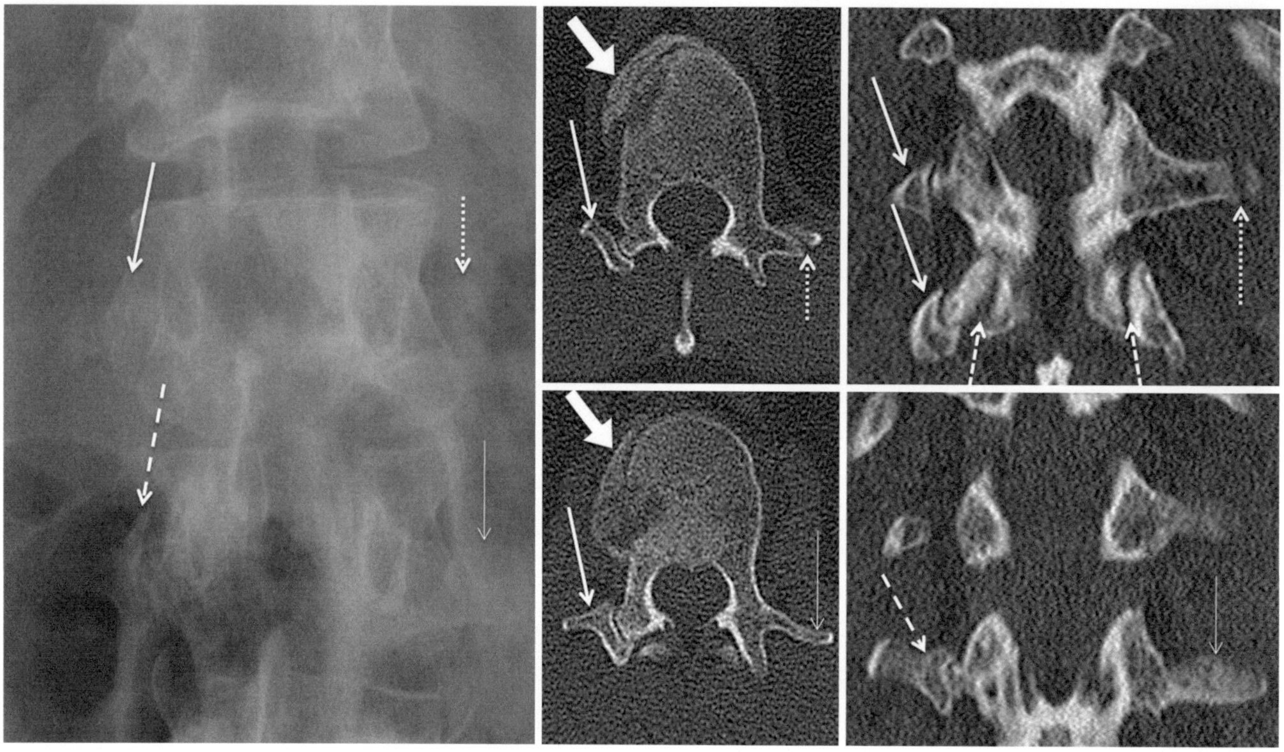

Fig. 7.29 Comparison case of multiple lumbar fractures. A 30-year-old male with back pain after a motor vehicle crash. An anteroposterior lumbar plain film (*left*) demonstrates a subtle transverse process fracture on the left at L1 (*dotted arrow*), with nonfused transverse processes on the right at the levels of L1 and L2 (*white arrow* and *dashed arrow,* respectively), and a normal left L2 transverse process (*thin white arrow*). An axial NECT bone window image at the level of L1 (*top middle*) demonstrates the nonfused transverse process on the right (*white arrow*), a slightly displaced left L1 transverse process fracture (*dotted arrow*), and an anterior segment fracture (*fat arrow*). Lower down at the level of L2, an axial NECT image (*bottom middle*) depicts a normal left transverse process of L2 (*thin arrow*), an incompletely fused right L2 transverse process (*white arrow*), and fracture fragments from a superior endplate compression fracture (*fat arrow*). Coronal reformats of the NECT (*top right, bottom right*) demonstrate the same findings at L1 and L2 (*arrow patterns as previously noted*) and the L1-L2 interfacet joints (*smaller dashed arrows*). The nonfused transverse processes do not have the same appearance as the rib articulations described in Figs. 7.27 and 7.28

7.21 Vertebral Hemangioma

Vertebral hemangiomas are the most common tumors of the spinal axis, having a prevalence in the range of 10–20% of adults, with multiple lesions visualized in 25–30% of those with vertebral body hemangiomas. These are benign vascular tumors consisting of thin-walled blood vessels and sinuses, and they are lined by endothelium interspersed among coarsened trabeculae and fatty matrix. They are usually focal and rounded but may replace the entire vertebral body. They are mainly asymptomatic, being routinely discovered as an incidental finding on imaging studies. There are three types of vertebral hemangiomas: cavernous, capillary, and venous hemangiomas. Some patients present with pain or neurologic symptoms; however, patients receiving spinal imaging studies often have other etiologies to explain the pain. On CT, most (but not all) hemangiomas display a corduroy appearance on plain films or sagittal/coronal reformatted cross-sectional images, and on axial images they have a "speckled" appearance. On MRI, hemangiomas are most commonly T1-hyperintense secondary to the fatty matrix and T2-hyperintense due to the high water content in the slowly moving blood within the lesion. Atypical hemangiomas vary in appearance but can be T1-hypointense, T2-hyperintense, and usually contain less fat and more vascular enhancing stroma. Aggressive hemangiomas, like atypical hemangiomas, contain more vascularity and less fat and should enhance avidly with contrast on postcontrast T1WI MRIs. They may become symptomatic with growth, which often occurs in pregnancy. Aggressive vertebral hemangiomas are most frequently located between the T3 and T9 levels and can uncommonly cause collapse of the vertebral body, with epidural or soft tissue extension and neurologic symptoms. As described above, atypical hemangiomas may enhance avidly or demonstrate no enhancement at all. When enhancing avidly or if simply demonstrating T1-hypointense and T2- or STIR-hyperintense signal on MRI, atypical or aggressive hemangiomas can simulate neoplasms, especially metastases. NECT can be the study of choice to confirm the typical corduroy (on sagittal/coronal images) or speckled appearance (on axial images) of a benign hemangioma when an atypical or aggressive hemangioma is suspected on MRI (Figs. 7.30, 7.31, 7.32, 7.33, 7.34 and 7.35).

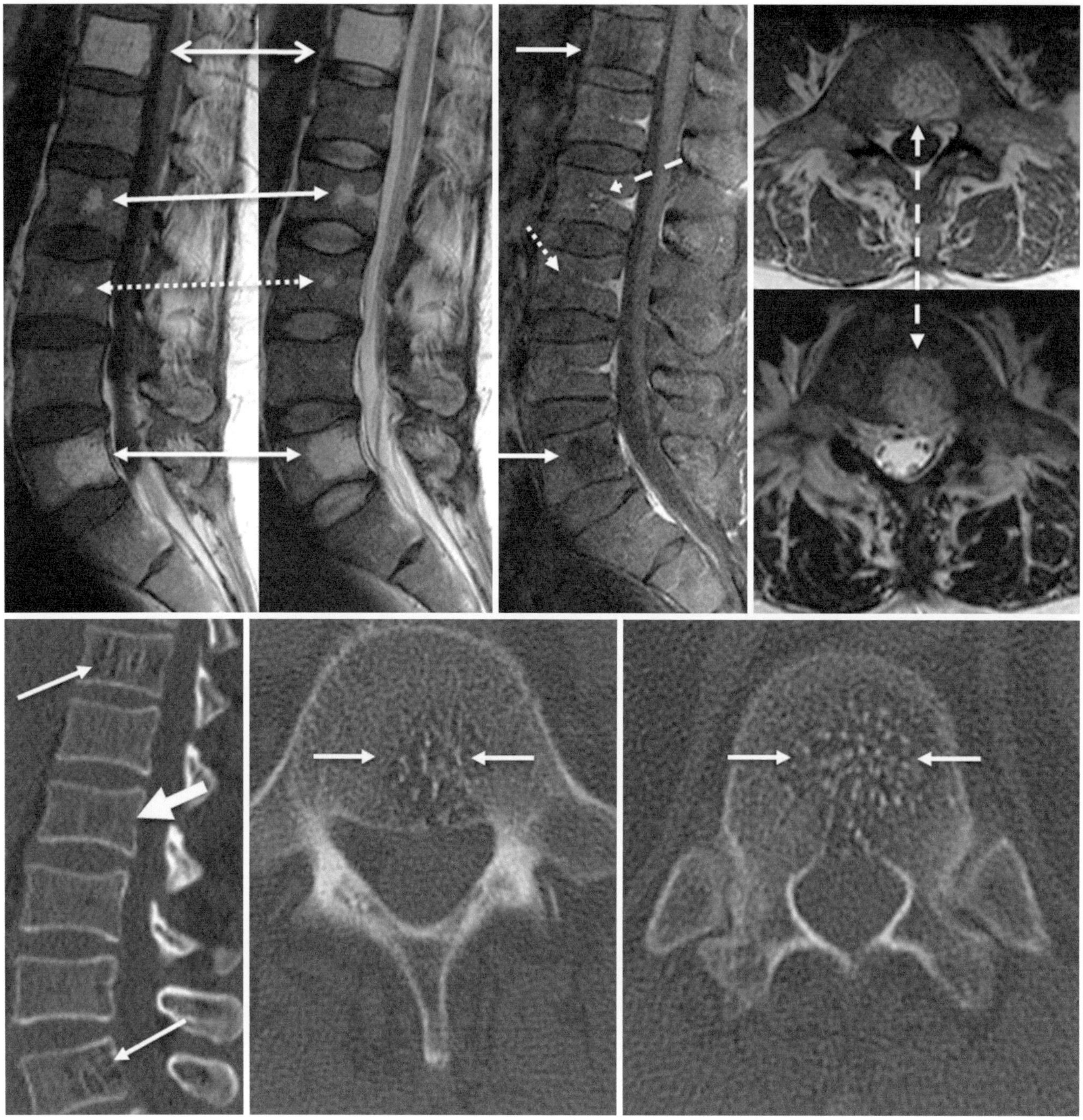

Fig. 7.30 A 25-year-old male with back pain. **Top row:** MRI sagittal SET1WI (*left*) and T2WI (*left middle*) images demonstrate hyperintense signal within the T12, L2, and L5 vertebrae (*double white arrows*); this is classic for typical hemangiomas. At L3, there is a tiny focus of hyperintensity (*dotted double arrow*) that probably is another hemangioma, given their multiplicity, but this could also represent focal fat deposition. On postcontrast FS SET1WI (*right middle*), there is no enhancement at T12 and L5 (*white arrows*), but there is subtle enhancement at L2 (*dashed arrow*), suggesting a slightly more vascular hemangioma; the tiny L3 lesion also does not enhance (*dotted arrow*). Axial SET1WI (*right, upper image*) and SET2WI (*right, lower image*) demonstrate the classic "salt-and-pepper" appearance with dark spots representing the thickened or coarsened trabeculae (*dashed double arrows*). **Bottom row:** On NECT bone algorithm windows with sagittal reconstruction (*left*), the classic corduroy appearance of the hemangiomas is noted at T12 and L5 (*white arrows*). This corduroy appearance is less evident at L2 but is still suggested (*fat white arrow*), particularly given the T1-bright precontrast SET1WI hyperintensity on MRI. Axial NECT images best demonstrate the "speckled" appearance that also confirms benign hemangiomas, as delineated at the levels of L5 (*white arrows, middle*) and T12 (*white arrows, right*)

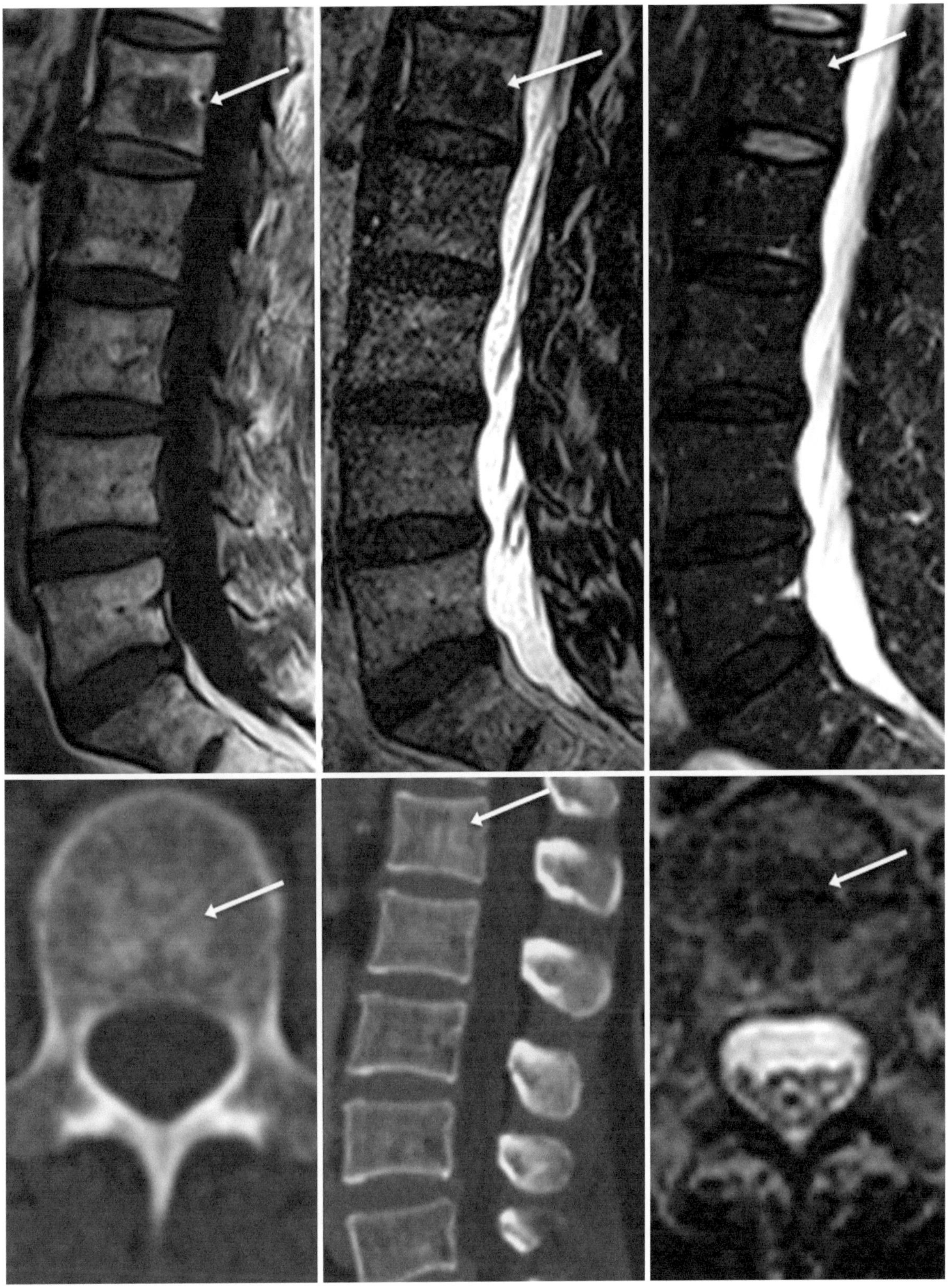

Fig. 7.31 A 78-year-old female with back pain and no history of malignancy. **Top row:** Sagittal SET1WI (*left*), SET2WI (*middle*), and STIR (*right*) demonstrate a rounded, hypointense lesion (*arrows*) within L1, which is barely visible on STIR and has a mildly hypointense periphery and slight T2 hyperintensity internally. This would be of concern for a sclerotic metastasis if no further imaging was available and no contrast medium had been administered, given the lack of a clinical history of tumor. **Bottom row:** Fortunately, an abdominal CECT had been obtained 3 years prior, on which comparison of the speckled, mildly sclerotic density on an axial reformat at the level of L1 (*left*), and corduroy-type density on a sagittal reformat (*arrows*, *middle*) was typical for hemangioma. Thus, the coarsened, thickened, and sclerotic trabeculae would be as expected for a hemangioma. The stability of this "don't touch" lesion over 3 years was confirmed following comparison of the axial CECT image with the T2-hypointense region on the axial SET2WI (*arrow, right*), being consistent with a benign hemangioma

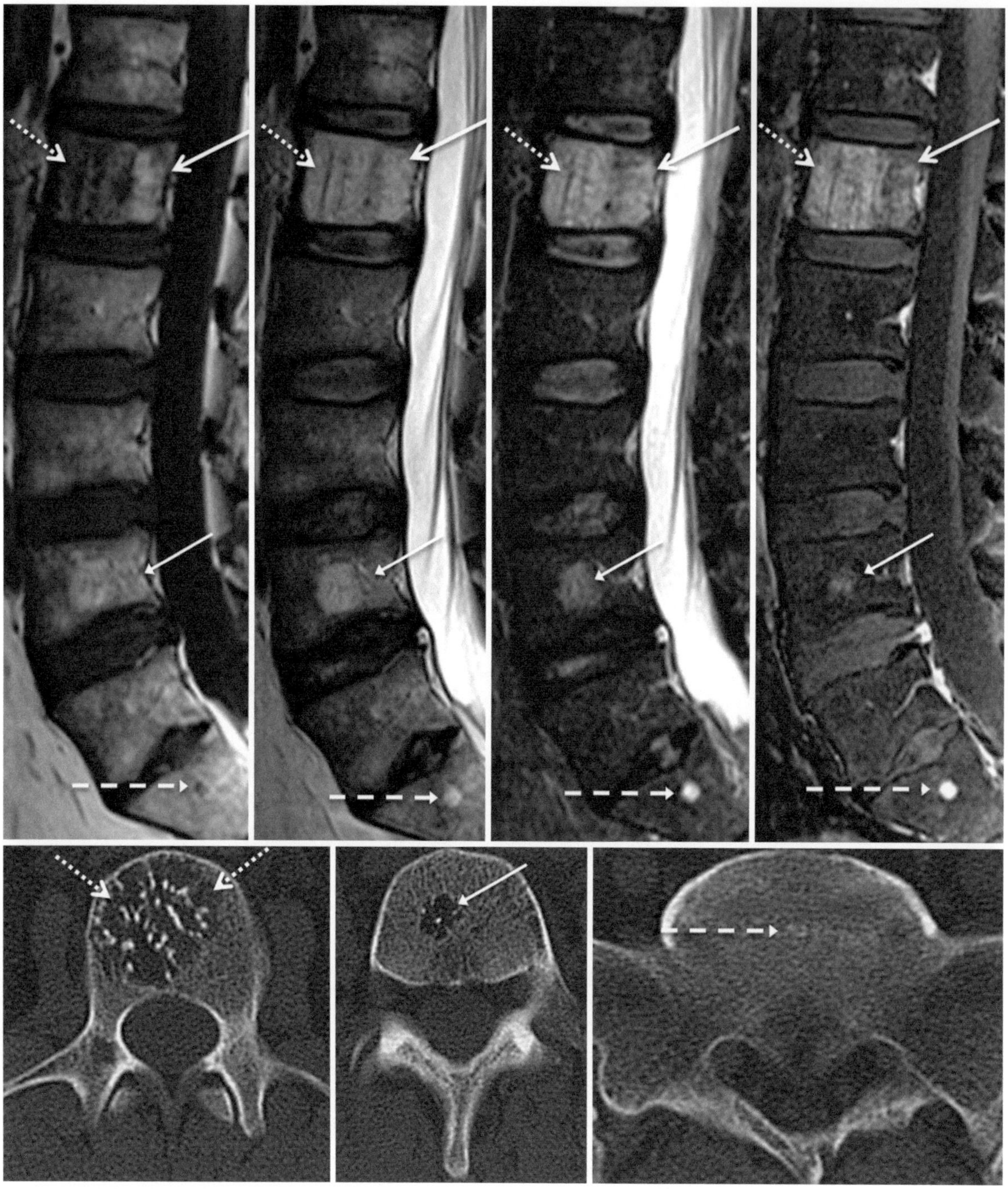

Fig. 7.32 A 42-year-old male with back pain. **Top row:** An MRI with SET1WI (*left*), SET2WI (*left middle*), and STIR (*right middle*) images shows a mixed signal intensity hemangioma replacing the entire anterior segment of the L1 vertebra, with T1-isointensity and T2-/STIR hyperintensity with the anterior portion of the lesion (*dotted arrows*) as well as T1-hyperintensity posteriorly within the lesion (*arrows*). On postcontrast FS SET1WI (*right*), the anterior portion of the lesion enhances avidly (*dotted arrows*), while the posterior portion enhances less so and more variably (*arrows*). Note the vertical hypointense lines as well in a corduroy pattern within the L1 hemangioma on each of these four sequences. Meanwhile, another hemangioma of the L4 vertebra (*thin arrows*) is similar to the signal characteristics of the posterior portion of the L1 lesion, having T1-bright signal prior to contrast (*left*) and mild enhancement on postcontrast FS SET1WI (*right*). Additionally, a subcentimeter T1-hypointense and enhancing focus within S1 (*dashed arrows*) is likely an "atypical" hemangioma, as it is not bright on T1WI prior to contrast. The sum of these findings suggests that the anterior portion of the L1 hemangioma has a higher vascularity and thus a lesser lipid component, while the posterior component has a higher lipid component and less vascularity. **Bottom row:** On three serial axial NECT images, the L1 lesion (*delineated by dotted arrows, left*) and L4 lesion (*thin arrow, middle*) both exhibit a similar appearance with coarsened/thickened trabeculae and intervening lucent areas. A rule of thumb is that if the area of T2 hyperintensity is also T1-isointense to a normal vertebral body's marrow, it is most likely a hemangioma. The vertical hypointense striations on the aforementioned MRI images are another clue (if present), but striations may not be visible if the hemangioma is not large. Regarding the lesion within S1 (*dashed arrow*), note that on the corresponding axial NECT image (*right*) there is no lytic or sclerotic focus that would be a sign of malignancy; thus, this hemangioma that enhanced on T1WI MRI is almost imperceptible on CT

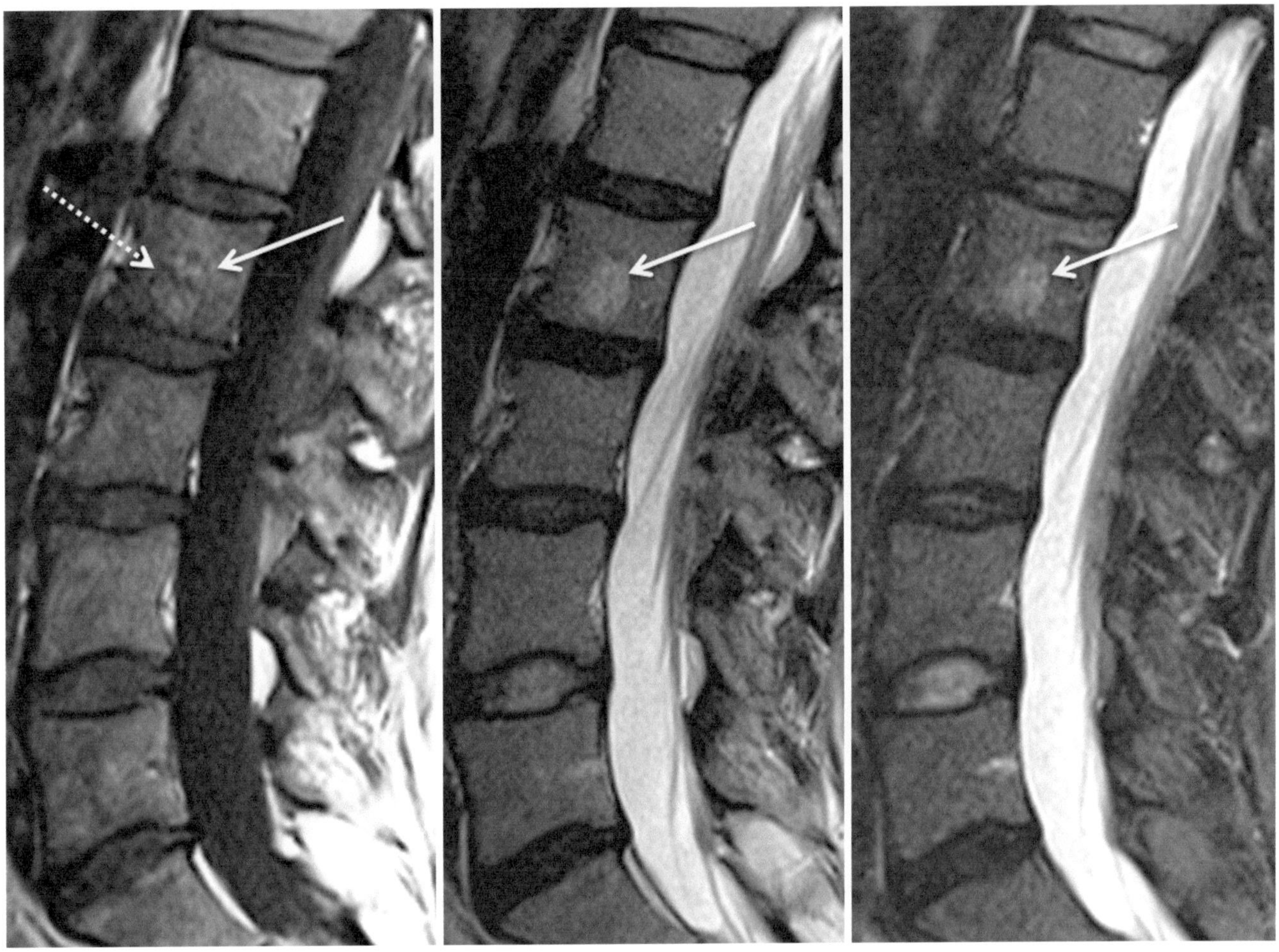

Fig. 7.33 A 30-year-old female with back pain. A sagittal SET1WI MRI (*left*) demonstrates another example of a hemangioma which is mostly T1 isointense to bone marrow but has a sclerotic rim (*arrow*). Instead of a corduroy pattern, there is a serpentine hypointensity centrally within the lesion on T1WI (*dotted arrow, left*). This presumably represents slow flow vasculature as this central hypointensity is not visible on the SET2WI (*middle*) or STIR (*right*) sagittal images, and the signal fades into the surrounding T2-hyperintensity (*arrows, middle and right images*)

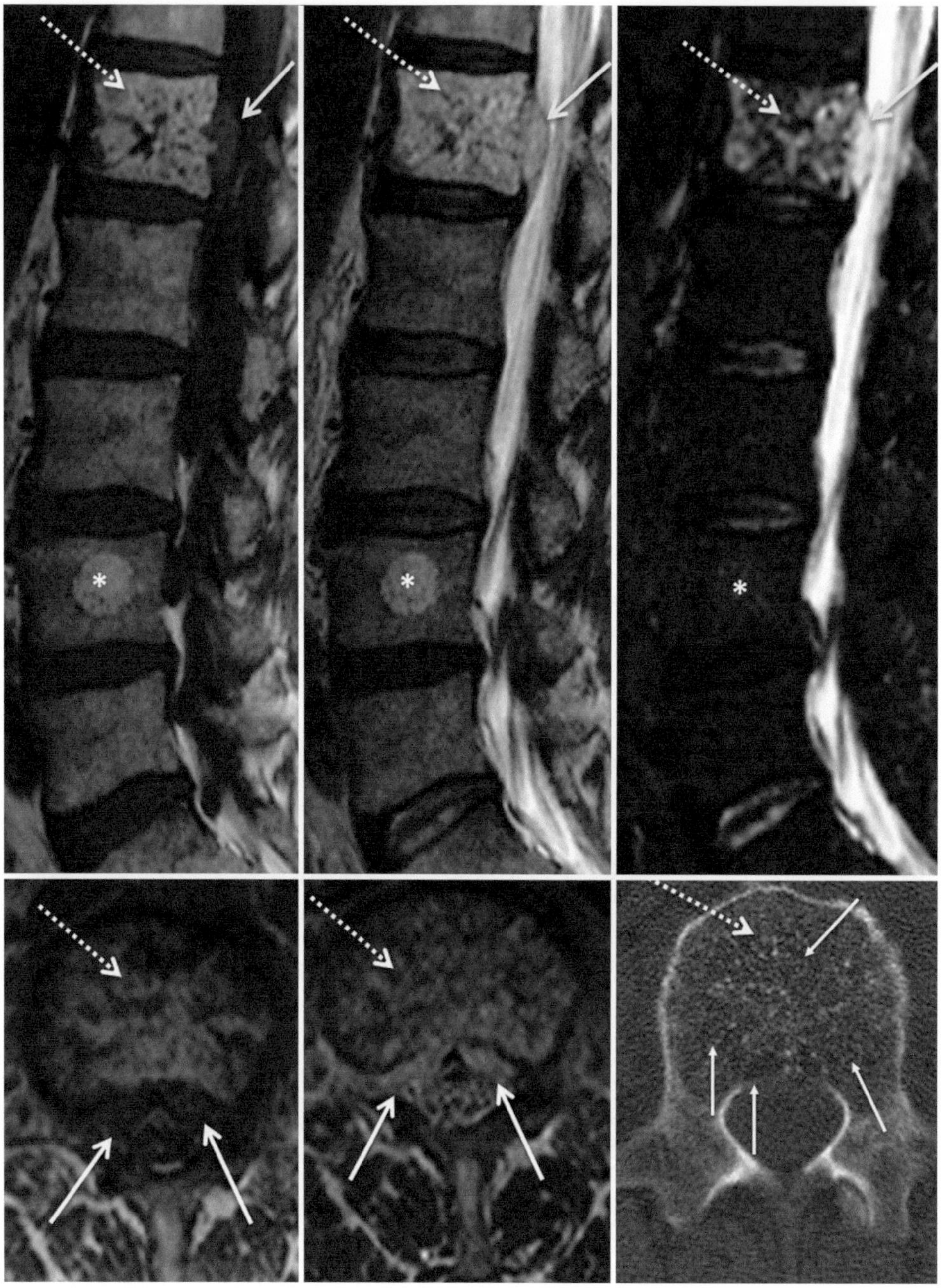

Fig. 7.34 A 57-year-old male with back pain radiating into the right hip. **Top row:** Sagittal SET1WI MRI (*left*) demonstrates a lesion within the L1 vertebra that is not well circumscribed and has a predominantly T1-hyperintense background (*dotted arrows*), with scattered hypointensities involving the entire vertebral body. On sagittal SET2WI (*middle*), there is a background of T2 hyperintensity with scattered hypointensity in that same region (*dotted arrow*). On STIR MRI (*right*), some of the L1 vertebral body is more hypointense than the rest, which is presumably an area with a greater concentration of fat that suppresses on STIR (*dotted arrow*); however, there is also an erosive process with posterior epidural extension and mass effect on the thecal sac (*white arrow*), which is T1-dark and T2-/STIR-hyperintense. Also, note an incidental, more typical T1-bright hemangioma of L4 in each image (*asterisks*). **Bottom row:** this mixed signal phenomenon of this atypical and aggressive-appearing L1 hemangioma is also demonstrated on noncontrast axial SET1WI (*left*) and SET2WI (*middle*), with the epidural extension depicted by the *white arrows* and the mixed trabecular signal intensity by the *dotted arrows* in both images. Note the salt and pepper appearance on these axial images, which in combination with the predominance of T1 hyperintensity are clues that this process represents an aggressive hemangioma and not a metastatic lesion. Axial NECT (*right*) confirms a diffusely speckled appearance (*dotted arrow*) due to coarsened trabeculae that are interspersed with patchy areas of relative lucency (*thin arrows*), being consistent with a benign hemangioma. Notably, the L1 epidural erosive process that had retropulsed into the ventral spinal canal was also related to this aggressive hemangioma, and was unchanged on repeat imaging over time (*not shown*)

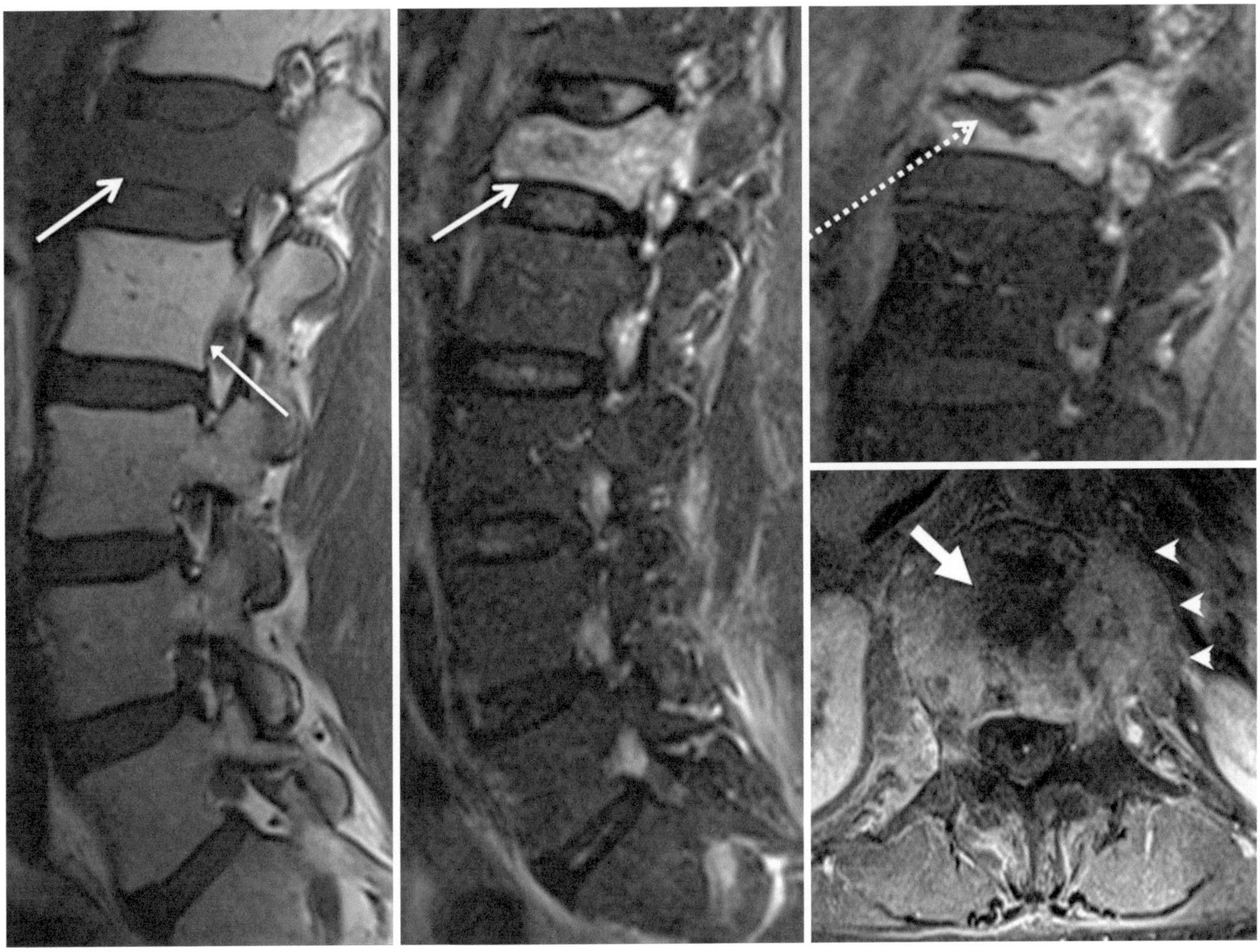

Fig. 7.35 Comparison case of metastasis. A 65-year-old female with a history of non–small cell lung carcinoma and back pain. Sagittal SET1WI (*left*) and STIR (*middle*) images demonstrate diffusely abnormal T1-hypointense and T2-hyperintense signals (*arrows*) replacing the entire anterior segment of the L1 vertebral body; there is also extension into the pedicle and an associated pathologic moderate compression deformity. Note the diffusely T1-hyperintense signal within some other vertebral bodies, indicative of fatty marrow conversion from prior radiation for previous metastatic disease (*thin arrow, left*). On postcontrast sagittal fat suppressed SET1WI (*right, upper image*), there is diffuse enhancement with a central area that is nonenhancing (*dotted arrow*), probably secondary to necrotic tumor. The axial postcontrast fat suppressed T1WI (*right, bottom image*) shows heterogeneous enhancement with a central nonenhancing focus (*fat arrow*). Note how this does not appear like the "salt and pepper" pattern that is typical of hemangiomas. Also, note the tumor extension into the left paraspinous tissues (*arrowheads, bottom right*)

7.22 Dependent Edema

Dependent edema within the posterior soft tissues is incidentally noted in approximately 40% of patients undergoing MR imaging of the lumbar spine, being typically T1-hypointense and T2- and STIR-hyperintense; there may be mild associated enhancement of this edema on postcontrast T1WI. Discrete fluid collections may even be seen as well in approximately 15–20% of cases. These are associated with increasing body mass and increasing age. The frequency and degree of edema tend to be greater in females and older patients. Clinical correlation is always recommended to exclude an underlying pathologic condition causing or contributing to the edema. This can mimic soft-tissue neoplasm or infectious processes such as cellulitis or abscess (Fig. 7.36).

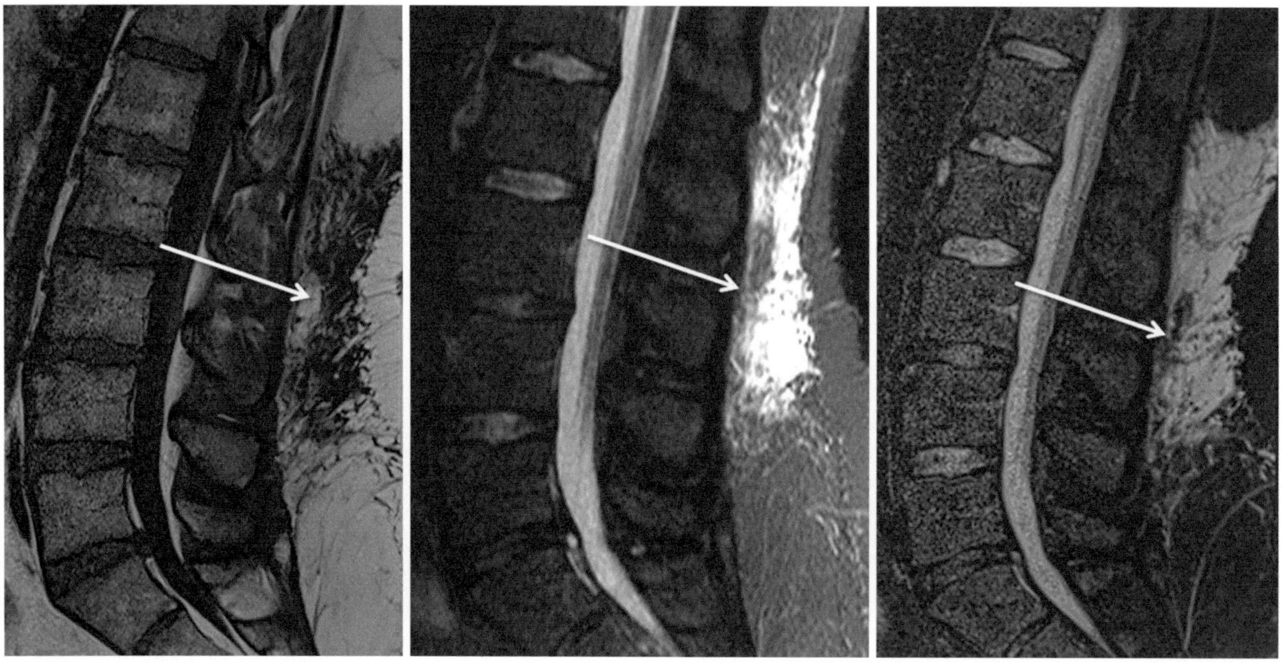

Fig. 7.36 A 45-year-old female with back pain. SET1WI (*left*), SET2WI (*middle*), and STIR (*right*) demonstrate T1-hypointense and T2-hyperintense subcutaneous tissue (*white arrows*) extending from the level of L1 to L5, consistent with dependent (and reversible) edema within the posterior soft tissues

7.23 Basivertebral Veins

The *vertebral venous plexus* includes the internal vertebral venous plexus, the external vertebral venous plexus, and the basivertebral veins. The basivertebral veins run horizontally within the vertebral bodies and receive drainage from numerous small venous channels. They are contained in large tortuous channels in the bone, which are analogous to the diploe in the cranium. These then drain into the anterior internal vertebral plexus between the superficial and deep layers of the posterior longitudinal ligament and the anterior external vertebral venous plexus in the paraspinous tissues anterior to the vertebral bodies through the vascular foramina. At the dorsal aspect of the vertebral body, the basivertebral veins converge and have a wedge-shaped and sometimes a slightly rounded appearance. The appearance of the basivertebral veins as they enter the anterior internal vertebral venous plexus can simulate an erosive lesion on CT or MRI along the dorsal surface of the central vertebral body, particularly when they appear slightly rounded (most often on axial or sagittal reformats). Occasionally, they can also simulate a fracture line in trauma patients as they exit the vertebral body anteriorly. They may also have slightly T2-bright signal on SET2WI and STIR imaging, with enhancement on postcontrast T1WI, which can cause them to simulate a neoplasm or metastasis. Knowledge of their different appearances is important when evaluating patients with back pain. On MRI in younger patients prior to marrow conversion, they will demonstrate a horizontal flow void surrounded by the increased signal of fat surrounding the basivertebral veins on sagittal T1-weighted images. On sagittal SET2WI and STIR images, the basivertebral veins are generally hyperintense owing to the high water content of slow-moving blood. In higher flow states, they may appear dark because of the flow void of fast-moving blood (Figs. 7.37, 7.38, 7.39 and 7.40).

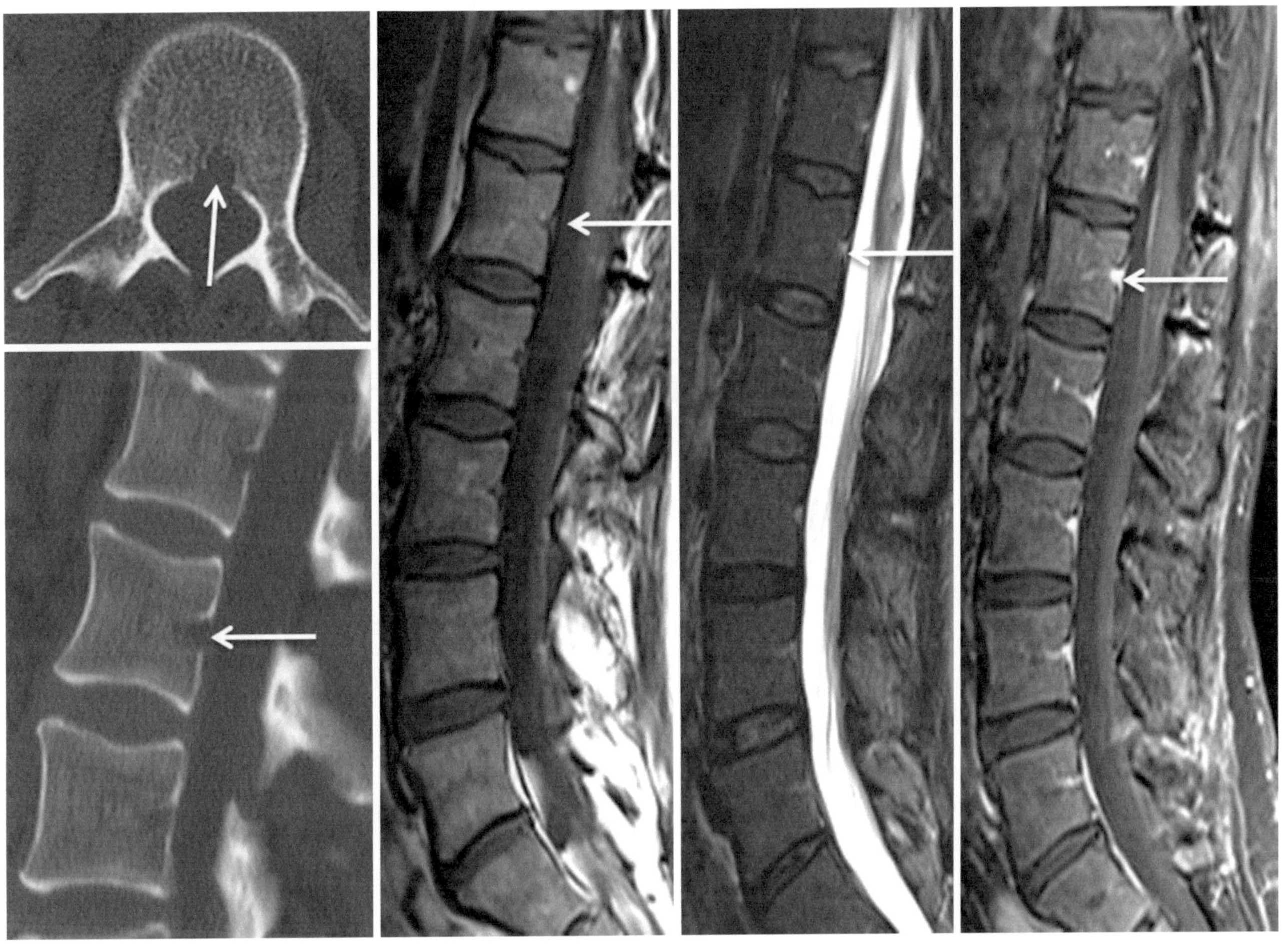

Fig. 7.37 A 30-year-old female with back pain. Sagittal (*left, top image*) and axial (*left, bottom image*) NECT with bone windows demonstrate what could be misconstrued as an erosive lesion in the middle of the posterior wall of the anterior segment of the vertebral body (*arrows*). SET1WI (*left middle*) depicts only a small hypointense focus (*arrow*), with a tiny focus of associated T2 hyperintensity on STIR (*right middle*). Sagittal postcontrast FS SET1WI (*right*) confirms typical linear enhancing basivertebral veins in that location (*arrow*)

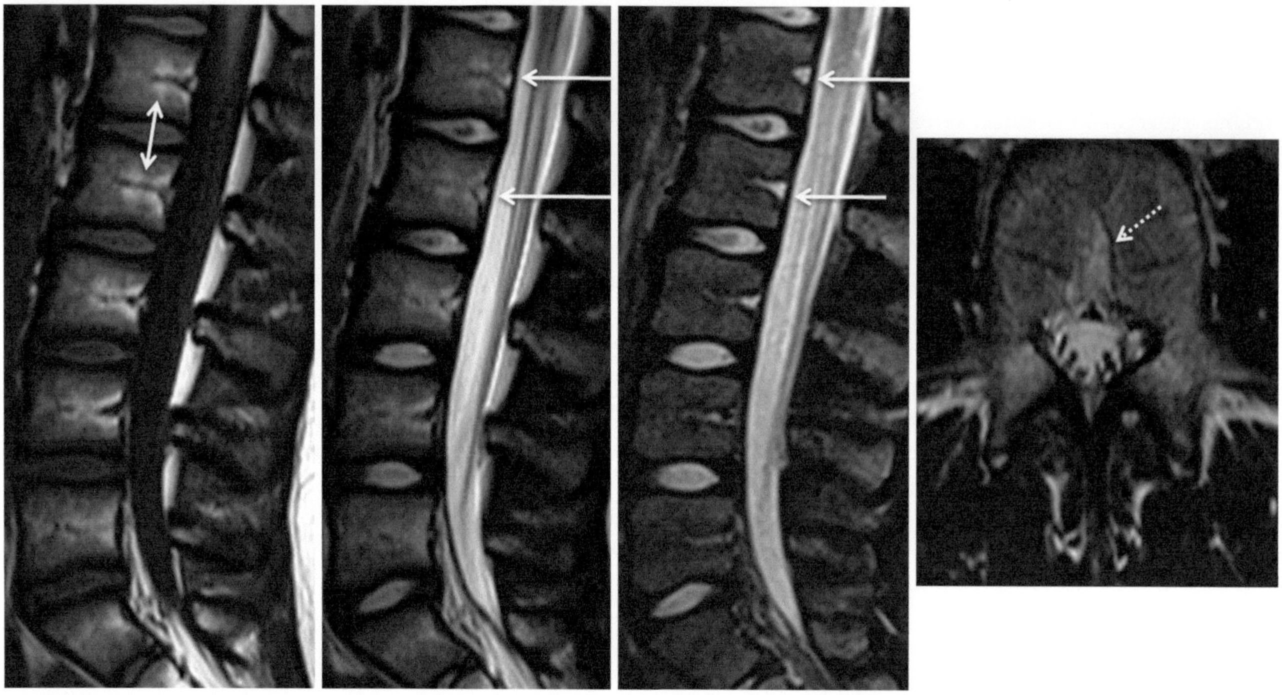

Fig. 7.38 A 13-year-old boy with back pain after trauma and a negative NECT (*not shown*). Sagittal SET1WI MRI (*left*) demonstrates hyperintense fat surrounding the flow void of the basivertebral veins (*double arrow*) in the background of predominantly red marrow (i.e., the remainder of the nonfatty marrow is darker on T1WI and T2WI). Sagittal T2WI (*left middle*) does not suppress the fat signal, where the basivertebral veins are hyperintense (*white arrows*). Sagittal STIR (*right middle*) saturates out the surrounding fat and only the T2-hyperintense signal is visible within the basivertebral veins (*white arrows*). Axial SET2WI (*right*) demonstrates T2 hyperintensity in a flame-like appearance (*dotted arrow*) at the confluence of the basivertebral veins

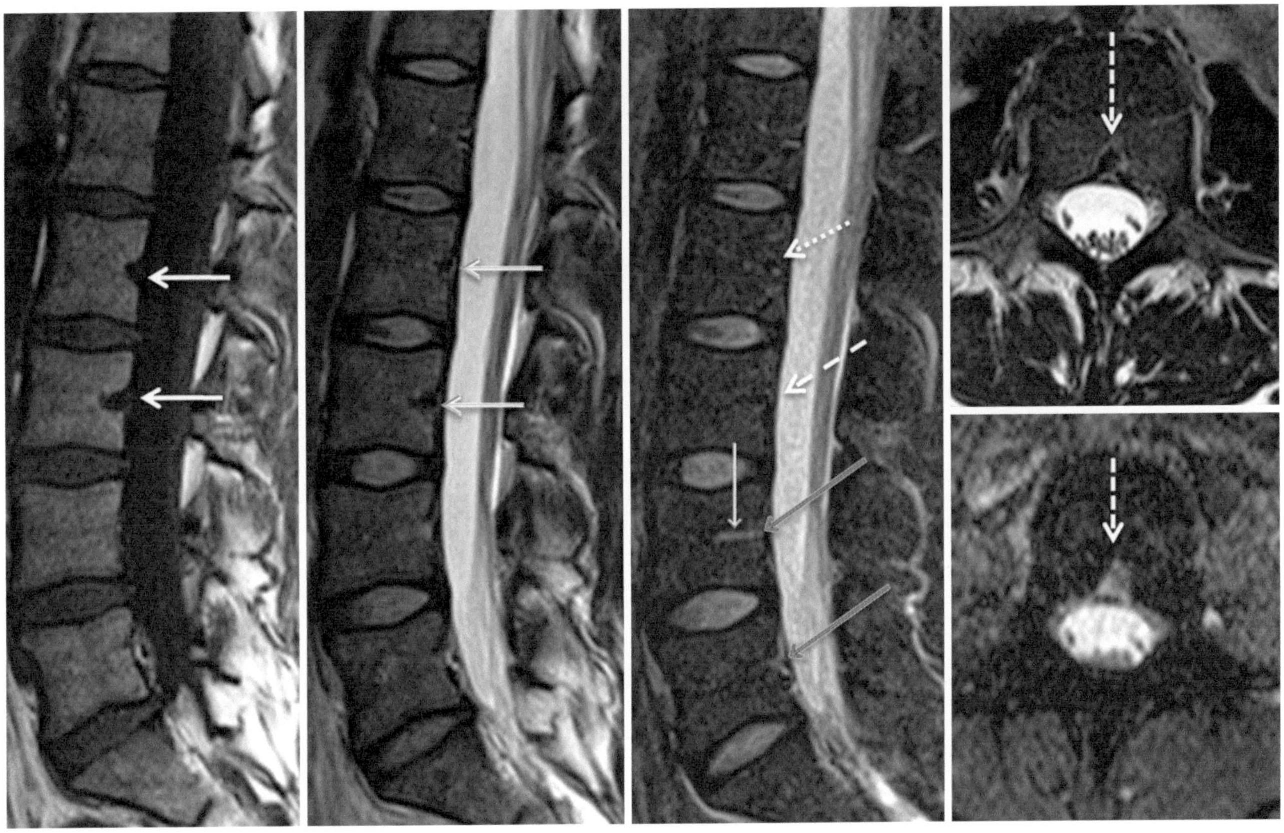

Fig. 7.39 A 25-year-old woman with back pain. Sagittal SET1WI (*left*) and SET2WI (*left middle*) MR images demonstrate hypointense signal (*arrows*) in the posterior basivertebral veins. These likely represent flow voids caused by the venous flow being mildly elevated (i.e., dark) relative to most patients. A sagittal STIR image (*right middle*) demonstrates a faint hypointense line in the basivertebral veins of L3 (*dashed line*), with a barely visible mixed signal in the L2 basivertebral veins (*dotted arrow*). However, the more normal basivertebral appearance of T2 hyperintensity is seen within the posterior aspects of the anterior segments of the L4 and L5 vertebrae (*gray beveled arrows*), presumably caused by a more typical flow rate; note the linear signal (*thin arrow*) from veins centrally within L4 draining posteriorly into the confluence of the basivertebral veins. The axial SET2WI image (*right, upper image*) at L3 again demonstrates a flow void (*dashed arrow*) with mild surrounding T2 hyperintensity, likely from laminar flow with the greatest velocity centrally and lesser velocity at the periphery. Axial GET2*WI (*right, lower image*) is a more rapid acquisition, thus being less susceptible to flow artifact and hence exhibits T2 hyperintensity (*dashed arrow*) within the confluence of the basivertebral veins of L3

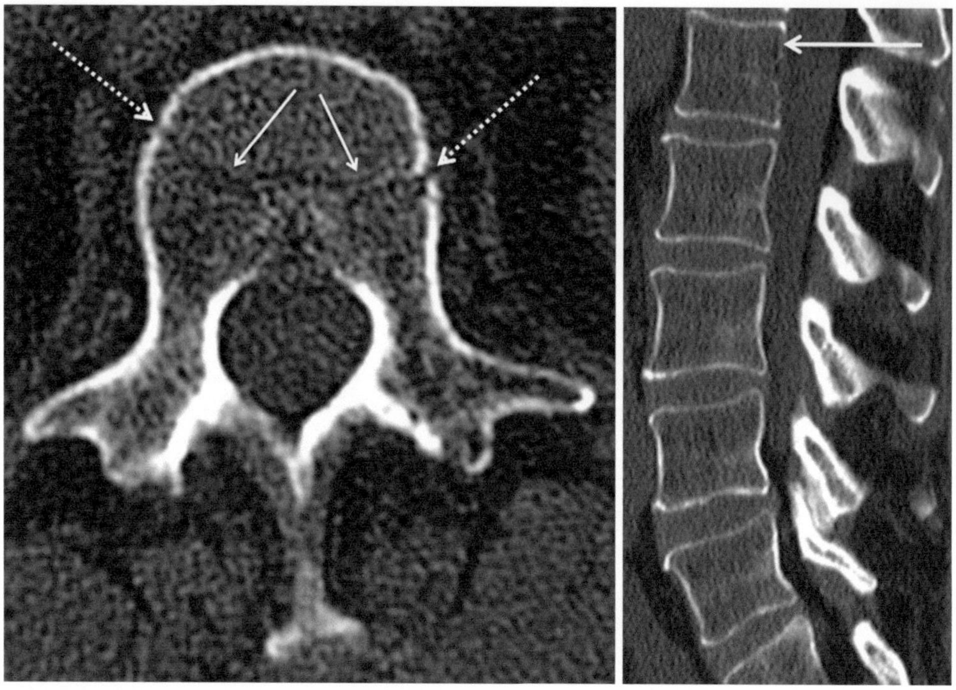

Fig. 7.40 A 30-year-old male with trauma and back pain. An axial NECT bone algorithm-windowed image at the level of L1 (*left*) demonstrates what appears to be cortical irregularity on both sides of the vertebral body (*dotted arrows*). There is an irregular lucent line (*thin arrows*) that connects the two cortical lucencies, thus simulating a fracture that caused alarm for the resident physician on call. This line was only visible on one axial image, and there was no evidence for fracture in that location within the L1 vertebra on the reconstructed sagittal image (*right*). The cortical "breaks" (*dotted arrows*) are not fractures but rather are normal vascular foramina through which the basivertebral veins (*thin arrows*) empty into the anterior external vertebral venous plexus

7.24 Prominent Anterior Internal Vertebral Venous Plexus

The *anterior internal vertebral venous plexus* is commonly thought to reside in the ventral epidural space; however, that is not truly the case anatomically. This anterior plexus resides in a space situated between the deep (ventral) and superficial (dorsal) layers of the posterior longitudinal ligament (PLL). These layers of the PLL are loosely attached to the posterior vertebral bodies and firmly attached to the annulus of the intervertebral disc. The *anterior internal vertebral venous plexus* is composed of two longitudinally oriented venous channels with numerous anastomotic interconnections. Overall, this plexus is part of the interconnected network of the vertebral venous plexus (VVP), which includes the internal vertebral venous plexus, the external vertebral venous plexus, and the basivertebral veins. Ultimately, the VVP network drains through the lumbar veins into the inferior vena cava. This venous system is valveless and permits vascular dilatation through retrograde flow. Thus, *engorgement of the vertebral venous plexus* can be secondary to numerous etiologies, including caval compression, caval blockage secondary to portal hypertension, or Budd-Chiari syndrome, vena cava thrombosis, or abdominal or thoracic malignancy. Engorgement can also be present in various physiologic states such as pregnancy, obesity, and even in patients with intracranial hypotension secondary to spontaneous or iatrogenic CSF leakage. Such patients with engorgement of the VVP may report radicular symptoms such as pain, paresthesias, or numbness of the lower extremities from venous nerve root compression or congestive venous ischemia of the nerve roots. On MRI, their appearance may mimic an epidural abscess/phlegmon or epidural hematoma (Figs. 7.41 and 7.42).

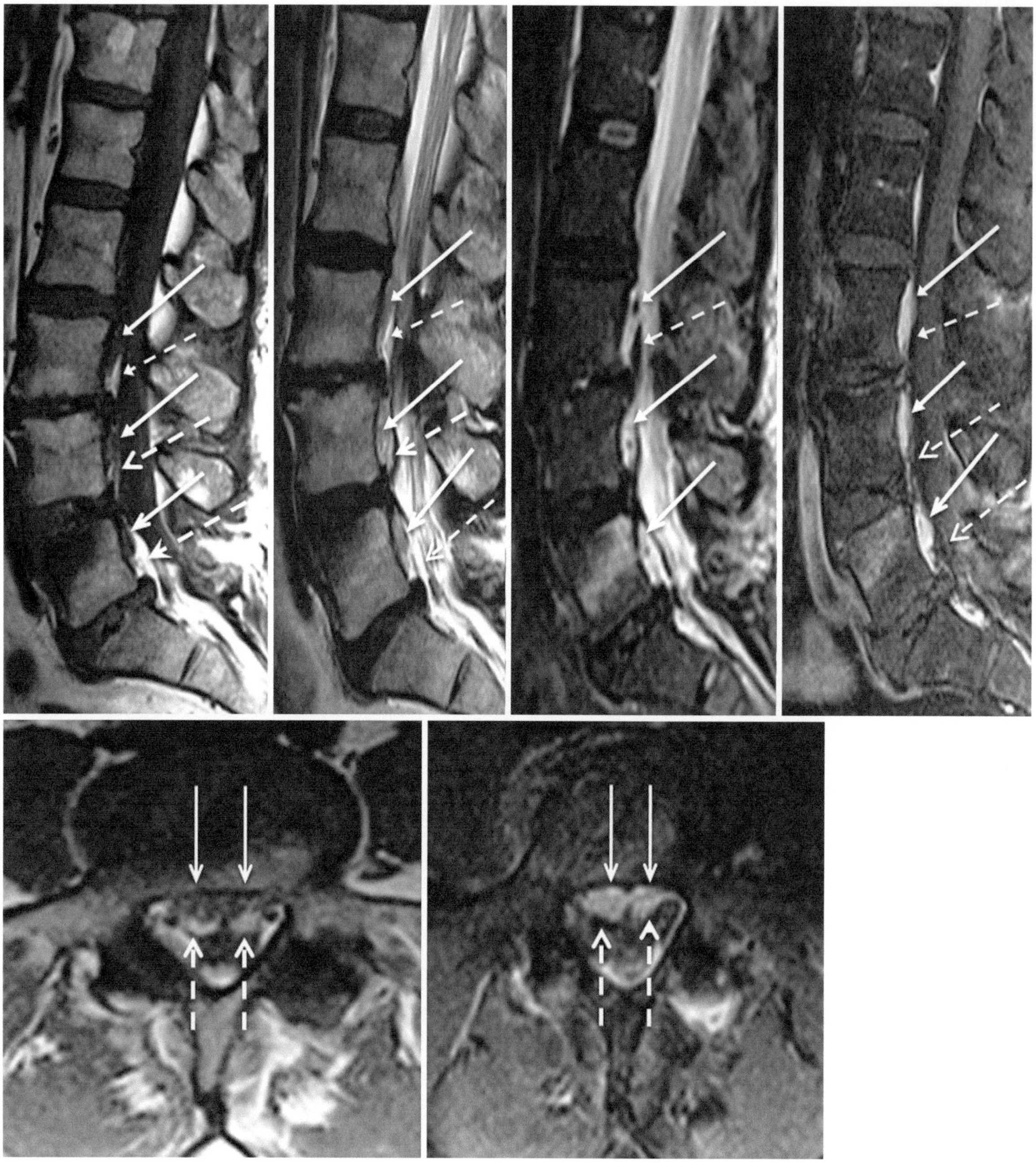

Fig. 7.41 A 57-year-old male with back pain. He had chronic pain and no fever and had initially undergone a routine, noncontrast MRI. The patient was brought back to receive intravenous MRI contrast agent because of the unusual appearance of the ventral epidural space and concern regarding possible fluid collection or abscess. **Top row:** SET1WI sagittal image *(left)* demonstrates dark signal, which represents vascular flow voids in the anterior internal vertebral venous plexus (AIVVP) in the region that would be expected to have hyperintense epidural fat at L3 (*white arrow*), L4 (*dashed arrow*), and L5 (*dotted arrow*). The T1-hyperintense epidural fat is displaced posteriorly at L3 (*thin arrow*), L4, and L5 *(arrowhead).* On SET2WI sagittal image *(left middle)* there is heterogeneous intermediate signal within the AIVVP at the level of L3 (*white arrow*), L4 *(dashed arrow) and L5 (dotted arrow),* with the T2 hyperintense epidural fat displaced posteriorly at the level of L3 *(thin arrow).* On sagittal STIR *(right middle),* the venous signal is T2-hyperintense throughout the AIVVP at the L3 to L5 levels (*labeling convention as above at each level*). The epidural fat saturates out (darkens) on STIR, which is best demonstrated at L3 *(thin arrow, right middle).* On sagittal postcontrast FS-SET1WI *(right),* there is contrast enhancement throughout the AIVVP at the level of L3 (*white arrow*), L4 (*dashed arrow*), and L5 *(dotted arrow),* with saturation (darkening) of the signal in the epidural fat at each level, best depicted at the level of L3 (*thin arrow*). **Bottom row:** At the level of L5, axial SET1WI *(left)*, SET2WI (*middle*), and axial postcontrast FS-SET1WI images *(right)* demonstrate similar characteristics to those seen on the sagittal images: dark T1, heterogeneous intermediate T2 and contrast enhancement of the AIVVP *(dotted arrows in each image),* which displaces the epidural fat posteriorly *(arrowheads).* Notice how the epidural fat is being lifted away from the posterior wall of the vertebral body. This is because the anterior internal vertebral venous plexus resides in the space between the two thin layers of the posterior longitudinal ligament (the ventral [deep] and dorsal [superficial] layers) and not in the epidural space. The posterior internal vertebral venous plexus (PIVVP) does reside in the epidural space. Also note that the enhancement has an elliptical shape, which narrows down at the intervertebral disc where the deep layer and superficial layers are firmly bound to the annulus. These factors help distinguish the prominence of the anterior internal vertebral venous plexus from a pathologic process such as an epidural phlegmon or abscess

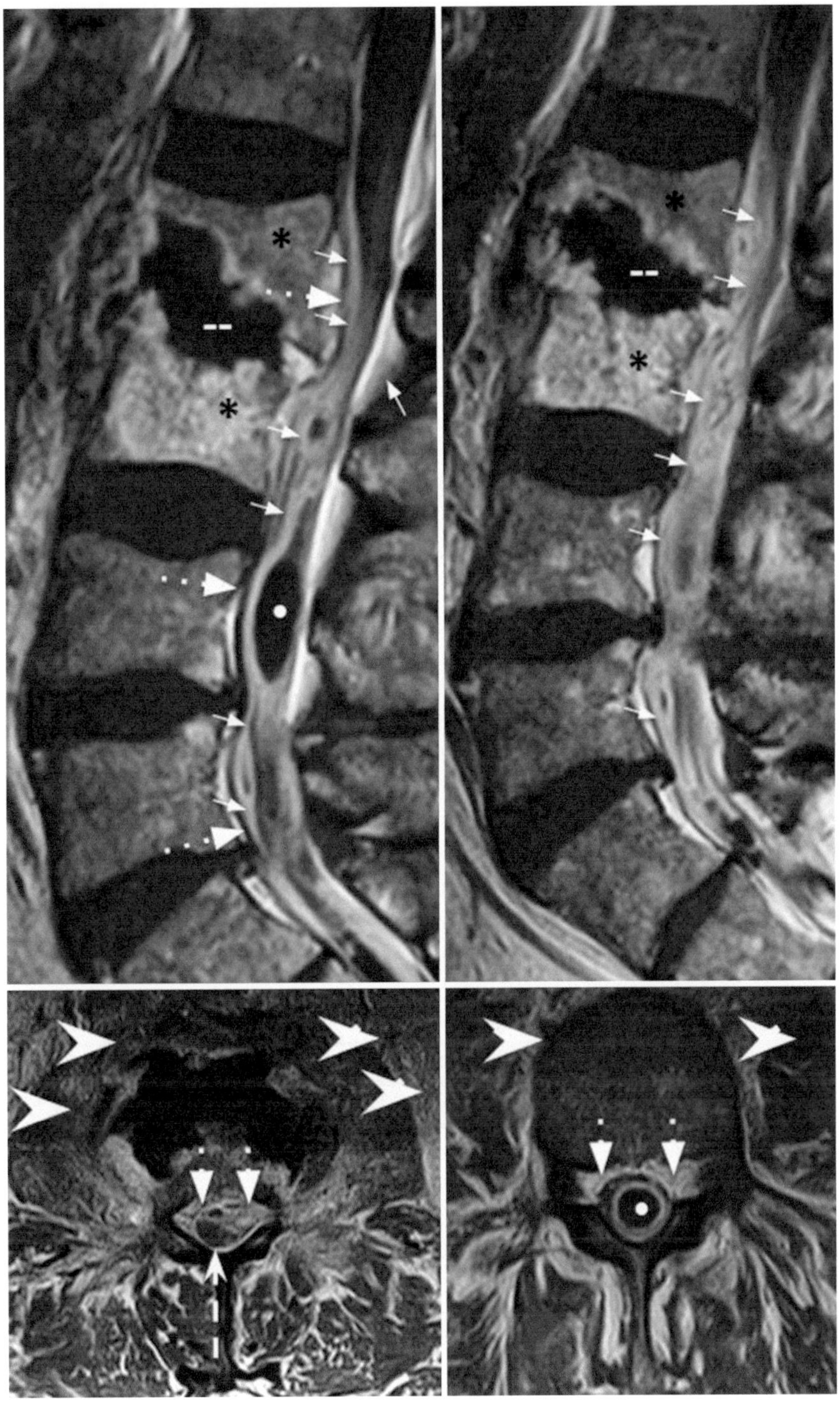

Fig. 7.42 Comparison case of osteomyelitis-discitis and epidural phlegmon. A 65-year-old male with slowly progressive back pain for over 6 weeks had low-grade fevers and an elevated white blood cell count. **Top row:** On an MRI from an outside institution, sagittal post-contrast nonfat suppressed SET1WIs (*left and right*) show diffuse enhancement of the L2 and L3 vertebral bodies (*asterisks*) with destructive endplate changes and partial collapse. The L2-L3 intervertebral disc space (--) is hypointense to the normal disc signal seen at L1-L2 and L3-L4 at levels above and below. The disc also contained fluid signal intensity on SET2WI and STIR images (*not shown*). Additionally, abnormal contrast enhancement is extensive throughout the epidural space (*tiny arrows*), with compression of the thecal sac, which is displaced posteriorly, and an intraspinal-intradural abscess as well (•). Note that the higher intensity anterior internal vertebral venous plexus enhancement is separated from the enhancing epidural phlegmon by the superficial layer of the posterior longitudinal ligament, which appears as cranio-caudally oriented linear dark signal (*dotted arrows, left*). **Bottom row:** At the level of L2-L3 (*left*) and the midportion of L4 (*right*), two axial postcontrast SET1WIs without fat saturation show abnormal paraspinous enhancement anteriorly within the psoas musculature bilaterally (*arrowheads*) and enhancing epidural phlegmon (*dotted arrows*). On the *left image*, the thecal sac is displaced posteriorly by the phlegmonous epidural tissue (*dotted arrows*). On the *right image*, in addition to the epidural phlegmon (*dotted arrows*), a large intraspinal/intradural abscess (•) compresses the entire spinal canal

7.25 Normal Age-Related Spine Changes

At birth and in infancy vertebral marrow is essentially all hematopoietic red marrow. Fat content slowly increases with age via a process known as marrow conversion. There are known signal patterns that correspond to the fat concentration (T1-hyperintense) and water content (T1-hypointense). These patterns can also be seen on turbo SET2WI sequences. The intervertebral disc has an intermediate T2 signal at birth, appears larger centrally than the vertebral body, and has a rounded appearance. The intervertebral disc quickly becomes T2-hyperintense after infancy, and the bone marrow signal on T1WI is hypointense to the intervertebral disc up to about the age of 1 year. The vertebral body forms from the fusion of two sclerotomes and initially appears T2-hyperintense with a dark horizontal band correlating with the cartilaginous plates at the point of fusion. The point of vertebral body fusion also incorporates the venous channels that will become the basivertebral veins. The vertebral body has a biconcave shape at this point.

The vertebral body develops a more "squared-off" appearance over the first years of life as the intervertebral discs decrease in relative size and become more flattened. Various patterns of bone marrow signals have been described by both Ricci and Sebag (please see "*Suggested Reading*" section). The rate at which there is *marrow conversion* is variable, as can be demonstrated in Ricci's patterns 1, 2, and 3. In pattern 1, the bone marrow has a uniformly low signal intensity on T1WI attributable to the hematopoietic red marrow, with the exception of linear areas of high T1 signal fatty marrow superior and inferior to the basivertebral veins. This pattern can be seen in patients up to about 30 years of age, with a few outliers over the age of 30. While the vast majority of patients with higher concentrations of fatty marrow (i.e., patterns 2 and 3) are seen over 40 years of age, these patterns can be seen in 14 and 24% in patients under the age of 40 years. Adult and elderly patients can also have red marrow reconversion, such as can be present in endurance athletes, heavy smokers, certain respiratory conditions, conditions related to chronic anemia, and patients treated with hematopoietic growth factors (such as postmarrow transplantation) (Figs. 7.43, 7.44, 7.45, 7.46, 7.47, 7.48, 7.49 and 7.50).

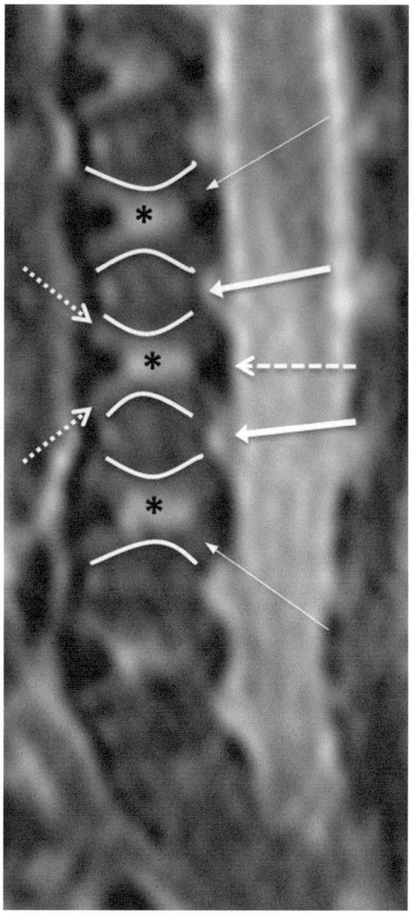

Fig. 7.43 A 13-day-old infant with a normal spine MRI. On sagittal SET2WI (the sagittal T1WI sequence was markedly degraded by motion), the intervertebral disc is relatively larger and rounded in appearance and has vertical striations (*white arrows*). On SET2WI, the vertebral body (*thin white arrows*) has a biconcave appearance (endplates represented by the *curved lines*), with central hyperintensity (*asterisks*) and a horizontal dark band representing the cartilaginous plates at the fusion point of the two sclerotomes that form each vertebral body (*dashed arrows*). At this age of the patient, the dark band is receding as the sclerotomes fuse. The endplates have an intermediate intensity (*dotted arrows*) lying subjacent to the curved lines

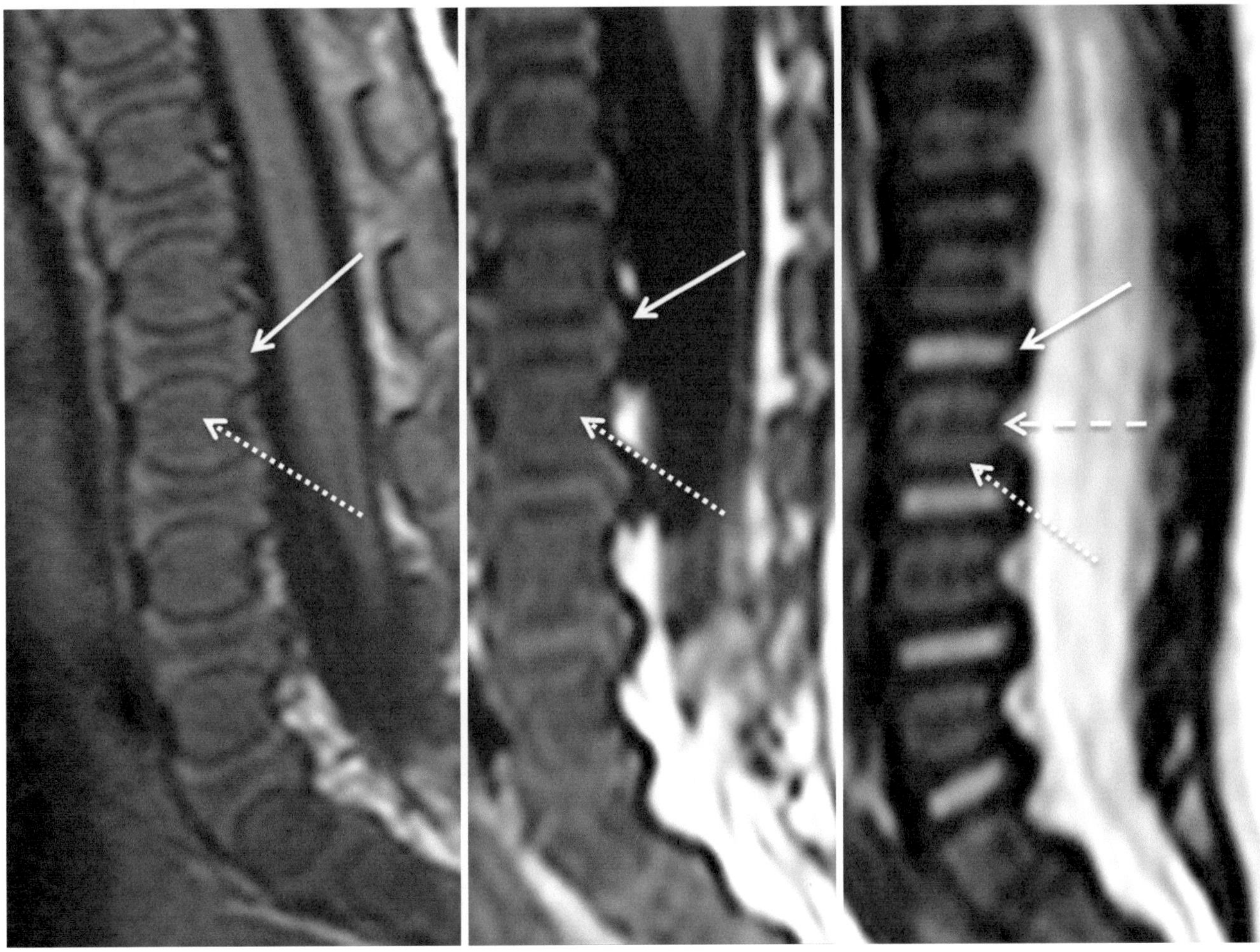

Fig. 7.44 A 2-month-old (*left*) and 6-month-old child (*middle, right*) with normal spine MRIs, with MR sequences. ***Left:*** On a sagittal SET1WI image from the 2-month-old, the vertebral marrow that is hematopoetic red marrow at this stage is hypointense (*dotted arrow*) compared with the intervertebral disc signal (*white arrow*). Note: the developing vertebral bodies now have a more rounded appearance compared to the intervertebral discs, which are becoming more flattened. ***Middle and Right:*** On a sagittal SET1WI (*middle*) image from the 6-month-old, the intervertebral disc (*white arrows*) has signal intensity slightly higher than the vertebral marrow (*dotted arrows*). On sagittal SET2WI from the 6-month- old (*right*), there is a hyperintense disc (*white arrows*) and intermediate signal vertebral body (*dotted arrows*) with a dark horizontal band that represents the basivertebral veins (*dashed arrow*), being incorporated at the point of fusion of the sclerotomes. The vertebral bodies appear more squared in the 6-month-old child

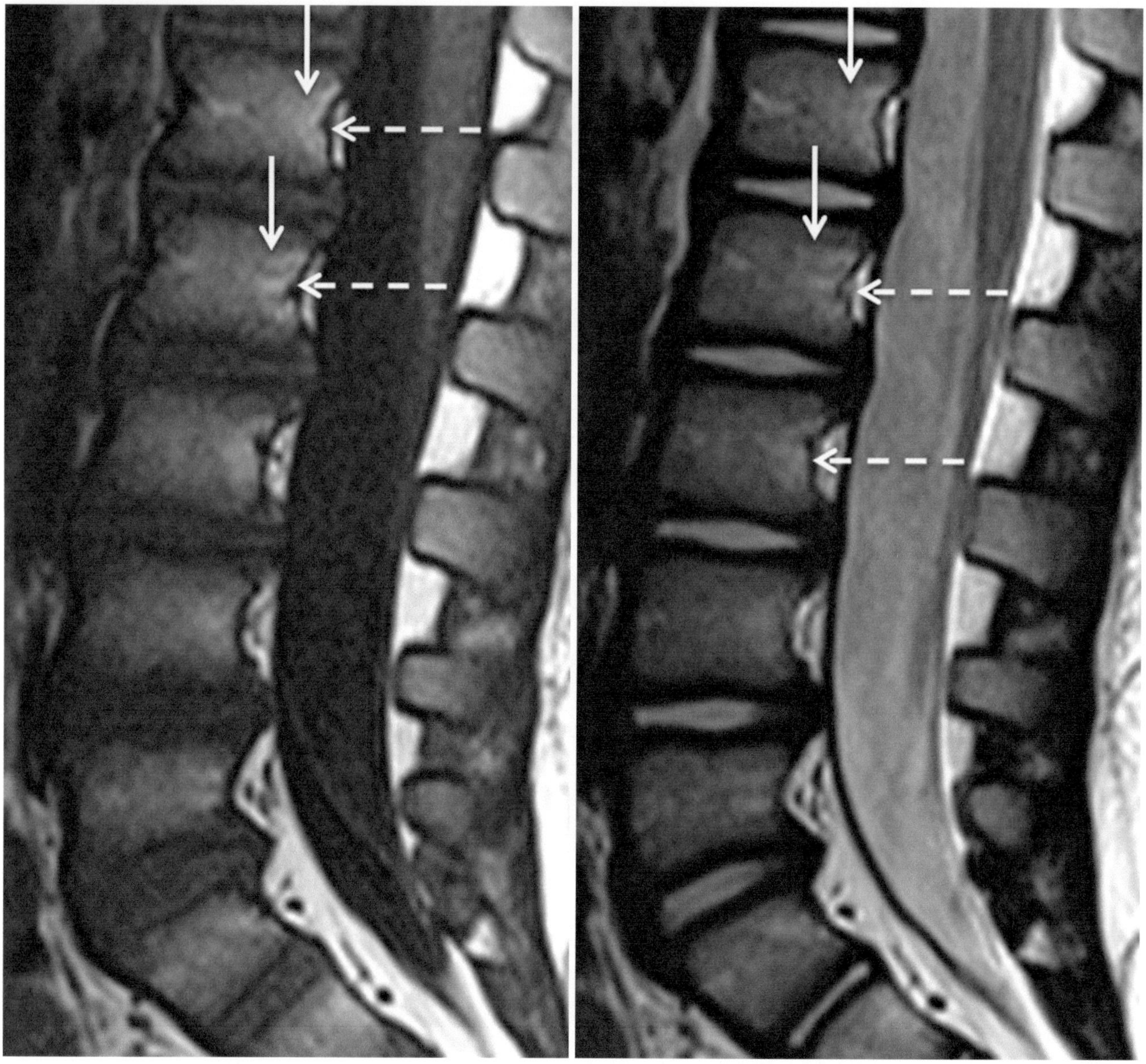

Fig. 7.45 Normal spine MRI in a 2-year-old child. The sagittal SET1WI (*left*) and SET2WI (*right*) MRI images demonstrate a background of hypointense marrow with central horizontal and faintly hyperintense signal (*arrows*) along the basivertebral veins (*dashed arrows*) in a nearly triangular formation; this triangular-shaped region in both images posteriorly (*arrows*) is at the confluence of the basivertebral veins at the posterior edge of the anterior segment of the vertebral body. Again, the vertebral bodies appear more squared as children age

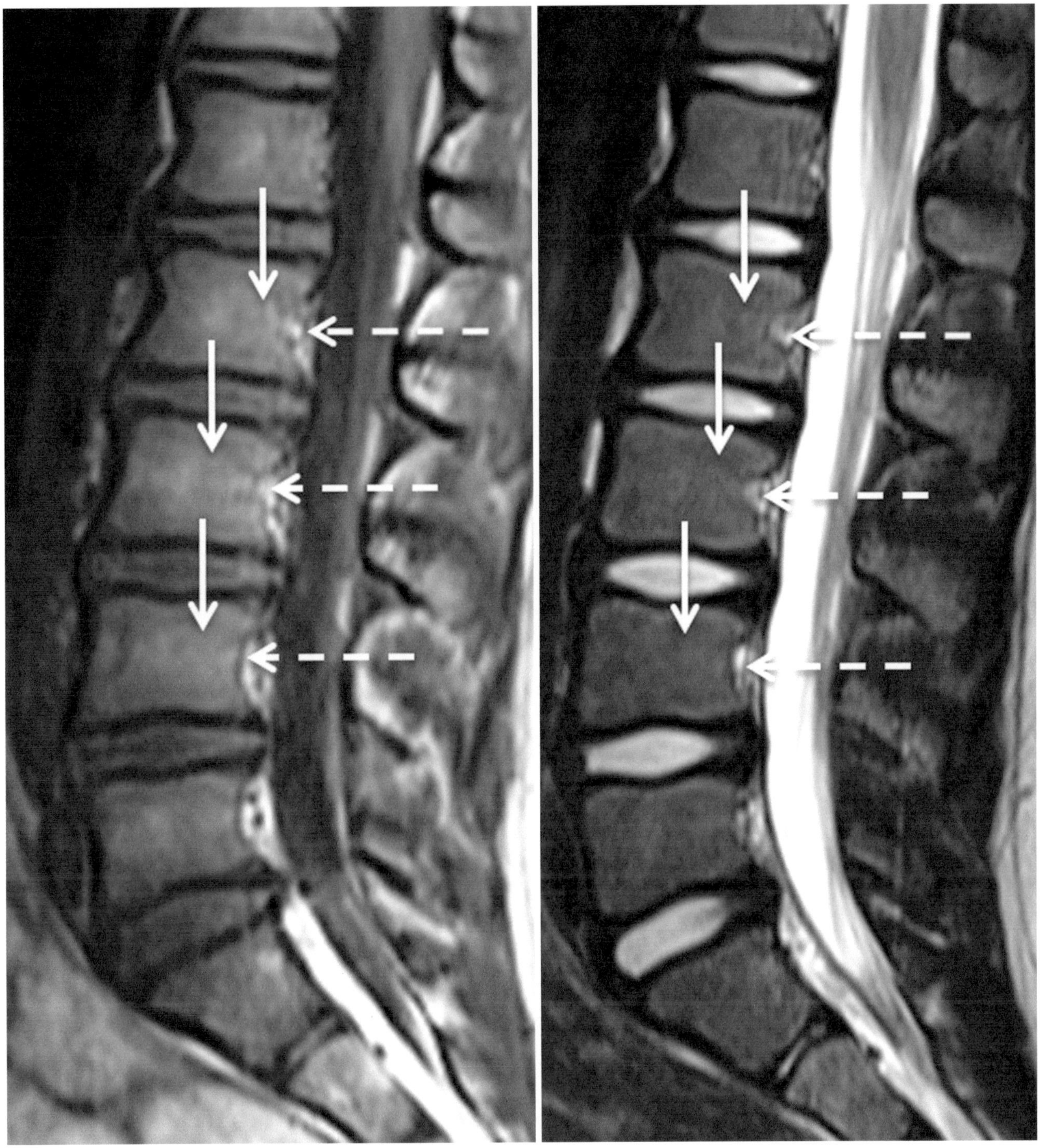

Fig. 7.46 Normal spine MRI in a 6-year-old child. A sagittal SET1WI MRI (*left*) demonstrates that the vertebral marrow at several levels has faint and centrally located hyperintense signal (*arrows*) that is horizontal and transversely oriented along the course of the basivertebral veins as they proceed towards the confluence (*dashed arrows*) that is located at the posterior margin of the anterior segment of the vertebra. Surrounding these faintly hyperintense central regions is an intermediate signal that is relatively isointense to the intervertebral disc signal. On a sagittal SET2WI image (*right*), there is intermediate marrow signal in those central locations (*arrows, right*), with mildly hyperintense basivertebral veins at the confluence (*dashed arrows*) and T2-hyperintense intervertebral discs

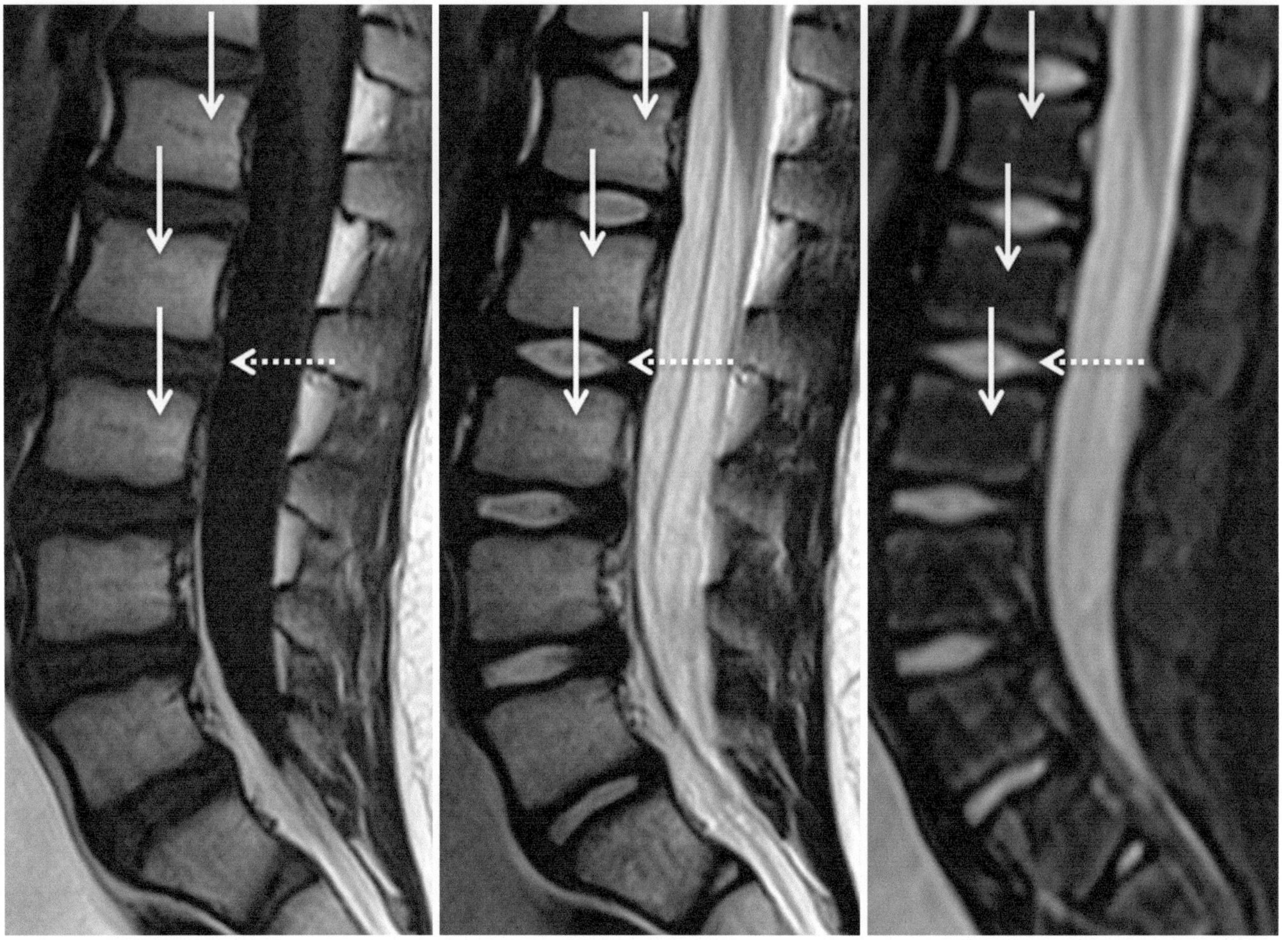

Fig. 7.47 Normal spine MRI in a 10-year-old child. On sagittal SET1WI (*left*), the marrow is becoming more diffusely mildly hyperintense (*arrows*), not just within the central regions. The marrow has now become clearly more hyperintense than the intervertebral disc (*dotted arrow*). On sagittal SET2WI (*middle*), the marrow appears faintly hyperintense as well (*arrows*) and saturates out on STIR (*arrows, right*). The intervertebral disc is hyperintense on T2WI and STIR (*dotted arrows, middle and right*)

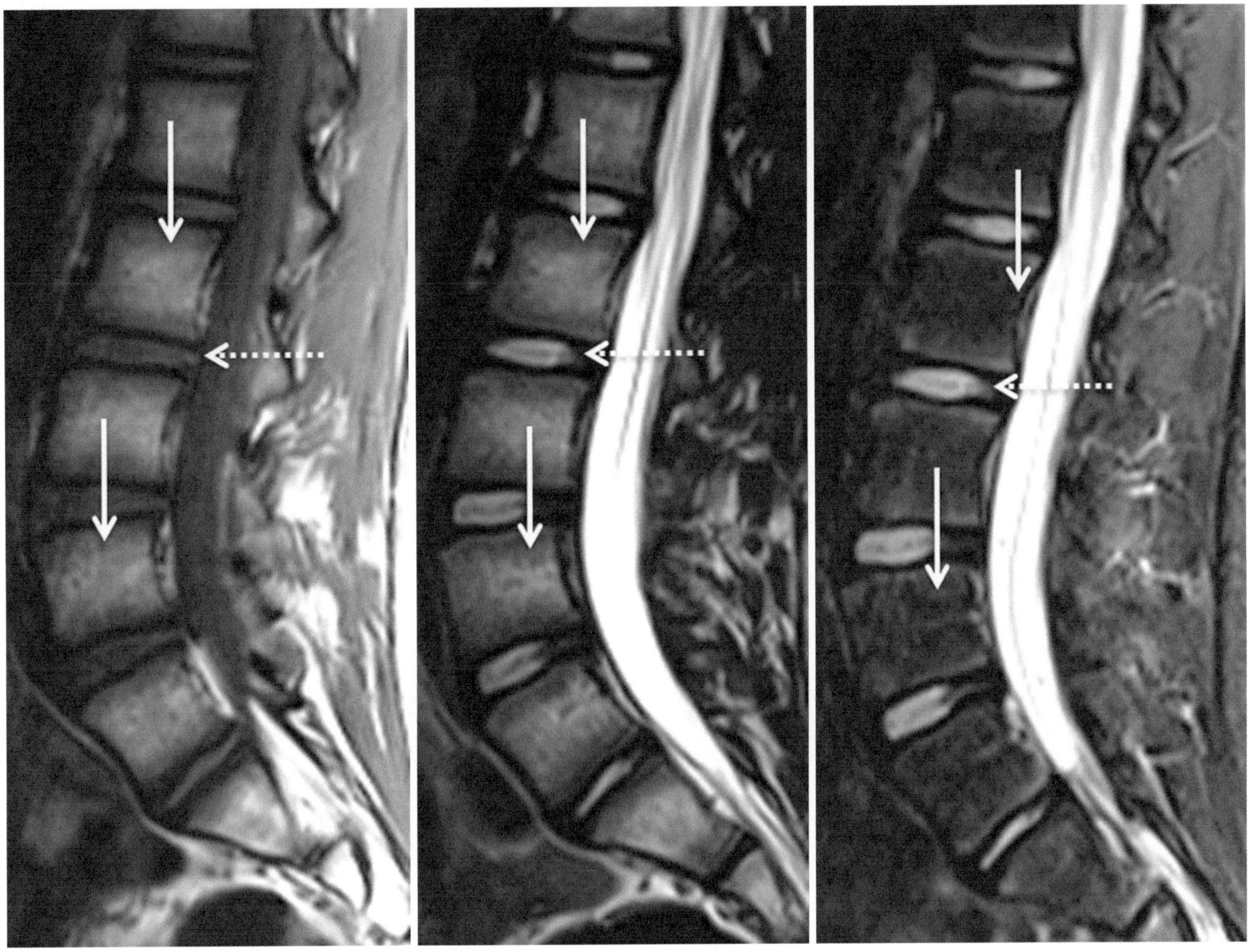

Fig. 7.48 Normal spine MRI in a 15-year-old. Progressive and increasingly hyperintense marrow signal (*arrows*) is noted centrally within the lumbar vertebrae, using L2 and L4 as examples in this patient (*arrows in each image*). The T1-hyperintense marrow is extending toward the periphery on SET1WI (*left*) and SET2WI (*middle*), which suppresses/darkens on STIR (*right*). Note that the intervertebral disc (*dotted arrows*) is of lower signal intensity than the vertebral marrow on the SET1WI image (*left*), while being brighter than the vertebral marrow on SET2WI (*middle*) and STIR (*right*)

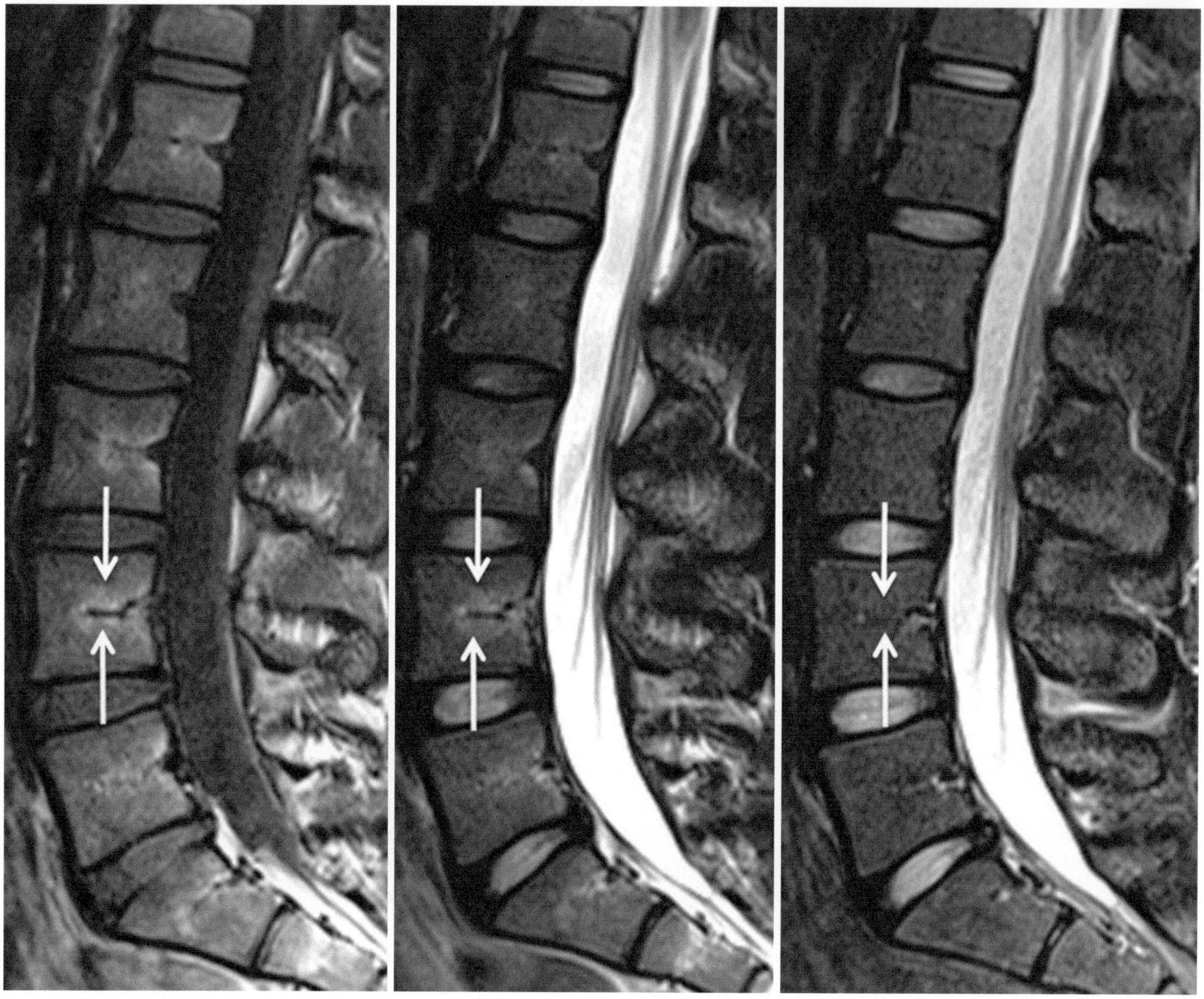

Fig. 7.49 Normal spine MRI in an 18-year-old. This is considered the Ricci Pattern 1, in which there is hyperintensity more focally on sagittal SET1WI (*left*) and SET2WI (*middle*); this suppresses on STIR (*right*) and is located only above and below the basivertebral veins (*arrows*). The remainder of the vertebral body is uniformly of relatively low intensity on each sequence. This pattern can actually be noticed in all age groups, but the majority are less than 40 years old

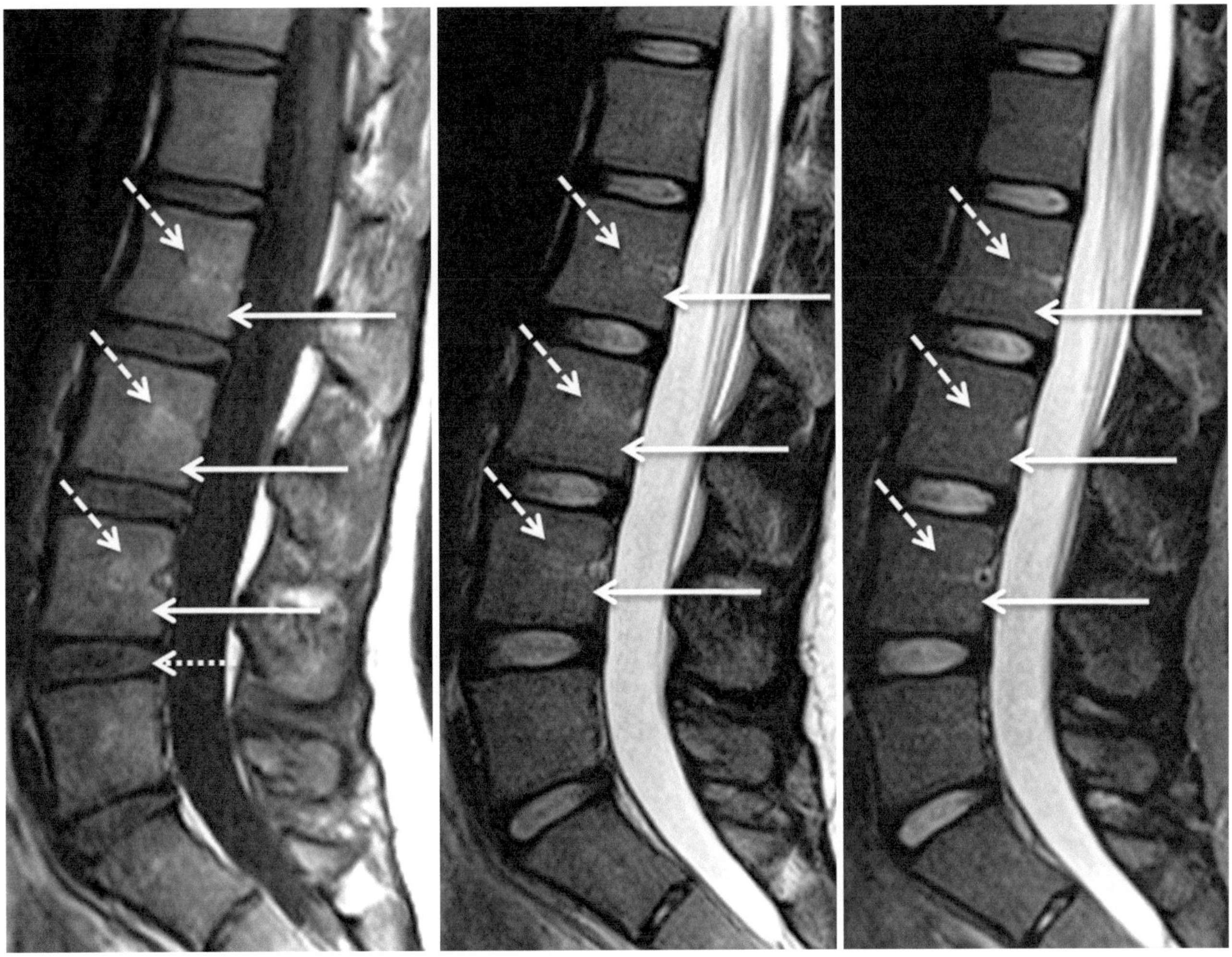

Fig. 7.50 Normal spine MRI in a 19-year-old endurance athlete but with a predominance of red marrow. On sagittal SET1WI MRI (*left*), the vertebral marrow (*arrows*) is nearly isointense to the intervertebral discs (*dotted arrows*), indicating a high concentration of red marrow; this is compatible with the patient's clinical history. On sagittal SET2WI (*middle*) and STIR (*right*) images, the marrow (*arrows*) appears nearly the same when comparing both sequences, as there is very little fat to suppress/saturate on STIR. Only a faint amount of hyperintense fatty marrow (*dashed arrows in all three images*) is seen centrally within the L3 vertebra on SET1WI (*left*) and SET2WI (*middle*), which suppresses/darkens on STIR (*right*)

7.26 Sacral Fat Deposition

As hematopoietic bone marrow converts to fatty marrow, the signal increases on T1-weighted and T2-weighted turbo spin echo (TSE) sequences. There are often focal areas of increased T1 and T2 signals in axial bone marrow that correlate with *focal fat deposition*. This is not gender related but is correlated with increasing age. In a study by Hajek et al. (1987), only 13% of those with focal fat deposition were between 0 and 10 years of age, whereas 52% of patients aged 31–40 years had areas of focal fat, as did 93% of patients aged 51–60 years. In my anecdotal experience, focal fat deposition seems to occur in the sacrum and coccyx earlier than other areas of the spine, but this may not be well-documented in the literature per this author's knowledge (Figs. 7.51, 7.52 and 7.53).

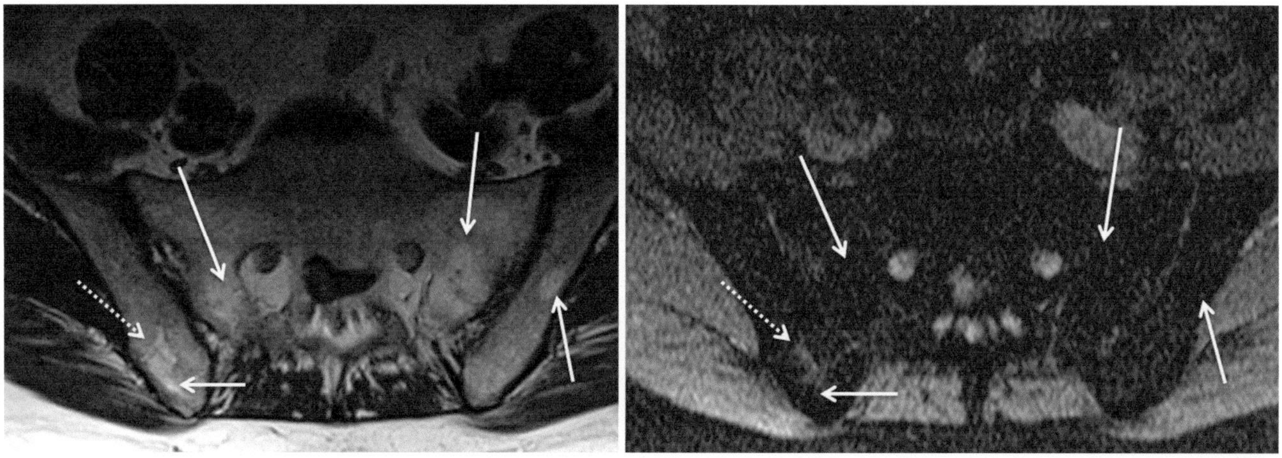

Fig. 7.51 Normal spine MRI in a 74-year-old male with back pain and radiculopathy. Axial SET2WI (*left*) through the sacrum and iliac bones demonstrates multifocal T2 hyperintensities (several are indicated by the *arrows*), which could be interpreted as focal fat deposition or edema secondary to a pathologic process. An axial GET2*WI sequence with fat-suppression (*right*) suppresses the fat signal, where that sequence would exhibit edema as hyperintensity. On this GET2*WI sequence, the aforementioned T2-hyperintense foci now have hypointense signal (*arrows*), confirming multifocal fat deposition. The branching structure in the right ilium (*dotted arrows*) would be consistent with an intraosseous vascular channel, as it has bright signal on the SET2WI (*left*) that does not suppress (i.e., stays bright) on GET2*WI (*right*)

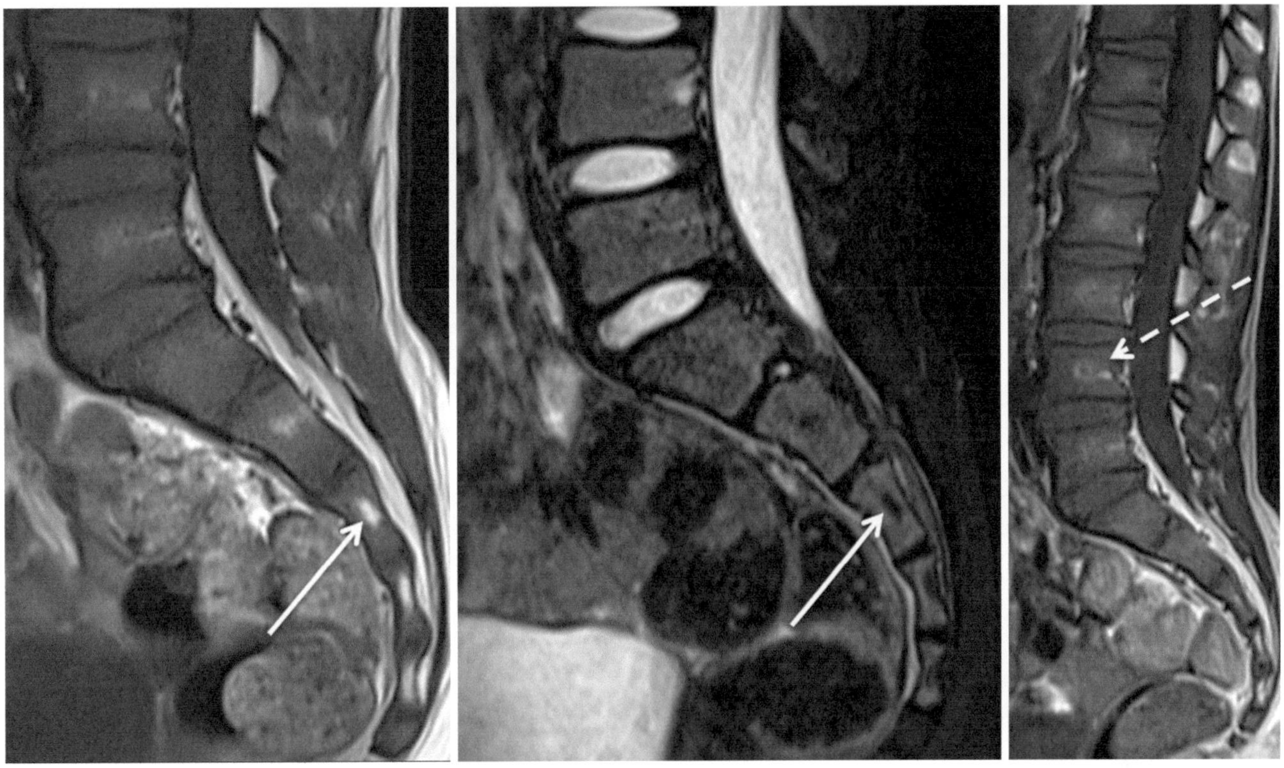

Fig. 7.52 Normal spine MRI in a 7-year-old male with encopresis. A sagittal SET1WI of the sacrum (*left*) demonstrates T1-hyperintense focal fat deposition (*arrows*) within the S3 vertebra, also present within each vertebra from the levels of S2 to S5. This suppresses on a sagittal STIR image (*arrow, middle*). Also, note the Ricci pattern 1 of the vertebral marrow signal throughout the remainder of the lumbar spine on the sagittal SET1WI (*right*), where there is focal hyperintensity that is centrally located (*dashed arrow, right*) and situated along the course of the basivertebral veins

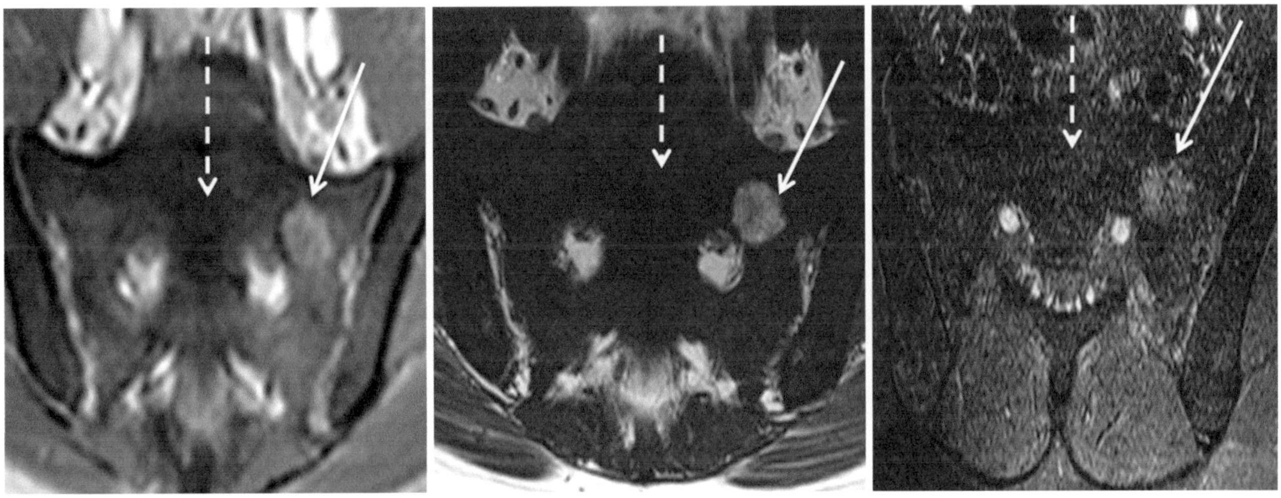

Fig. 7.53 **Comparison case of marrow abnormalities from prior bone infarcts in sickle cell anemia.** A 25-year-old male with sickle cell anemia and back pain underwent an MRI, with coronal SET1WI (*left*) and SET2WI (*middle*), which demonstrated a hyperintense rounded focus with a faint salt-and-pepper appearance (*arrows*) within the left side of the sacrum. This focus did not completely saturate on FS SET2WI (*arrow, right*) and was felt to be a hemangioma with mildly increased vascularity. It should be noted that most hemangiomas will completely suppress on FS images but a minority will not (i.e., atypical hemangiomas). Also, note the diffusely dark bone marrow on T1WI (*left*) and T2WI (*middle* and *right*), most notably centrally within the sacrum (*dashed arrows*) attributable to the patient's underlying anemia. The lumbar spine's marrow was also hypointense on T1WI when compared with that of the intervertebral discs (*not shown*)

7.27 Retrodural Space of Okada

First described by Okada in 1981, the retrodural *space* is a potential space that runs posterior to the ligamentum flavum and forms a communication between the interfacet joints on either side of the spine. Dr. Okada's work found that at the level studied, 80% of the cervical interfacet joints communicated with the contralateral interfacet joint, interlaminar region, interspinous region, and extradural space via this potential space. This space exists at all levels of the spine, including the lumbar levels. Later reports have indicated communication between pars interarticularis defects with the adjacent and contralateral interfacet joints through this space. There can be communication between the interfacet joint and the adventitial bursa formation between the spinous processes (i.e., Baastrup disease). Infectious or inflammatory processes can also spread through this retrodural space (Fig. 7.54).

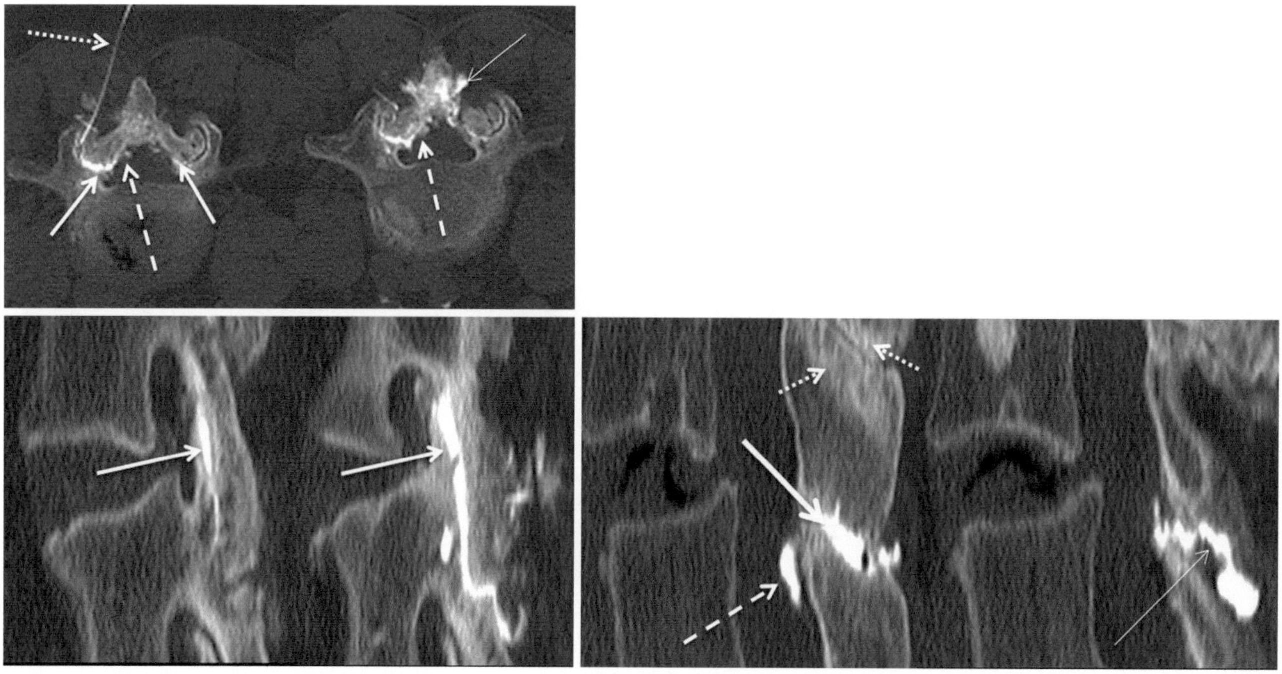

Fig. 7.54 An 81-year-old male with interfacet joint injection for back pain. **Top Row:** Sequential axial NECT images at L3-L4 with the patient prone for the interfacet injection procedure demonstrate the spinal needle entering the left interfacet joint (*dotted arrow, left*). There is contrast seen in the left interfacet joint and a small amount in the right joint (*white arrows, left image*). A couple of foci of contrast material are seen in the retrodural space (*dashed arrow, left*). In the *right image*, the retrodural space is better opacified with contrast agent (*dashed arrow*). There is also interlaminar extension of contrast, which has collected in the paraspinous region (*thin white arrow*). **Bottom row:** Sagittal NECT reformations demonstrate contrast in the left interfacet joint (*left, white arrow*), right interfacet joint (*middle left, white arrow*), interspinous adventitial bursa (*middle right, white arrow*), the retrodural space of Okada (*middle right, dashed arrow*), and the interlaminar space (*right, thin white arrow*). Note the sclerosis of the adjoining spinous processes at L2-L3 (*middle right, dotted arrows*), which, like the interspinous adventitial bursa at L3-L4, is also seen in Baastrup disease

7.28 Conjoined Root

A *conjoined root* (or *conjoined nerve root*) is the most common nerve root variant, being present in roughly 2–30% of the population undergoing lumbar disc surgery (the larger number being cadaveric studies, but in the clinical population on MRI or surgery is more likely in the 2–5% range). This variant is composed of two adjacent nerve roots that combine within or share a common dural sheath/envelope as they exit the thecal sac, typically extending into the neural foramen. These typically present at the level of L5-S1 and involve that neural foramen in >95%. While these are more likely to be incidental and asymptomatic, they can present with radiculopathy or nerve root claudication secondary to compression of the conjoined root by focal subarticular zone (lateral recess) stenosis and/or foraminal stenosis. Treatment in such cases involves decompression surgically by foraminotomy and/or laminectomy, if symptomatic, to create space for the exiting conjoined root.

The clinical diagnosis is typically made by noncontrast MRI (or CT myelography), by the presence of 3 signs: a "*fat crescent*" (extradural fat interposed between the conjoined root and dura, present in about 50% of patients), a "*parallel sign*" (visualization of the course of the nerve root in parallel at the level of the disc, present in about 66.6% of patients), and a "*corner sign*" (the anterolateral corner of the sac appears asymmetric, present in nearly all). The differential diagnosis in such cases is *disc herniation* (does not have CSF signal) or *schwannoma* (enhances with contrast, and lacks CSF signal) (Fig. 7.55).

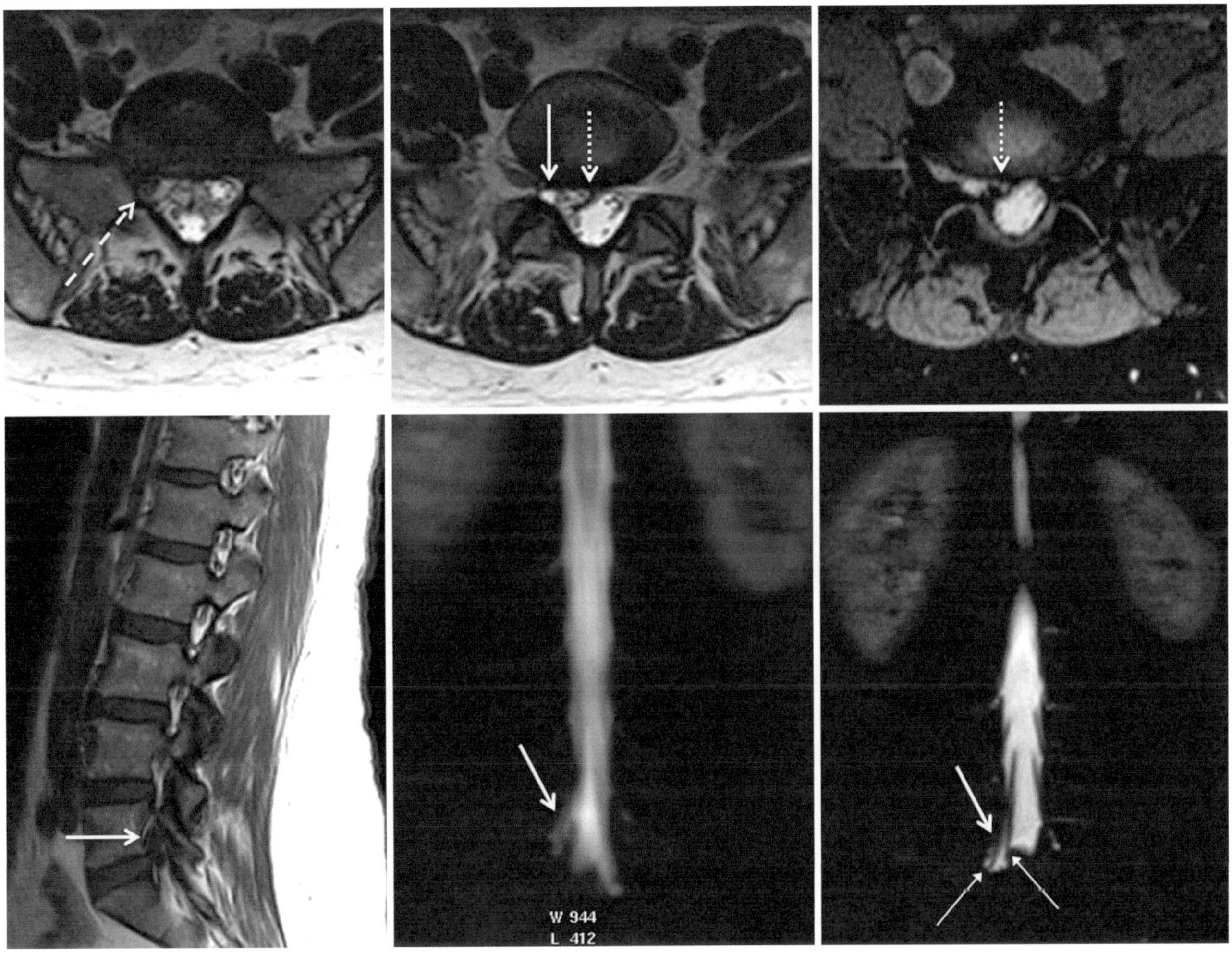

Fig. 7.55 In a 45-year-old female, a lumbar spine MRI was ordered for right lower extremity pain. **Top row:** On axial MRI images, a "*corner*" sign of a common dural sheath (*dashed arrows,* where the anterolateral corner of the sac appears asymmetric) and a "*fat crescent*" sign (extradural fat interposed between the conjoined root and dura, *dotted arrows, middle and right*) are noted on axial SET2WI (*left and middle*) and on FS-GET2*WI (*right*, showing fat suppression of the "fat crescent," *dotted arrows*), indicating a conjoined root within a common dural sheath. The *solid arrow* (*middle*) denotes the common dural sheath of the conjoined L5-S1 root, being T2-bright on all three of these T2WI sequences. **Bottom row:** On sagittal SET1WI of the right side (*left*), the common sheath is again noted with CSF signal intensity (*solid arrows*, being dark on T1WI), which demonstrates why a conjoined root may simulate an extraforaminal/foraminal disc herniation at first glance. On a 30 mm thickness coronally reconstructed 3D T2WI MR myelogram (*middle*), the common dural envelope is also defined (*solid arrows*), whereas on 1 mm thickness source images for the MR myelogram (*right*), the individual L5 and S1 roots (each denoted by the *thin arrows*) are noted within the common dural sheath, confirming a conjoined exiting root. The patient's symptoms improved after right-sided foraminotomy and decompression of the conjoined root at this level

Suggested Reading

Alfawareh M, Alotaibi T, Labeeb A, Audat Z. A symptomatic case of thoracic vertebral hemangioma causing lower limb spastic paresis. Am J Case Rep. 2016;17:805–9.

Al-Omari MH, Eloqayli HM, Qudseih HM, Al-Shinag MK. Isolated lipoma of the filum terminale in adults: MRI findings and clinical correlation. J Med Imaging Radiat Oncol. 2011;55:286–90.

Aly I, Chapman JR, Oskouian RJ, Loukas M, Tubbs RS. Lumbar ribs: a comprehensive review. Childs Nerv Syst. 2016;32:781–5.

Brooks BS, Duvall ER, El Gammal T, Garcia JH, Gupta KL, Kapila A. Neuroimaging features of neurenteric cysts: analysis of nine cases and review of the literature. Am J Neuroradiol. 1993;14:735–46.

Chengetanai S, Nchabeleng EK, Bacci N, Billings BK, Mazengenya P, Mazengenya P. Supernumerary lumbar ribs: a rare occurrence of an adult African male skeleton. Anat Cell Biol. 2017;50:155–8.

Chotigavanich C, Sawangnatra S. Anomalies of the lumbosacral nerve roots. An anatomic investigation. Clin Orthop Relat Res. 1992;278:46–50.

Cools MJ, Al-Holou WN, Stetler WR Jr, Wilson TJ, Muraszko KM, Ibrahim M, et al. Filum terminale lipomas: imaging prevalence, natural history, and conus position. J Neurosurg Pediatr. 2014;13:559–67.

Cramer GD, Darby SA. Clinical anatomy of the spine, spinal cord, and ANS. 3rd ed. St. Louis: Elsevier; 2014.

Diel J, Ortiz O, Losada RA, Price DB, Hayt MW, Katz DS. The sacrum: pathologic spectrum, multimodality imaging, and subspecialty approach. RadioGraphics. 2001;21:83–104.

DiPietro MA. The conus medullaris: normal US findings throughout childhood. Radiology. 1993;188:149–53.

Donmez FY, Qanadli SD. Epidural venous plexus engorgement: what lies beneath? Case Reports Radiol. 2015;965106:3.

Eubanks JD, Cheruvu VK. Prevalence of sacral spina bifida occulta and its relationship to age, sex, race, and the sacral table angle: An anatomic osteologic study of three thousand one hundred specimens. Spine. 2009;15:1539–43.

Fassett DR, Schmidt MH. Spinal epidural lipomatosis: a review of its causes and recommendations for treatment. Neurosurg Focus. 2004;16:E11.

Foley WJ, Whitehouse WM. Supernumerary thoracic ribs. Radiology. 1969;93:1333–4.

Ghelman B, Freiberger RH. The limbus vertebra: an anterior disc herniation demonstrated by discography. Am J Roentgenol. 1976;127:854–5.

Greenspan A. Bone island (enostosis): current concept—a review. Skeletal Radiol. 1995;24:111–5.

Greenspan A, Stadainik RC. Bone island: scintigraphic findings and their clinical application. Can Assoc Radiol J. 1995;46:368–79.

Haijiao W, Koti M, Smith FW, Wardlaw D. Diagnosis of lumbosacral nerve root anomalies by magnetic resonance imaging. J Spinal Disord. 2001;14:143–9.

Hajek PC, Baker LL, Goobar JE, Sartoris DJ, Hesselink JR, Haghighi P, Resnick D. Focal fat deposition in axial bone marrow: MR characteristics. Radiology. 1987;162:245–9.

Hjermstad BM, Helwig EB. Tailgut cysts: report of 53 cases. Am J Clin Pathol. 1988;89:139–47.

Kadish LJ, Simmons EH. Anomalies of the lumbosacral nerve roots. An anatomical investigation and myelographic study. J Bone Joint Surg Br. 1984;66:411–6.

Kolessar DJ, Everline CA. Differentiating osteopoikilosis from osteoblastic metastases: understanding this radiographic entity alleviates anxiety and minimizes testing. J Musculoskel Med. 2008;25:387.

Kriss VM, Kriss TC, Babcock DS. The ventriculus terminalis of the spinal cord in the neonate: a normal variant on sonography. Am J Radiol. 1995;165:1491–3.

Kumar R, Guinto FC, Madewell JE, Swischuk LE, David R. The vertebral body: radiographic configurations in various congenital and acquired disorders. RadioGraphics. 1988;8:455–85.

Kwaku AK, Than KD, Wang AC, Rahman SU, Valdivia-Valdivia JM, La Marca F, Park P. Schmorl's nodes. Eur Spine J. 2012;21:2115–21.

Laredo JD, Assouline E, Gelbert F, Wybier M, Merland JJ, Tubiana JM. Vertebral hemangiomas: fat content as a sign of aggressiveness. Radiology. 1990;177:467–72.

Mellado JM, Larrosa R, Martín J, Yanguas N, Solanas S, Cozcolluela R. MDCT of variations and anomalies of the neural arch and its processes: Part 1-Pedicles, pars interarticularis, laminae, and spinous process. Am J Radiol. 2011;197:W104–13.

Mendel E, Lese GB, Gonzalez-Gomez I, Nelson MD, Raffel C. Isolated lumbosacral neurenteric cyst with partial sacral agenesis: case report. Neurosurgery. 1994;35:1159–62.

Murthy NS, Maus TP, April C. The retrodural space of Okada. Am J Radiol. 2011;196:W784–9.

Nardo L, Alizai H, Virayavanich W, Liu F, Hernandez A, Lynch JA, et al. Lumbosacral transitional vertebrae: association with low back pain. Radiology. 2012;265:497–503.

Negi RS, Manchanda KL, Sanga S, Chand S, Goswami G. Osteopoikilosis—spotted bone disease. Med J Armed Forces India. 2013;69:196–8.

Netter FH. Atlas of human anatomy. Summit, NJ: Ciba-Geigy Corp; 1994. Veins of Spine: Plate 159.

Okada K. Studies on the cervical facet joints using arthrography of the cervical facet joint. Nippon Seikeigeka Gakkai Zasshi. 1981;55:563–80.

Pfirrmann CW, Resnick D. Schmorl nodes of the thoracic and lumbar spine: radiographico-pathologic study of prevalence, characterization and correlation with degenerative changes of 1650 spinal levels in 100 cadavers. Radiology. 2001;219:368–74.

Prashad B, Jain A, Dhammi I. Tarlov cyst: Case report and review of literature. Indian J Orthop. 2007;41:401–3.

Ricci C, Cova M, Kang YS, Yang A, Rahmouni A, Scott WW Jr, Zerhouni EA. Normal age-related patterns of cellular and fatty marrow distribution in the axial skeleton: MR imaging study. Radiology. 1990;177:83–8.

Ross JS. Hemangioma. Diagnostic imaging:spine. Salt Lake City, UT: Amirsys; 2007. IV 1 14–16.

Rufener S, Ibrahim M, Raybaud C, Parmar H. Congenital spine and spinal cord malformations--pictorial review. Am J Radiol. 2010;194:S26–37.

Salfuddin A, Burnett SJ, White J. The variation of position of the conus medullaris in an adult population. A magnetic resonance study. Spine. 1998;23:1452–6.

Schettino C, Horner N, Knightly J. Distended epidural varix. Applied Radiol. 2012;41:5D.

Schrock WB, Wetzel RJ, Tanner SC, Khan MA. Aggressive hemangioma of the thoracic spine. J Radiol Case Rep. 2011;5:7–13.

Sebag GH, Dubois J, Tabet M, Bonato A, Lallemand D. Pediatric spinal bone marrow: assessment of normal age related changes in the MRI appearance. Pediatr Radiol. 1993;23:515–8.

Shi H, Schweitzer ME, Carrino JA, Parker L. MR imaging of the lumbar spine: relation of posterior soft-tissue edema-like signal and body weight. Am J Radiol. 2003;180:81–6.

Shimizu S. "Epidural" vertebral venous plexus. Am J Neuroradiol. 2006;27:7.

Singh I, Rohilla S, Kumar P, Sharma S. Spinal dorsal dermal sinus tract: an experience of 21 cases. Surg Neurol Int. 2015;6:S429–34.

Song SJ, Lee JW, Choi JY, Hong SH, Kim NR, Kim KJ, et al. Imaging features suggestive of a conjoined nerve root on routine axial MRI. Skeletal Radiol. 2008;37:133–8.

Suh SH, Chung TS, Lee SK, Cho YE, Kim KS. Ventriculus terminalis in adults: unusual magnetic resonance imaging features and review of the literature. Korean J Radiol. 2012;13:557–63.

Sze G, Baierl P, Bravo S. Evolution of the infant spinal column: evaluation with MR imaging. Radiology. 1991;181:819–27.

Sze G, Bravo S, Baierl P, Shimkin PM. Developing spinal column: gadolinium-enhanced MR imaging. Radiology. 1991;180:497–502.

Tuna S, Ozdemir T, Ece H. Limbus vertebra presenting with inflammatory low back pain: a case report. J Clin Diagn Res. 2016;10:YD01–2.

Ulano A, Bredella MA, Burke P, Chebib I, Simeone FJ, Huang AJ, et al. Distinguishing untreated osteoblastic metastases from enostoses using CT attenuation measurements. Am J Radiol. 2016;207:362–8.

Walker HS, Lufkin RB, Peacock WJ, Kangarloo H. Magnetic resonance imaging of the pediatric spine. RadioGraphics. 1987;7:1129–52.

Index

A. McKinney et al., *Atlas of Head/Neck and Spine Normal Imaging Variants*, https://doi.org/10.1007/978-3-319-95441-7

MIX
Papier aus verantwortungsvollen Quellen
Paper from responsible sources
FSC® C105338

If you have any concerns about our products,
you can contact us on
ProductSafety@springernature.com

In case Publisher is established outside the EU,
the EU authorized representative is:
Springer Nature Customer Service Center GmbH
Europaplatz 3, 69115 Heidelberg, Germany

Printed by Libri Plureos GmbH
in Hamburg, Germany